Health of the Nation

Health of the Nation

Perspectives for a New India

Edited by

Ali Mehdi and S. Irudaya Rajan

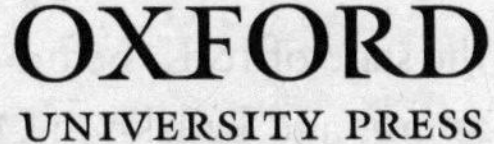

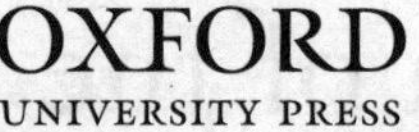

Oxford University Press is a department of the University of Oxford. It furthers the University's objective of excellence in research, scholarship, and education by publishing worldwide. Oxford is a registered trademark of Oxford University Press in the UK and in certain other countries.

Published in India by
Oxford University Press
22 Workspace, 2nd Floor, 1/22 Asaf Ali Road, New Delhi 110002, India

First Edition published in 2020

ISBN-13: 978-0-19-949983-0
ISBN-10: 0-19-949983-7

Typeset in 11/13 Adobe Garamond Pro
by Tranistics Data Technologies, Kolkata 700 091
Printed in India by Rakmo Press, New Delhi 110 020

This volume refers to Jammu and Kashmir as the state of J&K, before it was reorganized into the union territories of Jammu & Kashmir and Ladakh in October 2019.

Contents

Part V: Health Sector Regulation

Foreword

The Prime Minister gave a clarion call for establishing a 'New India' by 2022 to mark and celebrate our 75th anniversary of independence. To operationalize the Prime Minister's vision, we, at the NITI Aayog, developed the 'Strategy for New India @ 75' document, with a focus on 41 priority themes under 4 categories—drivers, infrastructure, inclusion, and governance. While 5 of these 41 themes pertained directly to health under the category of inclusion—public health management and action, comprehensive primary healthcare, human resources for health, universal health coverage, and nutrition—several other themes are either determinants of/dependent on the health of the nation. The first theme, growth, is a classic example. Drastic improvements in health are critical for enhancing the human capital and employability of India's rapidly expanding working-age population, reaping the demographic dividend, promoting economic growth and averting sociopolitical crises. Without growth, on the other hand, we may not have the resources to reduce financial hardships of citizens and expand universal health coverage and other interventions to improve the health of the nation. Other themes in the document related directly to health include, inter alia, Swachh Bharat Mission, sustainable environment, balanced regional development, and data-led governance and policymaking.

Since health is a state subject, the NITI Aayog instituted an annual Health Index in 2017, together with the Ministry of Health and Family Welfare (MoHFW) and World Bank, to rank and focus the attention of states/union territories on achieving better health outcomes. The Health Index is a weighted composite index based on 23 indicators grouped into 3 domains—health outcomes, governance and information, and key inputs/processes—with close to 75 per cent of weightage attached to health outcomes, signaling Government of India's shift towards outcome-oriented policymaking. On 9 October 2019, the MoHFW brought out its 'Health System Strengthening: Conditionality Report of States 2018–19', with the performance of health systems in states/union territories on 29 indicators—23 of which are from NITI Aayog's Health Index, with 40 per cent overall weightage—for results-based financing under Government of India's flagship National Health Mission (NHM). Both these annual exercises are based on available data, which suffers from its own set of limitations, conceptual as well as empirical. Conceptually speaking, let me quote the famous libertarian economist, Friedrich August von Hayek, from his lecture, 'The pretence of knowledge', delivered on receiving the 1974 Nobel Memorial Prize in Economic Science:

> Unlike the position that exists in the physical sciences, in economics and other disciplines that deal with essentially complex phenomena, the aspects of the events to be accounted for about which we can get quantitative data are necessarily limited and may not include the important ones. … the superstition that only measurable magnitudes can be important has done positive harm in the economic field.

Empirically speaking, our health data suffers from severe challenges, and I am glad Ali and his team at the Indian Council for Research on International Economic Relations (ICRIER) are reviewing it as part of a study commissioned by the NITI Aayog.

I am also glad that Ali independently took the initiative of bringing out a comprehensive 'Health of the Nation' report, offering perspectives by some of the world's topmost health experts for a New India, together with Prof. S. Irudaya Rajan from Centre for Development Studies (CDS), Trivandrum. This volume is distinctive in more ways than one:

1. There is no single volume that touches upon various aspects of health in India in a style which is, at once, lucid, analytical and practical. It will serve as a reference for all those interested in the status of health in India and its structural as well as immediate determinants.
2. It is the first volume with a dedicated section on health sector regulation, a theme that is highly important given the predominance of private health sector in India and largely ignored in terms of health sector discussions and legislation.
3. It not only covers a wide range of issues to analyse the status of health in India, but also brings in a wide variety of perspectives by some of the world's leading experts on India's health sector.

Some time before I took over as Director and Chief Executive of ICRIER, it prepared the first *India Health Report*, which was published by the Oxford University Press in 2003. Another one followed in 2010, prepared by Indicus Analyticus, published by Business Standard, and yet another in 2015, prepared and published by the Public Health Foundation of India (PHFI) and the International Food Policy Research Institute (IFPRI), focused on nutrition. However, none offered as comprehensive a view of the status, determinants, challenges as well as perspectives for improving health in India as this volume, with an interesting balance of theoretical, empirical and analytical discussions and a much wider appeal, in sync with the spirit of the social determinants of health.

Putting together 25 chapters by such a diverse and distinguished set of authors is no mean task, and I must conclude with congratulations to Ali, Prof Rajan as well as the Oxford University Press for their brilliant work as well as the suggestion that they should continue this on a regular basis, as an independent assessment of the direction and determinants of health in India, to complement the annual assessments of NITI Aayog and MoHFW to improve the health of the nation—@75 and beyond.

Rajiv Kumar, Vice Chairman, NITI Aayog, Government of India

Preface

'Healthy citizens are the greatest asset any country can have.'—Winston Churchill, BBC Broadcast, 21 March 1943

The lack of citizen-centric focus in public policy and practice continues to be, from our perspective, one of the biggest challenges facing Indian society and polity. Independence was expected to bring that about. However, despite substantial achievements, inequities between the potentials of citizens and their actual realizations—in addition to usually focused inequities in their respective actual realizations—have continued to be enormous and kept the nation back, by implication, from realizing its potential. A democratic polity should, as a matter of first and non-negotiable principle, be committed to the welfare and well-being of its citizens. A democratic society should demand this as a matter of its most basic right from its elected and non-elected representatives at various levels.

Health being a centrally constitutive element of well-being and human capital, and healthy citizens being the greatest asset of a nation (as Churchill stated in the midst of the Second World War, and something which we have known very well for a very long time), the *Health of the Nation* series is conceived to enhance the significance of health in India's public policy and discourse through an evidence-based, independent assessment of the status of health in the country on a regular basis by some of the leading experts from around the world. Since challenges to health are multi-faceted and discussions on health have largely been fragmented in the country, the first volume in the series is a comprehensive reference, which begins with a set of arguments on why health should be prioritized in India's public policy and then goes on to analyse historical and emerging burdens of disease and disability along with the structural and health sector determinants and regulatory challenges that have shaped the prevailing scenario. The composition of this volume informs on all relevant aspects of health, encompassing its various facets from prioritization to provisioning to regulation. There is explicit recognition of the changing population dynamics and the ensuing health transition while commenting on the response of the health system and strategies in operation. To make the analysis actionable, chapters end with a series of the most important workable policy recommendations to improve the health of the nation. While most existing reports tend to focus on data—and data does carry the potential to influence people—we also need cutting-edge analysis and actionable recommendations for promoting the health agenda.

While most of us would agree about the challenges that affect the health of citizens, our analysis of these challenges and solutions to address them would inevitably vary. In the spirit of pluralism and democracy, we have been careful as editors to provide space to a variety of—even conflicting—perspectives and leave it to the to readers decide which of them appeal to them the most. Undoubtedly, there are ideological groups in academic, policy, and civil society circles and, when it comes to ensuring the welfare and well-being of citizens are concerned, it is important to come together based on what we agree rather than fall apart over what we do not. We need such objectivity, tolerance, and respect for divergent viewpoints in this as well as other pursuits. Pluralism and democracy are the defining features of our nation rather than an embarrassment—and so they are for this volume. Needless to say, the views expressed in various chapters are those of the respective author(s) rather than ours.

On our part, we are most thankful to all the contributors who agreed and took out the time to write and revise their chapters for this volume. Our special thanks is also due to the Indian Council for Research on International Economic Relations (ICRIER), New Delhi, for being the host institution for the preparation of this volume as well as to the team at its Health Policy Initiative—particularly, Divya Chaudhry and Priyanka Tomar, research associates, whose contribution is as enormous as our debt to them; Aashna Arora, former research assistant, who provided immense support in the initial stages; and Rajesh Chaudhary, who formatted all the papers quite painstakingly as per the guidelines. The team at the Oxford University Press was very encouraging from the beginning, for seeing value in the proposed series and providing extraordinary support throughout the process of publication. Last but not least, we would like to thank our family members for their continuous support throughout the process.

Abbreviations*

3PL	Third party logistics
AAP	Ambient air pollution
ABPI	Association of British Pharmaceutical Industries
ACE	Angiotensin-converting enzyme
ADR	Alternative dispute resolution
AES	Acute encephalitis syndrome
AHS	Annual health survey
AIIMS	All India Institute of Medical Sciences
ALRI	Acute lower respiratory infection
AMR	Antimicrobial resistance
ANDA	Abbreviated new drug application
ANM	Auxiliary nursing midwife
APMP	Ambient particulate matter pollution
ARB	Angiotensin receptor blockers
ARI	Acute respiratory infection
ARPOB	Average revenue per occupied bed
ASHA	Accredited social health activist
AWW	Anganwadi worker
BPL	Below poverty line
CAG	Comptroller and Auditor General
CAGR	Compound annual growth rate
CDPC	Central Drug Procurement Corporation
CDSCO	Central Drugs Standard Control Organization
CEA	Clinical Establishments Act
CEDAW	Convention on the Elimination of All form of Discrimination Against Women
CES	Consumer expenditure survey
CHC	Community health centre

* This list consolidates abbreviations used in the book. There may be instances of duplication of an abbreviation by virtue of a difference in its full form. Readers are advised to refer to the list contextually.

CHD	Coronary heart disease
CII	Confederation of Indian Industries
CKD	Chronic kidney disease
CLTS	Community-led total sanitation
CMNND	Communicable, maternal, neonatal, and nutritional disease
CMO	Chief medical officer
COPD	Chronic obstructive pulmonary disease
CRM	Common Review Mission
CRO	Contract research organization
CSDH	Commission on Social Determinants of Health
CSG	Concrete service guarantees
CSO	Civil society organization
CSS	Centrally sponsored scheme
CT	Computerized tomography
CVD	Cardiovascular disease
DALY	Disability-adjusted life years
DAVA	Drugs authentication and verification application
DCA	Drugs and Cosmetics Act
DCR	Drugs and Cosmetics Rules
DCGI	Drug Controller General of India
DGFT	Directorate General of Foreign Trade
DGHS	Directorate General of Health Services
DLHS	District level household survey
DMC	Delhi Municipal Corporation
DMC	Dayanand Medical College and Hospital
DPCO	Drug Price Control Order
DPIP	District project implementation plan
DPMU	District programme manager unit
DSF	Demand side financing
EAG	Empowered Action Group
EC	Ethics committee
EHR	Electronic health record
EMR	Electronic medical record
EPI	Expanded Programme on Immunization
EU	European Union
FDA	Food and Drug Administration
FDI	Foreign direct investment
FSSAI	Food Safety and Standards Authority of India
FOS	Fortis Operating System
FY	Fiscal year
GBD	Global burden of disease
GCP	Good clinical practice
GDP	Good distribution practice
GDP	Gross domestic product
GDI	Gender development index
GMC	General medical council
GMP	Good manufacturing practice
GST	Goods and services tax
GTIN	Global trade item number
HALE	Health-adjusted life expectancy

HAP	Household air pollution
HDI	Human development index
HFA	Health for all
HHI	Herfindahl–Hirschman Index
HIS	Hospital information system
HLEG	High level expert group
HPV	Human papilloma virus
HRBA	Human rights-based approach
HRDG	Health-related development goal
HSM	Hub-and-spoke model
IAP	International advisory panel
ICDS	Integrated Child Development Services
ICF	Informed consent form
ICMR	Indian Council of Medical Research
ICSSR	Indian Council of Social Science Research
ICRIER	Indian Council for Research on International Economic Relations
ICT	Information and communications technology
IDSP	Integrated disease surveillance project
IFC	International finance commission
IEC	Information, education, and communication
IHDS	India Human Development Survey
IHHL	Individual household latrine
IHME	Institute of Health Metrics and Evaluation
IMA	Indian Medical Association
IMF	International Monetary Fund
IMR	Infant mortality rate
IP	Investigational product
IPHS	Indian Public Health Standard
IQ	Intelligence quotient
IRDA	Insurance Regulatory and Development Authority
IRDAI	Insurance Regulatory and Development Authority of India
ISO	International Organization for Standardization
IT	Information technology
ITeS	Information technology enabled services
JCI	Joint Commission International
JE	Japanese encephalitis
JMP	Joint monitoring programme
JSA	Jan Swasthya Abhiyan
LLP	Limited liability partnership
LMIC	Lower- and middle-income country
LPCD	Litres per capita per day
LPG	Liquified petroleum gas
MCI	Medical Council of India
MDG	Millennium development goal
MDRTB	Multidrug-resistant tuberculosis
MGNREGA	Mahatma Gandhi National Rural Employment Guarantee Act
MMR	Maternal mortality ratio
MoHFW	Ministry of Health and Family Welfare
MPCE	Mean (monthly) per capita consumer expenditure
MPI	Multi-dimensional poverty index

MRI	Magnetic resonance imaging
MRP	Maximum retail price
NAC	National Advisory Council
NABH	National Accreditation Board for Hospitals
NABL	National Accreditation Board for Testing and Calibration Laboratories
NCD	Non-communicable disease
NCEUS	National Commission for Enterprises in the Unorganised Sector
NCR	National Capital Region
NDA	New drug applications
NDAC	New drug advisory committee
NDRA	National Drug Regulatory Authority
NFHS	National Family Health Survey
NHEC	National Health Entitlement Card
NHP	National Health Policy
NHPS	National Health Protection Scheme
NHRC	National Human Rights Commission
NHA	National Health Accounts
NIC	National Informatics Centre
NITI Aayog	National Institution for Transforming India Aayog
NLEM	National List of Essential Medicines
NMC	National Medical Council (Bill)
NMR	Neonatal mortality rate
Non-SSI	Non-small scale industry
NPPA	National Pharmaceutical Pricing Authority
NRHM	National Rural Health Mission
NSSO	National Sample Survey Office
NTE	New therapeutic entities
OBC	Other Backward Classes
ODF	Open defecation free
OECD	Organisation for Economic Co-operation and Development
OOP	Out-of-pocket
ORGI	Office of the Registrar General of India
PDS	Public distribution system
PGIMER	Postgraduate Institute of Medical Education and Research
PHC	Primary health centre
PMS	Provincial medical service
PMUY	Pradhan Mantri Ujjwala Yojana
PPP	Public–private partnership
PRI	Panchayati Raj Institution
QP	Qualified persons
RAS	Rajiv Arogyasri Scheme
RBI	Reserve Bank of India
RCH	Reproductive and child health
RDOD	Rare diseases and orphan drugs
R&D	Research and development
RKS	Rogi Kalyan Samiti
RNTCP	Revised National Tuberculosis Control Programme
RRR	Responsibility, resources, and regulation
RSBY	Rashtriya Swasthya Bima Yojana

RTI	Right to Information
SADR	Serious adverse drug reaction
SAE	Serious adverse event
SAM	Swasthya Adhikar Manch
SBA	Swachh Bharat Abhiyan
SC	Scheduled caste
SDG	Sustainable development goal
SDH	Social determinants of health
SDH	Structural determinants of health
SDI	Social development index
SDPPC	State domestic product per capita
SDRA	State drug regulatory authority
SEC	Subject expert committee
SES	Socioeconomic status
SF	Substandard and falsified
SGRH	Sir Ganga Ram Hospital
SHP	State health policy
SNCU	Special newborn care unit
SRS	Sample registration system
ST	Scheduled tribe
STEMI	ST-elevation myocardial infarctions
TB	Tuberculosis
TCS	Tata Consultancy Services
TFP	Total factor productivity
TFR	Total fertility rate
TN	Tamil Nadu
TPA	Third party administrator
TRC	Technical review committee
TRIPS Agreement	Agreement on Trade Related Intellectual Property Rights
TSC	Total Sanitation Campaign
U5MR	Under-five mortality rate
UHC	Universal Health Coverage
ULB	Urban local bodies
UN	United Nations
UNDP	United Nations Development Programme
UNHRC	United Nations Human Rights Council
UP	Uttar Pradesh
UPA	United Progressive Alliance
UT	Union territory
VA	Verbal autopsy
VHNSC	Village health nutrition and sanitation committee
WASH	Water, sanitation, and hygiene
WBCERC	West Bengal Clinical Establishment Regulatory Commission
WDR	World Development Report
WHO	World Health Organization
WSP	Water and Sanitation Programme
WTO	World Trade Organization
YLD	Years lived with disability
YLL	Years of life lost

Introduction

Ali Mehdi and S. Irudaya Rajan

Irrespective of our backgrounds and goals in life, one of our first and strongest aspirations is to be able to lead a decently long and healthy life. A long and healthy life is not only valuable in itself, it determines the degree to which we can pursue other goals or aspirations in life (Sen 1992, 1998). A central reason why developing countries and their citizens are unable to realize their potential is their shortcoming on this count. India is a classic example. It has been independent and a democracy for more than 70 years now. From being one of the world's poorest, it is now among its top 10 economies. Its healthcare industry has been one of the largest contributors to its growth, both in terms of revenue and employment.[1] It is the world's leading provider of generic medicines,[2] and is often referred to as the 'pharmacy of the developing world'. Its healthcare providers have earned an international reputation for themselves—the highest number of foreign-origin doctors in OECD countries are from India, while its world-class private hospitals have been attracting patients from, and opening branches in, a number of developing and developed countries. Yet, survival and health for many Indians—including, in some respects, for the most privileged—continue to be precarious. No wonder, then, that the highest number of migrants (17 million) are also from India (UN 2017).

The highest number of deaths in the world continue to happen in India—in 2016, there were 9.8 million deaths, equivalent to 18 per cent of all deaths in the world (Global Burden of Disease 2016). Sometimes, it feels like we are surrounded by a whole range of risk factors on all sides and there is a competition on what kills us first—communicable, maternal, neonatal, and nutritional diseases claim the highest numbers of lives in India (2.7 million), so do injuries (1.1 million), and we are just behind China on deaths due to noncommunicable diseases (6 million). More worrisome is the fact that a high percentage of these deaths have been premature (that is, under the age of 70 years)—62 per cent of total deaths. China has had a larger population, yet its number of deaths have been slightly lower (9.7 million) and premature deaths far lower (39 per cent) in comparison. In Japan, a mere 17 per cent of deaths were premature. China and Japan are the world's second and third largest economies, and Indian policymakers

[1] Make in India. 'Sector Survey: Medical Devices'. Available at http://www.makeinindia.com/article/-/v/sector-survey-medical-devices, last accessed on 12 May 2018.

[2] IBEF. Indian Pharmaceutical Industry. Available at https://www.ibef.org/industry/pharmaceutical-india.aspx, last accessed on 12 May 2018.

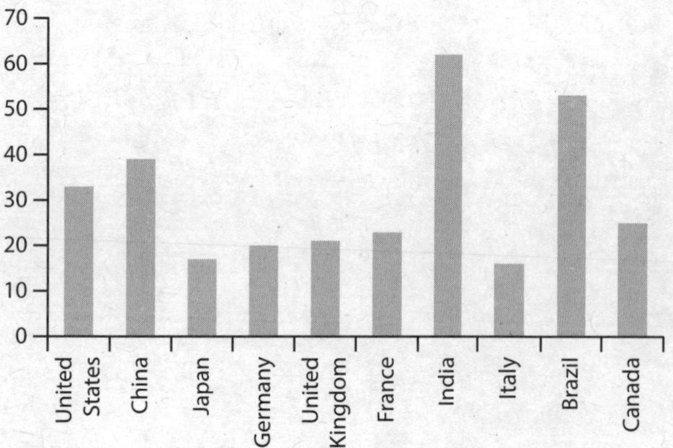

Figure I.1 Premature Deaths (as percentage of total deaths) in Top 10 Economies of the World, 2015–20

Source: UN DESA (2017).

argue that India will be among the top three in the next 25 years. With more than 42 per cent of deaths in the country happening within its working-age population (15–64 years)—which also indicates that the health condition of the survivors is not that great either—how exactly is that going to happen is not clear. Beyond bare survival, a child born in India can expect a healthy life expectancy of 59 years in comparison to 68 years in China and Sri Lanka and 73 in Japan (Global Burden of Disease 2016). One can argue that if Indian citizens were able to lead decently long and healthy lives, India might have already been among the top 10 economies, thanks to the increasing significance of human capital in global economic competitiveness.

The survival and health of its citizens is, probably, the biggest paradox of India's democracy and economy. Why has the world's largest democracy and one of its top 10 and most rapidly growing economies been unable to ensure a decently long and healthy life for its citizens? Citizens and their welfare should have been a top priority of public policy from the perspective of political legitimacy as well as human and economic growth and development. But this has not happened. If the survival and health of citizens is taken as a measure of 'the success of India's democracy'—to borrow the title of a wonderful book by Atul Kohli (2001)—we are afraid the answer is not going to be encouraging. If we are to take 'mortality as an indicator of economic success and failure', to borrow the title of an acclaimed paper by Amartya Sen (1998), we are afraid, this answer is not going to be encouraging either. What do India's democracy and economic growth, then, mean for the vast majority of its citizens?

Democracies are built on the promise of equality of opportunity, yet inequalities in such primordial opportunities as survival continue to be enormous. For instance, under-five mortality rate (U5MR) is 7 in Kerala and 78 in Uttar Pradesh (UP)—India's most populous state and majorly responsible for the non-realization of the global, and not just the national, target of reducing child mortality by two-thirds between 1990 and 2015 as part of the fourth Millennium Development Goal (MDG). It is 23 among the richest and 72 among the poorest in the country (Demographic and Health Survey [DHS] 2015–16). As a result, aggregate progress in survival and health was low even compared to some of the poorest regions in the world. For instance, gap in under-five death rates in sub-Saharan Africa and India narrowed substantially during the MDG period. U5MR among the richest in India (39) was higher compared to the poorest in Maldives (28) during their respective DHS surveys in 2005–6 and 2009. Survival inequality in Maldives is very low—U5MR was 21 among the richest and 28 among the poorest back then—and it is, therefore, no surprise that it was also the world's best performer in terms of percentage decline (90 per cent) as far as MDG 4 is concerned. China's was 80 per cent, if Maldives is too tiny, while India stood at 62 per cent. This is despite the fact that China is a dictatorship and there is a democracy in Maldives and other neighbouring countries, most of which have performed better than India on survival and health. India's state continues to be precarious. Voter turnout data between 2009 and 2014 general elections in India reveals that the poor and lower middle classes—comprising 74 and 53 per cent of India's population in these elections respectively—continue to repose faith in Indian democracy (Sridharan 2014). This is, probably, because the quest for equality 'remains, in diverse ways, the driving force in the *survival* of democracy' in India (Alam 2004: 5; emphasis as per original). Only time will tell whether the equality of opportunity vis-à-vis the survival and health of citizens will emerge as one of the central themes in Indian democracy.

We would also like to bring attention to another vulnerable population group in India—the elderly, aged 60 and above—although 'premature ageing' is also a major concern in countries like India. The demographic structure of India's population has undergone a shift with the number of elderly tipping the balance of the scale. India had nearly 140 million elderly persons (voters) or 10 per cent of its total population in 2019. The UN defines a country as ageing when the proportion of people over 60 years reaches 7 per cent of total population (Rajan et al. 2014; Rajan and Sunitha 2015)—as such, India is, officially, an ageing nation. During the period 1970–75, males and females aged 60 years could expect to live another 13.4 and 14.3 years respectively. Their life expectancy increased by 17.3 and 18.9 years respectively during the 2012–16 period. A similar pattern could be observed in previous periods as well (Figure I.2). Although the pattern seems similar across states, there is substantial variation in the case of females across states—females in Kerala could hope to live 4 more years at age 60 vis-à-vis their counterparts in Bihar (Figure I.3). Interestingly, male differentials were not that pronounced. Policy options to tackle ageing in India would have to be sensitive to differentials such as these as well as by other background characteristics.

It would be worth mentioning here that improvement in longevity does not imply that well-being or healthy living of older people could extend to a longer period. Indeed, the challenges and issues that have emerged from this situation have mounted in the country in the context of lack of sufficient social security and social transition of families from joint to nuclear. As longevity increases, there is an increase in the span of the morbid state. From a morbidity point of view, many of them acquire chronic diseases, multiple disabilities and a notable number of elderly are bedridden (1.6 per cent, according to National Sample Survey 2014). According to Kerala Ageing Survey 2013, one out of ten elderly had more than three chronic illnesses, while one out of four elderly had at least two chronic illnesses. According to Census 2011, there were 26.8 million disabled living in India. Among these, 20.2 per cent were elderly – most them being females (Rajan and Sunitha 2015). Higher life expectancy for females is not that cheerful after all. About 5 per cent of the elderly have some sort of physical disability. The main problem of the elderly is vision, followed by movement and hearing impairment. About one-ninth of the elderly aged 60 and above, and one-fifth of the elderly aged 80 and above, have multiple disabilities. Presently, around 2.1 million elderly are bedridden (Rajan and Balagopal 2017). Managing home-based care for these elderly is a challenge for care providers because they need care from multiple service providers for varied health issues. Also, health insurance coverage is largely limited to hospitalization.

Considering the earlier generation where there were higher fertility and mortality rates and lower migratory tendencies, living arrangements for the elderly were not much of a problem. However, with reductions in fertility and mortality rates and increases in migratory tendencies, the pattern of living arrangements has changed over the years. In 2001, there were 314 million migrants, which rose to 454 million in 2011. It is projected that, as of now, there are 600 million internal migrants and 20 million international migrants in India. In the light of the status of the elderly in India, we should reflect on the impact on the care economy, insurance coverage among the elderly, current incentives, and promotion of universal basic income for the elderly in India.

In the meantime, the current volume brings together some of the world's leading experts to analyse some of

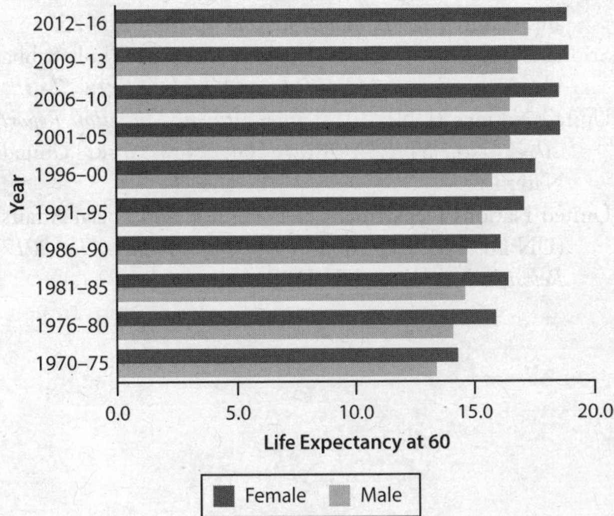

Figure I.2 Life Expectancy in the Elderly, 1970–75 to 2012–16

Source: Census of India, Vital Statistics, SRS abridged life tables 1970–75 to 2012–16, Registrar General of India.

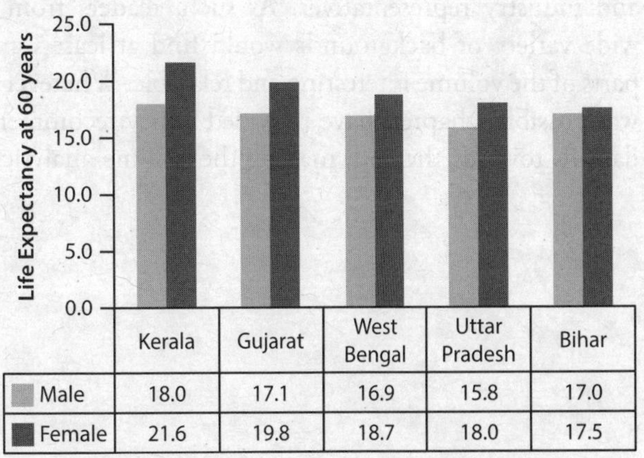

	Kerala	Gujarat	West Bengal	Uttar Pradesh	Bihar
Male	18.0	17.1	16.9	15.8	17.0
Female	21.6	19.8	18.7	18.0	17.5

Figure I.3 Life Expectancy across States, 2009–13

Source: Census of India, Vital Statistics, SRS abridged life tables 1970–75 to 2012–16, Registrar General of India.

the most complex challenges facing survival and health in India and what it would take to address them. It is an attempt to enhance the significance of health in the context of India's public policy and discourse for, without the latter, health will most likely not become a core concern for the former. Being the inaugural issue in a periodic series on the *Health of the Nation* volumes, it starts out with demographic, legal and constitutional, human rights, epidemiological, and ethical perspectives for the prioritization of health in India. It, then, goes on to present and analyse data on the burden of disease and disability in the country. The factors responsible for the current status of health are discussed in the next sections, ranging from the economic, social, spatial, and the environmental to the more immediate health sector determinants and resources. Health sector regulation has become a key area of concern for the protection and promotion of public health in the country in the context of the dramatic rise of the private sector in health care. A separate section has been dedicated to it.

This is the only volume on the state of health in India which not only covers a wide range of issues, but also brings in a wide variety of perspectives. Given the complexity surrounding health in India, and in keeping with the Indian tradition of pluralism, we thought it important to allow space for various, even if conflicting, points of views and let the reader decide what appears reasonable from his/her own particular perspective. Efforts have also been made to let the views of various stakeholders in the healthcare sector be represented—though most of the chapters have been written by academics (demographers, sociologists, epidemiologists, economists, environmentalists, so on), some have been written by retired policymakers and lawyers, doctors, and industry representatives. As such, readers from a wide variety of backgrounds would find at least some parts of the volume interesting and relatable. Wherever it was possible, chapters have provided policy recommendations towards the end, making the volume analytical as well as actionable. Finally, enhancing the variety of perspectives, some authors have leveraged their understanding of the international context to bring in insights and potential lessons for the particular Indian context.

Beyond highlighting these shared features of the volume, we purposely decided against summarizing various chapters in the introduction, as is the usual practice—it is better if the reader engages with the author(s) on a one-to-one basis rather through the medium of the editors.

REFERENCES

Alam, Javeed. 2004. *Who Wants Democracy?* New Delhi: Orient Longman.

Kohli, Atul. 2001. *The Success of India's Democracy*. Cambridge: Cambridge University Press.

Rajan, S.I. and Gayathri Balagopal 2017. 'Caring India: An Introduction', Chapter 1 in *Elderly Care in India: Societal and State Responses*, edited by S. Irudaya Rajan and Gayathri Balagopal. Singapore: Springer Nature.

Rajan, S.I., V. Kurusu, and S. Sunitha 2014. 'Demography of Ageing in India'. Chapter 2 in *Text Book of Geriatric Medicine: Under the Aegis of Indian Academy of Geriatrics*, edited by Pratap Sanchetee, pp. 6–18. Hyderabad: Paras Medical Publisher.

Rajan, S.I. and S. Sunitha. 2015. 'Demography of Ageing in India – 2011–2101', *Helpage India Research and Development Journal* 21(2).

Sen, Amartya. 1992. *Inequality Reexamined*. New York: Oxford University Press.

———. 1998. 'Mortality as an Indicator of Economic Success and Failure', *The Economic Journal* 108(446): 1–25.

Sridharan, E. 2014. 'Class Voting in the 2014 Lok Sabha Elections'. *Economic and Political Weekly* 49(39): 72–6.

United Nations (UN). 2017. *International Migration Report 2017*. No. ST/ESA/SER.A/404. New York: United Nations.

United Nations Department of Economic and Social Affairs (UN DESA). 2017. *World Population Prospects: The 2017 Revision*. New York: UN DESA.

Part I
Prioritizing Health

1

Right to Health

Legal and Constitutional Perspectives

N.R. Madhava Menon

In order to appreciate the status of right to health under the Indian Constitution and the laws it is necessary to have an understanding of the nature of the concept of rights under law and the definition of 'health' as a right. In simple terms, 'right' is an interest recognized and protected under law. The law which protects the right defines its scope and provides the remedies for its violation. Since all interests, however justifiable, are not recognized and protected by law, one cannot assume that basic needs like health, education, housing, work et cetera are part of all legal systems and the state is obliged to deliver the benefits implied under the so-called basic needs. Of course, one can create health rights for oneself by entering into enforceable contracts with health providers. Such private rights are enforceable only against the duty holders with whom the contract was entered into for consideration. This is part of private law, law of obligations.

When one talks about right to health as a common right available to citizens generally, the assumption is that the state and its agencies have undertaken the responsibility to provide the services of acceptable standards to enable citizens enjoy health essential to live a life with dignity and well-being. This is ordinarily done through legislation stipulating the rights and duties and identifying the mechanism for its delivery. There are many health-related laws in the Indian Statute Book,[1] some of them dating back to the colonial period. However, none of them provides right to health the way it is defined by health experts including the World Health Organization (WHO). What is provided in international human rights instruments is 'the highest attainable state of health', a loose expression difficult to capture by the language of rights. The Covenant on Economic, Social and Cultural Rights (1966) adopted by the UN puts the following obligation on State parties:

> Article 12 (i) The State Parties to the present Covenant recognize the right of everyone to the enjoyment of the highest attainable standard of physical and mental health.
>
> (ii) The steps to be taken by the States Parties to the present Covenant to achieve the full realization of this right shall include:
>
> (a) provision for the reduction of the stillbirth rate and of infant mortality and for the healthy development of the child;

[1] The Indian Statute Book is the collection of laws passed by Parliament or legislators.

(b) improvement of all aspects of environmental and industrial hygiene;

(c) prevention, treatment, and control of epidemic, endemic, occupational, and other diseases;

(d) creation of conditions which would assure to all medical service and medical attention in the event of sickness.

What then is the core content of right to health internationally? The WHO in the Alma Ata Declaration in 1978 identified six essential components of any programme aimed to achieve 'the highest attainable standard of health'. They include:

(a) preventive health services such as immunization, family planning, and sanitation;
(b) emphasis on maternal and child healthcare;
(c) education of people on health issues;
(d) people's participation in planning and implementation of healthcare services;
(e) priority in healthcare to vulnerable and high-risk groups; and
(f) provision for equal access to individuals to healthcare at affordable cost.

Should one were to articulate the obligation of the Indian State as a signatory to the Covenant, on the one hand, the policies of the State should not increase the health risks the people are exposed to, while on the other, it should create conditions to promote health status of the people and ensure equal access to all the health services available.

HEALTH AND THE INDIAN CONSTITUTION

As health is integral to life and the right to life is a guaranteed fundamental right under Article 21 of the Constitution, one can argue that the right to health is part of the Bill of Rights in India even though it is not expressly so acknowledged in the Constitution. The problem, however, is in the absence of legislative support, which one finds difficult to articulate the content of the right, the circumstances in which one can claim remedies for its violation, the nature of obligations it puts on the duty holders.

Health is given a prominent place in the chapter on directive principles of state policy (Part IV) of the Constitution, which are declared by the Constitution itself as fundamental in governance of the country that bind the State to make laws according to those principles (Article 37). Therefore, to find the status of right to health under the Constitution, one needs to examine the relevant provisions of Directive Principles which are reproduced below:

> Article 38. State is obliged to secure a social order for the promotion of welfare of the people.
>
> Article 39. The State shall, in particular, direct its policy towards securing–
>
> (e) that the health and strength of workers, men and women, and the tender age of children are not abused and that citizens are not forced by economic necessity to enter avocations unsuited to their age or strength;
>
> Article 41. The State shall, within the limits of its economic capacity and development, make effective provision for securing the right to work, to education and to public assistance in cases of unemployment, old age, sickness and disablement, and in other cases of undeserved want.
>
> Article 47. The State shall regard the raising of the level of nutrition and the standard of living of its people and the improvement of public health as among its primary duties and, in particular, the State shall endeavour to bring about prohibition of the consumption except for medicinal purposes of intoxicating drinks and of drugs which are injurious to health.
>
> Article 48-A. The State shall endeavour to protect and improve the environment and to safeguard the forests and wild life of the country.

It is interesting to note that the drafters of the Constitution used the language of rights (Article 41) even when they were reluctant to put it among judicially enforceable fundamental rights. However, an activist judiciary ever willing to expand basic rights of citizens has used its interpretative logic to adopt harmonious construction of fundamental rights with directive principles to read several aspects of health rights in the guaranteed right to life and liberty. The court reasoned to conclude that right to life is indeed right to live with dignity and not to live a vegetative life. Though the right to live with dignity would depend on the economic capacity and development of the country, 'in any view of the matter it would include the bare necessities of life and also the right to carry on such activities as constitute the bare minimum expression of the human self'.[2]

In a series of decisions, the Supreme Court further gave meaning and content to the right to life and

[2] *Francis Coralie Mullin* v *The Administrator, Delhi* (1981) 2 SCR 516.

livelihood by invoking the bare minimum of health rights into Article 21 read with Article 14 (Right to Equality). In *Parmanand Katara* v *Union of India,*[3] the court said that the right to access to emergency medical treatment is part of right to life. In *Consumer Education and Research Centre* v *Union of India,*[4] the court ruled that just and humane conditions of work and leisure to workmen are a part of the meaningful right to life of workers. In *Paschim Banga Khet Mazdoor Samiti* v *State of West Bengal,*[5] the court declared that non-availability of services in government health centres amounted to a violation of right to life under Article 21. This was a case where the patient was refused treatment at eight state-run medical institutions because of non-availability of beds or insufficient technical capacity. While declaring emergency medical care as a core component of right to health, the court awarded compensatory relief to the person who had to seek medical help at great cost in a private hospital.

Based on this logic, the Supreme Court and high courts exercising their writ jurisdiction have enlarged the content of right to health to include duty on the part of the State to maintain the quality and safety of blood banks, ensure the establishment of primary health centres in villages, ban of hazardous drugs, control the unhealthy condition in state-run care homes and custodial institutions, prohibit smoking in public places and sale of tobacco products, prevent discrimination in treatment to HIV positive patients, control pollution from cars in cities, tighten medical negligence standards in assessing deficiency of service by doctors and hospitals. Given the fact that the law declared by the Supreme Court shall be binding on all courts (Article 141), these rulings of the court can be taken as part of the corpus juris binding on all state authorities at the central, state, and local levels. These decisions not only remind the executive and the legislature of their constitutional obligations in respect of right to health of citizens but also empowers citizens for seeking remedies through constitutional courts pending appropriate legislative enactments on health rights. As happened in the evolution of right to education from a mere directive principle (Article 45) to that of a fundamental right[6] and later followed by the Right to Education Act, 2009, the time has come for the right to health to assume a similar status. In fact, the National Health Bill, 2009, evolved by a group of social action groups was under the active consideration of the Ministry of Health, even though it did not get the attention it deserved from the government and Parliament.

Constitutional perspectives in respect of health will not be complete without mention of the scheme of health governance that the constitution-makers have meticulously articulated under the federal framework the country has adopted. Under the distribution of legislative powers in the Seventh Schedule, entries relating to public health are included in all the three Lists. The Union List (List I) on which Parliament alone can make laws includes entries such as (i) treaties and agreements and their implementation (Entry 14); (ii) quarantine and marine hospitals (Entry 28); (iii) patents, inventions and trader marks (Entry 49); (iv) labour safety in mines and oil fields (Entry 55); (v) manufacture and distribution of salt and opium (Entry 58–59); (vi) professional and vocational training (Entry 65); (vii) interstate migration and interstate quarantine (Entry 81).

Health-related entries in the Concurrent List (List III) on which both parliament and state assemblies can make laws include items such as (i) lunacy and mental deficiency (Entry 16); (ii) adulteration of food stuffs and other goods (Entry 18); (iii) drugs and poisons (Entry 19); (iv) economic and social planning (Entry 20); (v) population control and family planning (Entry 20A); (vi) social security (Entry 23); (vii) welfare of labour (Entry 24); (viii) education including medical education (Entry 25); (ix) medical profession (Entry 26); (x) prevention of contagious diseases (Entry 29); (xi) price control (Entry 34); and (xii) factories and boilers (Entries 36–37).

On the State List (List II) are such important health subjects such as (i) public health, sanitation, hospitals and dispensaries (Entry 6); (ii) manufacturing and sale of intoxicating liquors (Entry 8); (iii) relief of the disabled (Entry 9); (iv) local self-government and village administration (Entry 5); (v) water supplies and drainage (Entry 17); (vi) industries (Entry 24). Furthermore, items in the State and Concurrent Lists on which state legislatures are empowered to make laws are expected to be implemented by the panchayats, and state governments are duly empowered for the purpose by the Constitution under the Eleventh and Twelfth Schedules. These two Schedules empowers panchayats and municipalities to devote their resources and powers

[3] AIR 1989 SC 2039.
[4] AIR 1995 SC 940.
[5] AIR 1996 SC 2426.
[6] Article 21-A introduced through the Constitutional Amendment Act, 2002.

for promotion of public health through management of water resources to make clear drinking water available to everyone, reduction of poverty conditions, ensuring health and sanitation through hospital, primary health centres and dispensaries, take special care of weaker sections including women, children, disabled, and the elderly. In short, the constitutional scheme makes a practical design of a three-level governance to ensure reasonable healthcare for all citizens across the country to be operationalized through laws and regulations by appropriate governments.

LEGISLATIVE PERFORMANCE IN PROMOTING PUBLIC HEALTH

Though there was no constitutional compulsion during the colonial era, many of the health-related laws in the Indian Statute Book dates back to the British period. Perhaps they were enacted more to protect the health of British citizens working in the country rather than that of Indians. Yet, they contributed to create a health jurisprudence particularly to control communicable diseases, occupational risks of workers in plantation and mines, and organizing institutions and services under modern medicine in the colony.

Soon after adoption of the Constitution, Parliament enlarged the health obligation of the state by enacting a host of legislations intended to improve standards of public health. These were mostly based on specific objectives identified under the development-oriented Five-Year Plans. They were directed towards creating an environment involving minimum of health risks and providing a right to have access to health services that can prevent or alleviate suffering and treat diseases. Health-related laws perform several functions in terms of policy development and public administration. From an individual's perspective, health laws create rights and entitlements for delivery of health services. From the perspective of the people at large, health laws prohibit conduct involving unacceptable levels of risks and regulate the use of products and processes that may be injurious to health. Health laws further set standards on medical experimentation on human beings, on health hazards arising from food and drugs. Some aspects of these standards get incorporated as part of ethical codes for health professionals to follow in delivery of services. Since right to equality and non-discrimination is a constitutional guarantee, all health laws have to abide by it subject, of course, to affirmative action in favour of disadvantaged sections of people.

In the legislative history of the health sector, the Bhopal gas leak disaster of December 1984 played a crucial role in as much as the Parliament was forced to adopt policy changes in the matter of industrial safety, environmental protection, mass disaster responses for social justice, and functioning of regulatory systems.

The human rights regime, which received greater attention of the legislature and the judiciary influenced policy development across all sectors of governance including public health. A serious attempt to look at public health comprehensively in its inter-relatedness to other sectors of governance got underway leading to long-term agenda for legislative action. The Consumer Protection Act, 1986; the Mental Health Act, 1987; the Prevention of Illicit Traffic in Narcotic Drugs and Psychotropic Substances Act, 1988; the Protection of Human Rights Act, 1993; the Pre-natal Diagnostic Techniques (Prohibition of Sex Selection) Act, 1994; the Transplantation of Human Organs Act, 1994; and the Food Safety and Standards Act, 2006 are some of the laws that have enriched the Indian Statute Book on healthcare services. Mechanisms like public hearing, social audit, civil society participation, compensatory reliefs for defective services, health education, and compliance requirements on the regulatory front have made a difference in the organization and delivery of healthcare services.

RECOMMENDATION OF THE EXPERT GROUP ON UNIVERSAL HEALTHCARE

An expert committee appointed by the Planning Commission in 2011 made a detailed report for ensuring quality of healthcare services and making its access universal to the Indian consumer. The focus of the report was securing the right to health of citizens highlighting the gaps in the legislative framework and institutional arrangements. It is important to briefly examine the key recommendations of this committee as it was made after a situational analysis, constitutional promises and advances in health services. The object as articulated by the committee is to ensure equitable access for all citizens to affordable health services of assured quality as well as public health services addressing the wider determinants of health delivered to individuals with the government being the guarantor and enabler, although not necessarily the only provider of health-related services. This is what universal health coverage (UHC) is meant to convey in policymaking. Among the recommendations were a few new initiatives proposed for UHC to become a reality. These include:

(i) Every citizen will be issued an IT-enabled National Health Entitlement Card (NHEC) that will ensure cashless transactions, allow for mobility across the country, and contain personal health information.
(ii) Universal health coverage can be achieved only when sufficient attention is paid to health-related areas like nutrition and food security, water and sanitation, social inclusion to address concerns of gender, caste, religious and tribal minorities, housing, clean environment, employment and work security, occupational safety, and disaster management.
(iii) Healthcare services to all citizens will be made available through the public sector and contracted-in private facilities participating in the UHC programme. Citizens are free to supplement free-of-cost services (both inpatient and outpatient care) offered under the UHC system by paying out-of-pocket or directly purchasing voluntary medical insurance.
(iv) Financing the proposed UHC system will require public expenditures on health to be stepped up from around 1.2 per cent of the gross domestic product (GDP) as of 2019 to 3 per cent by 2022.
(v) The UHC system should focus on reduction of the burden of disease along with early disease detection and prevention. The emphasis is on investing in primary care networks and holding providers responsible for wellness outcomes at the population level. Through high quality primary care network, UHC is likely to reduce the need for secondary and tertiary facilities.
(vi) The district hospital has a critical role to play in healthcare delivery, which should be well attuned to the needs of the particular district. It can be backed up by contracting-in of regulated private hospitals that should meet the healthcare needs of over 90 per cent of the population in the district. This will require the upgrading of district hospitals as high priority over the next few years.
(vii) Adherence to Indian Public Health Standards by all public and contracted-in private health facilities at the starting point of quality assurance in healthcare services delivery. Such a move should include licensing, accreditation, and public disclosure of accreditation status of all public and private health facilities participating in the UHC system.
(viii) A national council for human resources in health should be set up at the national level to prescribe, monitor, and promote standards of education of health professionals.
(ix) For ensuring effective and affordable access to medicine, vaccines, and appropriate medical technologies, the government should enforce price control on essential drugs, adopt a centralized national and state procurement system and strengthen the public sector capacity of domestic drug and vaccines industry.

Given the importance of health services in the scheme of accelerated development, as envisaged by the present dispensation taking advantage of the demographic dividend in the Indian workforce, it is imperative that legislative policymakers take note of some of the policy options proposed by the expert committee. It is a challenge for the proponents of cooperative federalism to take the states on board for future development of healthcare policies and share the expenses involved in the UHC system for the country.

NATIONAL HEALTH BILL, 2009

An initiative of a Working Group under the sponsorship of the Ministry of Health and Family Welfare in 2009 came up with a draft bill to introduce a National Health Policy providing for right to health and for achieving the goal of health for all conducive to living a life of dignity. The bill acknowledged the fact that the exercise of all other human rights is intricately linked with getting health recognized as a fundamental human right, and there is a need to have an overreaching legal framework and common set of standards, norms and values to facilitate the government's stewardship of private sector as a partner in future public health-related laws to be enacted at the central and state levels. The obligations of the government in this regard flow from right to equality and non-discrimination (Articles 14 and 15), the right to life (Article 21), prohibition of employment of children (Article 23) as well as the Constitutional Directives in respect of public health under Articles 38, 39, 41, 42, 47, and 48A. Furthermore, the Union of India is obliged under Article 253 to give effect to the international treaties in which the Union Government has undertaken to provide right to health, such as Article 12 of the International Covenant on Economic, Social, and Cultural Rights, Article 24 of the Convention on the Rights of the Child, Article 12 of the Convention on the Elimination of All Forms of Discrimination Against Women, Article 25 of the UN Convention on Rights of Persons with Disabilities, the Millennium Development Goals (2000), Declaration of Commitment on HIV/AIDS (2001), WTO Doha Deceleration on TRIPS Agreement and Public Health (2001), WHO Framework Convention on Tobacco Control (2005), and similar other declarations and Conventions.

Given the fact that nearly 60 per cent of the total family income of an average Indian household is spent on health-related expenditure and not even 10 per cent of Indians have some form of health insurance, it is imperative for governments to address the problem of health inequalities as a priority. In this context the legislative proposal under the National Health Bill should be revived and pushed forward. The bill does take into account the inter-relationship between health outcomes and related issues like water, nutrition, sanitation, and environment. The rights-based, inclusive approach adopted in the bill aims for a broad-based legal framework to bring the public, private, and voluntary sectors together.

For a rights-based health scheme, it is important to identify the duty holders and set their obligation upfront. This is what the bill does in the second chapter under the title 'Obligations of Governments in Relation to Health'. The duties are categorized under three heads namely, general obligation, core obligation, and specific public health obligations. There are negative obligations too, in the sense that the State and its agencies are expected to refrain from actions extinguishing or interfering with the enjoyment of existing health-related rights in the name of development.

The bill articulates the right to health as a bundle of independent rights some of which are individually held, while others are collectively enjoyed. Individual rights include right to receive quality healthcare services; right against discrimination in delivery of services; right to dignity, privacy, and confidentiality; right to access health information; right to give consent and refuse treatment; among others. Of course, those providing healthcare services also have rights which the users of such services are expected to respect.

The redressal mechanism for health rights stipulated in the bill apart from the usual civil and criminal remedies include dispute resolution through public hearings and dialogues as well as through in-house complaints forums at the institutional level using Alternative Dispute Resolution (ADR) methods.

The implementation mechanism contemplated in the bill includes national and state public health boards and decentralized implementation authorities at the village, block, and district levels. Monitoring implementation is the responsibility of both government and community-based organizations. There is to be an independent health information system to be put in place.

As a measure to project the legislative agenda for a rights-based approach in healthcare delivery, the draft bill provides a starting point for discussion among states and the Union. Unfortunately, in the changing political and economic scenario prevailing in the country, the bill seems to have been shelved at least for the moment.

THE ASSAM PUBLIC HEALTH ACT, 2010

The state of Assam came forward to legislate a modified version of the draft national health policy in 2010 under the title The Assam Public Health Act, 2010. Section 5 of the act empowers every person with the right to health including:

(a) appropriate healthcare, ambulance services, trained medical personnel, and essential drugs;
(b) reproductive health services with special emphasis for women and girls;
(c) registration of births and deaths and other vital statistics for health, food safety;
(d) safety availability and accessibility of drugs;
(e) regulation of health establishments as per rules;
(f) immunity from heath nuisances and bio-medical waste;
(g) safe drinking water in hospitals and health establishments;
(h) sanitation and environmental hygiene;
(i) effective measures for control of epidemics and effective mechanism in public health emergencies;
(j) right to specified standards for safety and quality assurance of all aspects of healthcare;
(k) right to education and access to information on public health issues; and
(l) right to efficacious medicines.

Sections 6, 7, 8, and 9 incorporate users' right to information on healthcare facilities and services—right to be fully informed about his/her health status including implications of refusal to healthcare, right to obtain a second opinion from another health service provider, right to have the complete medical records, right to consent as a pre-requisite for any healthcare proposed for him/her, right to refuse or halt a medical intervention, right to direct that all information about his/her health status must be kept confidential, even after his/her death.

The obligations of the state government in relation to health are vested by the act in the Department of Health and Family Welfare under Chapter II of the act. Section 3 contains the following obligations:

1. The general obligations under the section are subject to the limits of available resources and are directed towards the progressive realization of the health and well-being of every person in the state and include (a) undertaking adequate budgetary measures to satisfy the obligations and rights under the act; (b) provide access to healthcare services and to ensure no denial of services to anyone by any healthcare service provider, public or private, by laying down minimum standards and appropriate regulatory mechanism; (c) prioritizing the most vulnerable and marginalized persons and groups, and ensuring them the minimum conditions of healthcare.
2. In order to meet its obligations, the department will coordinate with other relevant departments for access to the minimum essential food which is nutritionally adequate, adequate supply of safe drinking water, sanitation through pollution control systems, sewage and drainage systems, waste disposal systems, and access to basic housing and other essential facilities.
3. The Health and Family Welfare Department will also be responsible, in order to safeguard health-related rights, to take effective measures to prevent and control epidemics, lay down standards and norms for safety and quality assurance of all aspects of healthcare within government, private, and other non-government sectors, provide education and access to information on health issues, provide best available preventative measures against infectious diseases, and to meet public health emergencies.

Section 4 obligations talk about review and enactment of public health-related laws, rules, and orders to specifically address inter alia the following:

(i) fixing responsibility of concerned departments in case of repeated outbreaks of communicable, viral, and water-borne diseases found to be due to failure to improve sanitation and safe drinking water facilities;

(ii) public health emergencies, vital statistics for health, food safety in hospitals and health establishments, safety and availability of drugs, regulation of health establishments, health impact assessment of all new development projects, lifestyle-related diseases, mental illness;

(iii) specify the class or group of patients who will be given free treatment in private health establishments;

(iv) formation of patient welfare societies in health institutions and presenting remedial measures in case a patient fails to receive attention at a government hospital because of absence of medical staff; and

(v) prescribe suitable schedule of inspection of government/private health institutions by various health functionaries.

Implementation of the obligations under the Assam Public Health Act, 2010 is to be done through the state and district public health boards constituted by the government as stated in the act. Section 17 promises to bring about an 'intensive accountability framework' through monitoring under the health information system by both the government (mandatory audits by government agencies as well as through surveys done by engaging autonomous professional bodies) and communities using human rights-based approaches and methods.

Interestingly Section 20 of the act provides for immunity of the government and government personnel for performance of duties/functions under the act and shall not be held liable for the death or injury caused to any individual or damage to property or violation of any kind. Furthermore, the section makes it explicit that even private sector partners of the state shall also be immune to any liability for acts done under the act. No superior officer can be held vicariously liable except in cases of gross negligence and being directly responsible to guarantee against the occurrence of the violation.

It will be interesting to study the implementation of the act and the rules made over the last six years in Assam and its impact on healthcare services delivery to the public to make an assessment of the model for developing legislative framework for the country as a whole.

LITTLE ACHIEVED, MUCH YET TO BE DONE

A report card on health laws and right to health is difficult to make, given the complex nature of issues involved and the nature of developments happening in society, technology, and governance. Nevertheless, public health, understood as conditions which enable people to live healthy or attain the highest attainable state of health, is engaging the attention of changing governments with varying degrees of emphasis. Meanwhile, right to health, understood as the right to an environment involving the minimum risks to health and the right to have access to healthcare services that can prevent or alleviate suffering of diseases, has grown under a human rights jurisprudence based on life with dignity and social justice founded on equity and equality. The developments in this regard can be captured in a dozen categories of legislative and executive action. Thus health-related legislations at the central and state levels have:

(a) conferred individual rights and entitlements to keep oneself healthy;
(b) regulated hazardous products and processes;
(c) organized preventive services promotive of public health;
(d) financed health education, research, and training;
(e) ensured quality control in healthcare services delivery;
(f) maintained equality in access and equity through affirmative action;
(g) promoted people's participation in planning and delivery of services;
(h) evolved special programmes for high risk groups including women and children;
(i) developed inter-sectoral cooperation in management of health services;
(j) established accountability systems at different levels of government; and
(k) built institutional capacities through research and development.

Given the multi-level law-making bodies and processes existing in the federal scheme of governance and divided responsibilities thereunder, it is impossible to present a comprehensive view of the status of right to health in this country. The laws themselves are too numerous to count. Added to these are the ever-increasing regulations, rules, and orders by the central and state administrations. Despite all the progress made in economic development, health inequalities prevail and the poor shoulder the burden of disease disproportionately.

Economic liberalization and globalization have widened the health divide aggravating the inequities. The government has tried to address the issue through two equity enhancing programmes—the National Rural Health Mission, and National Urban Health Mission. However, a more comprehensive approach to reduce health inequities is warranted and the National Health Bill proposed in 2009 is the way forward to make the right to health meaningful to citizens.

In short, as on date, it is difficult to claim access to healthcare as an individual right. Improvements in drinking water supply and sanitation, nutrition and environment, housing and employment have been far more beneficial for health status enhancement than preventative and curative healthcare services.

Development of human rights standards in healthcare is important. Better norms of medical ethics could also help a lot; but unless investment in health sector is substantially increased and comprehensive legislative framework outlining obligations is put in place, inequities in healthcare are not likely to end as the Constitution envisages. International law-making to reduce health hazards and promote capacities of individuals and communities to cope with them is a work in progress influencing domestic law making. The all-encompassing notion of health in modern times has helped in standard setting in relation to the human right to health. The obligation of the State in healthcare services is being continuously debated all over the world and there is no uniform pattern discernible in this regard. In its general comment on the right to life, the UN Human Rights Council (UNHRC) articulated the role of the state limited to undertaking measures for eliminating epidemics and malnutrition.[7] It is not clear from this comment as to when the State can be made responsible for breach of its obligation in curbing malnutrition. Due to the absence of an enforceable claim upon a government for allocation of a specific amount to health, the amount a nation can afford in this respect remains what it chooses to spend.

There is no doubt that ultimately in rule of law jurisdictions, it is necessary to have laws to reduce/prevent health hazards and to improve the prospects of

[7] General Comment 6- UN Document A/37/40, para 5 of Annexure III.

individuals and communities to cope with health hazards. Laws in respect of reducing health hazards have been there for long and the process is continuing. There are clear legal norms already available in this field. However, in the matter of claiming health as a right of individuals and communities, the advent of UN declarations and state-level constitutions incorporating fundamental human rights opened a new chapter even though it remains incomplete in detail. In clarifying rights and duties and setting standards and accountability, the State needs to legislate and fill the gaps if the right to health is to become a judicially enforceable legal right.

2

Towards Health Equity

Operationalizing a Human Rights-based Approach*

Abhijit Das

THE PURSUIT OF HEALTH EQUITY

The issue of equity has become an important policy concern at the international level in the last decade or so. The World Development Report of 2006 addressed equity and development, the World Health Organization (WHO) through its Commission on Social Determinants of Health (CSDH) report *Closing the Gap in a Generation* (CSDH 2008), as well as the UN through its Sustainable Development Goals (SDG) adopted at the UN Summit in September 2016 underlined this concern. Health equity is a matter of crucial concern in a country like India which has wide variations and differences between people. 'Equity' is concerned with whether these differences are fair and 'inequity' refers to differences which are both 'avoidable' and 'unjust'. Thus, differences between groups of people, be they social, economic, demographic or geographic, which cause people in these groups to be treated differently depriving them of opportunities, constraining them from achieving their full human potential compared to others, are inequitable. This inequity causes individuals from such groups to be deprived of dignified and remunerative livelihood opportunities or have greater chances of catching a disease and lesser opportunities for receiving appropriate treatment or have lesser chances to survive childbirth. There is an emerging consensus that such differences are unjust and unacceptable and, as a society, we need to find ways to remedy these differences.

Human rights are closely related to equity because they lay down the fundamental and irrevocable condition of equality among all human beings. The human right to healthcare usually means the satisfaction of certain conditions like access, availability, acceptability, and quality in the provision of healthcare. It includes creating legal or policy imperatives to address and redress inequities. A practical approach for doing so could be through identifying health inequities and finding specific ways to remedy the disparities. In this chapter various dimensions of health inequities in India are identified and the SDH framework is applied to understand the interaction of different social and cultural factors within a complex health policy paradigm. The chapter also outlines

* I would like to acknowledge my discussions with Abhay Shukla (SATHI, Pune, Maharashtra), Edward Pinto (CHSJ, New Delhi), V.R. Raman (Wateraid, New Delhi), and Jashodhara Dasgupta (NFI, New Delhi) on this subject.

Table 2.1 Infant Mortality Rate across Different Social Groups

State	Avg. State IMR	Urban IMR	IMR where the Mothers had No Schooling	IMR where the Mothers have 10 or More Years of Schooling	SC	ST	Muslim
Assam	47.7	28.3	59.4	26.8	41.3	41.6	51.5
Karnataka	27.7	19.5	39.8	21.6	33.0	37.7	24.2
Kerala	5.6	5.8	*	4.8	*	*	4.5
Maharashtra	23.9	23.5	19.5	21.1	31.7	32.8	28.5
MP	51.4	43.9	55.7	38.3	54.3	58.9	48.4
Rajasthan	41.3	30.7	45.4	28.6	50.2	39.5	42.5
UP	63.3	51.9	69.7	47.1	67.7	40.8	59.4

* Data not available.

Source: All data for this table has been drawn from the respective state reports of NFHS 4, 2015–16.

key elements of a 'right to health approach' that already exist and concludes with a set of practical recommendations that may be adopted to reduce health inequities in India. Most of the practical examples used in this chapter have been drawn from the reproductive and child health domain, reflecting both my own field of practice as well as a key domain of health policymaking in India.

IDENTIFYING HEALTH INEQUITY IN INDIA

It is not difficult to identify differences in the health status of different groups in India. Whenever health indicators are computed, it is standard practice to present the data stratified both by state and by urban and rural situation. There has been a consistent difference in health and socio–economic indicators between the northern–central belt of states compared to the southern, western, and northern states that led demographers to coin the term BIMARU states, which was aimed at comparing the erstwhile undivided states of BI(har), MA(dhya Pradesh), R(ajasthan), U(ttar Pradesh) with a sick person (*bimar* in Hindi).[1] The Ministry of Health and Family Welfare extended the group by adding Odisha, Assam, and Himachal Pradesh to create the category of 'high-focus states' when it launched the National Rural Health Mission (NRHM) in 2005. In order to track the health programme's performance in this identified geography, the ministry also commissioned a new Annual Health Survey (AHS) for 284 high-focus districts. Unfortunately, the new sampling method adopted was unable to provide information about the reality of marginalized social groups such as scheduled tribes (ST), scheduled castes (SC), and Muslims who have different health indicators from the general or caste Hindu population (Das 2017a).

In the last decade or so there has been a huge decline in mortality rates among children and mothers. Maternal mortality as a whole has reduced from 556 per 100,000 live births in 1990 to 167 in in 2011–13. Similarly, under-five mortality rate (U5MR) has reduced from 126 per 1,000 live births to 49 in 2013. However, India could not reach the MDG[2] targets set for either of these domains.

Table 2.1 shows wide differences in infant mortality rates (IMR) among a set of states in India. The table shows differences both across and within states, between urban and rural populations, as well as based on mothers' schooling. A similar difference is evident in social groups such as SC, ST, and Muslims and here the status varies in different states. In some states like Karnataka, Kerala, Madhya Pradesh, and Uttar Pradesh the IMR among Muslims is lower than that of the state as a whole. However, in most states and in most marginalized groups the IMR is well above 30 or 29 which was the target the country had set itself both through the NRHM and the MDG respectively.

Table 2.2 provides an analysis of 'no vaccination' among children aged between 12 and 23 months and here it is clear that in addition to the differences between social groups, the situation in different districts is vastly

[1] The term was coined by demographer Ashish Bose. See Sharma (2015).

[2] MDG refers to the Millennium Development Goals, a set of eight goals for development set by the UN for countries with poor socio-economic indicators. These goals were to be met by 2015.

Table 2.2 Status of Non-Vaccination among Children in Age Group of 12–23 Months

State	Overall	Male	Female	District Highest	District Lowest	SC	ST	Muslim
Assam	13.8	12.7	15.0	0	35.1	6.6	9.3	19.7
Karnataka	6.2	7.3	5.1	0	17.8	2.1	21.1	5.3
Kerala	1.7	2.1	1.2	0	4.9	0	NA	3.9
Maharashtra	6.1	6.0	6.1	0	20.3	5.1	10.2	4.4
Madhya Pradesh	8.2	7.7	8.6	0	21.7	8.1	12.1	12.9
Rajasthan	7.4	7.9	6.9	0	21.6	5.9	9.1	17.3
Uttar Pradesh	8.7	7.8	9.7	0	46.9	7.6	20.9	13.6

Source: All data for this table has been drawn from the respective state reports of NFHS 4, 2015–16.

different. This begs the question whether this locational disadvantage is the result of multiple adversities like social grouping along with living in remote locations like hills or forests where health systems are poor. The SDH framework (WHO 2010) presented in Figure 2.1 allows for this analysis. The key point to note is that despite immunization of children being an important thrust area of the government's health policy since the late 1970s when the Expanded Programme of Immunization (EPI) was started, today, 50 years later, there are large sections of the population who still remain excluded.

The SDH approach provides a useful framework to understand the interactions between different factors which affect access to healthcare and health status as a whole. Figure 2.1 indicates how the different factors interact with each other to influence health and well-being. The arrows in the diagram indicate pathways of

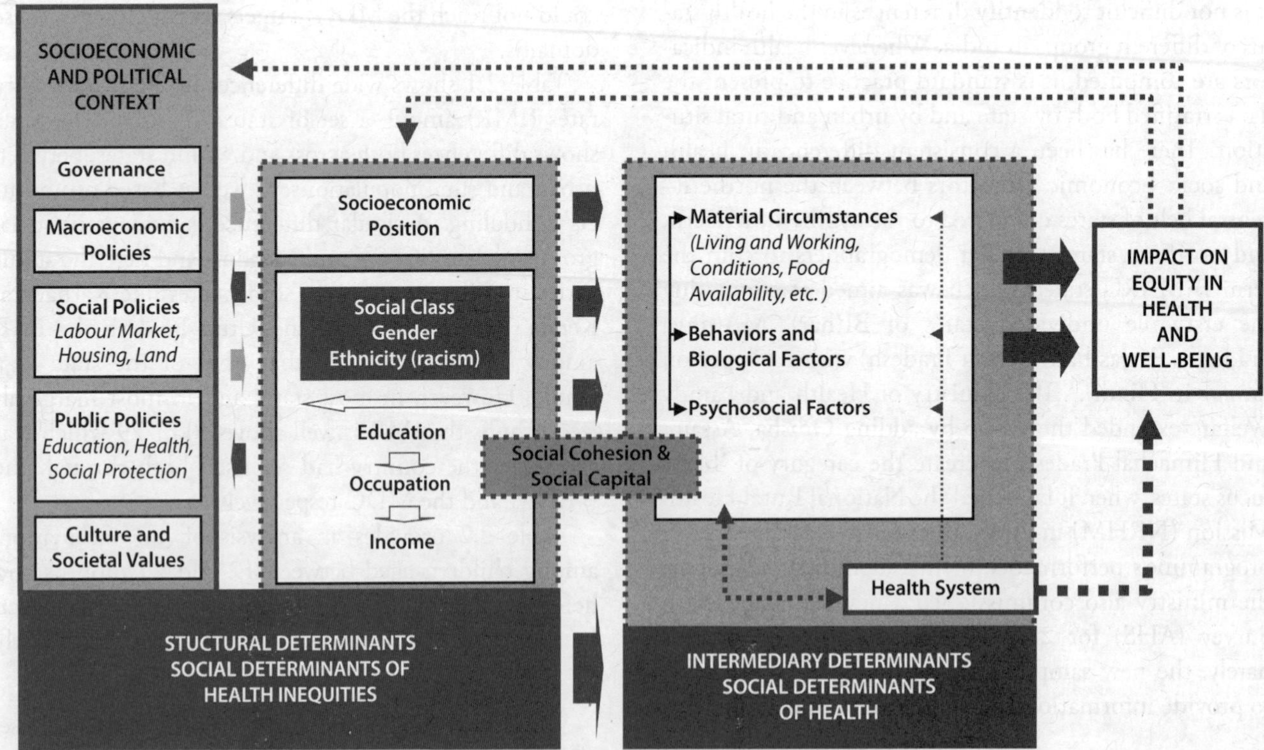

Figure 2.1 Social Determinants of Health Framework

Source: World Health Organization (2010).

influence and interaction. It is important to note that social factors like gender and ethnicity along with educational status or income reinforce each other, magnifying their combined influence. These are further influenced by psychosocial as well as behavioural issues influencing a person's or a community's ability to seek services and ability to lead a healthy life. In a recent study of health-seeking for maternal care among tribal communities in Odisha, it has been reported (Contractor and Das 2015) that the health system was completely ignorant of the health-related beliefs and practices of the tribal community in the district. The provisions that had been made available were not in consonance with the worldviews and practices of the forest-dwelling indigenous tribes. Their food habits, ways of living, and health belief systems were very different from the rural people of the same district. As a result, these forest-dwelling communities were not seeking services, and a sense of frustration had set in among providers. I have also witnessed a similar situation during a fact-finding mission into the unusually large numbers of maternal deaths reported among tribal communities in Badwani district of Madhya Pradesh (AGCA 2011) and Godda District of Jharkhand (NAMHHR and Torang Trust 2014). There is a need to recognize the different health belief systems of marginalized tribal communities if 'we' from the mainstream are to design and implement health systems useful for such communities. If, however, we consider them 'ignorant' and 'naïve', our intervention may not be successful.

I was involved in a review of 140 maternal deaths from the states of Jharkhand, Odisha, Uttar Pradesh, and West Bengal (NAMHHR and SAHAYOG 2016) and the experience highlighted a different set of issues around inequity around the relationship of the public provider with poor and marginalized communities. Communication between the public system functionaries and Dalit, tribal or Muslim communities was found to be wanting in many cases. In some instances it was found that the functionaries not only did not speak the indigenous language of these communities, but more importantly, harassed, indulged in abusive behaviour as well as delayed and refused to provide necessary treatment.

India has a highly structured society with caste hierarchies, tribal populations, and religious divisions. Social subordination also includes ideas of both exclusion and pollution which were earlier manifested as 'untouchability'. Even though illegal, shades of exclusion based on social hierarchies are evident in the way some health functionaries interact with marginalized communities. Matters are further complicated by the notion of ritual pollution and physical exclusion which are implicated in the process of childbirth in some Indian communities (Pinto 2008). Discriminatory mindsets, both social and patriarchal, are found among functionaries of the health system, influencing their attitude and behaviour towards patients from marginalized communities. In such a situation it is difficult to provide 'affirmative' healthcare support without a sociocultural analysis.

There are also situations where marginalized women readily accept extremely poor-quality services because they may not know of any other possibility. This was seen in the sterilization camp at Kaparfora, Bihar (Bannerjee 2012) where the camp was conducted in a school building with little concern for surgical standards. The women were from extremely backward classes and when interviewed later said that they were willing to take the risks of undergoing surgery in extremely difficult and distressing circumstances because they were extremely keen to limit their childbearing and this was the only option that they were aware of.

These examples show how a social determinants' approach, which helps to understand the relationship of social status of the patient, his/her material conditions, as well local health functionaries' attitudes and actions towards the patient along with the health belief systems and practices of the community, its levels of self-confidence and expectation, influence the ultimate health outcome of certain individual and communities. Detailed qualitative studies including ethnographic studies of the community as well as health system may be necessary to understand areas which need specific intervention. This understanding is essential for the appropriate design, delivery, and monitoring of health services.

RECONCILING HEALTH EQUITY AND HEALTH RIGHTS

Health inequity has a close relationship with health rights, including the additional dimension of redressal. The right to health has been considered an integral part of human rights since the Universal Declaration of Human Rights (UN 1948), however operational advice was provided by the Office of the High Commissioner on Human Rights through the General Comment 14 only in 2000. The General Comment clarifies that the rights include both freedoms and obligations. Freedoms include freedom from torture, freedom from non-consensual treatment, and right to one's decision regarding medical treatment, and the right over one's own body. On the other hand, the obligation of the State is to provide a health system that allows equal opportunity for all to enjoy the highest attainable standard of health. The instances of maternal health and family planning described in the earlier section on health inequity can easily be seen within a health rights' framework.

The issue of non-consensual sterilization has been documented for a long time, and in many places across the world (Patel 2017) including in India (Choudhury, Lairenlakpam, and Das 2012; Das, Rai, and Singh 2003; Pal, Singh, and Shakya n.d.). The Supreme Court of India had taken cognizance of the right of women to consensual and quality sterilization services and highlighted the need for the health department to follow standards laid down by the Government of India first in the case *Ramakant Rai and another* v *Union of India*[3] and reinforced again in the case of *Devika Biswas* v *Union of India.*[4] In Africa, the issue of non-consensual sterilization of HIV positive women has been raised in Namibia, South Africa, Zambia, and the Democratic Republic of Congo (Smith 2009). In Eastern Europe, marginalized Roma communities have been targeted. In Namibia and Slovakia, the courts have provided judgments in favour of the women acknowledging their rights have been violated (Patel 2017). In the *Devika Biswas* case, the Supreme Court notes that the right to life, right health and right to reproductive health have been violated. The Supreme Court has further asserted that the right to reproductive health has been established in India as a part of right to life through cases such as *Suchita Srivastava* v *Chandigarh Administration*[5] as well as through international jurisprudence such as *Ms AS* v *Hungary*[6] where the Committee on the Elimination of Discrimination Against Women found Hungary to have violated certain articles of CEDAW,[7] which is an international treaty akin to law.

General Comment 14 of the UN Committee on Economic Social and Cultural Rights (CESCR) identifies four key elements of health services—availability, accessibility, acceptability, and quality which are necessary to make it rights compliant. In India, the courts have, through a number of cases, for example, *Ramakant Rai* case, *Sandesh Bansal* v *Union of India and others,*[8] *Laxmi Mandal* v *Deen Dayal Harinagar Hospital and Others,*[9] *Jaitun* vs *Maternity Home, MCD, Jangpura & Others,*[10] referred to these parameters as being essential to state responsibility for healthcare and have called upon the state to comply. The Supreme Court has also indicated what the core obligations of the state are in terms of service provision as well as results or outcomes.

ELEMENTS AND INDICATORS OF A RIGHTS-BASED APPROACH

While courts have seen the obligations of conduct and obligations of outcome as core obligations of the state to comply with right to health and made these justiciable, it is not possible for all marginalized groups or individuals to seek the intervention of courts for perceived violations of their health rights. To address this challenge the human rights-based approaches (HRBA) to policymaking was adopted by the UN mechanism in 2003[11] and also applies to the domain involving health. This approach recognizes that health outcomes are a result of inequalities, discriminatory practices, and unjust power relations which have been illustrated with specific examples earlier. The key actors are divided into 'rights holders' or the community and 'duty bearers' or the health system functionaries as well as other members of government including policymakers. To take measures to respect, protect, and fulfill the right is the key obligation of duty bearers. Participation and inclusion, equality and non-discrimination, and accountability are elements included within HRBA. Recognizing that neither duty bearers nor rights holders are intrinsically competent to fulfill their functions due to existing social circumstances, mobilizing and empowering communities to recognize and claim their health rights and building capacity among duty bearers to fulfill their obligations are also included as components of a HRBA.

The HRBA allows the equity analysis to be taken a step further by adding the dimensions of participation, accountability, and remedy, and specifies obligations for the state to take operational measures to redress inequities. However, policymaking guidelines for this purpose

[3] WP(C) no. 209 of 2003.

[4] WP(C) no. 95 of 2012.

[5] (2009) 9 SCC 1.

[6] Comm. 2/2003, U.N. Doc.

[7] CEDAW or Convention on the Elimination of All form of Discrimination Against Women is an international treaty that was adopted by the UN in 1979 and ratified by India in 1994.

[8] WP no. 9061 of 2008.

[9] WP(C) no. 8853 of 2008.

[10] WP no. 10700 of 2009.

[11] For additional details, please see the HRBA portal at http://hrbaportal.org/.

are not readily available. Experts (Backman et al. 2008) have identified some 'right to health' features of a health system and elaborated a list of 72 indicators. Legal Recognition is seen as an important feature, but without other follow-up mechanisms it is hollow. Standards are considered as key because they outline what can be expected by way of health-related services and facilities through aspects like regulations, protocols, guidelines, and codes of conduct associated with healthcare practice. Quality, participation, equity, equality and non-discrimination, and transparency are obviously seen as important features. Respect for cultural differences is seen as an important feature and includes sensitizing the providers and managers to be aware of cultural differences and include this in their approach. Monitoring and accountability provide opportunities for the community to participate and include provisions for redress in case of mistakes and mishaps.

The practice of quality, evidence-based, and ethically sound medicine is increasingly becoming the norm, and forms an important component of a rights-based approach. Ethical standards are aimed at protecting patients from irresponsible actions and potentially harmful consequences. Protocols, guidelines, and checklists are useful to improve effectiveness and reduce cost of treatments. The WHO provides global guidance on these and individual countries as well as professional bodies of physicians and other specialists prepare them for their specific needs. Indian courts have made repeated reference to these standards and protocols in their orders and judgments described earlier. Expert bodies like the National Institute of Clinical Excellence (NICE) in the UK and similar bodies in countries such as Spain, Germany, Australia and others prepare these guidelines (Legido-Quigley et al. 2008). Patient rights or what is owed to the patient by the physician, hospital, and the state form the third key dimension that closes the loop of rights related to health. These rights have been defined slightly differently in various settings and countries and may also include legal liability provisions.

RIGHT TO HEALTH FEATURES IN INDIA

There have also been several occasions where the Government of India has acknowledged the right to health, even though it is not a constitutional right. The implementation framework of the NRHM (MoHFW 2005) acknowledged this in the sections on accountability, role of NGOs, and community action. It asserted that the 'right to health is recognized as inalienable right of all citizens as brought out by the relevant rulings of the Supreme Court as well as the International Conventions to which India is a signatory. As rights convey entitlement to the citizens, these rights are to be incorporated in the monitoring framework of the Mission. Therefore, providing basic Health services to all the citizens as guaranteed entitlements will be attempted under the NRHM.' Unfortunately, the accountability component of NRHM and subsequently the National Health Mission remained relatively less explored. Community-based accountability mechanisms were piloted and continue to be implemented unevenly in different states.[12] Maharashtra is one state where community-based planning and monitoring mechanisms have been implemented with some earnestness[13].

Twelve years after the introduction of the NRHM, the Government of India announced the National Health Policy, 2017 (NHP 2017), and this policy is in a dilemma over 'whether we have reached the level of economic and health systems development so as to make this a justiciable right—implying that its denial is an offense.' It goes on to place a number of practical barriers to legislating a right to health and ends with the proposal for a 'progressively incremental assurance based approach, with assured funding to create an enabling environment for realizing healthcare as a right in the future' (MoHFW 2017). The implementation framework for the NHP 2017 has still not been formulated and it remains to be seen the nature of assurances along with the accountability mechanisms that will get adopted. The draft of a national health bill 2009 had been publicly circulated but the fate of the bill and the inputs received remain unclear since it was not placed before Parliament.[14]

While policy articulations are still non-committal, there are several 'right to health' features that exist in the country. The Clinical Establishments Act, 2010, makes it mandatory for all medical institutions to be registered. Unfortunately, few states have enacted this law or framed the appropriate rules and hence this law remains unimplemented. Also, most hospitals, nursing homes, clinics, and laboratories function without any regulation or sometimes follow the National Accreditation Board for Hospitals (NABH) and National Accreditation Board

[12] For further details see www.nrhmcommunityaction.org.

[13] For further details see www.cbmpmaharashtra.org.

[14] A copy of the draft National Health Bill 2009 is available online at http://www.prsindia.org/uploads/media/Draft_National_Bill.pdf .

for Testing and Calibration Laboratories (NABL)[15] accreditation, which are voluntary. The centre–state schism is an important feature of health-related policymaking in the country. The Constitution of India places 'health' in the state list, while 'public health' and 'family planning' are in the Central and Concurrent lists respectively. However, the national government does exert its influence on healthcare provisioning in the state through a number of national health programmes, which have differential funding support from the national and state governments. The Government of India has made a beginning in developing such standards and guidelines for various national health programmes. The Concrete Service Guarantees (CSG) and the Indian Public Health Standards (IPHS) provide a framework for health entitlements at different levels of care. Among the states, the Chhattisgarh government has prepared a standard operating procedure for its hospitals. The Supreme Court of India in the case of *Devika Biswas*, directed the Union government to take all necessary steps to ensure that there is compliance of quality standards related to family planning programming.

In order to provide quality medical care at affordable costs to all, it is necessary to adopt a method which both guides rational therapeutic choices as well as use of low-cost generic medicines. Médecins Sans Frontières, a global healthcare nonprofit, has prepared its own standard treatment guidelines which is also approved by the WHO. In India, the Delhi Society for the Promotion of Rational Use of Drugs, an NGO working closely with the Delhi government, prepared a set of standard treatment guidelines (Sharma, Sethi, and Gupta 2009) appropriate for India. Some states have issued this standard treatment guidelines, but currently there are no mechanisms to ensure compliance. While junior doctors welcomed the idea, consultants were averse to it. Some of the opposition included fear of misuse by non-qualified practitioners, and limiting doctors' prescribing autonomy (Sharma 2015). There is also a concern whether such standard treatment guidelines can function without an essential medicines list. The WHO has advised countries to adopt such lists and the Indian government has adopted the National List of Essential Medicines in 2011 and revised it in 2015, resulting in the preparatory step being taken.

Another important component of right to health is the regulation of medical practice, both in the public and private sectors. In India the private sector is the main provider of health services. It is also characterized by high costs and inconsistent quality. The role of the Medical Council of India, regulating body for the practice of modern medicine, has been far from exemplary with its president having been prosecuted for corruption.[16] Currently it remains under the regulation of the Supreme Court of India. The Indian government has proposed a mechanism of a medical commission which will subsume the functions of the medical as well as nursing council, and while a bill to that effect has been drafted, it has not yet been formalized.

Another important 'right to health' feature in India includes the presence of national and state human rights commissions, or ombudsman organizations that engage with the right to health. The National Human Rights Commission (NHRC) has in the past issued guidelines for rights as well as taken up issues related to health such as mental illness and silicosis. The NHRC has a core group on health, which includes public health and health rights experts from the government, academia, and civil society. The presence of a vibrant civil society which actively engages in public policy formulation and monitoring is another feature of governance in India. The civil society has played an important role in drafting and pushing for the laws around the Right to Education, the Right to Information, the Protection of Women from Domestic Violence Act 2005 (PWDVA), Protection of Children from Sexual Offences (POCSO) Act 2012, the National Food Security Act 2013, and so on. Health rights have been an area of concern of civil society and various organizations concerned with this work together as the Jan Swasthya Abhiyan (Peoples' Health Movement) and various other networks.

Operationalizing a Rights-based Approach in India

Various elements of a right to health approach are present in India. The question is how can these be put together to create a viable framework for operation. During the preparation of the Twelfth Five-Year Plan (2012–17),

[15] NABH refers to the National Accreditation Board for Hospitals and NABL to National Accreditation Board for Testing and Calibration Laboratories that provide accreditation to hospitals and laboratories on their request.

[16] See http://indianexpress.com/article/india/india-others/indian-doctor-facing-corruption-charges-could-head-world-health-association/.

the government had set up a high-level expert group (HLEG) to advise the Planning Commission about how Universal Health Coverage (UHC) could be achieved. Some elements of the recommendations from the HLEG were incorporated into the Twelfth Plan. Subsequently the Planning Commission was disbanded in favour of the NITI Aayog (National Institution for Transforming India). The NITI Aayog has advised the current government in preparing a national health protection scheme, an insurance-based programme announced during the Annual Budget for 2018–19. Most experts are of the opinion that the budgetary outlay remains inadequate along with other issues. India has among the lowest public health investments in health at around 1.2 per cent of the GDP, despite several assurances to the contrary. It represents a little over 30 per cent of the entire health expenditure of the country, the rest of which is individual and out of pocket. Such high out-of-pocket (OOP) expenditures constrains health-seeking even among the not-so-poor, and is a major reason for impoverishment.

To complicate matters, the centre–state division of responsibilities and proportion of allocation makes it difficult in pinning down the locus of decision making in a diverse and federal country like India. The allocation to health by different states is vastly different, and states with poorer health indicators have lower allocations. Also, in recent years changes in the centre–state tax devolution mechanism have meant that a greater proportion of the revenue is now transferred to the state treasury for state-level decision making. However, the concomitant increases in allocation to health have not been visible in state budgets (CPR 2015). Thus, the somewhat simpler route to right to health through increased outlays either at the state or the central level is not easily available. Instead different components could be implemented separately by different stakeholders in the manner of trying to assemble pieces of a giant jigsaw puzzle.

State and National Level Health Bureaucracy

As has already been mentioned health is a state subject, and different states have varying levels of investments in health. The variation in the levels of state budgetary outlay is as high as 10 times between states. For example, it is roughly INR 600 per capita for Bihar and over INR 6,500 per capita for Mizoram, a state which is not among the richest in India (Bhattacharya and Kundu 2017). This means Mizoram is able to implement a state-wide health insurance scheme for all its citizens through the Mizoram State Health Care Scheme (Thanga 2015), arranging for treatment elsewhere when it does not have all the curative facilities in the state. Similarly, the state has adopted an essential medicines list, and is among the minority of states to have adopted the Clinical Establishments Act 2010 and formulated the rules. Karnataka, one of the more advanced states, has enacted the Karnataka Private Medical Establishment's Act 2007 to regulate the private sector, with instructions around standards and schedule of charges which have to be displayed. This law is currently being amended since some gaps were identified. The Maharashtra government has been implementing community monitoring within its national health mission systematically and regularly since 2007. These are a few examples to demonstrate that the state governments and even the bureaucracy at the national level have some level of flexibility of adopting and implementing different elements of a rights-based approach if they so wish.

District Level Health Managers

The Indian government has provided much guidance on standards of care through the IPHS as well as mechanisms for community engagement through the Rogi Kalyan Samitis (Patient Welfare Committees). Decentralized planning is expected during the annual planning process or preparation of the District Project Implementation Plan (DPIP). However, these mechanisms are seldom implemented, even though to do so is well within the jurisdiction of the district level managers. Participatory monitoring of the progress of the DPIP implementation is also possible under the mechanism of the community-based planning and monitoring processes. District health managers are in a position to take individual initiatives through these provisions, and these will improve the delivery of services.

Doctors

In recent times there have been increasing reports of patients' relatives and associates beating up doctors in public and private hospitals (Das 2017b). These incidents indicate a breakdown in the relationship between doctors and the patient community. Doctors are partly responsible for this erosion of respect as costs of care have risen exorbitantly and patients also perceive poor quality of care and a lack of empathy on the part of the doctors and healthcare workers. The medical community has also refused to accept regulations with state level protests by doctors' associations[17] against the Clinical Establishment's Act and other measures to introduce accountability as has happened in West Bengal and Karnataka.[18]

This situation of confrontation between doctors and patients, as well doctors' refusal towards regulation needs to change. As communities are becoming affluent, educated, and aspirational, they will expect better results and greater accountability from doctors. The medical community needs to anticipate this, and like in other 'developed' countries set up mechanisms for greater self-regulation. In countries such as the US and the UK, professional associations of specialists issue standards of care for their specialties. In India, healthcare providers need to take leadership to promote the practice of evidence-based medicine. This will require setting up guidance on standards of care and protocol for treatment as well as for monitoring their use. Doctors should also realize that healthcare costs are spiralling out of control. Some level of transparency and standardization of costs for treatment of different conditions and for conducting various procedures is absolutely necessary.

COURTS AND HUMAN RIGHTS COMMISSIONS

Mention has already been made of the progressive jurisprudence in the country which has made 'right to health' a de jure right even though it has not been explicitly included in the list of fundamental rights. The NHRC has the explicit mandate to review the human rights and has a core group on health, comprising eminent health professionals to advise it. It has taken a series of steps on particular issues like mental health, silicosis to help further a health rights approach. It has also worked closely with civil society groups like the Jan Swasthya Abhiyan in 2003–4 and 2015–16 to establish criteria for health rights violations and conducted several health-related public hearings across the country. Indian citizens can also independently approach the NHRC for arbitration in specific cases and they are known to issue directions to the particular government.

Legislators

Legislators, both at the state and the central levels, occupy the apex position where policymaking is concerned. The specific areas where legislators can intervene include the budget-making process, helping review health plans and policies through their participation in joint committees or select committees of the parliament at the state or central levels. Legislators can work individually or in groups to create an enabling environment increasing budgetary outlays that are known to be abysmal, or create greater legislative support for health-related laws and accountability. The idea of legislating a change in the position of health from being a subject of state jurisdiction to one on the concurrent list can go a long way to increasing the national government's interest and accountability in the state of health of its citizens. Every year the health plan and budget need to be passed through the legislature and, occasionally, the office of the comptroller and auditor general (CAG) prepares performance audits which are placed before the legislature. Legislators can also initiate action in their own constituency through their membership in the different district level committees as well as their ability to fund specific interventions through their discretionary funds. There are thus plenty of opportunities for the legislators to draw attention to key issues and to initiate action.

Civil Society

With the policymakers being reluctant in leading on rights-based policymaking, the civil society in India has been playing a crucial policy advocacy role. With increased economic growth, the need for civil society to provide services directly to deprived communities has reduced. The role of civil society is important in strengthening democratic governance by mobilizing 'active citizenship' among poor and marginalized communities. Many laws and policies in recent years have been the result of civil society campaigns like the Right to Food Campaign, Right to Information Campaign, campaigns against domestic violence, sexual violence and so on. In the realm of health there are a number

[17] UP Doctors to Protest Against Clinical Establishment's Act—https://timesofindia.indiatimes.com/city/agra/UP-doctors-to-protest-against-Clinical-Establishment-Act/articleshow/53304437.cms Clinical Establishment's Act: Doctors Observe Black Day—http://indianexpress.com/article/india/clinical-establishment-act-2017-doctors-observe-national-black-day-4631126/.

[18] Private Hospitals up in arms against KPME Act amendment—http://www.thehindu.com/news/national/karnataka/private-hospitals-up-in-arms-against-kpme-act-amendment/article19051222.ece.

of health advocacy groups including the Jan Swasthya Abhiyan members, who are involved in mobilizing communities to claim their rights and participate in spaces available in the current policy framework, for example, the Rogi Kalyan Samitis associated with hospitals and health centres and district and state level committees. Civil society groups are also engaged in community-based monitoring and planning in some states. Several other organizations are engaged in strategic litigation around health matters and some of these cases have been referred to in earlier sections. Though health is covered under the Consumer Protection Act, 1986, the presence of consumer groups or patients' groups in the country is still not widespread. More coordinated work along these lines, at the district, state, and national level in addition to linking this up with people's representatives can help in creating a political environment around health, which does not exist today.

* * *

The issue of health is increasingly emerging as an 'Achilles heel' in the glowing success story of India. Ensuring all citizens are able to access health services which is effective and of reasonable quality and also acceptable is at the core of a strong, self-reliant, and developed nation which occupies our imagination. Several practical steps have been outlined in this chapter that draw attention to ways in which a 'right to health' approach may be adopted through actions by different stakeholders in different places. This is possible because many of the components are already in place. A multi-stakeholder approach in drawing these elements together, including the participation of the community—those whose lives are at stake are important not only to be effective but to make these changes sustainable over time.

REFERENCES

Advisory Group on Community Action (AGCA). 2011. *Maternal deaths in Barwani district: Accountability, quality of care, referral systems AGCA team's visit to Barwani.* Available at https://nrhmcommunityaction.org/wp-content/uploads/2016/10/Microsoft-Word-Maternal-Deaths-in-Barwani-District-AGCA-visit-report-Final.pdf, last accessed on 4 October 2019.

Backman, Gunilla, Paul Hunt, Rajat Khosla, Camilla Jarmillo-Strauss, Belachew Mekuria FIkre, Caroline Rumble, David Pevalin et al. 2008. 'Health Systems and the Right to Health: An Assessment of 194 Countries'. *The Lancet*, December, vol 372: 2047–85.

Bannerjee, Soumojit. 2012. 'Barrack-room surgery in Bihar's Backwaters'. *The Hindu*, 23 January. Available at http://www.thehindu.com/todays-paper/tp-opinion/Barrack-room-surgery-in-Bihars-backwaters/article13377750.ece, last accessed on 4 October 2019.

Bhattacharya, Pramit and Tadit Kundu. 2017. 'How are State Governments spending on education, health and irrigation?' *Live Mint*, 26 April. Available at http://www.livemint.com/Politics/PGqjz0bMYX3uF2rZcIFd7H/How-are-state-governments-spending-on-education-health-and.html, last accessed on 4 October 2019.

Chowdhury, Jayeeta, Melissa Lairenlakapam, and Abhijit Das. 2012. 'Have the Supreme Court Guidelines made a difference? A study of Quality of Care of Women's Sterilisation in 5 States', in *Reaching the Unreached: Rapid Assessment Studies of Health Programmes Implementation in India*, edited by Amy Hagopian, Peter House and Abhijit Das. New Delhi: Nidhi Books.

Commission on Social Determinants of Health (CSDH). 2008. 'Closing the gap in a generation: Health equity through action on the social determinants of health'. Final Report of the Commission on Social Determinants of Health. Geneva: World Health Organization.

Contractor, Sana and Abhijit Das. 2015. 'Does one-size-fit-all? Re-evaluating the approach to address Maternal Health of Tribal Communities in India'. Paper presented at the 13th Development Dialogue, 'The ghosts of MDG: Unpacking the logics of development' at ISS, The Hague, November 4–5, 2015.

Das, Abhijit, Ramakand Rai and Dinesh Singh. 2004. 'Medical Negligence and Rights Violation'. *Economic and Political Weekly* 39(35): 3876–9.

Das, Abhijit. 2017a. 'The challenge of evaluating equity in health: Experiences from India's maternal health program'. In *Building Capacities to Evaluate Health Inequities: Some Lessons Learned from Evaluation Experiments in China, India and Chile*, edited by S. Sridharan, K. Zhao, & A. Nakaima. New Directions for Evaluation, 154: 91–100.

Das, Abhijit. 2017b. 'Challenge before the National Health Policy: Rebuilding trust between Patients and the Healthcare system'. *The Dialogue*, 29 March. Available at http://www.thedialogue.co/challenge-national-health-policy-rebuilding-trust-patients-healthcare-system/, last accessed on 4 October 2019.

Kapur Avni, Vikram Srinivas, and Priyanka R. Choudhury. 2015. 'State of Social Sector Expenditure in 2015–16'. Budget Brief, Accountability Initiative, Centre for Policy Research, New Delhi.

Legido-Quigley, Helena, Martin McKee, Ellen Nolte, and Irene A. Glinos. 2008. *Assuring the Quality of Health Care in the European Union: A Case for Action*. Copenhagen: WHO Regional Office for Europe.

Ministry of Health and Family Welfare (MoHFW). 2005. 'National Rural Health Mission: Framework for

Implementation 2005–2012', Ministry of Health and Family Welfare, Government of India. Available at http://nhm.gov.in/images/pdf/about-nrhm/nrhm-framework-implementation/nrhm-framework-latest.pdf, last accessed on 4 October 2019.

———. 2017. National Health Policy 2017. Ministry of Health and Family Welfare, Government of India, New Delhi.

National Alliance on Maternal Health and Human Rights (NAMHHR) and Torang Trust. 2014. *Maternal Health and Nutrition in Tribal Areas: Fact Finding Mission to Godda*. Ranchi, Jharkhand: NAMHHR India and Torang Trust.

Pal, Swarup, Bajrang Singh, and Shreeti Shakya. Undated. 'Continuing Concerns: An Assessment of Quality of Care of Female Sterilisation in Bundi District of Rajashtan in 2009–10'. Centre for Health and Social Justice New Delhi. Available at http://www.chsj.org/uploads/1/0/2/1/10215849/swarup_r_pal_bajrang_singh_shreeti_shakya-03-01-12.pdf, last accessed on 4 October 2019.

Patel, Priti. 2017. 'Forced sterilization of women as discrimination'. *Public Health Reviews* 38:15. doi:10.1186/s40985-017-0060-9.

Pinto, Sarah. 2008. *Where There is No Midwife: Birth and Loss in Rural India*. Berghahn Books, New York.

Sharma, Sangeeta, G.R. Sethi, and Usha Gupta. 2009. *Standard Treatment Guidelines: A Manual for Medical Therapeutics*, 3rd edition. New Delhi: B.I. Publications.

Sharma, Sangeeta, Gulshan R. Sethi, Usha Gupta, and Ranjit Roy Chowdhury. 2015. 'Developing standard treatment guidelines in India'. *WHO South-East Asia Journal of Public Health* 4(1): 86–91.

Sharma, V. 2015. 'Are BIMARU States still BIMARU', *Economic and Political Weekly* 50(18): 58–63.

Smith, David. 2009. 'African women with HIV "coerced into sterilization"'. *The Guardian*, 22 June. Available at https://www.theguardian.com/world/2009/jun/22/africa-hiv-positive-women-sterilisation, last accessed on 4 October 2019.

World Bank. 2005. *World Development Report 2006: Equity and Development*. Washington, DC: World Bank. https://openknowledge.worldbank.org/handle/10986/5988, last accessed on 4 October 2019.

World Health Organization. 2010. 'A Conceptual Framework For Action on Social Determinants of Health: Social Determinants of Health', Discussion Paper 2, World Health Organization, Geneva. Available at https://www.who.int/sdhconference/resources/ConceptualframeworkforactiononSDH_eng.pdf, last accessed on 4 October 2019.

3

Responsibility for Health

Ali Mehdi

There has been a fundamental lack of clarity and consensus in India regarding the nature of the State's responsibility for health. This is reflected in health governance, financing, and outcomes most particularly. According to India's National Health Policy, 2017 (NHP 2017), 'one of the most important strengths and at the same time challenges of governance in health is the distribution of responsibility and accountability between the Centre and the States.' While health is the constitutional responsibility of states, the Centre has, in practice, played a leading role at various levels, with several central departments not willing to give up their powers. This has led to a situation in which both the Centre (theoretically) and the states (practically) are able to disown responsibility for the health of citizens. The rise of the free market system and rising burden of so-called lifestyle-based diseases have encouraged the State to increasingly shift responsibility to individuals themselves—'Your health, your responsibility'; it is very intuitive and convincing, even for the affected citizens.

However, this has had implications for the country at various levels. Public expenditure pattern is a good indicator of practical priorities, irrespective of the rhetoric characteristic of public speeches and policies. As the NHP 2017 states, 'a policy is only as good as its implementation'. While government health expenditure—as a percentage of GDP or general government expenditure or current health expenditure—is the lowest, out-of-pocket expenditure incurred by citizens is the highest in India, both by huge margins vis-à-vis its economic peers (Figure 3.1). In terms of outcomes, India's healthy life expectancy is the lowest among the world's top 10 economies. In 2016, it was one year less in India than it was in China way back in 1990 (60 years), and has improved slower (16 per cent) than even sub-Saharan Africa (18 per cent) during this time (Global Burden of Disease [GBD]). That the Indian State has been more committed towards the wealth of the nation is evident from the fact that India is among the top 10 economies in the world; it aspires to be among the top three over the next quarter century (*Hindustan Times* 2018). Although the centrality of health for economic growth is now widely recognized in India's policy circles, there is no such aspiration for health—as we elaborate—even from an instrumentalist economic perspective.

In *Nicomachean Ethics* (written in 350 BC), Aristotle argued that 'the life of money-making is one undertaken under compulsion, and wealth is evidently not the good we are seeking; for it is merely useful and for the sake of something else'. Health, on the other hand, is useful in itself as well as, inter alia, for household and

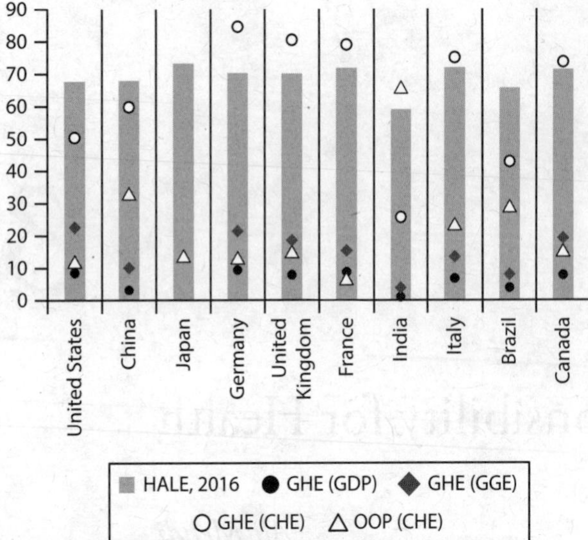

Figure 3.1 Health Life Expectancy and Levels of Health Expenditures in Top 10 Economies (2015/2016)

Source: HALE is from GBD, the rest from the World Development Indicators (WDI).

Notes: HALE stands for healthy life expectancy for birth (years), GHE for government health expenditure (percentage of whatever in brackets), GDP for gross domestic product, GGE for general government expenditure, CHE for current health expenditure, and OOP for out-of-pocket expenditure. All data is for 2015 unless mentioned otherwise.

national economy. One could argue that if there was as much commitment to health, the country might well have been among the top three economies by now, and without it, it might never be—thanks to the growing significance of human capital as a critical determinant of global economic competitiveness. A high OOP expenditure clearly reflects people's preference for health, even at the risk of impoverishment. Health appears to matter more to them than wealth.

In view of these implications, as well as to reap demographic and electoral dividends, the Centre and several states have been developing a host of healthcare schemes. The State is still not accepting responsibility for health, but rather adopting a welfarist route vis-à-vis health and other critical areas of concern, thanks to the shocking defeat of the 'India Shining' campaign in the 2004 general elections. The Centre has come up with several grand healthcare schemes ever since—the NRHM in 2005, the Rashtriya Swasthya Bima Yojana (RSBY) in 2008 and now the Ayushman Bharat National Health Protection Scheme (NHPS), announced in the Union budget 2018–19 and flaunted as the world's largest government-funded healthcare programme. Through the NHPS, the finance minister in his Budget speech for 2018–19,[1] promised to bring 'healthcare system closer to the homes of people' by means of 150,000 primary-care wellness centres and annual insurance cover of INR 500,000 for more than 100 million poor and vulnerable families for secondary/tertiary care hospitalization, and thereby build a 'New India 2022' which is characterized by 'enhanced productivity, well being' as well as minimized 'wage loss and impoverishment'. There was no commitment though to raise healthy life expectancy or government health expenditures even one notch up within the category of the top 10 economies, let alone among the top three. In health, we are fine to be in the company of sub-Saharan Africa; in wealth, nothing but the best.

The economic rationale for *investing* in citizens' health appears to be clear to Indian policymakers. A fundamental clarity on the issue of responsibility, however, remains absent. It has to be resolved, first and foremost, at the conceptual level and only then will there be clarity vis-à-vis governance, financing, and accountability with regards to outcomes. Therefore, in this chapter, I discuss the nature of the State's responsibility for health from epidemiological and ethical perspectives by first invoking the framework of types of responsibility outlined by Ronald Dworkin in his book *Justice for Hedgehogs* (2011). To offer more details, I highlight the determinants of health and their complexity to present an epidemiological rationale for the State's responsibility in Section 2. Unless the State is causally held responsible for a particular health outcome, the epidemiological rationale, by itself, does not make a normative case for the State's responsibility for health of citizens. This is why the ethical perspective is needed. In Section 3, therefore, I briefly make an ethical case for the State's duty and argue that the focus of public policy should be on health rather than determinants. Given a predominant focus on healthcare, along with incoherent commitments in national health policies and programmes towards health per se and broader determinants of health, a conceptual clarity on this issue is essential. Since health policies and programmes are prepared, and the national health discourse is dominated by technocrats, there has been little place for conceptual discussions on the subject. As a result, India's health sector continues to be marred by

[1] https://www.indiabudget.gov.in/budget2018-2019/ub2018-19/bs/bs.pdf, last accessed on 4 October 2019.

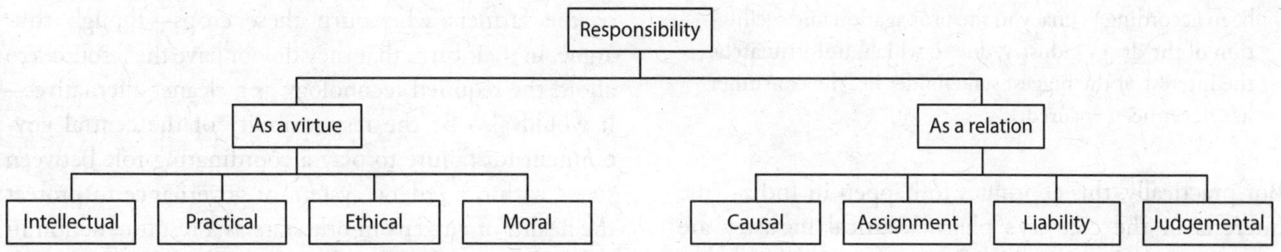

Figure 3.2 Types of responsibilities
Source: Developed by author from Dworkin (2011: 102–3).

unprincipled and unscientific policymaking, which itself is irresponsible of the State for the health of citizens. No wonder, the first type of responsibility that we discuss in the Dworkinian framework is intellectual.

While discussions here have been conducted with reference to the particular Indian context, they are conceptually relevant to other countries as well, where there is a lack of clarity and consensus vis-à-vis the nature of the State's responsibility. The US stands out as a classic example here—despite its per capita government health expenditure being the highest in the world, there has been a greater focus on individual responsibility—in health as in other spheres—compared to that in Europe or Canada, while the government's approach has been more welfarist in nature (Medicaid or Medicare). The result is health outcomes incommensurate with resources invested in healthcare. The US is also home to the world's most sophisticated health regulatory system. Yet, it seems that a State's sense of responsibility vis-à-vis health is a much better guarantor of good health outcomes. That is what matters at the end of the day as far as the concern for health goes. As Mirza Ghalib expressed in one of his Urdu couplets—'*ibn-e-mariyam huā kare koī, mere dukh kī davā kare koī*' ('let someone be the Son of Mary, let someone cure my pain').[2]

TYPES OF RESPONSIBILITIES

Although developed in the context of individuals, Dworkin's framework of types of responsibility (Figure 3.2) could be adapted for discussing the nature of the State's responsibility on the issue of health. Dworkin did not define his types in much detail, which allows us to take the liberty of defining them as per our own specific objective here, keeping within his overall framework.

All public policies and programmes to protect and promote the health of citizens should be developed as per the responsibilities characterized 'as a virtue'. For instance, all public policies and programmes pertaining to health should be based on sound evidence as part of the State's intellectual responsibility for health. This type of responsibility could also imply the promotion of research and development to understand and tackle the determinants of health, scientific approach to health sector regulation (particularly vis-à-vis drugs), et cetera. As part of its practical responsibility, its policies and programmes should be practical—in India, they are high in rhetoric, but rarely practical, which is one of the major reasons for a yawning gap between policies and programmes and their implementation and outcomes. Tackling issues related to implementation—for instance, ensuring that drug regulatory provisions are followed and medicines sold in the market meet the standards of safety, efficacy, and quality—is also an example of such responsibility. As per the 59th Report of India's Parliamentary Standing Committee on Health and Family Welfare (Parliament of India 2012), 'the state's responsibility to regulate the import, manufacture and sale of medicines so as to ensure that they are both safe, effective and of standard quality acquire almost sacrosanct dimensions'.

Our drug regulatory authorities—without singling out the drug regulator, who has not been sufficiently empowered to be blamed alone—have failed in their intellectual as well as practical responsibilities. An example of ethical responsibility is that all public efforts for health should have clear objectives. This may sound quite obvious, but consider this, once again, from the 59th Report:

> The Committee is of the firm opinion that most of the ills besetting the system of drugs regulation in India are mainly due to the skewed priorities and perceptions of CDSCO [drug regulator]. For decades together it has

[2] https://www.rekhta.org/ghazals/ibn-e-maryam-huaa-kare-koii-mirza-ghalib-ghazals (accessed on 4 October 2019). English translation by the author.

> been according primacy to the propagation and facilitation of the drugs industry, due to which, unfortunately, the interest of the biggest stakeholder i.e. the consumer has never been ensured.

But practically, this continues to happen in India—the interests of the country's pharmaceutical industry are supreme vis-à-vis the health of citizens, primarily because the former has been among the top five contributors to the nation's GDP and has brought international prestige to the country. And finally, an example of moral responsibility involves focusing on health *primarily* for intrinsic purposes—for instance, enabling citizens to enjoy a high quality of life and pursue ends that they deem desirable rather than for instrumental economic or other reasons. Protecting and promoting the health of citizens, discussed further in the chapter, is a central moral responsibility and one of the justifications for the legitimacy of the State. The performance of the Indian State has been grossly inadequate on all these counts.

Responsibilities 'as a relation' are with reference to causes and consequences of health/ill-health. For instance, if certain public policies, programmes or actions of the State affect the health of citizens, the State shall have causal responsibility for that particular health effect. Assignment responsibility relates to expected discharge of its duties in relation to the health of citizens. If the drug regulator, for instance, does not scrutinize registration applications with due care, he/she would default in the assignment responsibility. And if citizens die due to consuming substandard drugs, he/she would also be causally responsible for their death. Despite categorization, there can be significant overlaps in these responsibilities.

India has been fulfilling its liability responsibility to some degree by providing healthcare to the poor. Even if ill-health has not been caused as a result of a lapse in the State's responsibility of a causal or assignment type, the State will still be liable to address it since it failed to proactively protect the health of its citizens from various determinants of health. For instance, in 2016, ambient particulate matter pollution (APMP) led to 27.5 million years of life lost (YLL) and 2.3 million years lived with disability (YLDs) in India, the highest in the world, and more than 13 per cent of all deaths at the post-neonatal level (28–364 days after birth) (IHME 2016). Air pollution in Delhi, for instance, is largely said to be the result of crop burning in nearby states. The Delhi government, in this case, will have liability responsibility, despite not causing pollution. Beyond the individual responsibility of the farmers who burn these crops—though they argue, in their turn, that they do not have the resources to afford the required technology as a cleaner alternative—it would also be the responsibility of the central government for failure to play a coordinating role between states within a federal system of governance to protect the health of citizens in one state as a result of action in another. The inability of farmers to afford clean technology could also be, in some ways, State responsibility. In this case, the Delhi government should be able to claim compensation from both the concerned states where farmers are burning crops as well as the central government to fulfil its liability responsibility.

Finally, judgemental responsibility relates to State initiative even when it does not carry responsibility for the health of citizens from causal, assignment, or liability perspectives. This could be justified when the State accepts its responsibility for the health rather than merely the healthcare of citizens, and that too belonging to a particular category (welfarism).

Before closing this section, let me highlight that relational responsibilities of the State are not restricted to those who cannot afford healthcare, as has been the approach of governments since Independence, although the poor would enjoy precedence in terms of focus from a welfarist perspective. But State responsibility for health cannot be confined to welfare. At the general level, the State is responsible for the health of all citizens, which is what the term 'public health' implies. Air pollution has been referred to as a 'great equalizer'—it affects all sections of society, even if at different levels. The rich can afford to get treated to deal with its consequences for their health, but that does not mean that the government does not have relational responsibilities towards the rich on the issue of air pollution. It does, as an assignment as well as its liability responsibility. The *politics* of social justice has blinded the State to the principles of fairness and responsibility.

DETERMINANTS OF HEALTH—THE EPIDEMIOLOGICAL PERSPECTIVE

Several conceptual frameworks have been developed to depict multi-level determinants of health. Given the complexity and diversity in the definitions[3] and

[3] The most widely quoted is the one enshrined in the WHO constitution: 'health is a state of complete physical, mental and social well-being and not merely the absence of disease or infirmity'. I take this as my working definition here.

contextual determinants of health—both in terms of which ones affect which aspects of health in which population groups and through what sort of mechanisms and pathways—I decided to develop a non-specific and non-linear framework of my own keeping in mind such complexity. Despite a considerable level of universality in terms of the categories of determinants—not necessarily their sub-components or pathways though—every actionable account of determinants should be conceptually clear as well as contextually complex.

By invoking their complexity, I wish to distance myself from the deterministic tendencies inherent in the discourse on social or structural determinants of health (SDH). I do subscribe to the notion of SDH, which is also reflected in my proposal (Figure 3.3). However, I believe that just as there are health policies and countervailing policies which tend to circumvent the potential impact of the former or make a negative impact on health, the determinants of health interact in complex ways to impact or offset their respective impact on health, and it is therefore not appropriate to depict a specific or linear impact.

One can give several empirical examples to this effect. For instance, as far as the potential impact of international context and policies is concerned, despite being at the receiving end of international sanctions led by the US, Cuba and Iran have demonstrated how their potential impact could be offset through national commitment and political prioritization for their citizens'

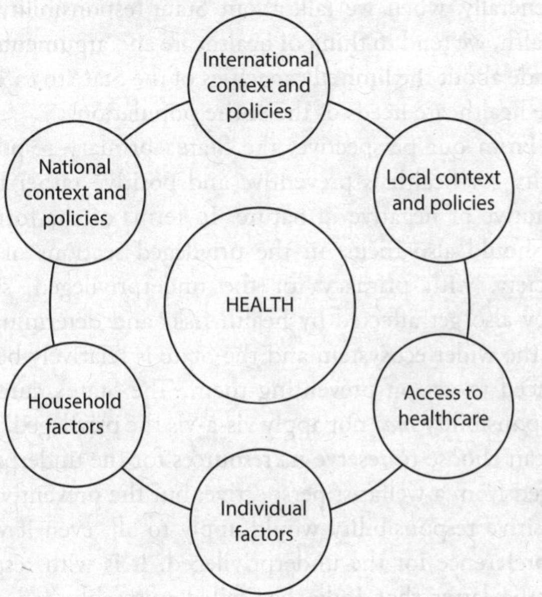

Figure 3.3 Determinants of Health

Source: Ali Mehdi.

health. Cuba's healthy life expectancy was 69.2 years vis-à-vis US' 67.7 (IHME 2016). Iran achieved the most rapid improvements in total fertility rate (TFR) in Asia *since* the sanctions; it was one of the top performers on MDG 4 (child mortality, 1990–2015), and is also among the top 10 performers generally on SDGs (2015–30). Second, despite poor national context and policies, Kerala (India) has been able to do well on health, comparable to some of the top performers in the world. Third, several countries in the developing world are trying to expand UHC for their poor populations in particular to offset the negative impact of household and individual characteristics on their health. And one may argue that if the preventive and primary aspects of healthcare are particularly efficient and equitable, we may not have to worry *as much* about the other determinants of health. There are powerful health sector stakeholders—policymakers, international organizations like the Bill and Melinda Gates Foundation, vaccine manufacturers, and so forth—who feel this way about vaccines for children in particular. While I believe in an evidence-based approach to vaccines, I do not share the enthusiasm (biomedical determinism) of these stakeholders regarding them. Finally, I have not attempted to explain pathways since there is already sufficient literature on them from a conceptual perspective. Beyond that, we will have to develop specific, complex accounts for various contexts and populations. For the purposes of this chapter, neither is required—our central concern is with the nature of responsibility of the State vis-à-vis health.

Given the examples of Cuba, Iran, and Kerala (India), the State in comparison to individuals and other health sector stakeholders possesses, even if relatively, greater capabilities to deal with the complexity of determinants and make the international, national, and local ecosystems for health as favourable as possible through positive action of its own as well as mitigating the negative impact of other determinants to the extent possible. The State's financial status is usually seen as defining the extent of its possibility for positive and negative action on determinants of health, but I would argue that, more importantly, it is its sense of responsibility, its commitment to make health a core concern of State policy in general that can stretch the limits of possibility to the furthermost limits. A resourcist approach to health needs to be balanced by the need for much wider action for health—for instance, comprehensive health sector regulation, which is woefully inadequate in countries such as India. However, resources and regulation will follow from the nature of the State's responsibility, which is why I argue that the latter is a more central notion as far as people's health is concerned. In contrast to the magic mantra of public–private partnership (PPP) that Indian policymakers like to invoke, I suggest responsibility, resources, and regulation (RRR) for improving the state of health in India.

Individual responsibility will come into force when there is a favourable ecosystem to make healthy choices. Choice and responsibility go hand-in-hand—for State, individuals, and other health sector stakeholders. Without real choices, there can be no responsibility. Given the complexity of the determinants and pathways of health, it is possible that in particular cases, even the State cannot be held responsible, when it might be beyond its capacity to act on them. Capabilities and choices define the limits of responsibility. Nevertheless, as we argue, even if the epidemiological or legal responsibility does not apply, the State will always be morally responsible for the health of its citizens and is obliged to make the best possible efforts to expand its relevant capacities. Do individuals not borrow, and get indebted and impoverished to take care of their health or their loved ones? Why can the State not do the same? Would it not in the case of war? The health crisis in developing countries such as India is nothing short of a war—the highest number of premature deaths happen in India (see IHME 2016). The International Monetary Fund (IMF), for instance, offered zero interest loans to low income countries in 2016 to achieve SDGs. The World Bank has invested in health systems strengthening for a very long time in several Indian states. With strong political will, India can leverage sufficient capacities at the domestic level to deal with various determinants of health and improve population health.

In practice, though, the State, particularly in India, prefers the relatively easier way of dealing with ill-health (focusing on healthcare), that too in a limited way, rather than trying to address other determinants or focus on prevention at the earliest levels. It shifts responsibility for health to individuals whose capacities and choice-sets to deal with complex determinants and pathways are far limited compared to that of the State's. With the emergence of so-called lifestyle-based diseases, data sources such as the GBD normatively classify several risk factors as 'behavioural'—for instance, malnutrition and dietary risks, two top risk factors for the disability-adjusted life years (DALYs)[4] at the global level. Policymakers have taken advantage of the epidemiological transition to shift health responsibility to individuals, and focus on behavioural change through information, education, and communication (IEC), yoga and so on. However, emerging pandemics like antimicrobial resistance (AMR) have made governments around the world acknowledge the need for a 'coordinated global response' (Berlin Declaration of G20 Health Ministers; G20 Germany 2017), but that too primarily based on their potential economic implications in the event of cross-border transmission rather than concern with the health of people in low- and middle-income countries per se. This makes it important to go beyond the epidemiological to the ethical case for underscoring the State's responsibility in relation to health at an international level too.

Before moving on to the next section, let me characterize two types of State responsibilities from an epidemiological perspective—preventive or positive responsibility (preventing/regulating health risks/determinants emanating from international, national, and local ecosystems), and curative or negative responsibility (dealing with consequences of health risks/determinants emanating from international, national, and local ecosystems). The discussion is largely focused on the latter, while the primary responsibility for health as far as the State is concerned is vis-à-vis the former because individuals cannot deal with or influence these ecosystems. Health is, first and foremost, a structural challenge and that is where the primary responsibility of the State lies. Generally, when we talk about State responsibility for health, we tend to think of healthcare and arguments are made about the limited capacities of the State to cater to the healthcare needs of the entire population.

From our perspective, the State's primary responsibility for health is preventive and positive rather than curative or negative in nature. In terms of the former, it should also focus on the privileged sections of the society, with primacy for the underprivileged, since they also get affected by health risks and determinants in the wider ecosystem and the State is relatively better placed to act on preventing them. The State's curative responsibility *may* not apply vis-à-vis the privileged, and it can choose to reserve its resources for the underprivileged from a welfarist perspective, but the preventive or positive responsibility would apply to all, even if with a preference for the underprivileged. It is with respect to the latter that India has failed miserably, reflected in massive levels of premature deaths in the country, especially among children under the age of five years,

[4] 'One DALY can be thought of as one lost year of "healthy" life.' See https://bit.ly/1eTnEqF, last accessed on 2 May 2018.

in whose case, India has been the world's largest contributor since 1953, the first year for which data for the country is available. By reducing the health narrative to a resourcist level, policymakers have been able to evade their primary responsibility (preventive or positive) for the health of India's citizens. They have rather taken the easy way of curative/negative responsibility with a welfarist approach.

DETERMINANTS OR HEALTH? THE ETHICAL PERSPECTIVE

Given the social determinants of health, which overlap with concerns of social justice, health has been analysed from an ethical perspective by public health scholars for a long time as well as political philosophers over the past few decades, although John Rawls, the greatest political philosopher of late twentieth century, saw health as a 'natural' rather than a social good, at least initially: 'Other primary goods such as health and vigor, intelligence and imagination, are natural goods' (Rawls 1971: 62). Later, however, he highlighted 'basic healthcare assured for all citizens' as one of the 'important requirements' which should be 'satisfied by the principles of justice of all liberal conceptions' (Rawls 1999: 50). Norman Daniels (1985, 2008), who has worked extensively at the intersection of health and justice, has expanded Rawls's theory of justice in the area of health.

Health could also be seen as an ethical issue from a religious–spiritual perspective—for example, karma as a determinant of health.[5] Yoga has become popular to address health from a holistic perspective and the current Indian government has been enthusiastically promoting it at national and international levels. While I feel that this line of research, at the intersection of health and religion, is worthy, I would prefer to focus on the public health and political philosophical arguments here. However, before moving on, let me say that even if we were to see health as determined, to some degree, by spiritual factors, we cannot shift responsibility on to individuals—culpability based on karma and cure based on yoga—and exonerate the State, which is what the present government intends to do by focusing on yoga as part of its effort to shift responsibility for health, inter alia, on to individuals.

The issue of responsibility, therefore, is a much wider concern than just health, especially as far as the present dispensation at the Centre is concerned. It made a pitch for lowering expectations from the State from the very start. Although it came to power by promising the moon, and still does in various elections, its ministers claim they cannot do magic; when stuck, they simply shift the blame and responsibility on to previous governments. This happens in the case of public health measures like sanitation too, under the Swachh Bharat Abhiyan (Clean India Mission), where the primary focus is on individuals rather than municipalities, especially vis-à-vis open defecation, which is largely treated as a cultural-cum-behavioural problem. When scores of children died within a few days in the hometown of the current chief minister of Uttar Pradesh—the largest and the most challenging Indian state vis-à-vis health and other developmental concerns—in mid-2017, he promptly blamed the children's parents for poor sanitation. Localities of disadvantaged groups, in general, are rarely cleaned by municipal authorities, while that of the dominant castes are—one can see this sort of disparity even in small villages, which are cleanly divided along caste lines. Muslims are regarded as having an advantage in child survival, but even professors of Aligarh Muslim University, Uttar Pradesh, live in their palatial houses in localities which are rarely cleaned, let alone Muslims living in poor ghettos. Communal segregation makes it easier to blame residents and their culture for sanitation, and by implication, absolve the State of its responsibility. This highlights that the issue of responsibility is not simply an epidemiological one—it is very political and, therefore, we need a normative engagement, from the perspective of the ought, based on principles of fairness.

From Dworkin's (2002: 1) viewpoint, 'no government is legitimate that does not show equal concern for the fate of all those citizens over whom it claims dominion and from whom it claims allegiance. Equal concern is the sovereign virtue of political community—without it government is only tyranny.' The question that we would like to deal with from an ethical perspective is what should the State focus on as a matter of 'equal concern' for its citizens in the sphere of health? Health itself, the determinants of health on which it can act, or narrowly on healthcare, that too of a basic type and from a welfarist perspective? The question of what should be equalized was raised and addressed initially by Rawls and also by Amartya Sen ('Equality of What', the title of his 1979 Tanner Lecture), and there has been a great deal of debate in political philosophy on this issue ever since.

[5] For a perspective on this, see 'Can Karma Cause Disease?'. Available at https://bit.ly/2jnRSta, last accessed on 3 May 2018.

Let us go back to Aristotle. Means (*wealth*; in our case, the determinants of health) are important for the sake of something else, and therefore a focus on means is not desirable from an ethical perspective. This could also be supported with reference to several religious–spiritual texts. In *Politics*, Aristotle says that 'it is evident that the best *politeia* (constitution) is that arrangement according to which anyone whatsoever might do best and live a flourishing life', and that 'it is the job of the excellent lawgiver to consider … how they will partake in the flourishing living that is possible for them'. The central focus is on flourishing living from an Aristotelian perspective. This is quite reasonable since our central concern will be with health, for instance, even if we are dealing with its determinants in a responsible way. The State's responsibility for health, as we argued from an epidemiological perspective, is complex and contextual—based on possibilities of action, although it should do everything, from a moral perspective, to extend the bounds of possibility as much as possible—and should primarily be concerned with the preventive or positive dimensions. Since its choices to act on health determinants are quantitatively and qualitatively higher, its responsibility for health is also higher compared to individuals'. The State should try its best to enhance the quality of life or flourishing of its citizens, the eventual aspect based on which its 'equal concern' for citizens should be judged. That is what the slogan of '*sab ka saath, sab ka vikaas*'[6] ('together with everyone, for everyone's development') should focus on. From this perspective, health becomes a part of a broader pursuit of flourishing of citizens by the State. Such a position of privilege cannot be granted to the determinants of health, let alone to healthcare.

***

The Indian State needs to take responsibility for the health of its citizens, whether we look at the issue from an epidemiological or ethical perspective. As far as the former perspective is concerned, the government should assume preventive or positive responsibility and ensure that health of citizens is secured from health risks emanating from international, national, and local ecosystems. Curative or negative responsibility comes later. From the perspective of the latter, it should ensure that citizens are able to lead flourishing lives, with health being one of its core constitutive elements. Resources do not carry intrinsic value, and therefore (a) health should get, at the least, as much focus as wealth in state policy; and (b) in terms of health, the focus should be on health rather than on the determinants of health, let alone narrowly on healthcare, and further on certain segments of the population. The responsibility of prevention and protection of health is inclusive because health risks in the wider ecosystems affect various segments of the population, even if differentially. Principles of fairness need to be followed in terms of facilitating the flourishing potential of citizens.

6 https://www.narendramodi.in/sabka-saath-sabkavikas-collective-efforts-inclusive-growth-3159, last accessed on 4 October 2019.

REFERENCES

Daniels, Norman. 1985. *Just Health Care*. Cambridge and New York: Cambridge University Press.

———. 2008. *Just Health*. Cambridge and New York: Cambridge University Press.

Dworkin, Ronald. 2002. *Sovereign Virtue*. Cambridge, MA: Harvard University Press.

———. 2011. *Justice for Hedgehogs*. Cambridge, MA: The Belknap Press of Harvard University Press.

G20 Germany 2017. 'Berlin Declaration of the G20 Health Ministers'. Available at http://www.g20.utoronto.ca/2017/170520-health-en.pdf, last accessed on 4 October 2019.

Institute for Health Metrics and Evaluation (IHME). 2016. Global Burden of Disease Study, data of 2016. Available at https://vizhub.healthdata.org/gbd-compare/, last accessed on 4 October 2019.

Hindustan Times. 2018. 'India to become one of three largest economies in 25 years: Jaitley'. 23 January. Available at https://www.hindustantimes.com/business-news/india-to-become-one-of-three-largest-economies-in-25-years-jaitley/story-Y3WBFW3Q8dqfkdZjRvNdLL.html, last accessed on 4 October 2019.

Parliament of India. 2012. 'Department- Related Parliamentary Standing Committee on Health and Family Welfare'. Fifty-Ninth Report on the Functioning of the Central Drugs Standard Control Organisation (CDSCO). Presented to the Rajya Sabha on 8th May 2012. Available at http://164.100.47.5/newcommittee/reports/englishcommittees/committee%20on%20health%20and%20family%20welfare/59.pdf, last accessed on 4 October 2019.

Rawls, John. 1971. *A Theory of Justice*. Cambridge, MA: The Belknap Press of Harvard University Press.

———. 1999. *The Law of Peoples*. Cambridge, MA: Harvard University Press.

Sen, Amartya. 1979. 'Equality of what?' The Tanner Lecture on Human Values. Delivered at Stanford University, 22 May. Available at https://tannerlectures.utah.edu/_documents/a-to-z/s/sen80.pdf, last accessed on 4 October 2019.

Part II
Burden of Disease and Disability

4

Health Transition in India

The Demographic Argument

Leela Visaria

Several developing countries around the world are passing through different stages of demographic transition from high mortality and high fertility to low mortality and low fertility. Over the course of the demographic transition, declines in fertility and mortality cause important changes in a population's age composition. At the initial stage after the decline in mortality level, when fertility also begins to fall with a time lag, the working-age population grows at a greater rate than the total population resulting in the increase in their share in the population. This is referred as 'demographic dividend' that can lead to economic growth if populations take advantage of the opportunities inherent due to the increase in the population in the working ages. However, economic growth to a large extent would depend on investments in human resource through good quality and skill-based education, creating employment opportunities, and investing in infrastructure as discussed by many (see for example: Acharya 2004; Bloom et al. 2010; Chandrasekhar, Ghosh, and Roychowdhury 2006; James 2008; Kurian 2007).[1] However, failure to take advantage of the opportunities inherent in demographic change can lead to economic stagnation or despair (Bloom 2011).

Along with demographic transition, many countries are also going through the epidemiological transition and health transition. They are experiencing decline in the share of communicable diseases and an increase in chronic and degenerative diseases. However, India's epidemiological transition is characterized by the dual burden of communicable diseases and non-communicable diseases (NCDs). This is evident when aggregated data for the country is examined. The structural changes in the pattern of diseases, culture, and social factors that shape health behaviour and interact with other determinants of health, along with changes in the age structure of population, can explain the presence of the dual

[1] Rapid economic growth of several East Asian countries is attributed to demographic transition during which their age structure became favourable for economic growth. The cohort of children became smaller enabling countries to divert resources from investing in children to investing in physical capital, job training, and technological progress. Also, with decline in fertility, greater number of women entered workforce. The increase in savings by the working force further boosted the accumulation of physical and human capital and technological innovation.

burden (Caldwell 1993; Yadav and Arokiasamy 2014). But the link between changing age and sex composition of population and changes in the causes of mortality and morbidity are not adequately studied. Different age groups have different health issues and disease profile. The changing age structure would affect the share of various age-specific burdens of diseases in the total disease burden. For example, with steady decline in fertility, the proportion of children in the total population declines and consequently, the share of childhood ailments among the total causes of ailments will also decline. It is therefore important to understand and estimate the quantum of change in the disease profile and in age-specific burdens of various diseases due to the changing age structure. This chapter aims to unravel this linkage between changing age structure of India's population and the shifts in the disease profile.

DATA PRESENTED IN THE CHAPTER

First we have data on changing age and sex composition of India's population since 1981 available from the Indian censuses. The chapter reviews the size, growth, and structure of India's population in historic and comparative perspective. Since the demographic transition has progressed at different paces across India, data is presented for three distinct regions. One region consists of states where the onset of decline in both mortality and fertility started early in the mid-1980s; the second group includes states where fertility decline started about two decades later; and the third group of states where fertility decline has started very recently. The population of the three groups of states has been projected to 2030 to explore the likely changes in their age structure. Information on fertility and mortality is collated mainly from the Sample Registration System (SRS) supplemented by the National Family Health Surveys (NFHS).

Next, data on cause of death is presented to discern the trends and patterns over time. The Government of India introduced the Registration of Births and Deaths Act in 1969, but its coverage, reporting, and quality of information continued to be unreliable. Since the scheme covered only the deaths occurring in urban medical institutions, for obtaining the data on rural deaths, most of which take place at home, the Survey of Causes of Death was launched in sample villages of selected primary health centres. This had its serious limitations. Barely 10 to 20 per cent of all possible deaths were recorded and to barely 30 to 40 per cent of the recorded deaths causes could be assigned.[2] So, from 1999, a system of verbal autopsy was introduced in the SRS covering both rural and urban areas. Since 2001 all the deaths recorded by SRS are scrutinized using a detailed verbal autopsy tool.[3] With the introduction of the new system, data on the causes of death is available for more than one million deaths for four time periods: 2001–3, 2004–6, 2006–9 and 2010–13. These are discussed to discern the shifts in the causes of death or epidemiological transition that India as a whole and the regions have gone through in the last one decade.[4]

This is followed by a discussion of the association between India's changing age structure and the changing mortality patterns and a discussion of the determinants of health transition. The chapter concludes with listing policy issues and measures needed to improve the well-being of people at all ages.

POPULATION STRUCTURE

The figures of India's population by broad age groups from 1981 until the Census of 2011 are presented in Table 4.1. The table highlights how India's age composition has changed during the 30-year period. Although the total population of the country increased from 683 million in 1981 to 1211 million in 2011 or by 77 per cent, this increase is not uniform across all ages. The child population aged 0–4 years and 5–14 years increased by 33 and 45 per cent respectively in the 30 years. But this increase has declined very rapidly; in fact, in the last decade of 2001–11, the increase in child population was marginal or 2.4 per cent only. It is predicted that with the continuous fertility decline, the

[2] The available data on cause of death from 1970 to 1995 has been analysed by few scholars to discern broad indications of changes in disease pattern and therefore is not discussed here (Aparajita and Ramanakumar 2004; Joshi et al. 2006; Reddy et al. 2005; Visaria 2004).

[3] The SRS field staff has been trained extensively to collect information on symptoms, signs, and key circumstances leading to death using a two-page structured form with a brief narrative in local language. The assignment of causes of death is done through a medical evaluation by two independent trained physicians, who examine the field reports (see for details: Office of the Registrar General 2009).

[4] While acknowledging the limitations of the rural cause of death statistics, their examination over a long period of 1966–95 did show a change in disease pattern. The share of communicable diseases in rural India's cause of death profile fell and that of NCDs increased (Visaria 2004: 42–6).

Table 4.1 Population of India by (a) Broad Age Groups, and (b) Decadal Growth for 1981–2011 (in million)

(a) Broad Age Groups

Year/Age group	1981		1991		2001		2011	
	Number	Share	Number	Share	Number	Share	Number	Share
All ages	665.3	100.0	838.6	100.0	1028.7	100.0	1210.9	100.0
0–4	83.5	12.6	102.4	12.2	110.4	10.7	112.8	9.3
5–14	179.6	27.0	210.0	25.0	253.2	24.6	259.6	21.4
15–59	358.7	53.9	464.8	55.4	585.6	56.9	730.1	60.3
60+	43.2	6.5	56.7	6.8	76.6	7.4	103.8	8.6
Ages not known	–	–	4.7	0.6	2.7	0.3	4.7	0.4

(b) Decadal Growth

Inter-censal change (%)	1981–91	1991–2001	2001–11
All ages	26.0	22.7	17.7
0–4	22.6	7.8	2.2
5–14	16.9	20.6	2.5
15-59	29.6	26.0	24.7
60+	31.3	35.1	35.5

Sources: *Socio and cultural tables*, C series, Census of India, 1981, 1991, 2001, and 2011.

growth in child population will become negative in the coming decades. In other words, each successive cohort of children will be smaller in number compared to the previous cohort.

On the other hand, the population in the prime age group of 15–59 more than doubled from 359 million to 730 million in this 30-year period. This bulging of the population is called demographic dividend, raising the hope among policymakers and the political class of economic growth. The number of people in the advanced ages of 60 years and over increased even faster or by 140 per cent; albeit at 6.8 per cent in 1981 and 8.6 per cent in 2011, they constitute a much smaller share of the total population.

This shift in the age composition of India's population in the recent decades is mainly due to the decline in fertility. Table 4.2 and Figure 4.1 show that the total fertility rate (TFR) or the number of children born to a woman almost halved between 1976–80 and 2010–15 or fell from 4.5 to 2.3. The steady decline in fertility rates shrinks the base of the population pyramid such that the share of the young in the population becomes smaller and decreases the young dependency ratio (the ratio of population aged 0–14 to the population aged 15–59, expressed per 100). In India this ratio fell from 23.3 in 1981 to 15.4 in 2011. Fewer children mean that both the nation and households can invest more in health and education per child, which in the long term is expected to pay off in reducing poverty and bring about prosperity.

Table 4.2 Trends in Total Fertility Rate, Infant Mortality Rate, Life Expectancy at Birth (male and female separately), All India, 1976–2016

Year/ Indicator	Total Fertility Rate	Infant Mortality Rate	Life Expectancy at Birth	
			Males	Females
1976–80	4.5	124	52.5	52.1
1981–5	4.5	104	55.4	55.7
1986–90	4.0	91	57.7	58.1
1991–5	3.5	76	59.7	60.9
1996–2000	3.3	71	61.2	62.7
2001–5	3.0	61	63.1	65.6
2006–10	2.6	53	64.6	67.7
2011–15	2.3	41	65.8*	69.3*

* Life expectancy estimates are for the period 2009–13.

Source: SRS estimates.

Table 4.2 also gives some data on two mortality indicators—infant mortality rate (IMR) and life expectancy at birth shown separately for males and females. A decline in IMR from 125 per 1000 live births in 1976–80 to just about a third of that level or 41 in 2011–15 is indicative of significant achievement in healthcare provision and utilization (Figure 4.2). However, there is considerable scope for further reduction in the overall

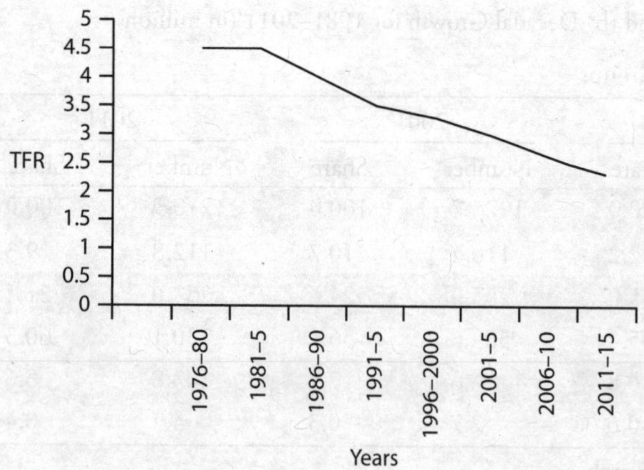

Figure 4.1 Total Fertility Rate, All India, 1976–2015

Source: Office of the Registrar General, *Sample Registration System* (SRS) (various years).

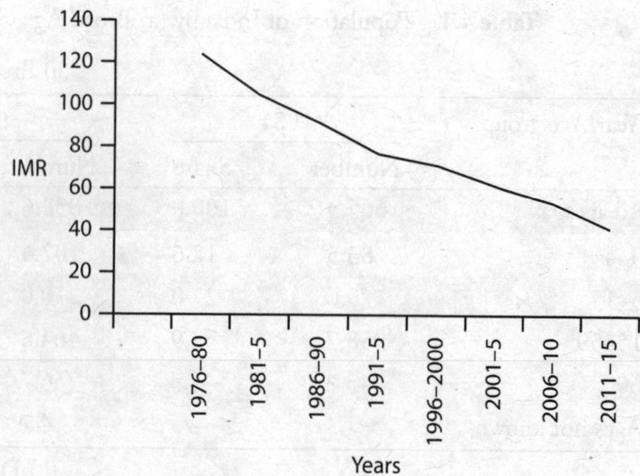

Figure 4.2 Infant Mortality Rate, all India, 1976–2015

Source: Office of the Registrar General, *Sample Registration* Bulletin (various years).

IMR level that is much higher than reported by some of the neighbouring countries like Sri Lanka and even Bangladesh. Also, within India the state-level variations in IMR continue to be very large.

The fall in IMR is often attributed to the efforts at provision of immunization and various public health measures. However, it needs to be recognized that the steady decline in fertility also helps to improve the average survival chances of infants and young children. Risk of mortality is much higher at higher parities and with fewer births taking place at high parities, infant mortality would fall to that extent.

In Table 4.2, estimates of life expectancy at birth are given separately for males and females. Life expectancy is the mean number of years a cohort of people might expect to live according to the current age-specific mortality rates. Although the trends over time in the same population indicate a decline in mortality and gain in years of living, it is relatively indifferent to changes in age structure.

Decline in fertility along with steady increase in life expectancy transforms the age pyramid of the population. The most important change is the transition towards older population structure. It increases the old age dependency ratio. In India, female life expectancy was lower than that of males until about the mid-1980s but since then, there has been a slow reversal of the trend and according to the 2009–13 life expectancy estimates, women will live 3.5 years longer than men, as Figure 4.3 shows. This implies that there will be more women at older ages than men. Given the prevailing social custom that Indian women do not generally remarry, a significant proportion of old women would be widows. Furthermore, today's

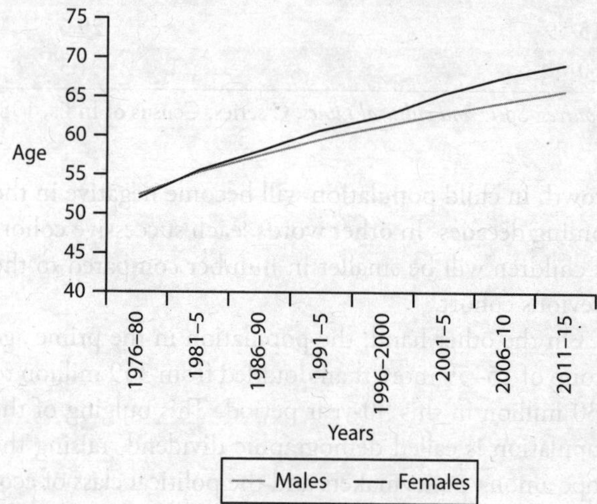

Figure 4.3 Life Expectancy at Birth by Sex, All India, 1976–2015

Source: Office of the Registrar General, *SRS Based Abridged Life Tables* (various years).

old women would have been born in the 1940s and the 1950s when a very small proportion of them were educated. These social disadvantages along with the reality of little or no savings make old Indian women quite vulnerable. Policy recommendations emanating from this phenomenon are discussed in a later section.

STATE-LEVEL VARIATIONS IN POPULATION STRUCTURE

India's diversity is evident in the variations in the demographic transition of different states. The states can be grouped into three broad categories based on the timing of the onset of fertility decline and the level of TFR according to the 2015 data from the SRS. The data is presented for three years 1971, 1991, and 2011 to show the change over time in each group's share in the population. The first group consists of all the four southern states (Karnataka, Kerala, the erstwhile undivided state of Andhra Pradesh, and Tamil Nadu) along with Maharashtra, Punjab, Himachal Pradesh, and West Bengal that have also attained TFR below replacement level. The second group of states has TFR between 2.2 and 2.4 and includes Gujarat, Odisha, Haryana, Assam, and Jammu & Kashmir. The large northern states of undivided Madhya Pradesh, Bihar, Uttar Pradesh, and Rajasthan form the third group where TFR is above 3.

Table 4.3 shows that early onset of fertility decline has reduced the share of the first group in India's total population from 45 per cent in 1971 to 40 per cent in 2011. The average annual increase in their population declined from 2.5 per cent during 1971–91 to 1.6 per cent in 1991–2011. Maharashtra, in this group, recorded higher growth partly because its urban areas, especially cities like Mumbai and Pune, attract sizeable in-migration from other states of India. There has

Table 4.3 Population of Three State Groups, Decadal Growth, and Changing Share in Total Population, 1971–2011, India (in million)

States	Total Population (in million)				Increase in 1971–91		Increase in 1991–2011	
	1971	1991	2011	2031	No.	Average Annual %	No.	Average Annual %
States with TFR at replacement or below replacement level in 2015								
Kerala	21.3	29.1	33.4	38.2	7.8	1.8	4.3	0.7
Tamil Nadu	41.2	55.9	72.1	73.0	14.7	1.8	16.3	1.4
Andhra Pradesh	43.5	66.5	84.6	97.4	23.0	2.6	18.1	1.4
Karnataka	29.3	45.0	61.1	70.1	15.7	2.7	16.1	1.8
Maharashtra	50.4	78.9	112.4	137.6	28.5	2.8	33.4	2.1
Punjab	13.6	20.3	27.7	32.4	6.7	2.5	7.5	1.8
Himachal Pradesh	3.5	5.2	6.9	7.9	1.7	2.4	1.7	1.6
West Bengal	44.3	68.1	91.3	104.9	23.8	2.7	23.2	1.7
Subtotal	247.1	368.9	489.5	561.5	121.8	2.5	120.6	1.6
Percentage of total population	45.1	43.6	40.4	36.9				
States with TFR ranging between 2.2 and 2.4 in 2015								
Gujarat	26.7	41.3	60.4	71.9	14.6	2.7	19.1	2.3
Odisha	21.9	31.7	42.0	47.4	9.7	2.2	10.3	1.6
Haryana	10.0	16.5	25.4	34.2	6.4	3.3	8.9	2.7
Jammu & Kashmir	4.6	7.8	12.5	13.8	3.2	3.5	4.7	3.0
Assam	14.6	22.4	31.2	39.3	7.8	2.7	8.8	2.0
Subtotal	77.9	119.7	171.5	206.6	41.8	2.7	51.8	2.2
Percentage of total population	14.2	14.1	14.2	13.6				
States with TFR above or around 3.0 in 2015								
Undivided Bihar	56.4	86.4	137.1	188.5	30.0	2.7	50.7	2.9
Undivided Madhya Pradesh	41.7	66.2	98.2	125.1	24.5	2.9	32.0	2.4
Undivided Uttar Pradesh	88.3	139.1	209.9	296.6	50.8	2.9	70.8	2.5
Rajasthan	25.8	44.0	68.5	97.0	18.2	3.5	24.5	2.8
Subtotal	212.1	335.7	513.7	707.2	123.6	2.9	178.0	2.7
Percentage of total population	38.7	39.7	42.4	46.4				
All India	548.2	846.4	1210.6	1522.6	293.8	2.7	364.1	2.2

Source: Office of the Registrar General, Censuses of India for 1971, 1991, and 2011; Population figures for 2031 are from Visaria and Visaria (2003).

Table 4.4 Population of Three Regions of India by Broad Age Groups, 1971–2011 (number in million)

States	1971		1991		2011	
	Number	Per cent Share	Number	Per cent Share	Number	Per cent Share
Region 1: States with TFR at replacement or below replacement level in 2015						
0–4	34.6	14.0	58.9	16.0	38.4	7.8
5–14	65.8	26.6	69.1	18.7	87.7	17.9
15–59	129.1	52.2	213.3	57.8	313.6	64.1
60+	14.8	6.0	26.2	7.1	48.2	9.8
Age Not stated	2.8	1.1	1.3	0.4	1.5	0.3
All Ages	247.1	100.0	369.0	100.0	489.5	100.0
Region 2: States with TFR ranging between 2.2 and 2.4 in 2015						
0–4	11.8	15.1	19.6	17.6	16.1	9.4
5–14	21.4	27.4	21.8	19.5	35.4	20.6
15–59	40.7	52.0	62.4	55.9	105.6	61.6
60+	4.3	5.5	7.4	6.6	14	8.2
Age Not stated	0.0	0.0	0.4	0.4	0.4	0.2
All Ages	78.2	100.0	111.6	100.0	171.5	100.0
Region 3: States with TFR above or around 3.0 in 2015						
0–4	31.9	15.0	68.0	20.3	55.0	10.7
5–14	58.3	27.5	66.9	19.9	129.3	25.2
15–59	108.9	51.3	175.8	52.4	287.7	56.0
60+	13.1	6.2	22.3	6.6	39.2	7.6
Age Not stated	0.0	0.0	1.6	0.5	2.5	0.5
All Ages	212.2	100.0	335.7	100.0	513.7	100.0
All India	548.2		846.4		1210.6	

Source: Office of the Registrar General, Censuses of India for 1971, 1991, and 2011.

been no change in the share of the middle category of five states; it has remained constant at 14.2 per cent throughout the 1971–2011 periods. The population grew at 2.7 per cent per annum during 1971–91 and at 2.2 per cent during 1991–2011. Conversely, the share in the total population of India of the large north Indian states increased from 38.7 to 42.4 per cent between 1971 and 2011. Also, its growth rate declined only marginally from 2.9 to 2.7 per cent per year. These states have started experiencing decline in their fertility only recently.

By 2031, and beyond that for at least two decades, the differences in the share of each region's population in India's total population, and their age structures will deepen and will create widening disparities. As shown in Table 4.3, by 2031 the share of population of the group with low fertility will further reduce to 37 per cent and that of the northern core states will increase to 46.4 from 42.4 per cent. In fact, by 2041, almost half of India's population will live in this region. This likely scenario has, from time to time, given rise to the debate and raises doubts about the rationale for freezing the number of seats in India's Parliament on the basis of the1971 Census population data.[5]

The variation in the onset of fertility decline affects the age composition of the population. This is evident from Table 4.4, which shows that different regions of India have now very varied age structures. Table 4.4 gives the population of the three regions described above by broad age groups for three time periods—1971, 1991,

[5] The freeze has been extended up to 2026 further creating discontent among political leaders from the states whose population share has increased. It implies that each elected member of the Parliament from faster growing states represents a larger population compared to the states with slower growth in population. It implies that they have fewer members than what they should have if allocation were based on their population size.

and 2011. As is to be expected, the share of children aged 0–14 years in the population of the region that has experienced fertility transition for two decades or so (Kerala, Tamil Nadu, Andhra Pradesh) has decreased from 40.6 per cent in 1971 to 25.7 per cent in 2011 or by 37 per cent in 40 years. In fact, in spite of nearly doubling of the total population during 1971 and 2011, the absolute number of children aged 0–4 years increased only marginally from 34.6 to 38.4 million or by only 2 per cent. Compared to that, the share of children aged 0–14 years in the total population in the core northern states (Uttar Pradesh, Bihar, Rajasthan, and Madhya Pradesh) decreased from 42.5 per cent in 1971 to 35.9 per cent in 2011 or by barely 18 per cent. The absolute number of children aged 0–4 years increased during this period from 32 to 55 million or by 72 per cent.

In every region of the country, the number of aged in the population tripled in 30 years between 1981 and 2011, although the share of the aged varied significantly between the regions. The share of aged in the first group increased from 6 to nearly 10 per cent between 1971 and 2011 and the absolute number of aged increased by more than three times in the three decades or from nearly 15 million to 48 million. In the third group, the increase in the aged population was from 6.2 per cent to 7.6 per cent or only marginal. However, increase in the absolute number of aged in this region was from 13 million to 39 million.

These different regional age structures affect the health transition and change the burden and incidence of different diseases in different regions of India since a large number of diseases are age (and sex) related. These in turn have implications for the programmes, priorities, and allocation of resources by the states. For example, the states where the proportion of young children is relatively high would have to invest much more in the provision of immunization coverage to ensure that children are protected against vaccine preventable diseases. States with a high share of elderly population would have to create facilities to provide long-term healthcare to treat chronic ailments. Health in India is a state subject and so it is important that the states be informed about not only the current disease burden but also about the likely burden in coming decades and plan to address it. Combating many ailments require fairly long-term planning, training of personnel, creating and investing in facilities along with creating awareness among people. Many diseases are a result of lifestyle changes and therefore awareness about healthy living will also have to be part of the efforts.

Table 4.5 Population of Three Regions of India by Broad Age Groups, 2031

State Groups	Total Population (in million)	% in Ages 0–14	% in Ages 15–64	% in Ages 65+
Group 1 states	561.5	20.1	69.4	10.5
Group 2 states	206.6	22.1	69.1	8.3
Group 3 states	707.2	29.7	64.3	6.0
All India	1522.6	24.9	67.1	8.0

Source: Based on the data presented in Table 4.3.

In Table 4.5, estimates of population by broad age groups and their share in the total population of the three regions are shown for 2031. It must be acknowledged that the broad age groups are not the same as shown in Table 4.4. They are, nonetheless, indicative of the likely scenario in the coming 10–12 years and of the widening of disparities between the three regions. As against only 20 per cent of the total population in low fertility states will be in the age group of 0–14 years in 2031, close to 30 per cent will be in the young age group in the large north Indian states. This implies that in the third group of states those in the working ages will have greater burden of young dependents compared to the other two groups.

CAUSE OF DEATH

The data on cause of death at country-wide level presented in Table 4.6 is examined next since they form the core of any health planning strategy. As indicated earlier, since the data for the decades earlier than 2001 was notoriously incomplete, information available since 2001 is discussed. Data for four time periods—2001–3, 2004–6, 2007–9, and 2010–13 indicative of the time trend over a decade suggests that the share of deaths due to communicable diseases in all causes of death has steadily declined from close to 30 per cent in 2001–3 to 21 per cent by 2010–13. Conversely, the share of deaths due to NCDs has increased from 42 per cent to 49 per cent. The share of deaths due to maternal and perinatal conditions had remained more or less stagnant for the period 2001–9; only in the last reporting period of 2010–13 a sizeable decrease has been noted. Possibly, increase in institutional deliveries, efforts to address anemia through various programmes undertaken with some vigour in recent years may have contributed to the decline. On the other hand, within the injury category, the share of deaths due to vehicular

Table 4.6 Causes of Death in India, 2001–13

Causes of Death/Year	2001–3		2004–6		2007–9		2010–13	
	No.	%	No.	%	No.	%	No.	%
Communicable diseases								
Tuberculosis	6,810	19.9	6,705	18.3	6,312	20.2	6,845	17.7
Diarrhoeal diseases	9,246	27.1	9,254	25.2	8,698	27.9	9,361	24.3
Respiratory infections	7,051	20.6	7,021	19.2	6,861	22.0	7,155	18.6
Malaria	3,494	10.2	3,223	8.8	3,148	10.1	3,621	9.4
Other infectious diseases and fevers of unknown origin	7,563	22.1	10,398	28.4	6,198	19.8	11,582	30.0
Total of communicable diseases	34,164	100.0	36,601	100.0	31,217	100.0	38,564	100.0
% share of communicable diseases in all causes		29.8		28.2		21.8		21.1
Maternal, perinatal, and nutrition diseases								
Maternal & perinatal conditions	8,072	87.5	9,764	90.0	10,418	90.0	10,921	89.8
Nutritional deficiencies	1,154	12.5	1,078	10.0	1,154	10.0	1,235	10.2
Total	9,226	100.0	10,842	100.0	11,572	100.0	12,156	100.0
% share of maternal conditions in all causes		8.0		8.4		8.1		6.6
Non-communicable diseases								
Cardiovascular	21,374	44.4	25,825	43.9	29,665	43.2		47.3
Respiratory diseases	9,905	20.6	9,680	16.4	11,666	17.0	13,984	15.5
Malignant and neoplasms	6,476	13.4	8,190	13.9	8,636	12.6	11,201	12.5
Digestive diseases	3,694	7.7	6,220	10.6	7,467	10.9	8,993	10.0
Diabetes	1,746	3.6	1,984	3.4	2,846	4.1	4,172	4.6
Genito-urinary diseases	2,186	4.5	3,157	5.4	3,878	5.6	4,797	5.3
Others (neuro-psychiatric, congenital, etc.)	2,789	5.8	3,793	6.4	4,488	6.5	4,290	4.8
Total	48,170	100.0	58,849	100.0	68,646	100.0	89,961	100.0
% share of non-communicable diseases in all causes		42.0		47.2		48.0		49.2
Injuries								
Vehicular injuries	2,084	19.1	2,857	21.3	3,535	23.5	5,373	27.5
Other unintentional injuries	5,559	51.1	6,699	49.8	7,003	46.5	8,625	44.1
Intentional injuries (suicide,	3,247	29.8	3,887	28.9	4,522	30.0	5,565	28.4
Total	10,890	100.0	13,443	100.0	15,060	100.0	19,563	100.0
% share of injuries in all causes		9.5		10.8		10.5		10.7
Symptoms, Signs, & Ill-defined Conditions (senility & others)	12,242	10.7	9,839	7.9	12,017	8.4	22,583	12.4
No. of deaths (Total)	**114,692**		**129,574**		**142,930**		**182,827**	

Source: Office of the Registrar General, India (various years).

accidents and injuries has increased substantially over the decade.

Apart from the explanatory factors such as effective public health measures contributing to lowering the incidence of communicable diseases and the changing lifestyle of Indians causing increase in diseases such as heart attacks, cancers, and so on, the changing age structure of population is also a contributory factor. Death is an inevitable fact of life, and the factors leading to it are, to a great extent, age related. When the share of young in the population is large, the share of those causes of death that affect children would also be high. At young ages, communicable diseases such as diarrhoeal diseases and respiratory infections, especially pneumonia, are major causes of death. At older ages people succumb to cardiovascular ailments, cancers, and diabetes.

The SRS has been able to collect information on causes of more than one million deaths, but that number is not large enough to provide state-level data. Therefore, it has been collating and presenting data for Empowered Action Group (EAG) states including Assam as one group and all the other states as another group. In addition, data is also compiled separately for six zones. The demarcated zones are contiguous geographical entities.[6] They are not exactly the same three broad groups in which we have divided the states based on their current total fertility level. Despite this anomaly, the data available for the six zones, on the share of a few specific causes of death and changes in their share over time as well as across zones, is quite revealing. Data for two time periods (2001–3 and 2010–13) is shown in Table 4.7. The table is compiled from the available data on 10 top causes of death in each zone, which accounts for 70 to 80 per cent of all deaths occurring in these places. We have selected five causes that represent the communicable, non-communicable, and maternal conditions. The selected diseases are: diarrhoeal diseases (which are communicable diseases and mostly lead to death among children) and tuberculosis. The maternal conditions largely account for deaths among women in reproductive ages and also include deaths among new born. The cardiovascular causes, malignant, and neoplasm fall in the category of NCDs lead to death mostly at middle or old age.

Broadly, the six zones can be categorized as our three fertility regions as follows: North zone and West zone include states that fall in the middle-level fertility category, East and Central zone together include the states with high fertility and the South zone includes the states with low fertility. The first essential takeaway from the table is that the two communicable diseases—diarrhoeal diseases and tuberculosis—appear among the list of top causes of death throughout the country, although the

Table 4.7 Share of Specified Causes of Death by Zone, 2001–3 and 2010–13

Specific Causes of Death	North Zone		North-East Zone		East Zone		Central Zone		West Zone		South Zone	
	2001–3	2010–13	2001–3	2010–13	2001–3	2010–13	2001–3	2010–13	2001–3	2010–13	2001–3	2010–13
Diarrhoeal diseases	6.4	3.7	9.2	5.3	10.4	8.1	9.8	10.4	6.1	3.5	5.0	3.9
Tuberculosis	5.2	NA	6.5	4.1	5.4	3.5	7.2	4.6	6.2	4.9	5.1	NA
Maternal condition	3.9	4.8	6.1	5.2	7.0	7.0	7.9	9.0	7.3	4.7	4.1	NA
Cardiovascular	22.3	26.1	15.7	18.3	18.3	23.9	12.1	13.8	22.9	24.2	25.1	28.6
Malignant and neoplasm	7.3	7.2	6.7	8.1	NA	4.9	4.3	4.7	6.4	8.2	7.3	6.9

Source: Office of the Registrar General, India (various years).

[6] The North zone includes Chandigarh, Delhi, Haryana, Himachal Pradesh, Jammu & Kashmir, Punjab, and Uttarakhand. The Northeast zone comprises the six small states of the region and Assam. The East zone comprises Bihar, Jharkhand, Odisha, and West Bengal. The Central zone comprises Chhattisgarh, Madhya Pradesh, Rajasthan, and Uttar Pradesh. The West zone includes Gujarat, Maharashtra, Goa, and the two small union territories in the region. The Southern zone includes Andhra Pradesh, Karnataka, Kerala, Tamil Nadu and the union territories in the region.

share of deaths due to these diseases has decreased in every region of the country. Given the non-availability of dependable morbidity data, one cannot infer that the incidence of these ailments has also decreased. Along with the southern zone, where tuberculosis is no longer among the top 10 causes of death, it does not also figure in the list of top 10 causes of death in the North zone during 2010–13. This is a bit surprising. It is likely that the tuberculosis deaths are included in the ill-defined category especially because of the stigma attached to it and people may report it as fever, which gets classified as other symptoms or ill-defined causes.

The second noteworthy point is that the overall decline in the share of deaths due to maternal condition in the country as a whole during 2010–13 is largely because of its significant decline in the West and South zone. In the other three large zones—North, East, and Central—maternal conditions continue to be an important cause of death. In the Southern zone, this condition does not appear among the top 10 causes of death. The nearly universal practice of institutional deliveries in all the states in this region along with better education among women is very likely responsible for this. In fact, interestingly, it is the only region that in 2010–13 reported genito–urinary diseases among the top 10 causes of death—diseases that affect older people to a large extent. Elsewhere such deaths are clubbed with the general category of all other remaining causes.

Deaths due to NCDs, especially cardiovascular problems, have increased in every region of the country and form the leading cause of deaths. However, there are very large regional variations in its share in the total profile of deaths. In the Southern region, among the reported deaths, one in three deaths was due to cardiovascular ailments or malignancy at some site. The figures reflect the fact that the southern states have higher proportion of older people in their population because it is the elderly who suffer from such chronic ailments and eventually die due to them. In the Central region comprising Chhattisgarh, Madhya Pradesh, Rajasthan, and Uttar Pradesh, these two NCDs account for around 18 per cent of the top 10 causes.

We acknowledge the fact that the different regions are at different stages of health transition and also the overall socio-economic development vary between them that would account for, and explain to a certain extent, the prevalence of certain behavioural risk factors that result in certain disease profile and the capacities of health system to respond to specific disease challenges (Agrawal 2015). At the same time, the demographic phenomenon or the large variations in the age structures of their populations do determine the variations in the burden of different diseases that lead to death.

POLICY IMPLICATIONS

The changing age structure is increasingly recognized as a critical dimension of population dynamics. However, most of the literature and studies related to this have focused on the increase in the share of working-age population in the total population as a result of decline in fertility and mortality. In the context of developed countries, the increase in the proportionate share of elderly and the issues around their health, care needed, economic security, financial cost to support them, and such factors have received a lot of attention. Since the elderly in India still constitute a small share of the population and majority of them continue to stay with their children, their health and other needs thus far have received little attention. It is time we recognize that given India's diverse population structure across regions, its health transition is at different stages. As shown in the previous section, there are regions which continue to experience sizeable communicable diseases and there are states which are experiencing old-age related health concerns.

In the context of the diverse demographic scenario, one uniform policy prescription cannot address specific health issues. Health is a state subject and the states will have to devise programmes and invest resources to address their specific health problems keeping in focus the changing age structure of their population. For example, Kerala would have to address the old-age related chronic ailments in near future and invest resources in the training of geriatric nurses. Uttar Pradesh and Bihar, on the other hand, will have to continue to invest financial and human resources in combating childhood ailments for several years, and in providing service to address reproductive health problems and simultaneously invest in dealing with chronic health problems as life expectancy is also increasing and will do so in the coming decades in the more backward states.

There is an urgent need to collect morbidity data. While recognizing that it is difficult to both ascertain ailment if people are unwilling to report or to assign accurate cause to self-reported morbidity, the rationale for data is well worth the effort. Apart from understanding the disease-specific burdens, costs associated with their treatment both on the household and the health system, the information would help in devising measures to lower the incidence of several communicable diseases and NCDs through targeted programmes. Also, such data would enable to design disease-appropriate material, training, and messages.

There is currently almost a vacuum with respect to institutions and policies to address ageing-associated challenges in India in general, and of elderly women in particular. In view of the recent increase in life expectancy of women at a greater rate compared to that of men in India, women's health and well-being in old age merits serious attention from policymakers. Beside higher life expectancy, differences in the ages at which men and women marry as well as differing proportions of older men and women who remarry are significant causes responsible for one-tailed skewed sex ratio among older adults (Agrawal and Keshri 2014). The growing proportion and size of older widows thus poses critical challenges to tackle multiple problems of their health and well-being in India. While morbidity is reported to be higher among widows compared to that among widowers, the level of healthcare utilization by as well as expenditure on healthcare is substantially lower among elderly widows in contrast to elderly widowers or married older persons.[7] There is an urgent need for old age homes especially for old women who have no one to turn to and who become victims of social and economic marginalization; homes that are well managed and well-endowed for women in the twilight years of their life.

Like elderly women, socially marginalized and disadvantaged population groups also need attention. They suffer much more from ill health compared to the others due to their poor nutritional status, the nature of their work, and environment of their places of residence. Compared to 5 per cent of households in India in which at least one member had any kind of health insurance according to NFHS-3 (2005–6) (IIPS and Macro International 2007), the percentage went up to around 29 in 2015–16 (Shijith and Sekher 2013; NFHS-4 2017: 370). However, inequities between social groups persist in spite of the introduction of Rashtriya Swasthya Bima Yojana (RSBY) in 2008 to cover the hospitalization expenses of below poverty line (BPL) families. In spite of that the insurance cover reported by the lowest quintile of respondents in 2015–16 was only 16 and 17 per cent among women and men, respectively.

A number of NGOs have been implementing the community health insurance schemes, but their reach is very limited and therefore after closely examining various models, the Indian government launched the Ayushman Bharat scheme in 2018, which plans to offer universal health coverage to about 500 million beneficiaries (100 million vulnerable families or nearly 40 per cent to 45 per cent of the country's population). The scheme is yet to be rolled out but envisages to provide cover up to INR 500,000 to every family for medical treatments. Insurance would be extended through the universal health coverage of the NHPS. This scheme is targeted at secondary and tertiary care hospitalization in both public and private hospitals that are empanelled. In addition, the government has also announced the setting up of 150,000 health and wellness centres for primary care and women's health, and to distribute essential drugs and provide basic diagnostic services. The intention to provide healthcare to vulnerable sections of society is indeed laudable. One hopes that the schemes are implemented efficiently, honestly, and reach to those for whom they are intended. Since states are expected to partner by contributing their share with the centre and through setting up of state nodal agencies, the scheme should not be allowed to falter in states that find excuses not to implement these schemes.

Child health interventions are both cost-effective in saving lives and preventing disabilities in the short run, and in the long run can result in major cost savings to health systems and can accelerate national development by improving the health and productivity of children when they become adults. In this context, the slow transition to safe sanitation is of demographic concern. Poor public hygiene and widespread open defecation, especially in rural areas, is posing threats to the survival, physical growth, and cognitive development of children (Coffey et al. 2015; Spears and Lamba 2016). In addition to building and achieving the targets of toilets under the Swachh Bharat Abhiyan, there is an urgent need to understand and address the ideas about pollution and purity and cultural meanings of latrine and open defecation that govern the behaviour of people. More detailed and nuanced research is needed to tackle the resistance to use toilets even when they are built with government subsidy.

[7] An analysis of data from the two rounds of NSSO (1999–2000 and 2009–10) showed that out of the total healthcare expenditure on the widowed, almost 90 per cent was spent on elderly widowers and only 10 per cent on widows in 1999–2000 in spite of widows who were found to suffer more from chronic ailments compared to widowers. Over time, the inequality was found to have slightly increased and not decreased (Maharana 2017).

REFERENCES

Acharya, Shankar. 2004. 'India's Growth Prospects Revisited', *Economic and Political Weekly* 39(41): 4537–42.

Agrawal, G. 2015. 'Health Transition in India: Does Data on Causes of Death Reveal Trends, Patterns and Determinants?', *International Journal of Human Rights in Healthcare* 8(2): 92–109. doi:10.1108/IJHRH-11-2014-0030.

Agrawal, G. and K. Keshri. 2014. 'Morbidity Patterns and Health Care Seeking Behaviour among Older Widows in India', *PLOS ONE* 9(4): e94295. doi:10.1371/journal.pone.0094295.

Aparajita, C. and A. Ramanakumar. 2004. 'Burden of Disease in Rural India: An Analysis through Cause of Death', *The Internet Journal of Third World Medicine* 2(2).

Bloom, D.E. 2011. 'Population Dynamics in India and Implications for Economic Growth', Working Paper No. 65, Harvard Initiative for Global Health, Program on the Global Demography of Aging.

Bloom, D.E., A. Mahal, L. Rosenberg, and J. Sevilla. 2010. 'Economic Security Arrangements in the Context of Population Ageing in India', *International Social Security Review* 63(3–4): 59–89.

Caldwell, J. 1993. 'Health Transition: The Cultural, Social and Behavioural Determinants of Health in the Third World', *Social Science & Medicine* 36(2): 125–35.

Chandrasekhar, C.P., J. Ghosh, and A. Roychowdhury. 2006. 'The "Demographic Dividend" and Young India's Economic Future', *Economic and Political Weekly* 41(49): 5055–64.

Coffey, D., A. Gupta, P. Hathi, D. Spears, N. Srivastav, and S. Vyas. 2015. 'Culture and the Health Transition: Understanding Sanitation Behaviour in Rural North India', Working paper, April, International Growth Centre, London School of Economics.

International Institute for Population Sciences (IIPS) and ICF. 2017. *National Family Health Survey (NFHS-4), 2015–16*. Mumbai: IIPS.

International Institute for Population Sciences (IIPS) and Macro International. 2007. *National Family Health Survey (NFHS-3), 2005–06, India*, Volume I. Mumbai: IIPS.

James, K.S. 2008. 'Glorifying Malthus: Current Debate on "Demographic Dividend" in India', *Economic and Political Weekly* 43(25): 63–9.

Joshi, R., M. Cardona, S. Iyengar, A. Sukumar, C.R. Raju, K.R. Raju, K.S. Reddy, et al. 2006. 'Chronic Diseases Now a Leading Cause of Death in Rural India—Mortality Data from the Andhra Pradesh Rural Health Initiative', *International Journal of Epidemiology* 35(6): 1522–9. doi:10.1093/ije/dyl168.

Kurian, N.J. 2007. 'Widening Economic and Social Disparities: Implications for India', *Indian Journal of Medical Research* 126(October): 374–80.

Maharana, B. 2017. 'Disparity in Healthcare Expenditure between Elderly Widows and Widowers in India'. Paper presented at the 28th IUSSP International Population Conference, Cape Town, South Africa, 29 October to 4 November.

Office of the Registrar General, India. Various years. *Report on Causes of Death in India*, years 2001–3, 2004–6, 2007–9, and 2010–13. New Delhi: Ministry of Home Affairs.

Reddy, K.S., B. Shah, C. Varghese, and A. Ramadoss. 2005. 'Responding to the Threat of Chronic Diseases in India', *Lancet* 366(9498): 1744–9. doi:10.1016/S0140-6736(05)67343-6.

Ramana, N.V., G. Sastry, and D. Peters. 2002. 'Health Transition in India: Issues and Challenges', *The National Medical Journal of India* 15(1 Suppl.): 37–42.

Shijith, V.P. and T.V. Sekhar. 2013. 'Who Gets Health Insurance Coverage in India? New Findings from Nation-wide Survey'. Paper presented at the 27th IUSSP International Population Conference, Busan, Republic of Korea, 26 August to 31 August.

Spears, D. and S. Lamba. 2016. 'Effects of Early-life Exposure to Sanitation on Childhood Cognitive Skills: Evidence from India's Total Sanitation Campaign', *Journal of Human Resources* 51(2): 298–327.

Yadav, S. and P. Arokiasamy. 2014. 'Understanding Epidemiological Transition in India', *Global Health Action*. doi:10.3402/gha.v7.23248.

Visaria, L. 2004. 'Mortality Trends and the Health Transition'. In *Twenty-First Century India*, edited by T. Dyson, R. Cassen, and L. Visaria, pp. 32–56. New York: Oxford University Press.

Visaria, L. and P. Visaria. 2003. 'Long-Term Population Projections for Major States, 1991–2101', *Economic and Political Weekly* 38(45): 4763–75.

5

Burden of Disease

Traditional Areas of Concern

Sanjay K. Mohanty and Basant K. Panda

Maternal and child health, undernutrition, and communicable diseases have continued to be the central focus of national and international health-related development goals (HRDGs), both nationally and internationally (UN 2015). Improving maternal health (Goal 5), reduction of child mortality (Goal 4) and combatting HIV/AIDS, malaria and other infectious diseases (Goal 6) were part of the Millennium Development Goals (MDGs) (UN 2000). The Sustainable Development Goals (SDGs), launched in 2015, expanded the HRDGs and continued focus on these traditional areas of concern (targets 3.1 to 3.3 and 3.7). Given that global progress in these areas is still highly uneven, within as well as across countries (Bhutta and Black 2013; UN 2015), continued focus is warranted. This holds true for India where deaths due to communicable, maternal, neonatal, and nutritional diseases continue to be the highest in the world (2.7 million)—almost three times more than that in Nigeria, which is in the second spot (Dandona et al. 2017; James 2018). Policymakers in the country need to have a simultaneous focus on such traditional as well as emerging areas of concern.

Maternal and child care and child undernutrition are intertwined. Food, health, and care during and after pregnancy are key determinants of child undernutrition (UNICEF 2018). The chance of infectious diseases is more among undernourished children. Globally, about 26 per cent of under-five children are stunted, and 16 per cent are underweight, and undernutrition is the leading cause of under-five mortality (Black et al. 2013; UNICEF 2018). The burden of undernutrition is disproportionately higher in the South Asian region, particularly in India (Bommer, Vollmer, and Subramanian 2019).

The global share of maternal and child death and child undernutrition in India is higher than the share of its population. India accounts for about one-fourth of the world's maternal deaths (WHO 2012), one-fifth of under-five deaths, two-fifths of the world's undernourished children (UNIGME 2015; UNICEF 2013) and about one-fourth of tuberculosis patients (WHO 2015). The maternal mortality ratio (MMR)[1], Infant Mortality

[1] Maternal death is defined as 'the death of a woman while pregnant or within 42 days of termination of pregnancy, irrespective of the duration and site of the pregnancy, from any cause related to or aggravated by the pregnancy or its management but not from accidental or incidental causes' (WHO 2012).

Rate (IMR)[2] and child undernutrition in India is higher than that in other countries with a similar level of income. For example, the MMR in Sri Lanka was estimated as one-sixth of that in India (ORGI 2018; WHO 2012). Besides, these indicators vary largely across different states of India, among rural and urban areas, and by income/wealth of the household (IIPS and ICF 2017). However, process indicators such as institutional delivery, antenatal care, and child immunization have shown considerable improvement during the last decade, largely due to the implementation of the NHM. Institutional delivery had almost doubled from 38 per cent in 2005–6 to 79 per cent in 2015–16 (IIPS and ICF 2017). Progress has also been made in antenatal care and child immunization. Recent studies also suggest a significant reduction in out-of-pocket expenditure and catastrophic health spending in public health centres in the post-NHM period (Mohanty et al. 2019). Though the MMR and IMR continued to decline in the post-NHM period, it remained high in some states of India. Studies suggest that economic growth at a low-income level has a significant impact on the reduction of MMR (Joe et al. 2015; Mohanty and Kastor 2017). The recently released National Health Policy (NHP 2017), aims to reduce MMR to 100 per 100,000 live births by 2020, IMR to 28 per 1,000 live births by 2019, and neonatal mortality to 16 per 1,000 live births by 2025 (MoHFW 2017).

In this context, this chapter examines the progress of maternal and child health, contraception, child nutrition, and other communicable diseases in India, and accordingly offers a few policy recommendations.

DATA PRESENTED IN THE CHAPTER

Data for this chapter has been drawn from multiple sources—the Sample Registration System (SRS), the National Family Health Surveys (NFHSs), the India Human Development Survey (IHDS), the Reserve Bank of India (RBI) and other published sources. A panel data file was prepared with demographic, social, and economic and health indicators over a period of 25 years, from 1991 to 2015 for all states of India. Data on MMR for the major states of India for 2000, 2002, 2005, 2008, 2011, and 2012 were obtained from the Special Bulletin on Maternal Mortality, published by the Office of the Registrar General of India (ORGI 2013, 2009). The annual estimates of IMR and Total Fertility Rate (TFR) were collected from the compendium of fertility and mortality indicators, 1971–2013 published by the Sample Registration System (SRS) (ORGI 2014). The cause of death statistics at the state level was obtained from the report on medical certification of cause of death 2015 (ORGI 2017). The annual estimates of State Domestic Product Per Capita (SDPPC) at constant prices were collected from the RBI (2016). These estimates were converted to 2004–5 base year for comparability. The annual growth rate of SDPP was computed for the states of India. The mean year of schooling for the population aged 15 years and above, the percentage of children undernourished, and percentage of institutional delivery were computed from the NFHS-1 (1992–3), NFHS-2 (1998–9), NFHS-3 (2005–6). For 2011–12, the mean year of schooling was computed from the India Human Development Survey 2 (IHDS 2). The use of contraception and nutritional indicators were taken from the factsheet of fourth round of NFHS. Data on notified tuberculosis was obtained from the National Tuberculosis Report (DGHS 2017).

METHODS

Outcome Variable

Percentage of underweight children, MMR, IMR, and use of modern method of contraception are the main outcome variables in the analyses.

Covariates

We have used SDPP, growth rate of SDPP, TFR as covariates in time-series analyses. The mean years of schooling and institutional delivery are used as independent variables in cross-sectional analyses. While data on IMR, SDPP, the growth rate of SDPP and TFR were available annually for the states, the mean years of schooling and institutional delivery were compiled at data point closure to NFHSs time period (1993, 1998, 2005, and 2015).

Analytical Methods

We have used descriptive statistics, constructed composite indices, and performed econometric analyses. A brief description of the methods used is given below. A social development index (SDI) based on mean year of schooling, SDPP, and TFR has been computed along

[2] Infant mortality rate is defined as the number of deaths during the first one year of life per 1,000 live births in a given year or period.

the same lines as the human development index. Each of the variables has been converted to dimensional indices, and the geometric mean is used in computing the SDI. The upper limit of TFR was taken as 6 and lower limit as 1.6, while for the mean year of schooling the upper limit of 15 and lower limit of 0 is used. In case of SDPP, the logarithmic transformation was used, and the upper and lower limits were fixed at INR 6,257 and INR 137,401. The lower limit was the lowest observed value of SDPP in 1993, and the upper limit was the observed maximum value in 2013. We present the SDI on a scale of 0 and 100; the closer the values to 0, poorer is the state of SDI and closer the value to 100, better is the SDI. The correlation of IMR, MMR, change in IMR, and change in MMR were examined with SDI and other indicators.

The time-series analyses have been carried out for IMR and MMR. The regression model used is given as:

$$IMR_{i,t} = a + b_1 \times Time_i + b_2 \times ln\_SDPP_{i,t} + b_3 \times \Delta SDPP_{it} + b_4 \times TFR_{i,t+}\ i.state + e_{i,t}, \quad (1)$$

where $IMR_{i,t}$ is the IMR of *i*th state in time period *t*; Time is the Year; b_1, b_2, b_3, and b_4 are regression coefficients, and a is the intercept; $ln\_SDPP_{i,t}$ is the logarithmic transformation of SDPP; $\Delta SDPP_{it}$ is the growth rate of SDPP; and e is the error term.

The equation has been estimated for 1993–2013, pre-NHM (1993–2004) and post-NHM (2005–13). A similar model was estimated for MMR. Besides, we have used descriptive statistics and run the regression model at varying data points.

RESULTS

Table 5.1 presents the share of deaths due to communicable, maternal, perinatal, and nutritional conditions, labelled as deaths due to Group I causes in India, which account for one-third of the total deaths in India. Though the share of deaths due to Group I causes in India has declined over time, it varies largely across the states. During 2007–13, about half of the deaths in Odisha were due to communicable, maternal, and nutritional condition and it was 40 per cent or more in the states of Uttar Pradesh, Rajasthan, and Bihar (see Figure 5.1). The Empowered Action Group (EAG) states along with Andhra Pradesh and Gujarat had a higher share of deaths than the national average due to communicable, maternal, perinatal, and nutritional conditions. On the other hand, a desirable level of these deaths for each state would be that of Kerala that accounts for

Table 5.1 Cause of Death in India (%), for the period 2001–13

Cause of Death	2001–3	2004–6	2007–13
Communicable, maternal, perinatal, and nutritional conditions (Group I)	38.2	36.7	30.15
Non-communicable diseases (Group II)	42.4	45.4	48.69
Injuries (Group III)	9.6	10.4	10.59
Symptoms, and ill-defined causes	9.9	7.6	10.62
Total	100	100	100

Source: Cause of Death Statistics, 2001–13. ORGI.

9 per cent of all deaths in the state. Many states required strategic investment to reach the level of maternal and child health prevailing in Kerala.

Table 5.2 presents the MMR in India for the years 2000, 2005, and 2012. The MMR in India declined by half, from 327 per 100,000 live births in 2005 to 167 in 2012. In 2012, the MMR was highest in the state of Assam and lowest in Kerala. Figure 5.2 plots the MMR in 2005 (a level similar to pre-NHM) and change in MMR between 2005 and 2012 (a period of post-NHM) by Indian states. All the states had experienced a reduction in MMR during 2005–12. The states with a high level of MMR in 2005 had experienced a higher reduction in MMR during 2005–12. It may be mentioned that haemorrhage and hypertensive disorders are the leading

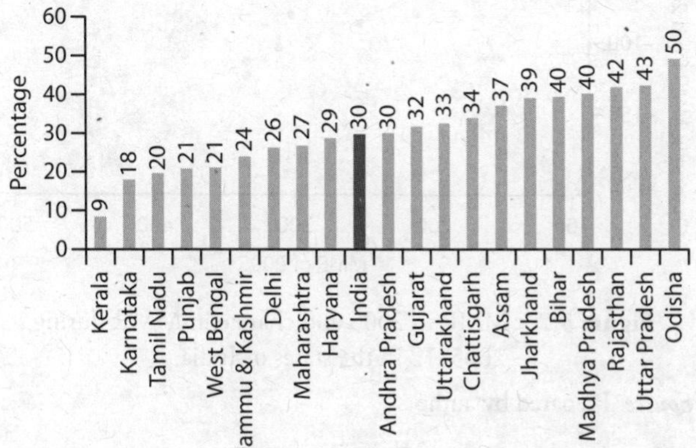

Figure 5.1 Percentage of deaths due to communicable, maternal, perinatal, and nutritional conditions in the states of India (Group I), for the period 2007–13

Source: Cause of Death Statistics, 2007–13. http://www.censusindia.gov.in/vital_statistics/VA_2007-13_Final.pdf, last accessed on 10 October 2019.

Table 5.2 Maternal Mortality Ratio, Institutional Delivery, and Social Development Index in the States of India, for the period 1998–2015

State	MMR per 100,000 Live Births (MMR)			Institutional Delivery in Percentage)			SDI		
	2000	2005	2012	1998–9	2005–6	2015–16	1998	2005	2012
Kerala	149	95	61	93.0	99.3	99.9	59.4	67.1	74.1
Maharashtra	169	130	68	52.6	64.6	90.3	52.9	62.1	71.7
Tamil Nadu	167	111	79	79.3	87.8	99.0	52.9	61.0	69.3
Andhra Pradesh	220	154	92	49.8	64.4	91.6	43.5	51.4	59.8
Gujarat	202	160	112	46.3	52.7	88.7	49.3	54.6	64.2
West Bengal	280	141	113	40.1	42.0	75.2	44.5	51.0	59.0
Haryana	176	186	127	22.4	35.7	80.5	47.7	56.2	66.1
Karnataka	266	213	133	51.1	64.7	94.3	49.7	55.0	62.4
Punjab	177	192	141	37.5	51.3	90.5	53.8	59.1	67.6
Jharkhand	400	312	208	14.6	18.3	61.9	12.1	38.4	49.9
Bihar	400	312	208	14.6	19.9	63.8	12.1	18.7	36.1
Chhattisgarh	407	335	211	20.1	14.3	70.2	33.4	39.6	51.1
Madhya Pradesh	407	335	221	20.1	26.2	80.8	33.4	37.4	48.0
Odisha	424	303	222	22.6	35.6	85.4	37.1	43.9	52.8
Rajasthan	501	388	244	21.5	29.6	84	33.5	38.1	49.4
Uttar Pradesh	539	440	285	15.5	20.6	67.8	23.8	33.2	44.9
Assam	398	480	300	17.6	22.4	70.6	38.3	44.4	53.3
All India	**327**	**254**	**167**	**33.6**	**38.7**	**78.9**	**42.3**	**49.1**	**58.4**

Source: MMR from ORGI 2016; ORGI 2007 ORGI 1999; Institution Delivery from IIPS and ICF 2007, IIPS and ICF 2005–6 and IIPS and ICF 2015–16; SDI is calculated by authors.

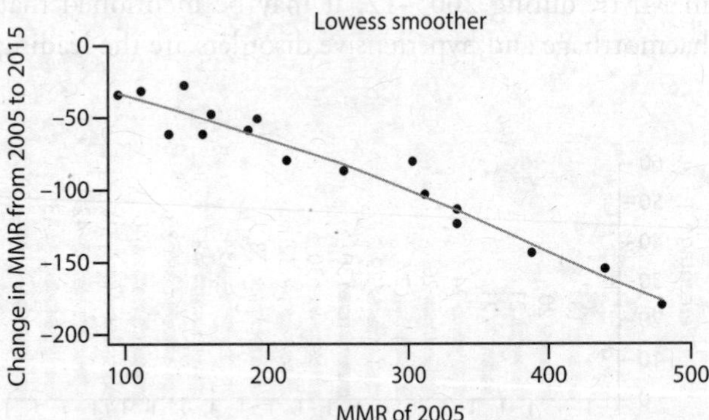

Figure 5.2 MMR in 2005 and change in MMR during 2005–12 in the states of India

Source: Prepared by authors.

causes of maternal mortality in developing countries (Say et al. 2014) and pre-term birth complication is the major cause of neonatal mortality (Liu et al. 2015).

One of the strategies employed to reduce MMR was to increase institutional delivery. The NHM had been successful in increasing institutional delivery across the states. Table 5.2 presents the MMR for the years 2000, 2005, and 2012 along with institutional delivery and SDI in the major states of India. MMR has declined, and the institutional delivery, and SDI have increased in all the states. In 2012, the MMR was lowest in Kerala (61 per 100,000 live births) and highest in Assam (300 per 100,000 live births). Institutional delivery had increased more than twofold in many states. In 2015–16, in six states, institutional delivery was more than 90 per cent. The mean SDI value of India increased from 42.3 to 58.4, and it varies across the states. In 2012, the SDI was highest in Kerala and lowest in Bihar. In general, states with high MMR have low SDI and relatively lower coverage of institutional delivery, while states with low MMR have higher SDI and higher coverage of institutional delivery.

Table 5.3 presents the association of change in MMR between 2005 and 2012 with a change in institutional delivery and SDI in the states. The correlation coefficient of change in MMR and institutional delivery is

Table 5.3 Correlation coefficient of Change in MMR, Change in Institutional Delivery and Social Development Index

Variables	Change in MMR during 2005–12	Change in ID during 2005–15	Change in SDI during 2005–15	Change in TFR during 2005–15	ID 2005	SDI at 2005	TFR 2005	MMR 2005
Change in MMR during 2005–12	1							
Change in ID during 2015 and 2005	−0.51	1						
Change in SDI during 2005 and 2015	−0.58	0.52	1					
Change in TFR during 2015 and 2005	0.69	−0.88	−0.75	1				
ID 2005	0.68	−0.94	−0.65	0.94	1			
SDI at 2005	0.78	−0.72	−0.85	0.84	0.82	1		
TFR 2005	−0.69	0.77	0.86	−0.93	−0.85	−0.91	1	
MMR 2005	−0.75	0.79	0.49	−0.78	−0.81	−0.77	0.78	1

Source: Prepared by authors.

Table 5.4 Result of Fixed Effect Regression Model with MMR as Dependent Variable with Time, Log SDPP, and Growth Rate of SDPP in India, 1997–2012

Variable	All (1997–2012)		1997–2004		2005–12	
	Coefficient	T-statistics	Coefficient	T-statistics	Coefficient	T-statistics
Time	−10.25	−3.23	−8.97	−1.23	−13.45	−4.10
Log State Domestic Product Per capita (SDPP)	105.79	2.20	94.55	0.47	108.98	−2.28
Growth rate of SDPP	−1.78	−2.08	−2.20	−1.20	−1.42	−2.15
Total Fertility Rate (TFR)	84.49	3.74	15.09	0.25	75.96	4.95
N	113		45		68	
R^2	0.92		0.94		0.98	

Source: Prepared by authors.

strong and positive (0.68). Similarly, the correlation coefficient of change in MMR and SDI is 0.78. Also, the correlation of change in MMR during 2005 and 2015 and MMR in 2005 is strong and negative.

We present the result of fixed effect regression model by pooling data of MMR at varying points in Table 5.4. Time, income, growth rate of income, and fertility in the states are the independent variables, and the state is the unit of analyses. Results are presented for 1997–2012, 1997–2004, and 2005–12. Results suggest that the average annual decline in MMR was 10 points during 1997–2012; 13 points during 2005–12 (post-NHM period) and 9 points during 1997–2004 (pre-NHM period). The coefficient was statistically significant suggesting that reduction in MMR was higher over time. The SDPP and growth rate of SDPP was significant in post-NHM period but not in the pre-NHM period. TFR was positively and significantly associated with MMR in post-NHM period. All models explain more than 90 per cent variation in MMR across states of India.

The regression coefficient of MMR with institutional delivery was −3.86 (se = 0.71) in 2005 and −4.55 (se = 1.13) in 2012. The coefficients were significant at both time periods, suggesting that institutional delivery is a significant predictor of MMR in India.

TRENDS IN INFANT MORTALITY RATE IN INDIA, 1993–2015

Figure 5.3a presents the trend in IMR and neonatal mortality rate (NMR)[3] in India since 1993. Both IMR and NMR have declined over time. IMR had declined by half from 74 per 1,000 live births in 1993 to 37 in

[3] Neonatal mortality rate is defined as the number of deaths during the first 28 completed days of life per 1,000 live births in a given year or period.

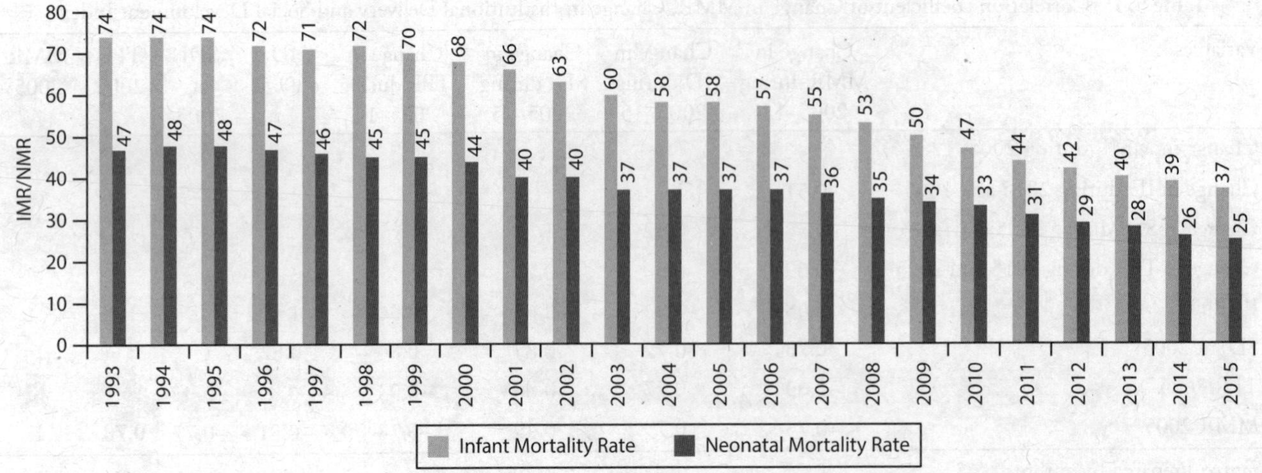

Figure 5.3a Trends in Infant Mortality Rate and Neonatal Mortality Rate in India, 1993–2015

Source: Office of the Registrar General and Census Commissioner (ORGI). 2014. Compendium of India's Fertility and Mortality Indicators, 1971–2013. Ministry of Home Affairs, Government of India. New Delhi. 2. *Sample Registration System Statistical Report 2014 and 2015.*

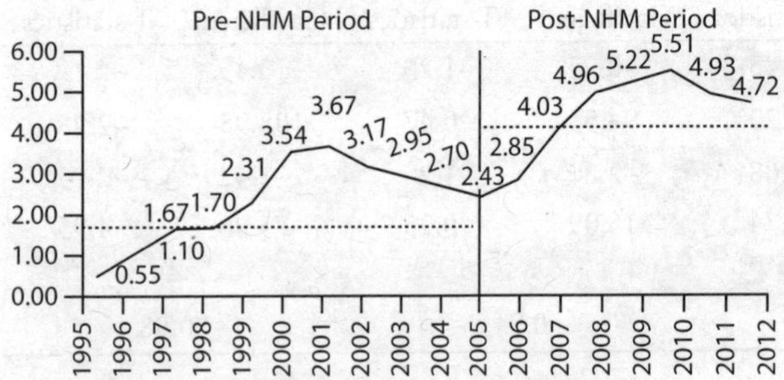

Figure 5.3b Annual Reduction in Infant Mortality Rate (percentage) in India, 1995–2012

Source: Prepared by authors.

2015, while NMR declined from 47 to 25 during the same period. Much of the reduction in IMR is due to the decline of post-neonatal mortality. NMR as a share of IMR has increased from 64 per cent in 1993 to 68 per cent in 2015. Further reduction in IMR depends on the reduction of NMR.

Figure 5.3b presents an annual reduction in IMR (percentage) over time. Reduction in IMR has been computed from a five-year moving average of IMR over 1995–2012. Reduction in IMR in the post-NHM period was higher than that in the pre-NHM period most of the time.

Prematurity and low birth-weight are the two main causes of neonatal mortality, and pneumonia and diarrhoeal diseases are the two main causes of death among children aged 1–59 months in India (MDS collaborator 2010).

Figure 5.4 presents the average decline in IMR (based on a five-year moving average) in the major states of India during 1993–2004 and 2005–15. IMR has declined in most of the states in the post-NHM period. A considerable decline in IMR during 2005–15 was in Odisha and Madhya Pradesh. Kerala had already a low level prior to 2005, and the level was almost the same in 2015. It is possible to attain the level of IMR similar to that in Kerala in the other states of India with additional investment, particularly in neonatal care.

Figure 5.5 plots the change in IMR and IMR during 2005–15. The rationale is to understand whether the reduction in IMR was higher in states with a high level of IMR in 2005. In general, states with a high level of IMR in 2005 had higher reduction between 2005 and 2015. These include Odisha, Madhya Pradesh, Rajasthan, and Uttar Pradesh. The only outlier was Kerala that already had a low level of IMR in 2005.

Table 5.5a presents the results of the fixed effect regression model with IMR as the dependent variable. The average reduction in IMR during 1993–2014 was 1.12 and 1.44 during 2005–12. Time was a significant predictor in all of the models. The coefficient of time was larger in the post-NHM period compared to the pre-NHM period suggesting that reduction in IMR was faster in the post-NHM period. Neither the SDPP nor the growth rates of SDPP were significant in any of the models. However, the TFR was positively and significantly associated with IMR in all the periods taken under observation.

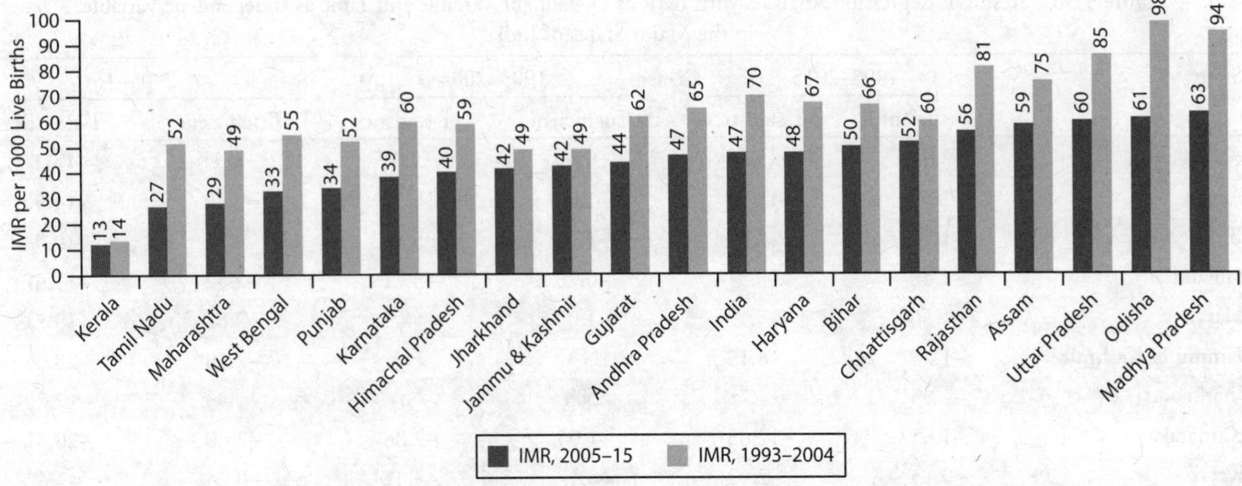

Figure 5.4 Infant Mortality Rate in pre- and post-NHM Periods in the Major States of India

Source: Prepared by authors using data from SRS annual reports.

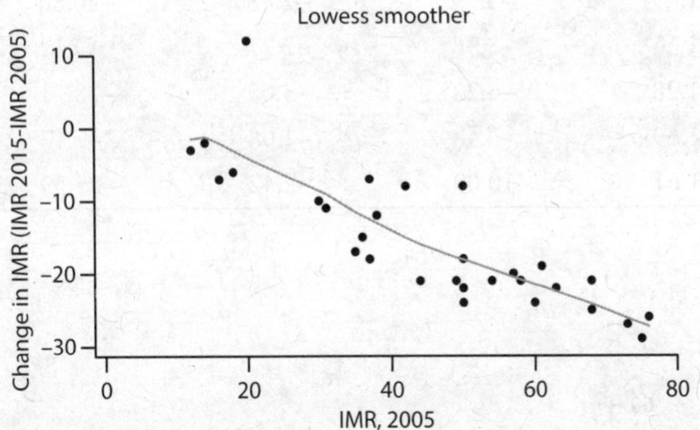

Figure 5.5 IMR in 2005 and Change in IMR during 2005–15 in the States of India

Source: Prepared by authors.

Table 5.5b presents the results of regression analyses with IMR as the dependent variable and time as an independent variable for 1993–2015, 1993–2004, and 2005–15 for each of the major states of India. Reduction in IMR during 1993–2015 was significant for all the states. The coefficient was largest in Odisha and smallest in Kerala. Kerala had the lowest IMR, and so the reduction was minimal. Reduction in IMR in the post-NHM period was significantly higher than that in the pre-NHM period in all the major states of India except West Bengal. The coefficient (absolute value) in the post-NHM period was higher than that in the pre-NHM period. At the national level, the average annual reduction in IMR was 2.4 in the post-NHM period compared to 1.6 in the pre-NHM period.

Table 5.5a Result of Fixed Effect Regression Model with IMR as Dependent Variable with Time, Log SDPP, and Growth Rate of SDPP in India, 1993–2012

Variable	All (1993–2012)		1993–2004		2005–12	
	Coefficient	T-statistics	Coefficient	T-statistics	Coefficient	T-statistics
Time	−0.55	−3.48	−1.12	−4.37	−1.44	−7.13
Log State Domestic Product Per capita (SDPP)	−1.57	−0.63	−1.27	0.27	1.27	0.48
Growth Rate of SDPP	0.058	1.32	−0.041	−0.68	0.043	1.21
Total Fertility Rate (TFR)	13.35	9.47	3.15	1.27	7.20	4.73
N		534		271		263
R^2		0.93		0.95		0.97

Source: Prepared by authors.

Table 5.5b Result of Regression Analyses with IMR as Dependent Variable and Time as Independent Variable in the Major States of India

State	1993–2015		1993–2004		2005–15	
	Coefficient	T-statistics	Coefficient	T-statistics	Coefficient	T-statistics
Andhra Pradesh	−1.49	−13.18	−0.60	−3.01	−2.35	−18.37
Assam	−1.37	−15.93	−1.06	−5.27	−2.20	−14.90
Bihar	−1.49	−13.57	−1.23	−5.14	−2.57	−10.98
Gujarat	−1.48	−13.51	−0.76	−3.71	−2.52	−19.67
Haryana	−1.66	−15.92	−1.00	−5.43	−2.62	−19.71
Jammu & Kashmir	−1.75	−8.13	NA	NA	−2.30	−28.06
Jharkhand	−1.69	−11.78	NA	NA	−1.93	−12.70
Karnataka	−1.63	−12.68	−1.05	−2.88	−2.60	−20.71
Kerala	−0.13	−2.42	−0.47	−3.41	−0.25	−2.42
Madhya Pradesh	−2.48	−32.68	−2.05	−9.93	−2.97	−23.28
Maharashtra	−1.66	−24.86	−1.46	−6.31	−1.73	−14.56
Odisha	−2.87	−28.37	−2.27	−7.54	−3.27	−24.07
Punjab	−1.50	−11.71	−0.55	−2.95	−2.75	−20.17
Rajasthan	−2.16	−20.87	−1.49	−5.79	−2.88	−20.80
Tamil Nadu	−2.07	−26.27	−1.55	−8.96	−2.27	−9.12
Uttar Pradesh	−2.02	−18.25	−1.28	−6.22	−3.05	−28.71
West Bengal	−1.68	−23.15	−1.69	−9.48	−1.08	−7.17
All India	−1.87	−30.32	−1.61	−10.09	−2.42	−25.39

Source: Prepared by authors.

TRENDS AND CHANGE IN THE USE OF MODERN CONTRACEPTION

India has made significant progress in achieving demographic targets, particularly in reducing the fertility level. The TFR has declined from over five children in the 1970s to 2.2 children in 2015, a level close to the replacement level of fertility (ORGI 2017). More than half of the states have reached the replacement level of fertility. Reduction in fertility levels in India is largely explained by two key proximate determinants—increase in the use of the modern methods of contraception and increase in age at marriage. The age at marriage in India has been increasing over time. However, the use of modern methods of contraception had shown a downward pattern during the last decade.

Figure 5.6 presents the use of any method, use of the modern methods of contraception, and type of method used in India for 1992–3, 1998–9, 2005–6, and 2015–16. The use of any modern method had increased from 36.5 per cent in 1992–3 to 48.5 per cent in

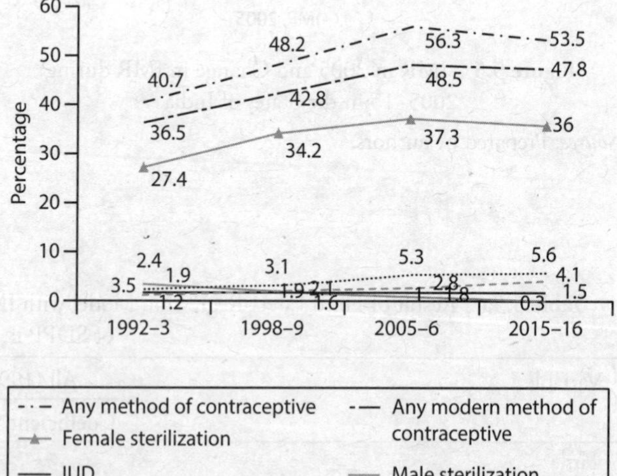

Figure 5.6 Trends of Contraceptive Use by Methods in India, 1992–2015

Source: International Institute for Population Sciences and ICF (1995, 2000, 2007, 2017); National Family Health Surveys, various rounds.

2005–6, but fell to 47.8 per cent in 2015–16. Female sterilization, the most dominant method of contraception, had also shown a decline in recent years. The use of the spacing method remained low over time. The decline in fertility rate in the absence of increase in modern contraception is puzzling to demographers. What explains the fertility reduction in the absence of an increase in the use of modern methods of contraception is a matter of further research. Induced abortion continued to be low and the duration of postpartum insusceptibility was relatively stable.

Table 5.6 presents the percentage of couples using any modern method and/or permanent method (female sterilization/ male sterilization) in the states

Table 5.6 Percentage of Women using any Modern Method of Contraception and Permanent Methods in the States of India, 2005–15

States	Modern Methods		Permanent Method		Total Fertility Rate	
	2005–6	2015–16	2005–6	2015–16	2005–6	2015–16
Andaman & Nicobar	NA	41.1	NA	39.9	NA	1.5
Andhra Pradesh	67.0	68.1	65.9	66.8	1.8	1.8
Arunachal Pradesh	37.3	23.5	22.6	11.2	3.0	2.1
Assam	27.0	38.4	13.2	9.6	2.4	2.2
Bihar	28.8	32.1	24.4	20.7	4.0	3.4
Chandigarh	NA	58.2	NA	21.9	NA	1.6
Chhattisgarh	49.1	57.3	44.2	46.9	2.6	2.2
Dadra and Nagar Haveli	NA	31.6	NA	31.7	NA	2.3
Daman and Diu	NA	30.2	NA	25.7	NA	1.7
Goa	37.2	31.6	25.9	16.3	1.8	1.7
Gujarat	56.5	41.2	43.5	33.7	2.4	2.0
Haryana	58.2	55.1	38.9	38.7	2.7	2.1
Himachal Pradesh	71.0	50.3	55.3	36.9	1.9	1.9
India	48.5	47.8	38.3	36.3	2.7	2.2
Jammu & Kashmir	44.9	56.0	28.9	24.8	2.4	2.0
Jharkhand	31.1	42.5	23.8	31.3	3.3	2.6
Karnataka	62.5	47.1	57.6	48.7	2.1	1.8
Kerala	57.9	50.6	49.7	45.9	1.9	1.6
Lakshadweep	NA	14.7	0.0	10.3	NA	1.8
Madhya Pradesh	52.8	49.0	45.6	42.7	3.1	2.3
Maharashtra	64.9	60.7	53.2	51.1	2.1	1.9
Manipur	23.5	12.9	8.6	3.2	2.8	2.6
Meghalaya	18.5	27.6	9.6	6.2	3.8	3.0
Mizoram	59.9	38.4	42.9	17.5	2.9	2.3
Nagaland	22.5	25.5	9.9	9.1	3.7	2.7
NCT of Delhi	56.4	47.2	23.8	19.6	2.1	1.7
Odisha	44.6	48.3	34.1	28.5	2.4	2.1
Puducherry	NA	61.5	NA	57.4	NA	1.7
Punjab	56.0	65.3	32.0	38.1	2.0	1.6
Rajasthan	44.4	57.9	35.0	40.9	3.2	2.4
Sikkim	28.8	32.1	24.4	20.7	2.0	1.2
Tamil Nadu	60.0	53.5	55.4	49.4	1.8	1.7
Telangana	NA	58.3	NA	55.8	NA	1.8

(*Cont'd*)

Table 5.6 (*Cont'd*)

States	Modern Methods		Permanent Method		Total Fertility Rate	
	2005–6	2015–16	2005–6	2015–16	2005–6	2015–16
Tripura	44.9	43.1	18.1	13.9	2.2	1.7
Uttar Pradesh	29.3	39.8	17.5	17.4	3.8	2.7
Uttarakhand	55.5	48.4	33.9	28.1	2.6	2.1
West Bengal	49.9	53.0	32.9	29.4	2.3	1.8

Source: International Institute for Population Sciences and ICF (2007, 2017); National Family Health Surveys,
* NA referees to not available as the survey is not conducted in the respective states in 2005–6.

during 2005–6 and 2015–16. The states are arranged in descending order of the use of the modern method of contraception in 2015–16. In 2015–16, the use of the modern methods of contraception was highest in Andhra Pradesh followed by Punjab, and lowest in Manipur and Lakshadweep. During 2005–16, the use of any modern method had declined in 16 out of the 36 states and union territories of India. Himachal Pradesh, Gujarat, and Mizoram had experienced a decline of 15 points or more in the use of the modern methods, though all these states had reached the replacement level of fertility.

Bihar had recorded only 3 per cent increase in the use of the modern methods of contraception, while Uttar Pradesh had recorded a 10 percentage point increase in the use of modern methods, though their fertility levels remained high. Two issues are pertinent with respect to contraceptive use—falling use of the modern methods of contraception in high fertility states and the low use of the modern spacing method. Table 5.7 presents the results of the regression model with TFR as the dependent variable. The coefficient of the modern methods of contraception was significant at both time periods. However, the coefficient was smaller in 2015–16 compared to that in 2005–6. About 66 per cent variation in TFR was explained in 2005–6, and 69 per cent variation explained in 2015–16.

CHILD UNDERNUTRITION AND OTHER COMMUNICABLE DISEASES

India accounts for about two-fifths of undernourished children globally. Though the country has maintained over 6 per cent growth rate of GDP in the last decade, reduced poverty by half, and increased educational attainment, reduction of undernutrition has been slow. The undernutrition of children is measured using underweight (weight-for-age), stunting (height-for-age), and wasting (weight-for-height) for children under-five years of age. Undernutrition severely affects the cognitive development of children and increases the chance of morbidity and mortality. Table 5.8 presents levels of underweight and stunting in Indian states for 1998–9, 2005–6, and 2015–16. The percentage of children underweight had declined from 48 per cent in 2005–6 to almost 36 per cent in 2015–16. In 2015–16, Mizoram had the lowest percentage of underweight children

Table 5.7 Result of the Regression Model with TFR as Dependent Variable and Contraceptive Use, Marriage, Female Schooling and State Domestic Product Per Capita as Independent Variables, 2005–15

Variables	2005–6		2015–16	
	Coefficient	T-statistics	Coefficient	T-statistics
Use of any modern method of contraception	−0.026	−4.12	−0.016	−3.8
Women aged 20–24 years married before age 18	0.005	0.54	0.002	0.23
Mean year of schooling, female	0.001	0.01	−0.031	−0.68
State Domestic Product per capita (log)	−0.471	−1.62	−0.401	−2.82
Constant	8.414	3.15	7.271	5.24
R^2	0.66		0.69	
N	28		31	

Source: Prepared by authors.

Table 5.8 Percentage of Children Underweight and Stunting in the States of India, 1998–2015

State/UT	Percentage of Children Underweight			Percentage of Children Stunting		
	1998–9	2005–6	2015–16	1998–9	2005–6	2015–16
Andaman & Nicobar Islands	NA	21.6	25.6	NA	23.3	27.7
Andhra Pradesh	37.7	NA	31.9	38.6	NA	31.4
Arunachal Pradesh	24.3	32.5	19.5	26.5	43.3	19.5
Assam	36.0	46.5	29.8	50.2	36.4	36.4
Bihar	54.4	55.6	43.9	53.7	55.9	48.3
Chandigarh	NA	NA	24.5	NA	NA	28.7
Chhattisgarh	60.8	47.1	37.7	57.9	52.9	37.6
Dadra & Nagar Haveli	NA	NA	38.9	NA	NA	41.7
Daman & Diu	NA	NA	26.7	NA	NA	23.4
Goa	28.6	25.0	23.8	18.1	25.6	20.1
Gujarat	45.1	44.6	39.3	43.6	51.7	38.5
Haryana	34.6	39.6	29.4	50.0	45.7	34.0
Himachal Pradesh	43.6	36.5	21.2	41.3	38.6	26.3
Jammu & Kashmir	34.5	25.6	16.6	38.8	35.0	27.4
Jharkhand	54.3	56.5	47.8	49.0	49.8	45.3
Karnataka	43.9	37.6	35.2	36.6	43.7	36.2
Kerala	26.9	22.9	16.1	21.9	24.5	19.7
Lakshadweep	NA	NA	23.4	NA	NA	27.0
Madhya Pradesh	55.1	60.0	42.8	51.0	50.0	42.0
Maharashtra	49.6	37.0	36.0	39.9	46.3	34.4
Manipur	27.5	22.2	13.8	31.3	35.6	28.9
Meghalaya	37.9	48.8	29.0	44.9	55.1	43.8
Mizoram	27.7	19.9	11.9	34.6	39.8	28.0
Nagaland	24.1	25.2	16.8	33	38.8	28.6
NCT of Delhi	34.7	26.1	27.0	36.8	42.2	32.3
Odisha	54.4	40.7	34.4	44.0	45.0	34.1
Puducherry	NA	22.0	18.7	NA	23.7	21.1
Punjab	28.7	24.9	21.6	39.2	36.7	25.7
Rajasthan	50.6	39.9	36.7	52.0	43.7	39.1
Sikkim	20.6	19.7	14.2	31.7	38.3	29.6
Tamil Nadu	36.7	29.8	27.1	29.4	30.9	23.8
Telangana	37.7	28.5	33.1	38.6	28.1	33.3
Tripura	42.6	39.6	24.1	44.4	35.7	24.3
Uttar Pradesh	51.7	42.4	39.5	55.5	56.8	46.3
Uttaranchal	51.7	38.0	26.6	55.5	44.4	33.5
West Bengal	48.7	38.7	31.5	41.5	44.6	32.5
India	47.0	48.0	35.7	45.5	42.5	38.4

Source: IIPS and ORC Macro 2000, IIPS and ICF 2007 and IIPS and ICF 2017.

* NA refers to not available as the survey was not conducted for the specific states.

followed by Manipur, Sikkim, and Kerala. It was highest in the state of Jharkhand followed by Bihar, Madhya Pradesh, and Chhattisgarh. Economically developed states like Maharashtra and Gujarat had a higher proportion of underweight children than the national average. The nutritional indicators have a strong gradient of income/wealth and educational attainment of the household.

Map 5.1 maps out the distribution of districts by the level of underweight children in 2015–16. Among 640 districts in India, data was not available for Chandigarh and Lakshadweep. Among 638 districts, 192 districts (16%) had less than 20 per cent of underweight children, and 162 districts (25%) had 20–30 per cent of underweight children. Districts with lower than 20 per cent of underweight children were mainly from Kerala, Northeastern states, Punjab, Haryana, and Jammu & Kashmir. A total of 171 districts (27%) had 30–40 per cent of underweight children and these districts are spread across many states of India. A total of 165 districts (26%) had underweight children of 40–50 per cent and 38 districts (6%) had underweight children above 50 per cent. Most of these districts are from Uttar Pradesh, Bihar, Jharkhand, Madhya Pradesh, and Chhattisgarh. The spatial pattern of underweight children is clear from the map suggesting targeted intervention in districts with high numbers of underweight children.

Diarrhoea and Acute Respiratory Infection in India

Diarrhoea is the single biggest cause of death among children worldwide. It is caused due to varying reasons including poor water, hygiene, and other morbidities. Table 5.9 presents the percentage of children suffering from diarrhoea and acute respiratory infection (ARI)—two common communicable diseases in India. The prevalence of diarrhoea in India has remained the same during the last decade at 9 per cent. In 2015–16, the prevalence of diarrhoea was highest in Uttaranchal (17%) and least in Sikkim. There is no specific pattern with reference to diarrhoea among states over time. The prevalence of ARI has declined from 5.8 per cent in 2005–6 to 2.7 per cent by 2015–16. Most of the states had recorded a decline in ARI during the last decade.

Prevalence of Tuberculosis in India

Tuberculosis (TB) is one of the key public health challenges in India. Despite concerted efforts by successive governments, India has the highest number of TB patients and the highest burden of disease worldwide (DGHS 2017). In 2016, about 1.74 million people in India were diagnosed with TB and over 28,000 were diagnosed with multidrug-resistant tuberculosis (MDR-TB). The Government of India had strengthened efforts to reduce the prevalence and incidence of TB. The revised national tuberculosis control programme (RNTCP) aimed to provide universal access to TB diagnosis and treatment free of cost. The monitoring mechanism of TB patients had been strengthened. About 90 per cent of the TB patients are registered in public health centres. The Indian government had targeted to eliminate TB by 2025 (DGHS 2017). Despite the fatal nature of the disease and effort for reduction of TB, we do not have the prevalence rate for individual states. The TB notification rate is much lower than the prevalence rate. By 2015, the TB prevalence rate was 217 per 100,000 population (declined from 289 in 2000) compared to 134 patients per 100,000 for TB notification rate.

Table 5.10 presents the number of TB cases and TB notification rates for India and its states for 2011 and 2016. Since there is no estimate of the prevalence rate, we use the case notification rate. The total number of TB cases notified in public and private health centres in India increased from 1,522,147 in 2011 to 1,754,957 in 2017. The TB notification rate has also increased from 129 in 2011 to 135 in 2017, possibly due to better coverage. The number of TB cases notified is proportional to the population size of the states. Bigger states such as Uttar Pradesh, Maharashtra, Madhya Pradesh, Bihar, and Rajasthan had notified a large number of TB patients. In 2016, the TB notification rate was highest in Delhi followed by Chandigarh, and lowest in Lakshadweep followed by Bihar. There are 19 states that have showed an increase in case notification and 16 states had shown a reduction in case notification.

STATE OF MATERNAL AND CHILD HEALTH: FINDINGS

We presented the state of maternal and child health in India using a set of indicators over a period of two decades. The analyses also focused on the change in some of these outcomes in pre- and post-NHM periods. Following are the main findings.

First, reduction in MMR was significantly higher in the post-NHM period compared to that in the pre-NHM period. Reduction in MMR was strongly

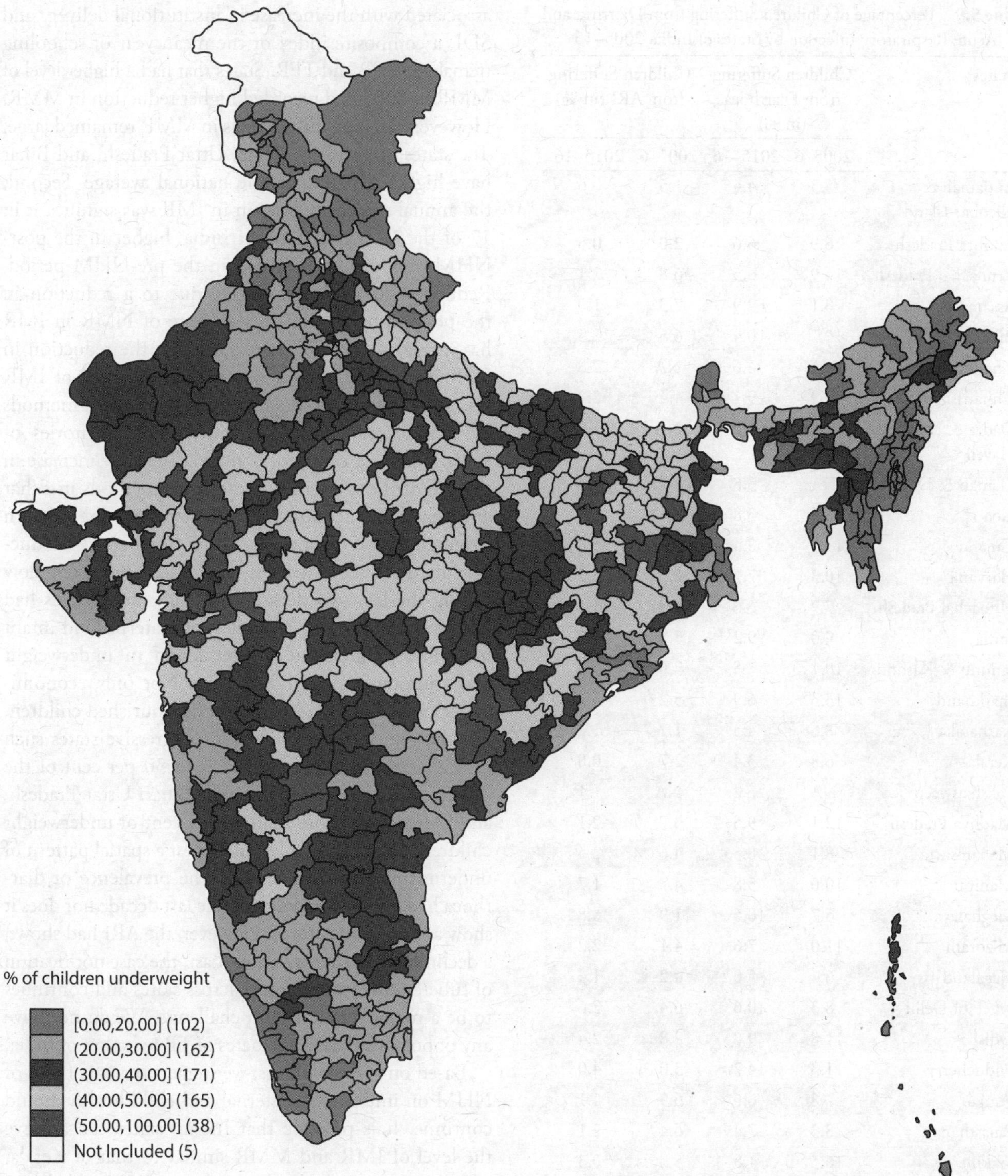

Map 5.1 Percentage of Underweight Children in the Districts of India, 2015–16

Source: Prepared by authors using NFHS 4 data.

Table 5.9 Percentage of Children Suffering from Diarrhea and Acute Respiratory Infection by States of India, 2005–15

States	Children Suffering from Diarrhoea (in %)		Children Suffering from ARI (in %)	
	2005–6	2015–16	2005–6	2015–16
Andaman & Nicobar Islands	5.3	4.4	1.5	0.6
Andhra Pradesh	6.9	6.6	2.0	0.5
Arunachal Pradesh	14.9	6.5	6.8	2.1
Assam	8.1	2.9	7.3	1.0
Bihar	10.7	10.4	6.8	2.5
Chandigarh	NA	4.6	NA	2.8
Chhattisgarh	5.2	9.1	4.4	2.2
Dadra & Nagar Haveli	NA	4.2	NA	1.9
Daman & Diu	NA	3.8	NA	0.6
Goa	6.8	3.8	3.6	1.4
Gujarat	13.1	8.4	4.7	1.4
Haryana	10.3	7.7	2.7	3.2
Himachal Pradesh	7.7	6.6	1.4	1.6
India	9.0	9.2	5.8	2.7
Jammu & Kashmir	10.1	7.5	7.6	5.4
Jharkhand	13.3	6.9	5.2	3.2
Karnataka	8.6	4.5	1.7	1.2
Kerala	6.8	3.4	2.7	0.8
Lakshadweep	NA	5.2	NA	1.1
Madhya Pradesh	12.1	9.5	3.7	2.1
Maharashtra	8.1	8.5	4.6	2.4
Manipur	10.0	5.8	4.7	1.7
Meghalaya	5.7	10.6	1.9	5.8
Mizoram	11.0	7.6	4.1	2.2
Nagaland	6.4	5.0	4.2	1.4
NCT of Delhi	8.3	10.6	6.4	2.6
Odisha	11.8	9.8	2.8	2.4
Puducherry	11.3	14.7	3.0	4.0
Punjab	7.8	6.6	6.9	4.1
Rajasthan	8.3	7.4	6.4	2.1
Sikkim	16.5	1.8	5.0	0.3
Tamil Nadu	5.4	8.0	3.7	2.8
Telangana	8.4	8.6	2.1	2.0
Tripura	8.4	4.9	14.2	2.6
Uttar Pradesh	8.1	15.0	7.1	4.7
Uttaranchal	12.8	17.0	4.3	4.6
West Bengal	6.5	5.9	13.0	3.3

Source: IIPS and ICF 2007 and IIPS and ICF 2017 National Family Health Surveys.

associated with the increase in institutional delivery and SDI, a composite index of the mean year of schooling (female), SDPP, and TFR. States that had a higher level of MMR in 2005 had recorded higher reduction in MMR. However, the state differentials in MMR remained large. The states of Assam, Odisha, Uttar Pradesh, and Bihar have higher MMR than the national average. Second, the annual average reduction in IMR was significant in 17 of the 18 major states of India, higher in the post-NHM period than recorded in the pre-NHM period. Reduction in IMR was largely due to a reduction in the post-neonatal period. The share of NMR in IMR has increased in many states. Though the reduction in IMR in the EAG states was higher, the level of IMR was still high. Third, reduction in the modern methods of contraception in some states/union territories of India remains a cause for concern. The slow increase in the use of the modern contraceptive methods in Bihar and Jharkhand requires urgent attention. The modern spacing method remained low over time. Fourth, reduction in the undernutrition of children remained slow during the last two decades. Though many states had performed well in the reduction of maternal and infant mortality, progress on the reduction in underweight and stunting has been very slow. Not only economically poorer states had higher undernourished children, but the rate was also higher in progressive states such as Maharashtra and Gujarat. About 30 per cent of the districts largely from Jharkhand, Bihar, Uttar Pradesh, and Odisha had more than 40 per cent of underweight children. The findings clearly suggest a spatial pattern of undernutrition in India. Fifth, the prevalence of diarrhoea had not declined during the last decade nor does it show any specific pattern. However, the ARI had shown a declining trend across states. Last, the case notification of tuberculosis varies largely across states and continues to be a major public health challenge. We do not have any population-based estimates of TB for states of India.

Based on these findings, we suggest that the focus of NHM on improving maternal and child health should continue. It is possible that Indian states can achieve the level of IMR and MMR similar to that of Kerala, which requires continued support to NHM and allocation of funds by the state government. The NHP 2017, had stipulated an increase in the current central government spending from 1.15 per cent of GDP to 2.5 per cent of GDP by 2015, which would help to intensify the programme. Second, we also suggest focusing on comprehensive care during pregnancy and strategies for reduction of neonatal infection to reduce neonatal mortality. Prematurity and low birth-weight are the

Table 5.10 Tuberculosis Cases by the States of India, 2011 and 2016

States	No. of TB Cases Notified, 2011	No. of TB Cases Notified, 2016	TB Case Notification Rate (per 100,000), 2011	TB Case Notification Rate (per 100,000), 2016	Change in Cases (in %)	Change in Rates (in %)
Andaman & Nicobar Islands	804	534	168	139	–33.6	–17.3
Andhra Pradesh	114,414	74,373	136	145	–35.0	6.6
Arunachal Pradesh	2,360	2,788	192	183	18.1	–4.7
Assam	39,788	40,851	132	123	2.7	–6.8
Bihar	78,510	97,001	81	84	23.6	3.7
Chandigarh	2,764	3,413	202	305	23.5	51.0
Chhattisgarh	28,658	39,484	120	138	37.8	15.0
Dadra & Nagar Haveli	397	552	118	133	39.0	12.7
Daman & Diu	293	487	113	166	66.2	46.9
NCT of Delhi	50,476	62,706	281	348	24.2	23.8
Goa	2,156	1,996	126	131	–7.4	4.0
Gujarat	77,839	126,665	134	193	62.7	44.0
Haryana	36,589	47,545	146	172	29.9	17.8
Himachal Pradesh	14,179	14,961	211	207	5.5	–1.9
Jammu & Kashmir	13,482	9,937	117	72	–26.3	–38.5
Jharkhand	39,465	39,515	127	108	0.1	–15.0
Karnataka	68,655	68,462	117	105	–0.3	–10.3
Kerala	26,255	47,293	77	139	80.1	80.5
Lakshadweep	13	23	17	35	76.9	105.9
Madhya Pradesh	87,823	129,915	124	164	47.9	32.3
Maharashtra	136,135	195,139	123	164	43.3	33.3
Manipur	3,652	2,393	151	81	–34.5	–46.4
Meghalaya	4,947	4,586	191	137	–7.3	–28.3
Mizoram	2,310	2,205	233	186	–4.6	–20.2
Nagaland	3,904	2,821	176	139	–27.7	–21.0
Odisha	49,869	43,851	123	99	–12.1	–19.5
Puducherry	1,437	1,421	108	103	–1.1	–4.6
Punjab	40,637	39,836	148	136	–2.0	–8.1
Rajasthan	112,987	106,756	169	143	–5.5	–15.4
Sikkim	1,664	1,539	272	241	–7.5	–11.4
Tamil Nadu	82,457	96,079	123	125	16.5	1.6
Tripura	2,850	2,374	80	61	–16.7	–23.8
Uttar Pradesh	277,245	297,746	141	137	7.4	–2.8
Uttaranchal	14,754	15,081	151	138	2.2	–8.6
West Bengal	102,397	89,656	115	93	–12.4	–19.1
All India	1,522,147	1,754,957	129	135	15.3	4.7

Source: Annual Report of Central Tuberculosis Division, MoHFW, 2017.

leading causes of neonatal deaths, which require care during and after pregnancy. Provisioning of hospital-based delivery alone cannot reduce these deaths to a large extent. Third, reduction of child undernutrition requires addressing the immediate cause (inadequate dietary intake), the underlying cause (household food insecurity, inadequate care and feeding practices, unhealthy environment, and inadequate health services) and basic causes (inadequate financial, human, physical, and social capital). Besides, child nutrition and maternal care during pregnancy are intertwined. Thus, comprehensive measures that focus on advice and nutrition supplements to mothers during and after pregnancy can improve neonatal survival and reduce child undernutrition. Fourth, reduction or slow increase in modern contraception in many states of India can be reversed by promoting contraceptive use as part of postnatal care. Last, TB continued to be the major public health challenge despite sustained efforts of the central government to prevent and limit it.

POLICY OPTIONS

1. Reduction in MMR and IMR in the post-NHM period was significantly higher than that in the pre-NHM period. Though many states had a significant reduction in MMR and IMR in the post-NHM period, the interstate differentials were large. Continued public investment in NHM is recommended.
2. The share of neonatal deaths in IMR has increased over time, and further reduction in IMR is possible by reducing neonatal deaths.
3. Despite the reduction in poverty level, undernutrition among children remains high. Comprehensive measures that focus on advice and nutrition supplements to mothers during and after pregnancy can improve neonatal survival and reduce child undernutrition.
4. Reduction in the use of modern contraceptive methods during 2005–16 in 16 states of India is puzzling and requires policy intervention.
5. Tuberculosis remains the major public health challenge in India.

REFERENCES

Bhutta, Zulfiqar A., and Robert E. Black. 2013. 'Global Maternal, Newborn, and Child Health—So Near and Yet So Far'. *New England Journal of Medicine* 369(23): 2226–35.

Black, R.E., C.G. Victora, S.P. Walker, Z.A. Bhutta, P. Christian, M. de Onis, M. Ezzati et al. 2013. 'Maternal and Child Undernutrition and Overweight in Low-Income and Middle-Income Countries', *The Lancet* 382(9890): 427–51.

Bommer, C., S. Vollmer, and S.V. Subramanian. 2019 'How Socioeconomic Status Moderates the Stunting-Age Relationship in Low-Income and Middle-Income Countries', *BMJ Glob Health* 4: e001175.

Dandona, L., R. Dandona, G.A. Kumar, D.K. Shukla, V.K. Paul, K. Balakrishnan, ... A. Nandakumar. (2017). 'Nations within a Nation: Variations in Epidemiological Transition across the States of India, 1990–2016' in the Global Burden of Disease Study. *The Lancet* 390(10111): 2437–60.

Directorate General of Health Services (DGHS). 2017. Revised National Tuberculosis Control Programme, Annual Status Report. Ministry of Health and Family Welfare, Government of India, New Delhi.

International Institute for Population Science (IIPS) and IFC. National Family and Health Survey 3, 2005–06. State Fact Sheet [Internet]. Mumbai.

———. 2016. National Family and Health Survey 4, 2015–16. State Fact Sheet [Internet]. Mumbai. Available at http://rchiips.org/nfhs/factsheet_NFHS-4.shtml, last accessed on 10 August 2019.

International Institute for Population Science (IIPS) and ORC Macro. 2000. National Family and Health Survey 2, 1998–99. Mumbai.

James, S.L., D. Abate, K.H. Abate, S.M. Abay, C. Abbafati, N. Abbasi, H. Abbastabar et al. 2018. 'Global, Regional, and National Incidence, Prevalence, and Years Lived with Disability for 354 Diseases and Injuries for 195 Countries and Territories, 1990–2017: A Systematic Analysis for the Global Burden of Disease Study 2017', *The Lancet* 392(10159): 1789–858.

Lim, Stephen S., Lalit Dandona, Joseph A. Hoisington, Spencer L. James, Margaret C. Hogan, and Emmanuela Gakidou. 2010. 'India's Janani Suraksha Yojana, A Conditional Cash Transfer Programme to Increase Births in Health Facilities: An Impact Evaluation'. *The Lancet* 375(9730): 2009–23.

Liu, Li, Shefali Oza, Daniel Hogan, Jamie Perin, Igor Rudan, Joy E. Lawn, Simon Cousens, Colin Mathers, and Robert E. Black. 2015. 'Global, Regional, and National causes of Child Mortality in 2000–13, with Projections to Inform Post-2015 Priorities: An Updated Systematic Analysis'. *The Lancet* 385(9966): 430–40.

Million Death Study Collaborators. 2010. 'Causes of Neonatal and Child Mortality in India: A Nationally Representative Mortality Survey'. *The Lancet* 376(9755): 1853–60.

Ministry of Health and Family Welfare (MoHFW). 2005. *Mission Document: National Rural Health Mission (2005–12)*. New Delhi: MoHFW.

———. 2012. Framework for Implementation of National Health Mission, 2012–17, MoHFW, New Delhi.

———. 2017. *National Health Policy 2017*. New Delhi: MoHFW.

Mohanty, Sanjay K., and Anshul Kastor. 2017. 'Out-of-pocket Expenditure and Catastrophic Health Spending on Maternal Care in Public and Private Health Centers in India: A Comparative Study of Pre- and Post-national Health Mission Period'. *Health Economics Review* 7(1): 31.

Office of the Registrar General and Census Commissioner (ORGI). 2009. Special Bulletin on Maternal Mortality in India 2004–06, Ministry of Home Affairs, Government of India, New Delhi.

———. 2013. Special Bulletin on Maternal Mortality in India, 2010–12, Ministry of Home Affairs, Government of India, New Delhi.

———. 2014a. Compendium of India's Fertility and Mortality Indicators, 1971–2013. Ministry of Home Affairs, Government of India. New Delhi.

———. 2014b. Special Bulletin on Maternal Mortality in India 2011–13, Ministry of Home Affairs, Government of India, New Delhi. Available at http://www.censusindia.gov.in/vital_statistics/mmr_bulletin_2011-13.pdf, last accessed on 15 August 2019.

———. 2016. *Sample Registration System Statistical Report 2015*. New Delhi: Ministry of Home Affairs, Government of India.

———. 2017. *Report on Medical Certification of Cause of Death 2015*. New Delhi: Ministry of Home Affairs, Government of India.

Patten, Scott B. and Mehdi Javanbakht. 2017. 'Global, Regional, and National Levels of Maternal Mortality, 1990–2015: A Systematic Analysis for the Global Burden of Disease Study 2015'. *Obstetrical and Gynecological Survey* 72(1): 11–13.

Paul, Vinod Kumar, Harshpal Singh Sachdev, Dileep Mavalankar, Prema Ramachandran, Mari Jeeva Sankar, Nita Bhandari, Vishnubhatla Sreenivas, et al. 2011. 'Reproductive Health, and Child Health and Nutrition in India: Meeting the Challenge'. *The Lancet* 377(9762): 332–49.

Reserve Bank of India (RBI). 2017. *Handbook of Statistics on Indian Economy*. Available at https://www.rbi.org.in/Scripts/PublicationsView.aspx?id=17785, last accessed on 20 August 2019.

Say, Lale, Doris Chou, Alison Gemmill, Özge Tunçalp, Ann-Beth Moller, Jane Daniels, A. Metin Gülmezoglu, Marleen Temmerman, and Leontine Alkema. 2014. 'Global Causes of Maternal Death: A WHO Systematic Analysis'. *The Lancet Global Health* 2(6): e323-e333.

United Nations. 2000. 'United Nations Millennium Declaration'. *United Nations General Assembly*.

———. 2015. 'UN Sustainable Goals Summit 2015'. New York City.

United Nations Inter-agency Group for Child Mortality Estimation (UNIGME). 2015. Level and Trends in Child Mortality, New York: UNICEF.

United Nations Children's Fund (UNICEF). 2018. Improving Child Nutrition: The Achievable Imperative for Global Progress. New York: UNICEF.

Whitehead, Margaret, Göran Dahlgren, and Timothy Evans. 2001. 'Equity and Health Sector Reforms: Can Low-income Countries Escape the Medical Poverty Trap?' *The Lancet* 358(9284): 833–6.

William, Joe, Suresh Sharma, Jyotsna Sharna, Manasa Shanta, Mala Ramanathan, U.S. Mishra, and Subha Sri. 2015. Maternal Mortality in India: A Review of Trends and Patterns. IEG Working Paper No 352. IEG, New Delhi.

World Health Organization, United Nations Population Fund (UNFPA). 2012. *World Bank: Trends in Maternal Mortality: 1990–2010*. Geneva: WHO, UNICEF.

World Health Organization and UNICEF. 2012. Trends in Maternal Mortality: 1990 to 2010: WHO, UNICEF, UNFPA and The World Bank estimates.

World Health Organization (WHO). 2015. *Global Tuberculosis Report 2015*. Geneva: WHO.

6

Burden of Disease and Disability

Emerging Areas of Concern

Shivani A. Patel, K.M. Venkat Narayan, D. Prabhakaran, Nikhil Tandon, Kenneth Thorpe, and Mohammed K. Ali

THE EPIDEMIOLOGIC TRANSITION IN INDIA

The early twenty-first century has been one of major progress in population health in India: life expectancy at birth increased from 64.55 years in 2006 to 68.55 years in 2016, while adult mortality for ages 15–45 years reduced from 331 to 265 deaths per 1,000 in the same time period (IHME 2017, 2018). These trends are thought to be driven by achievements across health, social, and economic sectors through factors such as enhanced maternal and child health interventions, improvements in population nutrition, and rising incomes and educational attainment in both urban and rural settings. These improvements in social and economic conditions, however, are also associated with the rising burden of non-communicable diseases (NCDs)—or chronic conditions such as cardiovascular diseases (CVDs), diabetes, cancers, respiratory disease, and depressive disorders—which collectively threaten continued improvements in population-level health and quality of life.

Despite the continued and unacceptably high burden of child mortality, 771 deaths per 100,000 (IHME 2017, 2018), the chronic diseases that predominantly affect adults have overtaken malnutrition and infectious diseases as the leading cause of disability and mortality in India even in rural areas (Joshi et al. 2006). The United Nations General Assembly acknowledged in 2011 that, 'the global burden and threat of non-communicable diseases constitutes one of the major challenges for development in the twenty-first century, which undermines social and economic development throughout the world and threatens the achievement of internationally agreed development goals' (United Nations 2011). Nevertheless, given that many of the major NCDs are treatable, and that many risk factors for NCDs are common across diseases and potentially preventable and treatable, appropriate leadership, inter-sectoral collaboration, and resource investments may go a long way in mitigating the impact of NCDs on the Indian public.

In this chapter, we draw on national data sources to report estimates of health burdens and temporal trends associated with high-priority NCDs such as CVDs, diabetes, cancers, chronic respiratory diseases, and mental disorders. We describe leading individual and environmental risk factors for NCDs, and identify important special populations that deserve further attention. We conclude with recommendations from a population-health perspective to address the emerging challenges entailed in addressing chronic diseases and injuries in the Indian population.

BURDEN OF MAJOR NON-COMMUNICABLE DISEASES

Table 6.1 summarizes the major NCDs discussed in this chapter and their contribution to the total burden of disease and mortality in India in 2016.

Diabetes

Diabetes is a metabolic disorder characterized by high levels of glucose in the blood. Diabetes accounted for 2.23 per cent of all Disability Adjusted Life Years (DALYs) and 23.13 deaths per 100,000 persons in India in 2016, which represents a greater than doubling of its contribution to the disease burden in 1990 (IHME 2017, 2018). India is home to nearly 80 million people with diabetes and is considered an epicentre of the global diabetes epidemic (International Diabetes Federation 2015). Of note, poorly controlled diabetes leads to atherosclerotic cardiovascular diseases (for example, coronary disease, strokes, and heart failure) (Grundy et al. 1999), eye diseases (for example, cataracts and retinopathy) (Fong et al. 2004), chronic kidney disease and failure (CDC 2014), neurovascular limb diseases (for example, foot ulcers and peripheral vascular disease [PVD]) (Adler et al. 1999), mental health or cognitive disorders (for example, depression, dementia) (Gudala et al. 2013; Pan et al. 2010), and physical disability (Bardenheier et al. 2016; Vos et al. 2015).

Although obesity/overweight is a major risk factor for diabetes in India and elsewhere, diabetes occurs at high rates even among the normal weight population in ethnic Indians (Gujral et al. 2013; Gujral et al. 2015). Diabetes tends to occur at younger ages and at lower body mass index in Indians as compared with other ethnic groups (Gujral et al. 2013; S.A. Patel et al. 2016; Unnikrishnan, Anjana, and Mohan 2014). Notably, a major community-based study that screened a representative sample of adults in urban and rural locales of 15 states of India showed that 7.3 per cent of adults in India are affected by diabetes (Anjana et al. 2017). The authors report that diabetes prevalence was twice as high in urban (11.2%) compared to rural populations (5.2%), a finding that cannot be explained by selective screening practices because of the objectively assessed diabetes status. The socioeconomic gradient related to diabetes is also evolving. States/union territories (UTs) in India with higher per capita GDP such as Chandigarh, Maharashtra, and Tamil Nadu have higher diabetes prevalence than states with the lowest GDP per capita such as Bihar, Manipur, and Jharkhand. However, in urban areas of the more affluent states, diabetes tends to be as or more prevalent in lower socioeconomic classes as well (Anjana et al. 2017), and this has also been seen in other urban cross-sectional studies (Ali et al. 2016). An additional

Table 6.1 The Contribution of Major NCDs to the Total Burden of Disease and Deaths in India, 2016.

Condition	Per Cent Contribution to Total DALYs in India	Number of Deaths per 100,000
Diabetes mellitus	2.23	23.13
Cardiovascular diseases		
Coronary heart disease	8.66	132.47
Stroke	3.51	52.75
Rheumatic heart disease	0.81	8.33
Cancers*		
Other neoplasm	0.54	5.66
Stomach cancer	0.45	5.86
Breast cancer	0.41	4.71
Tracheal, bronchus, and lung cancer	0.38	5.29
Lip and oral cavity cancer	0.36	4.50
Other pharynx cancer	0.34	4.37
Colon and rectum cancer	0.29	4.08
Leukemia	0.26	2.59
Cervical cancer	0.26	2.87
Esophageal cancer	0.22	2.92
Chronic kidney disease	1.65	17.89
Chronic obstructive pulmonary disease	4.81	64.45
Mental disorders		
Depression	1.29	0.00
Anxiety	0.87	0.00
Self-harm	2.50	17.50
Total of all NCDs shown in this table	**29.14**	**352.98**

* Top 10 cancers in men and women combined.
Source: GBD 2016.

10.3 per cent of India's adult population has prediabetes which likely equates to some 100 million people, and this portends continued increases in prevalence as prediabetes is associated with a 5–10 times higher incidence of diabetes than have normal fasting and post-prandial glucose levels.

The challenges posed by diabetes to India are at many levels. Those diagnosed with diabetes are recommended to adopt healthy, active lifestyles and to self-manage their conditions carefully in partnership with healthcare providers to lower the risk of fatal and often debilitating complications—delivering on these recommendations is complicated by economic, behavioural, and structural barriers. Individuals and their families contend with the daily and costly challenges of managing the disease to try and forestall complications of diabetes. Caring for diabetes can also become increasingly costly over time, requiring progressively more medications and affordable, well-coordinated healthcare to control one's blood sugar, blood pressure, cholesterol levels, and ensuring those affected are screened for early signs of diabetes complications. Up to 25 per cent (rural) and 35 per cent (urban) of household income can be consumed by diabetes-related expenditures among poor households in India (Ramachandran et al. 2007).

Physicians and allied health professionals have to contend with large volumes of patients. Several of these patients have limited resources to be able to access and adhere to treatments. Even in metropolises such as Delhi, less than 20 per cent of patients receive standard preventive exams such as dilated eye or foot exams (Shivashankar et al. 2016). Furthermore, policymakers may have to contend with the increased burdens of diabetes through lost productivity and premature mortality in years to come, as the disease occurs quite frequently among younger and working age adults.

Without intervention, diabetes and its related complications may cannibalize the demographic dividend that India currently enjoys. Further complicating this scenario is that diabetes in Asian Indians may have a somewhat different, possibly accelerated pathophysiology (Staimez et al. 2013). The implications of this are that traditional interventions such as low-fat diets and exercise that have been shown to decrease incidence of diabetes in other high risk populations in Europe and North America (Knowler et al. 2002; Tuomilehto et al. 1993) may not be as effective alone in reducing diabetes incidence in Asian Indians (Weber et al. 2016). More research to find focused interventions that can prevent and manage diabetes better are needed among Asian Indians. Furthermore, widespread efforts to lower costs of and increase access to medications and diagnostics are needed to help lower the growing direct medical costs (outpatient and inpatient care; medications; monitoring and diagnostics) of managing diabetes. Overall, diabetes in the general Indian population is a major concern for policymakers.

Cardiovascular Diseases

Cardiovascular diseases are a range of conditions related to the circulatory system and constitute the number one cause of rates of DALYs and death worldwide and in India (Kassebaum et al. 2016). Taken together, CVDs accounted for 14.1 per cent of total DALYs and 28.1 per cent of all deaths in 2016 in India (IHME 2017, 2018). At 399 and 291 deaths per 100,000 men and women, respectively, age-adjusted CVD mortality is two to three times higher in India than it is in the US (IHME 2017, 2018). Moreover, a large study reported that rates of major cardiovascular disease and fatal cardiovascular disease were 1.5 and 6 times higher, respectively, in adults in low-income countries (Bangladesh, India, Pakistan, and Zimbabwe) compared with adults in high income countries (Yusuf et al. 2014). India's high CVD mortality is understood as failures of social policy targeting behavioural risk factors (for example, tobacco use, high sodium intake, inadequate intake of fruits and vegetables), of health policy targeting management of biomedical risk factors (for example, blood pressure and glucose, lipids), and of the health system to provide quality acute and long-term care for CVD patients (Gupta, Mohan, and Narula 2016).

Coronary heart disease (CHD) is the most prevalent type of CVD globally and refers to a narrowing of the coronary arteries that results in reduced blood flow to the heart and may lead to angina or heart attack. CHD accounts for 9 per cent of DALYs and 132 deaths per 100,000 persons (IHME n.d.). The prevalence of CHD in the urban population is estimated to have increased by seven-fold since 1960 (Prabhakaran, Jeemon, and Roy 2016), while the current prevalence in the general population is estimated to be 2 per cent to 4 per cent (Gupta, Mohan, and Narula 2016). Important risk factors include tobacco use, high cholesterol, hypertension, diabetes, obesity, and family history of the condition. South Asians are on average eight years younger at the time of their first heart attack compared with non-South Asians; most of this younger age of first attack is attributed to worse risk factor profiles at younger ages

(Joshi et al. 2007). Heart attacks are subdivided based on their appearance in an electrocardiogram (ST-elevation myocardial infarctions or STEMI versus non-STEMI), which generally also is related to the severity of the heart attack. Indians are more likely to experience the more severe STEMI heart attacks, characterized by prolonged blockage to blood flow and therefore causing more damage to the heart muscle (Xavier et al. 2008). These STEMI heart attacks also require greater resources to treat, and available data indicate widespread shortcomings of urban hospitals to optimally manage these time-sensitive events (Prabhakaran, Jeemon, and Roy 2016). Lifestyle management and preventive pharmacotherapy is recommended to reduce the risk of complications among those with CHD; strategies include weight loss, smoking cessation, daily aspirin, and treatment of risk factors such as blood pressure. Medications such as beta blockers are also recommended after a person experiences a heart attack. Many of these evidence-based strategies are underutilized in India due to poverty (Xavier et al. 2008), though achieving consistent medication adherence is a challenge across socioeconomic spectrum.

Stroke is the next most common type of CVD. Stroke is characterized by acute brain dysfunction brought on by lack of blood flow to the brain. Haemorrhagic stroke is due to a haemorrhage, while ischemic stroke is due to blockage. Stroke accounts for 3.5 per cent of all DALYs (1.9 per cent haemorrhagic stroke, and 1.6 per cent ischemic stroke) and 52.8 deaths per 100,000 (25.4/100,000 due to haemorrhagic stroke, and 27.3/100,000 due to ischemic stroke) in India. Haemorrhagic (as compared with ischemic) stroke, which is related to hypertension, is more common in India than in high income countries (O'Donnell et al. 2010). Though relatively rare, strokes are extremely fatal and debilitating due to loss of motor and cognitive function. Stroke-related case fatality is higher across the board in India as compared with Western industrialized nations, and this is acutely apparent among women. Stroke disproportionately affects younger age groups in India relative to other countries (O'Donnell et al. 2010; Sridharan et al. 2009; Wasay, Khatri, and Kaul 2014). Within India, stroke is higher in urban (334–424 cases per 100,000) compared with rural areas (84–262 cases per 100,000). The chronic disability and dependency associated with stroke can be financially and socially devastating for patients, their families, and the society at large (Das et al. 2010; Kwatra et al. 2013; Rigby, Gubitz, and Phillips 2009). Health systems in India are unprepared to address the large and growing burden of stroke (Mehndiratta et al. 2013; Pandian et al. 2007; Pandian and Sudhan 2013). Delivery of post-stroke care in India has many challenges due to the shortage of physicians, physiotherapists, and organized inpatient- or outpatient-based rehabilitation facilities; the focus on motor rehabilitation through physiotherapy neglects cognitive domains (Pandian and Sudhan 2013). Additional challenges in accessing appropriate rehabilitation services are experienced by rural compared with urban patients due limited geographic access and financial barriers to afford costs of therapists. This inequity in accessing service manifests as a rural disadvantage in both post-stroke disability (Ferri et al. 2011) and short-term mortality (Sridharan et al. 2009).

Rheumatic heart disease arises from an abnormal autoimmune response to streptococcal infection usually in childhood or adolescence, termed Rheumatic fever, which causes permanent damage to the heart machinery by scarring cardiac valves. Rheumatic heart disease accounted for 1% of all deaths and <1 per cent of total DALYs in India in 2016 (IHME 2017, 2018). In 2015, India was the country with the highest number of deaths worldwide due to rheumatic heart disease (estimate: 119,100 deaths) and has one of the highest age-standardized rates of DALYs caused by the disease (Watkins et al. 2017). Rheumatic fever can be treated with penicillin, and it is virtually eliminated in high income countries, but remains an important cause of heart damage in low- and middle-income countries. In India and elsewhere, lower socioeconomic status is a risk factor for the condition (Marijon et al. 2012; Saxena et al. 2011). Women of childbearing age appear to have higher prevalence of rheumatic heart disease (Marijon et al. 2012), and those with the condition may suffer complications during pregnancy. As management of the condition is extremely expensive, efforts are directed towards prevention (Marijon et al. 2012).

Cancers

The aetiology of cancer is complex and varied based on the type of cancer, which also influences which cancers are most prevalent in different parts of the world and within regions of India (Goss et al. 2014). Cancers accounted for 5 per cent of total DALYs and 8.3 per cent of all deaths in India in 2016 (IHME 2017, 2018). Although genetics play an important role, preventable environmental exposures (for instance air pollution, arsenic), infections (such as human papilloma virus, hepatitis B and C), and behaviours (such as tobacco use, excess alcohol consumption, diet) are implicated in

India's cancer burden. Although the impact of cancer on health as measured by DALYs is similar for both women and men, the specific cancers with greatest impact on each gender differ in important ways. Breast cancer is the most common type in women and lip and oral cavity cancers are the most prevalent in men (Mallath et al. 2014). Breast cancer is the most common cancer among women worldwide, but Indian women have much higher prevalence of triple negative breast cancer, an aggressive subtype that tends to occur in younger women and advances rapidly (Sandhu et al. 2016). Oral and lip cancers are less frequent worldwide, and disproportionately occur among Indian men due to tobacco chewing. Lung, lip and oral, stomach, leukaemia, colorectal and other cancers are among the top 10 cancer contributors to total DALYs among both women and men. Among women, breast, cervical, ovarian, and gallbladder (in that order) figure in the top 10. Among men only, other pharynx, oesophageal, larynx, and liver cancer rank in the top 10 (IHME 2017, 2018).

Despite lower age-standardized incidence, India accounted for 1 million of 14 million new cancer cases in 2012 (Mallath et al. 2014). Compared to Western Europe, India has lower cancer incidence but as many cancer-related deaths after accounting for age (Mallath et al. 2014). Within India, the socioeconomically disadvantaged groups experience the highest cancer mortality (Chalkidou et al. 2014); groups with lower socioeconomic status (SES) suffer twice the cancer mortality of higher SES groups (Goss et al. 2014). Currently, cancer treatment is deemed unaffordable for the majority of Indian households (Goss et al. 2014). Of all of the NCDs, cancer was associated with the highest costs related to admissions and outpatient visits, and places families at high risk for catastrophic expenditures in India (Chalkidou et al. 2014). In addition to lack of affordability, limited cancer awareness and cancer-associated stigma may delay seeking proper diagnosis and treatment for cancer in India (Gupta et al. 2015; Nyblade et al. 2017). At the level of the health system, the inability to achieve progress in cancer outcomes has been described as a product of 'poor financing, access, availability, and quality of care' (Chalkidou et al. 2014). Past national policies have been critiqued as being inadequate to achieve greater awareness of cancer among the public or implement widespread screening for earlier diagnosis which is critical for ultimate prognosis (Chalkidou et al. 2014). In sync with evidence-based recommendations for screening and early detection of common cancers in India (Rajaraman et al. 2015), an Operational Framework for Screening and Management of Common Cancers has been developed for screening and management of oral, breast, and cervical cancers at the sub-centre and primary health centre level.

Chronic Kidney Disease

Chronic kidney disease (CKD) is defined as abnormal kidney structure or impaired kidney function lasting over three months. CKD was responsible for 1 per cent of DALYs and 1.59 per cent of deaths in 1990; both CKD-associated deaths and DALYs have increased by 75 per cent since then (IHME 2017, 2018). Estimates of the prevalence of CKD vary widely and range from 8 per cent to 20 per cent in rural and urban areas (Anand et al. 2015; Trivedi et al. 2016; Varma 2015). Diabetes, hypertension, and acute inflammation of the kidneys are the common immediate causes of CKD. The prevalence of CKD is expected to only rise as its precursors diabetes and hypertension rise in the population and as CVD patients survive with better medical management (Jagannathan and Patzer 2017; Singh et al. 2013). Important for India and other lower and middle income countries (LMICs), common infectious diseases such as malaria and tuberculosis may aggravate CKD or accelerate its progression (Jha and Prasad 2016). In addition to these factors, older age, smoking, alcohol and tobacco use, being overweight, and urban residence are also associated with CKD. There is also major concern regarding unconventional risk factors (Jagannathan and Patzer 2017), such as chemical exposures, and what has been termed 'CKD of unknown aetiology' (Reddy and Gunasekar 2013; Varma 2015). These chemical exposures include inorganic chemicals such as chromium and mercury, and organic chemicals such as chloroform and ethylene glycol (Reddy and Gunasekar 2013). Overall, through the first Indian CKD registry it was found that diabetic nephropathy was the most common cause of CKD, while unknown aetiology and hypertension followed as the second and third most common causes of CKD, respectively (Rajapurkar et al. 2012).

Complications of CKD include cardiovascular disease, anaemia, and bone disease. It is possible to treat risk factors for CKD to mitigate functional decline; medical interventions include prescription of Angiotensin-converting enzyme (ACE) inhibitors and angiotensin receptor blockers (ARBs), and generally controlling blood pressure and glucose levels among those with diabetes. End-stage renal disease, the final stage of CKD progression, is relatively rare—roughly 230 cases per million population after age-standardization—but life-threatening and extremely costly. The recommended renal replacement therapies only reach about 10 per cent of the population with end-stage renal disease (Modi and Jha 2006).

Chronic Obstructive Pulmonary Disease

Chronic Obstructive Pulmonary Disease (COPD) is characterized by difficulty in breathing due to inflammation-related damage to lung tissue. The condition is progressive, such that lung function tends to worsen over time, and is associated with complications such as respiratory failure and general disability. Chronic respiratory diseases were the second highest contributor to total DALYs and deaths in India in 2016. Specifically, COPDs account for 5.15 per cent of all DALYs and 8.71 per cent of deaths in 2016 (IHME 2017, 2018). While older data estimated COPD prevalence to be ~4 per cent nationally (Jindal 2006), a recent nationwide prevalence study of patients seen by primary healthcare practitioners across India, nearly 15 per cent of diagnoses were for obstructive airway diseases (including COPD and asthma) (Salvi et al. 2015). The burden of COPD is high in both absolute and relative terms. Compared with 1990, the absolute number of DALYs associated with COPD increased by 34 per cent. Whereas the age-standardized rate of DALYs declined by 30 per cent in 2015, the COPD-associated DALY rate in India is still among the highest in the world (GBD 2015 and Chronic Respiratory Disease Collaborators 2017). Furthermore, age-adjusted mortality from COPD is estimated to be over thrice as high in India as compared with the UK, for instance (Mannino and Buist 2007).

Major risk factors for COPD include smoking, occupational exposures (such as dust, chemicals, and fumes), and indoor and outdoor air pollution (Jindal 2006; Vogelmeier et al. 2017). Due to this risk factor profile, COPD is higher in men compared to women and in lower SES groups. Although symptoms of COPD can be treated, there are no medications that can prevent long-term decline in lung function among COPD patients.

Mental Disorders

Although the WHO defined health as 'a state of complete physical, mental, and social well-being and not merely the absence of disease or infirmity' as early as 1946 (Grad 2002), mental health has only in recent decades been placed on an even footing with physical health ailments by the international community (Prince et al. 2007). Depression and anxiety account for 1.29 per cent and 0.87 per cent of total DALYs in India, respectively (IHME 2017, 2018). Self-harm, including suicide, accounts for 2.5 per cent of total DALYs and 17.5 deaths per 100,000 persons (IHME 2017, 2018); the toll of self-harm in India is higher than the global average.

Data describing the prevalence, risk factors, and treatment associated with mental health issues remains limited. Estimates suggest that the burden of mental, neurological, and substance use disorders will grow by one-quarter from 2013 to 2025 (Charlson et al. 2016). While several other mental disorders such as schizophrenia and bipolar disorder (<1 per cent prevalence in men and women) have important health and social impacts in India, depression (prevalence of 4 per cent in men and 5 per cent in women) and anxiety (prevalence of 2 per cent in men and 4 per cent in women) are the most common (Baxter et al. 2016). As in high income countries, lower income and education is associated with common mental disorders (Cheng et al. 2016). Being married (among women) and older age are risk factors for common mental disorders in India, but the opposite is true in high income countries (Cheng et al. 2016).

Treatment coverage for mental health issues is inadequate: only 5 per cent to 12 per cent of those with common mental disorders have any contact with any healthcare provider (V. Patel et al. 2016). In general, India lags behind China in the healthcare system's response to mental disorders. Only 0.3 psychiatrists per 100,000 people exist, and 43 mental hospitals serve the entire country (V. Patel et al. 2016). Given this scenario, there is a major emphasis on integrating basic mental healthcare with primary healthcare. Treating depression is thought to be a cost-effective strategy to reduce the disease burden (<USD 440 per DALY prevented) (V. Patel et al. 2011). Moreover, evidence suggests a bidirectional relationship between depression and diabetes, and untreated depression may lead to the adoption of unhealthy behaviours placing one at risk for other chronic diseases, and for failure to adhere to medication.

MULTILEVEL DRIVERS OF THE NCD BURDEN

Following a socioecological model of disease causation, the development and prognosis of most NCDs entails a confluence of (a) individual pathophysiology; (b) lifestyle-related behavioural risk factors; (c) biomedical

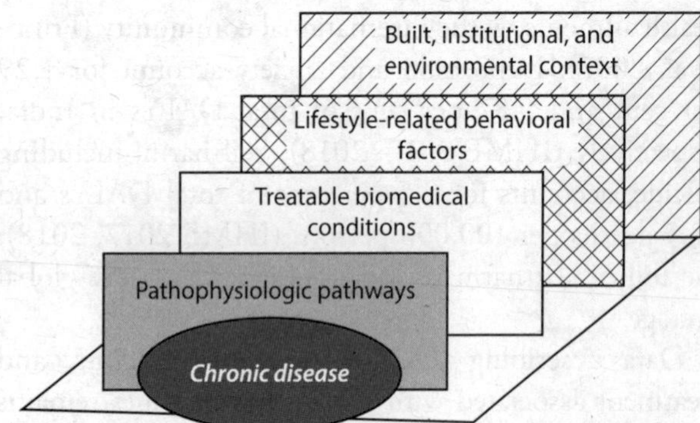

Figure 6.1 Socioecological Model of Disease Causation
Source: Adapted from Kaplan (2004).

risk factors that have known treatments; and (d) the built, institutional, and environmental factors that structure pathophysiology and other risks (see Figure 6.1). All these risk factors occur in the context of complex social and economic processes, which are discussed at length in other chapters of this volume. The leading NCDs share many common contributors across this multilevel and interconnected domain of causation. We briefly describe key shared contributors here, and Table 6.2 summarizes the contribution of typically measured behavioural, biomedical, and environmental risk factors to the NCD disease burden in India.

Table 6.2 Contribution of Behavioural and Biomedical Factors to the NCD Disease Burden in India, 2016

Risk factor	Per Cent of Total NCD DALYs	NCD DALYs per 100,000
Dietary risks	8.92	3159.4
High systolic blood pressure	8.47	3000.2
Air pollution	7.21	2555.7
High fasting plasma glucose	5.67	2008.7
Tobacco	4.93	1745.2
High total cholesterol	4.13	1463.8
High body-mass index	3.56	1261.5
Impaired kidney function	2.76	977.9
Occupational risks	2.32	823.8
Alcohol and drug use	2.18	771.7
Other environmental risks	1.01	357.8
Low physical activity	0.95	336.1
Unsafe sex	0.26	91.9
Sexual abuse and violence	0.21	75.0
Child and maternal malnutrition	0.01	2.5

Source: GBD data of 2016.

Distinct Pathophysiology

Notwithstanding the heterogeneity among India's ethnically diverse population, on average, at any given body mass index, resident Indians (S.A. Patel et al. 2016) and the diaspora (Anand et al. 2000; Creatore et al. 2010; McKeigue and Marmot 1988; McKeigue, Miller, and Marmot 1989) appear to be at higher risk for cardiometabolic disorders such as diabetes, hypertension, and CVDs compared to non-Indians. In addition, coronary heart disease and diabetes tends to occur at younger ages in South Asians compared with whites (Gujral et al. 2013; McQueen et al. 2008; Tillin et al. 2013). This propensity to develop cardiometabolic disorders, despite being relatively leaner, has been termed the 'South Asian phenotype' (Unnikrishnan, Anjana, and Mohan 2014). Shared environmental factors (long histories of malnutrition, dietary norms) and genetic predisposition may both be contributors to the high proportion of individuals with this lean but disease-prone phenotype. Moreover, current evidence suggests that although phenotype is distinctively high in South Asians, it is certainly not unique to South Asians (for example, glucose and lipid abnormalities may also develop in thin individuals in other ethnic groups [S.A. Patel et al. 2016]), nor is it universal in all South Asians (for instance, diabetes is more likely in heavier individuals, compared to thinner people, even among South Asians; diabetes prevalence is heterogeneous across ethnically Indian adults who reside within and outside India [Gujral et al. 2013]). The fact that Indians residing in the diaspora have among the longest life expectancies of any ethnic group—and far longer than Indians who continue to reside in India—suggests that broader living conditions and access to quality healthcare may indeed mitigate the mortality risks associated with ethnic predisposition to cardiometabolic disease.

Important for public health policy and action, the distinctive presentation of cardiometabolic disease in Indians has implications for optimal disease screening and treatment. The conditions embodied in the South Asian phenotype are themselves risk factors for other NCDs. High levels of blood pressure, fasting plasma glucose, and total cholesterol ranked as the second, fourth, and sixth leading risk factors for NCD-related DALYs in 2015. Each of these conditions is also heavily impacted by lifestyle-related behaviours described further.

Lifestyle-related Health Behaviours

Lifestyle-related health behaviours are perhaps the causes of NCDs that have received the most attention by the public health and medical communities alike. These behaviours include diet, physical activity, tobacco use, and alcohol and drug use, and are thought to be the backbone of the NCD epidemic. According to the GBD study, with the exception of tobacco, alcohol, and drug use, each of these behaviours was associated with a larger number of total DALYs per population in 2015 as compared to 1990 (IHME 2017, 2018). Focusing on the NCD disease burden specifically, dietary risks were the leading cause in 2016, accounting for 16 per cent of NCD-related DALYs (IHME 2017, 2018). Low consumption of whole grains, fruits, nuts and seeds, followed by high sodium consumption, are the major nutritional risk factors impacting NCDs (IHME 2017, 2018). These nutritional risk factors are also part and parcel of the nutrition transition, or the shift away from traditional diets high in unprocessed foods in favour of modern (globalized) diets high in processed, energy-dense foods—although gains in life expectancy have also accompanied this transition (Misra et al. 2011). Although India is not unique in this nutrition transition, the rapidity at which these dietary shifts are occurring may impact the pace of the NCD epidemic (Dehghan et al. 2017; Misra et al. 2011; 2017). Low physical activity ranks as the eleventh cause of NCD-related DALYs.

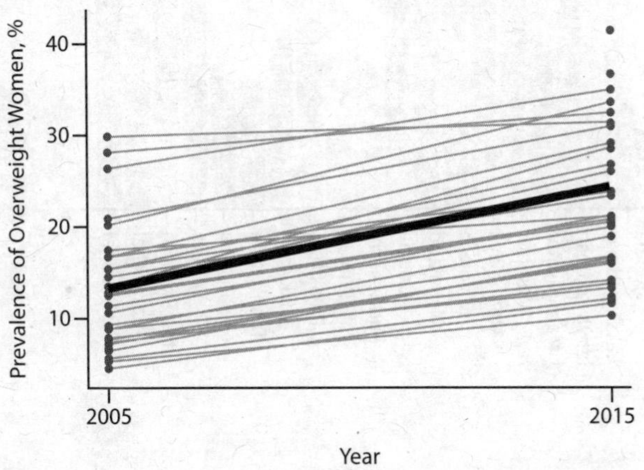

Figure 6.2 State-level trajectory of overweight (BMI ≥ 25 kg/m^2) among Indian women in 2005 and 2015

Source: National Family Health Surveys III and IV.

Each circle represents the prevalence of overweight in a single state; a line is drawn to connect the prevalence of overweight in a single state over time. The thick line shows the average increase in overweight from 2005 to 2015 in all states.

The welcome rise of efficient and affordable mechanized labour and transportation, and the unfortunate diminishing opportunities for physical activity in congested cities, has led to widespread concern around the impact of low physical activity in future generations.

Together, diet and physical activity play an important role in shaping energy balance, and in turn, overweight and obesity. High body mass index, the metric used to determine overweight and obesity, is the eighth leading risk factor for NCD-related DALYs. State-level numbers of overweight (BMI ≥ 25 kg/m^2) among women in 2005 and 2015 based on the NFHS state factsheets are mapped in Figure 6.2 (NFHS 2017). The numbers of overweight people rose in virtually every state, especially in women. States of Andhra Pradesh, Kerala, and Punjab had the highest proportion of overweights in both men and women, reflecting the vulnerability of those residents to NCDs such as diabetes, hypertension, heart disease, and breast cancer. Tobacco use ranks as the fifth leading risk factor for DALYs related to NCDs (IHME 2017, 2018). We show a map of state-level tobacco use in Figure 6.3. Tobacco use is much higher among men, and we find that the map is inverted compared with that of obesity. The highest tobacco-consuming states are Madhya Pradesh and the northeastern states.

Treatable Biomedical Risk Factors and the Treatment Gap

Hypertension, high plasma glucose, and high total blood cholesterol—in that order—are leading risk factors contributing to 6 per cent, 5 per cent, and 2 per cent of the NCD-associated DALYs in India. Each of these risk factors are chronic conditions in themselves and may be controlled through evidence-based treatment options. In fact, treating high blood pressure has been deemed as among the most cost-effective interventions per DALY averted (V. Patel et al. 2011). Seeking treatment for hypertension, however, requires awareness of one's blood pressure status (Chow et al. 2013; Khatib et al. 2014). Nationally, nearly one in three adults has hypertension (Anchala et al. 2014; Singh et al. 2011). In rural areas, where almost 70 per cent of the population resides, data suggest that only 25 per cent of those with hypertension are aware of their condition, 25 per cent of those with hypertension are treated for their condition, and only 10 per cent of those with hypertension achieve adequate blood pressure control (Anchala et al. 2014). Nationally, as many as 75 per cent of Indian adults have uncontrolled hypertension (Basu and Millett 2013).

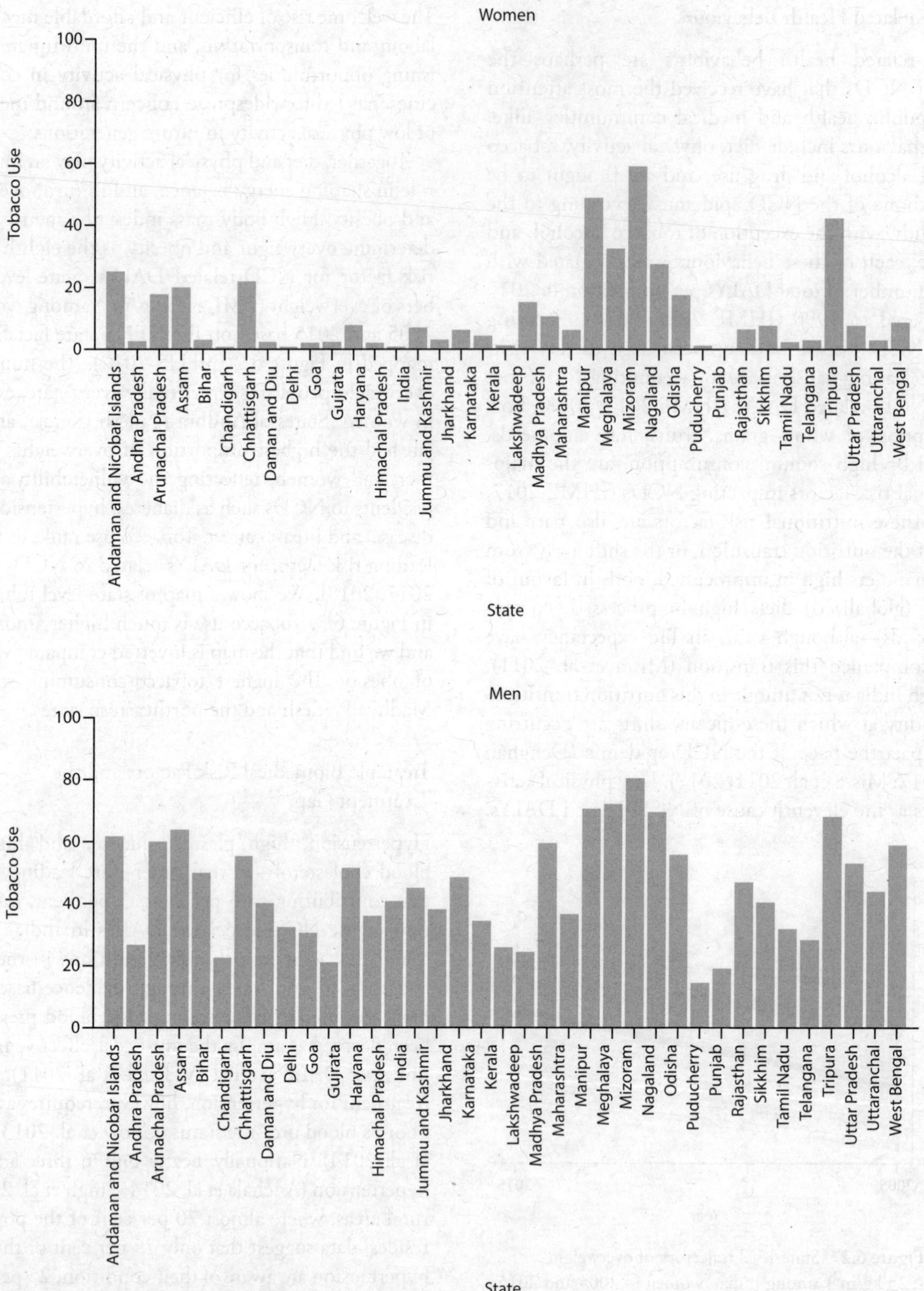

Figure 6.3 State-level tobacco use (per cent) in 2015 in India

Source: National Family Health Survey IV.

Besides hypertension, diabetes is one of the most prevalent and deadly of all chronic conditions in India (Anjana et al. 2011; Deepa et al. 2015; V. Patel et al. 2011). In the population-based Centre for Cardiometabolic Risk Reduction in South Asia (CARRS) Surveillance cohort (Nair et al. 2012), 42 per cent of persons with hypertension have comorbid diabetes, and 53 per cent of persons with diabetes have comorbid hypertension (authors' calculation from the CARRS data). Like hypertension, diabetes remains under-treated and poorly controlled, with only 20 per cent–25 per cent of persons with diabetes in Indian cities achieving glucose control (Deepa et al. 2015). With respect to cholesterol, expansion of treatment of high blood cholesterol is responsible for the decline in CVD mortality worldwide (Ford et al. 2007). In India, only half of patients with heart attacks in urban hospitals receive cholesterol-lowering medications (Xavier et al. 2008). South Asians are also more likely to have elevated apolipoprotein B_{100}/apolipoprotein A-I ratio than residents of other regions (Joshi et al. 2007). Healthcare systems play an important role in the screening and management of major NCDs.

As discussed throughout this chapter, there is a major treatment gap in the number of individuals with a controllable chronic condition and the number receiving treatment. This gap is reflected in poor health system performance in addressing preventable causes of death—such as CHD, stroke, and diabetes. The GBD's Healthcare Access and Quality Index reflects the unaddressed burden of preventable deaths; in 2015, India ranked below the global average (45 versus 54, respectively) and Myanmar (48) (Barber et al. 2017).

The Physical, Built, and Institutional Environments

Neither risk factors nor health outcomes develop in a vacuum. The broader physical, built, and institutional environments are those contextual features external to the individual that shape lifestyle, treatment-seeking behaviours, and pathophysiological pathways discussed earlier. While some of these 'upstream' environmental features constrain or facilitate 'downstream' health behaviours (for instance, availability of parks facilitates physical activity), other environmental features have a direct pathophysiological impact (such as exposure to air pollutants impacts cardiovascular function). These environmental features are crucial leverage points for improving population health because they—unlike individual behaviour—are often within the purview of policymakers.

The physical environment refers to the natural environment, such as air and water resources. Air pollution has been linked with cardiovascular disease, respiratory ailments, and cancers. In India, air pollution was ranked as the leading cause of disease and the third leading cause of NCD-related DALYs in India in 2015. Ambient particulate matter and household air pollution contribute to the total air pollution risk nearly equally, while ozone contributes a relatively smaller fraction (IHME 2017, 2018). Several large studies are underway to better understand the role of air pollution in the development of chronic diseases in large Indian cities.

The built environment includes human-made infrastructure such as housing, food outlets, and sidewalks. Urbanization is a major driver of the ever-evolving built environment globally. In comparison to rural areas, the road, commercial, and residential infrastructure needed to sustain densely populated urban areas often leads to limited space for physical activity and increased access to calorie dense foods. A study in New Delhi replicated findings from high income settings and suggests that fast food availability is related to obesity (O. Patel et al. 2017). In another related study, investigators found that the availability of large parks was associated with lower depressive symptoms among adults with chronic conditions (Mukherjee et al. 2017); they also found a marginally statistically significant link between walking over 150 minutes/week among those living near larger parks compared with those living near smaller parks, suggesting that green space may impact physical activity patterns.

We refer to the institutional environment as the public and private institutions providing services and generating policies relevant to health outcomes. These institutions include education, employment opportunities, welfare services, and the healthcare system—all of which are discussed at length in other chapters of this volume and fundamentally shape the resources needed to achieve good health.

Many of these environmental features are interrelated. For example, the production of fruits and vegetables relies on the natural environment and may be promoted (or thwarted) by agricultural policy. The distribution of such fruits and vegetables to consumers is impacted by the built environment. Given that fruits and vegetables are associated with lower mortality risk (Miller et al. 2017), it is a global tragedy that the global production of fruits and vegetables is insufficient to meet recommended consumption (Siegel et al. 2014) and that affordability limits consumption in LMICs (Miller et al. 2016).

SPECIAL POPULATIONS OF INTEREST

The Elderly

The relative contribution of NCDs to the disease burden varies by the stage of one's life course (Figure 6.4). Among children under the age of five, less than 20 per cent of total DALYs are due to NCDs; by age 65, this number goes up to over 80 per cent. Increased life expectancy and lower fertility contribute to the steady increase in the population of adults aged 65 and older in India, at ~6 per cent of the total population (PopulationPyramid.Net n.d.). The growing population of elderly has been referred to as the 'silver tsunami' the world over, and undoubtedly, India will have to find its path. Unsurprisingly, given that health declines with age, population ageing is a major factor driving the surge in NCDs in India (Chatterji et al. 2008). Moreover, negative health behaviours such as tobacco use (roughly two in five men are daily smokers) and physical inactivity (roughly one in five adults report inadequate activity) are prevalent in older adults in India (Chatterji et al. 2008). Among the elderly, chronic diseases in lower wealth quintiles, women, and rural residents disproportionately go undiagnosed (Basu and King 2013).

Older adults are also vulnerable to multimorbidity, or experiencing two or more conditions simultaneously (Arokiasamy, Uttamacharya, and Jain 2015; Banjare and Pradhan 2014; Pati et al. 2015). Multimorbidity is in turn associated with higher disability (Arokiasamy, Uttamacharya, and Jain 2015; Basu and King 2013) and higher healthcare utilization (Pati et al. 2014). The disabling and debilitating health effects and costs associated with the NCDs are compounded by multimorbidity (Basu and King 2013). Within families, caring for the elderly and especially those with multimorbidity takes a toll on caregivers, who are often women (Jamuna 1997). Within the health system, there is broad consensus that particularly in rural areas there is inadequate preparedness to address the NCD burden in the older population.

Women

While undernutrition among women has long been a relatively high-priority health and social issue, the burden of overweight is catching up to the burden of underweight in India. Nationally, the proportions of overweight and underweight women are increasingly comparable, with 21 per cent overweight (BMI ≥ 25 kg/m^2) and 23 per cent underweight (BMI < 18.5 kg/m^2). In cities, however, the prevalence of overweight exceeds the prevalence of underweight in women (31 per cent versus 16 per cent, respectively), and the prevalence of overweight is substantially higher in women compared to men (31 per cent versus 26 per cent, respectively; see Figure 6.5; NFHS 4). Prior national data indicates that the overweight disparity between urban and rural women and the overweight disparity between urban women and urban men is more pronounced with increasing age (Patel, Narayan, and Cunningham 2015). These trends raise concerns regarding the dual burden of disease among Indian women and their risk for cardiometabolic disease and physical limitations as they age. In addition, both overweight and underweight in women of reproductive age has intergenerational implications, increasing the risk of NCDs in the offspring.

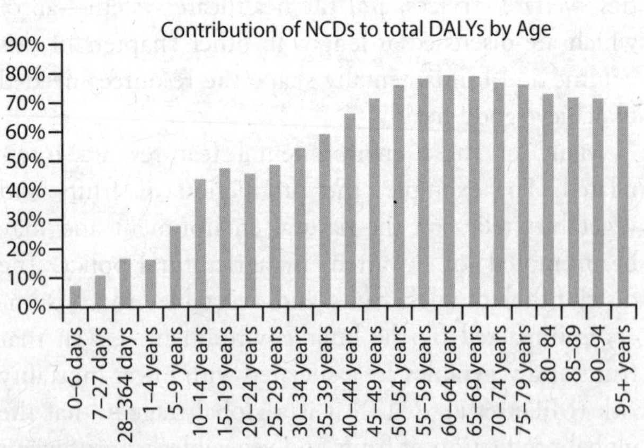

Figure 6.4 Relative contribution of NCDs to the disease burden varies by stage of the life course

Source: GBD 2016.

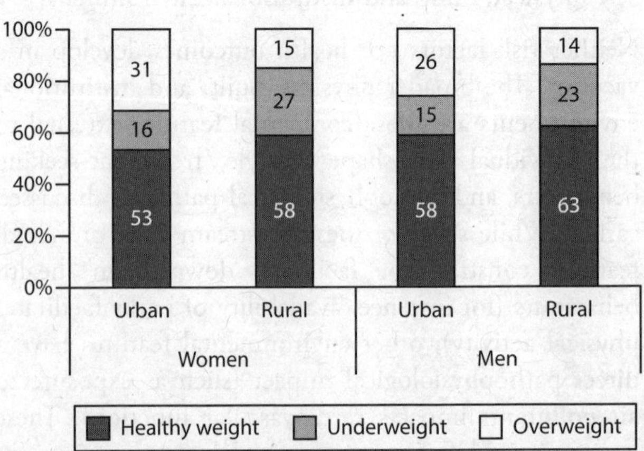

Figure 6.5 Healthy weight, underweight, and overweight in India by rurality in 2015

Source: National Family Health Survey IV.

There is growing appreciation for the impact of undernutrition during pregnancy on cardiometabolic disease. It is argued that underweight pregnant women physiologically prime their developing foetus for restrictive nutritional conditions; their infants go on to experience a 'thrifty phenotype' which favors conservation of fat and possibly to reduced beta cell function (Wadhwa et al. 2009; Yajnik 2002). In the context of economic development and the nutrition transition, many infants of underweight mothers in fact are exposed to nutritional conditions favouring weight gain in childhood (Yajnik 2004). South Asians who experienced rapid weight gain in infancy and childhood are more likely to develop cardiometabolic abnormalities in later life (Fall et al. 2008; Sachdev et al. 2005). In addition, higher body mass index is associated with worse pregnancy complications in South Asian women (Bryant et al. 2013). One such complication is gestational diabetes, which may be as high as 41 per cent in north India according to recently developed measurement guidelines (Gopalakrishnan et al. 2015). Our understanding of the prevalence and population-level impacts of gestational diabetes in India is limited, but studies outside of India indicate that gestational diabetes predisposes women for risk of diabetes (Feig et al. 2008) and is associated with severe obesity and risk of type 2 diabetes among her children (Flores and Lin 2013).

Rural Residents

Rural areas experience a dual burden of disease in which diseases of undernutrition and infectious origins persist at a high level alongside increasing vulnerability to NCDs. Despite having greater proportions of underweight individuals as compared to overweight (see Figure 6.5), the numbers afflicted with overweight and obesity have risen at the same or faster pace in rural areas as in urban ones and, by 2015, 15 per cent of women and 14 per cent of men in rural India were found to be overweight. Despite being relatively thin, metabolic morbidities are common in rural Indians. High triglycerides and high ratio of total cholesterol to high-density lipoprotein (HDL) cholesterol affect over 20 per cent of rural Indians, while hypertension affects nearly 20 per cent (Kinra et al. 2010). Although diabetes in rural compared to urban areas is about half as high (Anjana et al. 2011), diabetes has risen at a fast pace in the past decades, with the condition's prevalence in rural southern India being thrice as high in 2003 as it was in 1989 (Ramachandran et al. 2004).

In terms of addressing these burdens, there are several challenges. Only 37 per cent of rural residents had heard of diabetes compared with 58 per cent of urban residents (Deepa et al. 2014). Poor health behaviours are also prevalent. Low physical activity and low fruit and vegetable intake affect over 60 per cent of the population. Rural residents when compared to urban residents are more likely to use tobacco and have undiagnosed chronic conditions (Basu and King 2013). There are also very limited economic resources and infrastructure across the bulk of rural settings in India—in the context of rising chronic conditions, this lack of physical access imposes major challenges to the health system.

POLICY RECOMMENDATIONS

We summarize five key areas for development with regard to addressing the NCD burden from a population-health perspective: (a) promotion of data infrastructure and health research scientists; (b) focus on translation and implementation science; (c) multi-sectoral and multidisciplinary partnership; (d) investment in healthcare infrastructure and technology; and (e) development of the healthcare workforce.

Promotion of Data Infrastructure and Health Research Scientists

Simply importing and applying scientific findings from high income countries to the Indian population will likely be insufficient in addressing the NCD burden in a meaningful way, as disease patterns and manifestations vary in India. Moreover, several aspects of the broader Indian context must be considered in designing appropriate interventions and even medical dosing. For example, as we have discussed earlier, Indians may have unique pathophysiology when it comes to cardiometabolic disease. They are furthermore exposed to a distinct set of environmental pollutants, underlying infectious disease burdens, and nutritional conditions as compared with high income countries where most past research has been conducted. Promoting the health sciences within our borders is thus needed. Health sciences rely on high-quality data to address existing health issues and also innovatively investigate novel scientific questions pertinent to the Indian population. The primacy of data infrastructure is also highlighted in this volume in Rao's chapter ('The Policy Framework: A Critical Assessment'), describing policy deficits due to inadequacy of surveillance and health data at a more general level. As important as data are research scientists who are equipped to appropriately use data to answer pressing questions. Public and private funding towards the development of research scientists should be a high priority area.

Translation and Implementation Science

Effective healthcare delivery requires implementation science research to fine-tune best practices that improve the NCD continuum of care, or the process going from diagnosing a patient, to connecting the patient with appropriate care, to sustained and effective management of disease. Studies have demonstrated the feasibility and effectiveness of strategies using coordinated care and decision-support software to deliver high quality affordable care for people with chronic diseases such as diabetes (Ali et al. 2016); further studies are needed to promote scale-up. Because treatment is so closely linked with improved outcomes across the diverse spectrum of NCDs, understanding barriers to the process leading up to engaging with care is high priority (Krishnan et al. 2013). Implementation science can also provide insights into system inefficiencies and efficiencies, to prune the workforce appropriately.

Multi-Sectoral and Multi-Disciplinary Partnerships

Since NCDs are preventable and treatable, it is imperative that both prevention-oriented efforts are combined with healthcare-system-oriented efforts at improvement in care. Prevention of NCDs rests largely on improvements in living conditions, access to health promoting resources, and health behaviours—these rest outside the health system and require partnership across various ministries and stakeholders. The perspective of multiple disciplines, such as epidemiology, economics, behavioural science, and anthropology, would be useful in formulating a policy vision to enact. In addition, engagement with local communities to understand local needs and strengths better is a must.

Development of Healthcare Infrastructure and Appropriate Technology

First, healthcare infrastructure is not keeping pace with population growth. Even India's 153,655 sub-centres—the first line of defence—are stretched to serve a larger population than what was originally intended. Second, healthcare system was designed to primarily address maternal and child health and infectious diseases (Jamison et al. 2013), and must be reoriented to meet the needs of chronic conditions. Modern information technology systems, such as electronic health records, text messaging, and telemedicine, must be tested and leveraged appropriately to track and refer patients, and possibly evaluate impacts of health interventions.

Development of the Healthcare Workforce

There are progressively larger shortfalls of healthcare providers as we move up the healthcare system hierarchy; the shortfall—as the proportion of vacant posts among those sanctioned—is 5 per cent for nurses at the village level, 10 per cent for physicians at the primary healthcare centre level, but 81 per cent at community health centres. Reaching the population in need demands that there are sufficient numbers of healthcare providers, that they are well-trained, and that they remain in their posts for sufficient time to execute their responsibilities. Ongoing education of the healthcare workforce is necessary for providers to be familiar with a wide range of diagnostic modalities, standard treatment guidelines, and pharmaceuticals (Hasan, Zodpey, and Saraf 2012; Unnikrishnan, Anjana, and Mohan 2011).

REFERENCES

Adler, A.I., E.J. Boyko, J.H. Ahroni, and D.G. Smith. 1999. 'Lower-Extremity Amputation in Diabetes. The Independent Effects of Peripheral Vascular Disease, Sensory Neuropathy, and Foot Ulcers', *Diabetes Care* 22(7): 1029–35. doi:10.2337/diacare.22.7.1029.

Ali, Mohammed K., Kavita Singh, Dimple Kondal, Raji Devarajan, Shivani A. Patel, Roopa Shivashankar, Vamadevan S. Ajay, et al. 2016. 'Effectiveness of a Multicomponent Quality Improvement Strategy to Improve Achievement of Diabetes Care Goals: A Randomized, Controlled Trial', *Annals of Internal Medicine* 165(6): 399–408. doi:10.7326/M15-2807.

Anand, Shuchi, Roopa Shivashankar, Mohammed K. Ali, Dimple Kondal, B. Binukumar, Maria E. Montez-Rath, Vamadevan S. Ajay, et al. 2015. 'Prevalence of Chronic Kidney Disease in Two Major Indian Cities and Projections for Associated Cardiovascular Disease', *Kidney International* 88(1): 178–85. doi:10.1038/ki.2015.58.

Anand, Sonia S, Salim Yusuf, Vladmir Vuksan, Sudarshan Devanesen, Koon K Teo, Patricia A Montague, Linda Kelemen, et al. 2000. 'Differences in Risk Factors, Atherosclerosis, and Cardiovascular Disease between Ethnic Groups in Canada: The Study of Health

Assessment and Risk in Ethnic Groups (SHARE)', *The Lancet* 356(9226): 279–84. doi:10.1016/S0140-6736(00)02502-2.

Anchala, Raghupathy, Nanda K. Kannuri, Hira Pant, Hassan Khan, Oscar H. Franco, Emanuele Di Angelantonio, and Dorairaj Prabhakaran. 2014. 'Hypertension in India: A Systematic Review and Meta-Analysis of Prevalence, Awareness, and Control of Hypertension', *Journal of Hypertension* 32(6): 1170–77. doi:10.1097/HJH.0000000000000146.

Anjana, R.M., M. Deepa, R. Pradeepa, J. Mahanta, K. Narain, H.K. Das, P. Adhikari, et al. 2017. 'Prevalence of Diabetes and Prediabetes in 15 States of India: Results from the ICMR-INDIAB Population-Based Cross-Sectional Study', *Lancet Diabetes Endocrinol* 5(8): 585–96. doi:10.1016/S2213-8587(17)30174-2.

Anjana, R.M., R. Pradeepa, M. Deepa, M. Datta, V. Sudha, R. Unnikrishnan, A. Bhansali, et al. 2011. 'Prevalence of Diabetes and Prediabetes (Impaired Fasting Glucose and/or Impaired Glucose Tolerance) in Urban and Rural India: Phase I Results of the Indian Council of Medical Research–INdia DIABetes (ICMR–INDIAB) Study', *Diabetologia* 54(12): 3022–27. doi:10.1007/s00125-011-2291-5.

Arokiasamy, Perianayagam, Uttamacharya, and Kshipra Jain. 2015. 'Multi-Morbidity, Functional Limitations, and Self-Rated Health Among Older Adults in India', *SAGE Open* 5(1): 2158244015571640. doi:10.1177/2158244015571640.

Banjare, Pallavi, and Jalandhar Pradhan. 2014. 'Socio-Economic Inequalities in the Prevalence of Multi-Morbidity among the Rural Elderly in Bargarh District of Odisha (India)', *PLOS ONE* 9(6): e97832. doi:10.1371/journal.pone.0097832.

Barber, Ryan M., Nancy Fullman, Reed J.D. Sorensen, Thomas Bollyky, Martin McKee, Ellen Nolte, Amanuel Alemu Abajobir, et al. 2017. 'Healthcare Access and Quality Index Based on Mortality from Causes Amenable to Personal Health Care in 195 Countries and Territories, 1990–2015: A Novel Analysis from the Global Burden of Disease Study 2015', *The Lancet* 390(10091): 231–66. doi:10.1016/S0140-6736(17)30818-8.

Bardenheier, Barbara H., Ji Lin, Xiaohui Zhuo, Mohammed K. Ali, Theodore J. Thompson, Yiling J. Cheng, and Edward W. Gregg. 2016. 'Disability-Free Life-Years Lost Among Adults Aged ≥50 Years With and Without Diabetes', *Diabetes Care* 39(7): 1222–29. doi:10.2337/dc15-1095.

Basu, Sanjay, and Abby C. King. 2013. 'Disability and Chronic Disease Among Older Adults in India: Detecting Vulnerable Populations Through the WHO SAGE Study', *American Journal of Epidemiology* 178(11): 1620–28. doi:10.1093/aje/kwt191.

Basu, Sanjay, and Christopher Millett. 2013. 'Social Epidemiology of Hypertension in Middle-Income Countries Determinants of Prevalence, Diagnosis, Treatment, and Control in the WHO SAGE Study', *Hypertension* 62(1): 18–26. doi:10.1161/HYPERTENSIONAHA.113.01374.

Baxter, Amanda J., Fiona J. Charlson, Hui G. Cheng, Rahul Shidhaye, Alize J. Ferrari, and Harvey A. Whiteford. 2016. 'Prevalence of Mental, Neurological, and Substance Use Disorders in China and India: A Systematic Analysis', *The Lancet Psychiatry* 3(9): 832–41. doi:10.1016/S2215-0366(16)30139-0.

Bryant, M., G. Santorelli, D.A. Lawlor, D. Farrar, D. Tuffnell, R. Bhopal, and J. Wright. 2013. 'A Comparison of South Asian Specific and Established BMI Thresholds for Determining Obesity Prevalence in Pregnancy and Predicting Pregnancy Complications: Findings from the Born in Bradford Cohort', *International Journal of Obesity(2005)*, June. doi:10.1038/ijo.2013.117.

CDC (Centers for Disease Control and Prevention). 2014. 'National Chronic Kidney Disease Fact Sheet: General Information and National Estimates on Chronic Kidney Disease in the United States, 2014'. Available at http://www.cdc.gov/diabetes/pubs/factsheets/kidney.htm, last accessed on 31 August 2017.

Chalkidou, Kalipso, Patricio Marquez, Preet K. Dhillon, Yot Teerawattananon, Thunyarat Anothaisintawee, Carlos Augusto Grabois Gadelha, and Richard Sullivan. 2014. 'Evidence-Informed Frameworks for Cost-Effective Cancer Care and Prevention in Low, Middle, and High-Income Countries', *The Lancet Oncology* 15(3): e119–31. doi:10.1016/S1470-2045(13)70547-3.

Charlson, Fiona J., Amanda J. Baxter, Hui G. Cheng, Rahul Shidhaye, and Harvey A. Whiteford. 2016. 'The Burden of Mental, Neurological, and Substance Use Disorders in China and India: A Systematic Analysis of Community Representative Epidemiological Studies', *The Lancet* 388(10042): 376–89. doi:10.1016/S0140-6736(16)30590-6.

Chatterji, Somnath, Paul Kowal, Colin Mathers, Nirmala Naidoo, Emese Verdes, James P. Smith, and Richard Suzman. 2008. 'The Health of Aging Populations in China and India', *Health Affairs* 27(4): 1052–63. doi:10.1377/hlthaff.27.4.1052.

Cheng, Hui G., Rahul Shidhaye, Fiona Charlson, Fei Deng, Tanica Lyngdoh, Shengnan Chen, Sharmishtha Nanda, Kimberly Lacroix, Amanda Baxter, and Harvey Whiteford. 2016. 'Social Correlates of Mental, Neurological, and Substance Use Disorders in China and India: A Review', *The Lancet Psychiatry* 3(9): 882–99. doi:10.1016/S2215-0366(16)30166-3.

Chow C.K., K.K. Teo, S. Rangarajan, and et al. 2013. 'Prevalence, Awareness, Treatment, and Control of Hypertension in Rural and Urban Communities in High-, Middle-, and Low-Income Countries', *JAMA* 310(9): 959–68. doi:10.1001/jama.2013.184182.

Creatore, Maria Isabella, Rahim Moineddin, Gillian Booth, Doug H. Manuel, Marie DesMeules, Sarah McDermott, and Richard H. Glazier. 2010. 'Age- and Sex-Related Prevalence of Diabetes Mellitus among Immigrants to Ontario, Canada', *Canadian Medical Association Journal* 182(8): 781–89. doi:10.1503/cmaj.091551.

Das, Sujata, Avijit Hazra, Biman Kanti Ray, Malay Ghosal, Tapas Kumar Banerjee, Trishit Roy, Arijit Chaudhuri, Deepak K. Raut, and Shyamal Kumar Das. 2010. 'Burden among Stroke Caregivers: Results of a Community-Based Study from Kolkata, India', *Stroke; a Journal of Cerebral Circulation* 41(12): 2965–68. doi:10.1161/STROKEAHA.110.589598.

Deepa, M., A. Bhansali, R.M. Anjana, R. Pradeepa, S.R. Joshi, P.P. Joshi, V. K. Dhandhania, et al. 2014. 'Knowledge and Awareness of Diabetes in Urban and Rural India: The Indian Council of Medical Research India Diabetes Study (Phase I): Indian Council of Medical Research India Diabetes 4', *Indian Journal of Endocrinology and Metabolism* 18(3): 379–85. doi:10.4103/2230-8210.131191.

Deepa, Mohan, Mundu Grace, Bhaskarapillai Binukumar, Rajendra Pradeepa, Shivashankar Roopa, Hassan M. Khan, Zafar Fatmi, et al. 2015. 'High Burden of Prediabetes and Diabetes in Three Large Cities in South Asia: The Center for CArdio-Metabolic Risk Reduction in South Asia (CARRS) Study', *Diabetes Research and Clinical Practice*, September. doi:10.1016/j.diabres.2015.09.005.

Dehghan, Mahshid, Andrew Mente, Xiaohe Zhang, Sumathi Swaminathan, Wei Li, Viswanathan Mohan, Romaina Iqbal, et al. 2017. 'Associations of Fats and Carbohydrate Intake with Cardiovascular Disease and Mortality in 18 Countries from Five Continents (PURE): A Prospective Cohort Study', *The Lancet*, August. doi:10.1016/S0140-6736(17)32252-3.

Fall, Caroline H.D., Harshpal Singh Sachdev, Clive Osmond, Ramakrishnan Lakshmy, Sushant Dey Biswas, Dorairaj Prabhakaran, Nikhil Tandon, et al. 2008. 'Adult Metabolic Syndrome and Impaired Glucose Tolerance Are Associated With Different Patterns of BMI Gain During Infancy Data from the New Delhi Birth Cohort', *Diabetes Care* 31(12): 2349–56. doi:10.2337/dc08-0911.

Feig, D.S., B. Zinman, X. Wang, and J. E. Hux. 2008. 'Risk of Development of Diabetes Mellitus after Diagnosis of Gestational Diabetes', *Canadian Medical Association Journal* 179(3): 229–34. doi:10.1503/cmaj.080012.

Ferri, Cleusa P., Claudia Schoenborn, Lalit Kalra, Daisy Acosta, Mariella Guerra, Yueqin Huang, K. S. Jacob, et al. 2011. 'Prevalence of Stroke and Related Burden among Older People Living in Latin America, India and China', *Journal of Neurology, Neurosurgery, and Psychiatry* 82(10): 1074–82. doi:10.1136/jnnp.2010.234153.

Flores, G., and H. Lin. 2013. 'Factors Predicting Severe Childhood Obesity in Kindergarteners', *International Journal of Obesity* 37(1): 31–39. doi:10.1038/ijo.2012.168.

Fong, D.S., L. Aiello, T.W. Gardner, G.L. King, G. Blankenship, J.D. Cavallerano, F.L. Ferris 3rd, and R. Klein. 2004. 'Retinopathy in Diabetes', *Diabetes Care* 27(Suppl 1): S84-7.

Ford, Earl S., Umed A. Ajani, Janet B. Croft, Julia A. Critchley, Darwin R. Labarthe, Thomas E. Kottke, Wayne H. Giles, and Simon Capewell. 2007. 'Explaining the Decrease in U.S. Deaths from Coronary Disease, 1980–2000', *The New England Journal of Medicine* 356(23): 2388–98. doi:10.1056/NEJMsa053935.

GBD 2015 and Chronic Respiratory Disease Collaborators. 2017. 'Global, Regional, and National Deaths, Prevalence, Disability-Adjusted Life Years, and Years Lived with Disability for Chronic Obstructive Pulmonary Disease and Asthma, 1990–2015: A Systematic Analysis for the Global Burden of Disease Study 2015', 2017. *The Lancet Respiratory Medicine* 5(9): 691–706. doi:10.1016/S2213-2600(17)30293-X.

Gopalakrishnan, V., R. Singh, Y. Pradeep, D. Kapoor, A.K. Rani, S. Pradhan, E. Bhatia, and S.B. Yadav. 2015. 'Evaluation of the Prevalence of Gestational Diabetes Mellitus in North Indians Using the International Association of Diabetes and Pregnancy Study Groups (IADPSG) Criteria', *Journal of Postgraduate Medicine* 61(3): 155–58. doi:10.4103/0022-3859.159306.

Goss, Paul E., Kathrin Strasser-Weippl, Brittany L. Lee-Bychkovsky, Lei Fan, Junjie Li, Yanin Chavarri-Guerra, Pedro E.R. Liedke, et al. 2014. 'Challenges to Effective Cancer Control in China, India, and Russia', *The Lancet Oncology* 15(5): 489–538. doi:10.1016/S1470-2045(14)70029-4.

Grad, Frank P. 2002. 'The Preamble of the Constitution of the World Health Organization', *Bulletin of the World Health Organization* 80(12): 981–981.

Grundy, Scott M., Ivor J. Benjamin, Gregory L. Burke, Alan Chait, Robert H. Eckel, Barbara V. Howard, William Mitch, Sidney C. Smith, and James R. Sowers. 1999. 'Diabetes and Cardiovascular Disease: A Statement for Healthcare Professionals From the American Heart Association', *Circulation* 100(10): 1134–46. doi:10.1161/01.cir.100.10.1134.

Gudala, Kapil, Dipika Bansal, Fabrizio Schifano, and Anil Bhansali. 2013. 'Diabetes Mellitus and Risk of Dementia: A Meta-Analysis of Prospective Observational Studies', *Journal of Diabetes Investigation* 4(6): 640–50. doi:10.1111/jdi.12087.

Gujral, Unjali P., K.M. Venkat Narayan, R. Ghua Pradeepa, Mohan Deepa, Mohammed K. Ali, Ranjit M. Anjana, Namratha R. Kandula, Viswanathan Mohan, and Alka M. Kanaya. 2015. 'Comparing Type 2 Diabetes,

Prediabetes, and Their Associated Risk Factors in Asian Indians in India and in the U.S.: The CARRS and MASALA Studies', *Diabetes Care* 38(7): 1312–18. doi:10.2337/dc15-0032.

Gujral, Unjali P., R. Pradeepa, Mary Beth Weber, K.M. Venkat Narayan, and V. Mohan. 2013. 'Type 2 Diabetes in South Asians: Similarities and Differences with White Caucasian and Other Populations', *Annals of the New York Academy of Sciences* 1281(1): 51–63. doi.org/10.1111/j.1749-6632.2012.06838.x.

Gupta, Adyya, Preet K. Dhillon, Jyotsna Govil, Dipika Bumb, Subhojit Dey, and Suneeta Krishnan. 2015. 'Multiple Stakeholder Perspectives on Cancer Stigma in North India', *Asian Pacific Journal of Cancer Prevention: APJCP* 16(14): 6141–47.

Gupta, Rajeev, Indu Mohan, and Jagat Narula. 2016. 'Trends in Coronary Heart Disease Epidemiology in India', *Annals of Global Health*, Hypertension and Cardiovascular Disease in Low and Middle Income Countries, 82(2): 307–15. doi:10.1016/j.aogh.2016.04.002.

Hasan, Habib, Sanjay Zodpey, and Abhay Saraf. 2012. 'Diabetologist's Perspective on Practice of Evidence Based Diabetes Management in India', *Diabetes Research and Clinical Practice* 95(2): 189–93. doi:10.1016/j.diabres.2011.09.021.

IDF (International Diabetes Federation). 2015. *IDF Diabetes Atlas*. Brussels: International Diabetes Federation.

IHME (Institute for Health Metrics and Evaluation). n.d. 'GBD Compare | IHME Viz Hub',, GBD Comparative Data Visualization. Available at http://vizhub.healthdata.org/gbd-compare, data accessed separately on 27 August 2017 and 17 April 2018.

IIPS (International Institute for Population Sciences). 2017. '(NFHS) 4 State Level Factsheets: 2015–2016'. Mumbai: IIPS.Jagannathan, Ram, and Rachel E. Patzer. 2017. 'Urbanization and Kidney Function Decline in Low and Middle Income Countries', *BMC Nephrology* 18(August): 276. doi:10.1186/s12882-017-0685-4.

Jamison, Dean T., Lawrence H. Summers, George Alleyne, Kenneth J. Arrow, Seth Berkley, Agnes Binagwaho, Flavia Bustreo, et al. 2013. 'Global Health 2035: A World Converging within a Generation', *Lancet (London, England)* 382(9908): 1898–955. doi:10.1016/S0140-6736(13)62105-4.

Jamuna, D. 1997. 'Stress Dimensions among Caregivers of the Elderly', *The Indian Journal of Medical Research* 106(October): 381–88.

Jha, Vivekanand, and Narayan Prasad. 2016. 'CKD and Infectious Diseases in Asia Pacific: Challenges and Opportunities', *American Journal of Kidney Diseases* 68(1): 148–60. doi:10.1053/j.ajkd.2016.01.017.

Jindal, Surinder K. 2006. 'Emergence of Chronic Obstructive Pulmonary Disease as an Epidemic in India', *The Indian Journal of Medical Research* 124(6): 619–30.

Joshi, Prashant, Shofiqul Islam, Prem Pais, Srinath Reddy, Prabhakaran Dorairaj, Khawar Kazmi, Mrigendra Raj Pandey, et al. 2007. 'Risk Factors for Early Myocardial Infarction in South Asians Compared With Individuals in Other Countries', *JAMA* 297(3): 286–94. doi:10.1001/jama.297.3.286.

Joshi, Rohina, Magnolia Cardona, Srinivas Iyengar, A. Sukumar, C. Ravi Raju, K. Rama Raju, Krishnam Raju, K. Srinath Reddy, Alan Lopez, and Bruce Neal. 2006. 'Chronic Diseases Now a Leading Cause of Death in Rural India—Mortality Data from the Andhra Pradesh Rural Health Initiative', *International Journal of Epidemiology* 35(6): 1522–29. doi:10.1093/ije/dyl168.

Kassebaum, Nicholas J., Megha Arora, Ryan M. Barber, Zulfiqar A. Bhutta, Jonathan Brown, Austin Carter, Daniel C. Casey, et al. 2016. 'Global, Regional, and National Disability-Adjusted Life-Years (DALYs) for 315 Diseases and Injuries and Healthy Life Expectancy(HALE), 1990–2015: A Systematic Analysis for the Global Burden of Disease Study 2015', *The Lancet* 388(10053): 1603–58. doi:10.1016/S0140-6736(16)31460-X.

Khatib, Rasha, Jon-David Schwalm, Salim Yusuf, R. Brian Haynes, Martin McKee, Maheer Khan, and Robby Nieuwlaat. 2014. 'Patient and Healthcare Provider Barriers to Hypertension Awareness, Treatment and Follow Up: A Systematic Review and Meta-Analysis of Qualitative and Quantitative Studies', *PLOS ONE* 9(1): e84238. doi:10.1371/journal.pone.0084238.

Kinra, S., L.J. Bowen, T. Lyngdoh, D. Prabhakaran, K.S. Reddy, L. Ramakrishnan, R. Gupta, et al. 2010. 'Sociodemographic Patterning of Non-Communicable Disease Risk Factors in Rural India: A Cross Sectional Study', *BMJ* 341(1): c4974–c4974. doi:10.1136/bmj.c4974.

Knowler, W.C., E. Barrett-Connor, S.E. Fowler, R.F. Hamman, J.M. Lachin, E.A. Walker, and D.M. Nathan. 2002. 'Reduction in the Incidence of Type 2 Diabetes with Lifestyle Intervention or Metformin', *N Engl J Med* 346(6): 393–403. doi:10.1056/NEJMoa012512.

Krishnan, Suneeta, Emily Madsen, Deborah Porterfield, and Beena Varghese. 2013. 'Advancing Cervical Cancer Prevention in India: Implementation Science Priorities', *The Oncologist*, November. doi:10.1634/theoncologist.2013-0292.

Kwatra, Gagandeep, Paramdeep Kaur, Gagan Toor, Dinesh K. Badyal, Raminder Kaur, Yashpal Singh, and Jeyaraj D. Pandian. 2013. 'Cost of Stroke from a Tertiary Center in Northwest India', *Neurology India* 61(6): 627–32. doi:10.4103/0028-3886.125270.

Mallath, Mohandas K., David G. Taylor, Rajendra A. Badwe, Goura K. Rath, V. Shanta, C.S. Pramesh, Raghunadharao Digumarti, et al. 2014. 'The Growing Burden of Cancer in India: Epidemiology and Social Context', *The*

Lancet Oncology 15(6): e205–12. doi:10.1016/S1470-2045(14)70115-9.

Mannino, David M., and A. Sonia Buist. 2007. 'Global Burden of COPD: Risk Factors, Prevalence, and Future Trends', *The Lancet* 370(9589): 765–73. doi:10.1016/S0140-6736(07)61380-4.

Marijon, Eloi, Mariana Mirabel, David S. Celermajer, and Xavier Jouven. 2012. 'Rheumatic Heart Disease', *The Lancet* 379(9819): 953–64. doi:10.1016/S0140-6736(11)61171-9.

McKeigue, P.M., and M.G. Marmot. 1988. 'Mortality from Coronary Heart Disease in Asian Communities in London', *BMJ : British Medical Journal* 297(6653): 903.

McKeigue, P.M., G.J. Miller, and M.G. Marmot. 1989. 'Coronary Heart Disease in South Asians Overseas: A Review', *Journal of Clinical Epidemiology* 42(7): 597–609. doi:10.1016/0895-4356(89)90002-4.

McQueen, Matthew J., Steven Hawken, Xingyu Wang, Stephanie Ounpuu, Allan Sniderman, Jeffrey Probstfield, Krisela Steyn, et al. 2008. 'Lipids, Lipoproteins, and Apolipoproteins as Risk Markers of Myocardial Infarction in 52 Countries (the INTERHEART Study): A Case-Control Study', *The Lancet* 372(9634): 224–33. doi:10.1016/S0140-6736(08)61076-4.

Mehndiratta, Man Mohan, Aneesh B. Singhal, Seemant Chaturvedi, M.R. Sivakumar, and Majaz Moonis. 2013. 'Meeting the Challenges of Stroke in India', *Neurology* 80(24): 2246–47. doi:10.1212/WNL.0b013e318296e7c3.

Miller, Victoria, Andrew Mente, Mahshid Dehghan, Sumathy Rangarajan, Xiaohe Zhang, Sumathi Swaminathan, Gilles Dagenais, et al. 2017. 'Fruit, Vegetable, and Legume Intake, and Cardiovascular Disease and Deaths in 18 Countries (PURE): A Prospective Cohort Study', *The Lancet* 390(10107): 2037–49. doi:10.1016/S0140-6736(17)32253-5.

Miller, Victoria, Salim Yusuf, Clara K. Chow, Mahshid Dehghan, Daniel J. Corsi, Karen Lock, Barry Popkin, et al. 2016. 'Availability, Affordability, and Consumption of Fruits and Vegetables in 18 Countries across Income Levels: Findings from the Prospective Urban Rural Epidemiology (PURE) Study', *The Lancet Global Health* 4(10): e695–703. doi:10.1016/S2214-109X(16)30186-3.

Misra, Anoop, Neha Singhal, Bhattiprolu Sivakumar, Namita Bhagat, Abhishek Jaiswal, and Lokesh Khurana. 2011. 'Nutrition Transition in India: Secular Trends in Dietary Intake and Their Relationship to Diet-Related Non-Communicable Diseases', *Journal of Diabetes* 3(4): 278–92. doi:10.1111/j.1753-0407.2011.00139.x.

Misra, Anoop, Nikhil Tandon, Shah Ebrahim, Naveed Sattar, Dewan Alam, Usha Shrivastava, K. M. Venkat Narayan, and Tazeen H. Jafar. 2017. 'Diabetes, Cardiovascular Disease, and Chronic Kidney Disease in South Asia: Current Status and Future Directions', *BMJ* 357(April): j1420. doi:10.1136/bmj.j1420.

Modi, G.K., and V. Jha. 2006. 'The Incidence of End-Stage Renal Disease in India: A Population-Based Study', *Kidney International* 70(12): 2131–33. doi:10.1038/sj.ki.5001958.

Mukherjee, Debarati, S. Safraj, Mohammad Tayyab, Roopa Shivashankar, Shivani A. Patel, Gitanjali Narayanan, Vamadevan S. Ajay, et al. 2017. 'Park Availability and Major Depression in Individuals with Chronic Conditions: Is There an Association in Urban India?' *Health & Place* 47(September): 54–62. doi:10.1016/j.healthplace.2017.07.004.

Nair, Manisha, Mohammed K. Ali, Vamadevan S. Ajay, Roopa Shivashankar, Viswanathan Mohan, Rajendra Pradeepa, Mohan Deepa, et al. 2012. 'CARRS Surveillance Study: Design and Methods to Assess Burdens from Multiple Perspectives', *BMC Public Health* 12(1): 701. doi:10.1186/1471-2458-12-701.

Nyblade, Laura, Melissa Stockton, Sandra Travasso, and Suneeta Krishnan. 2017. 'A Qualitative Exploration of Cervical and Breast Cancer Stigma in Karnataka, India', *BMC Women's Health* 17(August). doi:10.1186/s12905-017-0407-x.

O'Donnell, Martin J., Denis Xavier, Lisheng Liu, Hongye Zhang, Siu Lim Chin, Purnima Rao-Melacini, Sumathy Rangarajan, et al. 2010. 'Risk Factors for Ischaemic and Intracerebral Haemorrhagic Stroke in 22 Countries (the INTERSTROKE Study): A Case-Control Study', *Lancet* 376(9735): 112–23. doi:10.1016/S0140-6736(10)60834-3.

Pan, A., M. Lucas, Q. Sun, R.M. van Dam, O.H. Franco, J.E. Manson, W.C. Willett, A. Ascherio, and F.B. Hu. 2010. 'Bidirectional Association between Depression and Type 2 Diabetes Mellitus in Women', *Arch Intern Med* 170(21): 1884–91. doi:10.1001/archinternmed.2010.356.

Pandian, Jeyaraj D., Velandai Srikanth, Stephen J. Read, and Amanda G. Thrift. 2007. 'Poverty and Stroke in India: A Time to Act', *Stroke* 38(11): 3063–69. doi:10.1161/STROKEAHA.107.496869.

Pandian, Jeyaraj Durai, and Paulin Sudhan. 2013. 'Stroke Epidemiology and Stroke Care Services in India', *Journal of Stroke* 15(3): 128–34. doi:10.5853/jos.2013.15.3.128.

Patel, Opal, Safraj Shahulhameed, Roopa Shivashankar, Mohammad Tayyab, Atiqur Rahman, Dorairaj Prabhakaran, Nikhil Tandon, and Lindsay M. Jaacks. 2017. 'Association between Full Service and Fast Food Restaurant Density, Dietary Intake and Overweight/Obesity among Adults in Delhi, India', *BMC Public Health* 18(July): 36. doi:10.1186/s12889-017-4598-8.

Patel, Shivani A., K.M. Venkat Narayan, and Solveig A. Cunningham. 2015. 'Unhealthy Weight among Children and Adults in India: Urbanicity and the Crossover in Underweight and Overweight', *Annals of*

Epidemiology, February. doi:10.1016/j.annepidem.2015.02.009.

Patel, Shivani A., Roopa Shivashankar, Mohammed K. Ali, R.M. Anjana, M. Deepa, Deksha Kapoor, Dimple Kondal, et al. 2016. 'Is the 'South Asian Phenotype' Unique to South Asians?' *Global Heart* 11(1): 89–96.e3. doi:10.1016/j.gheart.2015.12.010.

Patel, Vikram, Somnath Chatterji, Dan Chisholm, Shah Ebrahim, Gururaj Gopalakrishna, Colin Mathers, Viswanathan Mohan, Dorairaj Prabhakaran, Ravilla D Ravindran, and K Srinath Reddy. 2011. 'Chronic Diseases and Injuries in India', *The Lancet* 377(9763): 413–28. doi:10.1016/S0140-6736(10)61188-9.

Patel, Vikram, Shuiyuan Xiao, Hanhui Chen, Fahmy Hanna, A.T. Jotheeswaran, Dan Luo, Rachana Parikh, et al. 2016. 'The Magnitude of and Health System Responses to the Mental Health Treatment Gap in Adults in India and China', *The Lancet* 388(10063): 3074–84. doi:10.1016/S0140-6736(16)00160-4.

Pati, Sanghamitra, Sutapa Agrawal, Subhashisa Swain, John Tayu Lee, Sukumar Vellakkal, Mohammad Akhtar Hussain, and Christopher Millett. 2014. 'Non Communicable Disease Multimorbidity and Associated Health Care Utilization and Expenditures in India: Cross-Sectional Study', *BMC Health Services Research* 14(1). doi:10.1186/1472-6963-14-451.

Pati, Sanghamitra, Subhashisa Swain, Mohammad Akhtar Hussain, Shridhar Kadam, and Chris Salisbury. 2015. 'Prevalence, Correlates, and Outcomes of Multimorbidity Among Patients Attending Primary Care in Odisha, India', *The Annals of Family Medicine* 13(5): 446–50. doi:10.1370/afm.1843.

PopulationPyramid.Net. n.d. 'Population Pyramids of the World from 1950 to 2100'. https://www.populationpyramid.net/india/2016/, last accessed on 8 September 2017.

Prabhakaran, Dorairaj, Panniyammakal Jeemon, and Ambuj Roy. 2016. 'Cardiovascular Diseases in India', *Circulation* 133(16): 1605–20. doi:10.1161/CIRCULATIONAHA.114.008729.

Prince, Martin, Vikram Patel, Shekhar Saxena, Mario Maj, Joanna Maselko, Michael R. Phillips, and Atif Rahman. 2007. 'No Health without Mental Health', *The Lancet* 370(9590): 859–77. doi:10.1016/S0140-6736(07)61238-0.

Rajapurkar, Mohan M., George T. John, Ashok L. Kirpalani, Georgi Abraham, Sanjay K. Agarwal, Alan F. Almeida, Sishir Gang, et al. 2012. 'What Do We Know about Chronic Kidney Disease in India: First Report of the Indian CKD Registry', *BMC Nephrology* 13(March): 10. doi:10.1186/1471-2369-13-10.

Rajaraman, Preetha, Benjamin O. Anderson, Partha Basu, Jerome L. Belinson, Anil D'Cruz, Preet K. Dhillon, Prakash Gupta, et al. 2015. 'Recommendations for Screening and Early Detection of Common Cancers in India', *The Lancet Oncology* 16(7): e352–61. doi:10.1016/S1470-2045(15)00078-9.

Ramachandran, A., C. Snehalatha, A.D.S. Baskar, S. Mary, C.K. Sathish Kumar, S. Selvam, S. Catherine, and V. Vijay. 2004. 'Temporal Changes in Prevalence of Diabetes and Impaired Glucose Tolerance Associated with Lifestyle Transition Occurring in the Rural Population in India', *Diabetologia* 47(5): 860–65. doi:10.1007/s00125-004-1387-6.

Ramachandran, Ambady, Shobhana Ramachandran, Chamukuttan Snehalatha, Christina Augustine, Narayanasamy Murugesan, Vijay Viswanathan, Anil Kapur, and Rhys Williams. 2007. 'Increasing Expenditure on Health Care Incurred by Diabetic Subjects in a Developing Country: A Study from India', *Diabetes Care* 30(2): 252–56. doi:10.2337/dc06-0144.

Ranjit Unnikrishnan, I., R.M. Anjana, and V. Mohan. 2011. 'Importance of Controlling Diabetes Early--the Concept of Metabolic Memory, Legacy Effect and the Case for Early Insulinisation', *The Journal of the Association of Physicians of India* 59 Suppl(April): 8–12.

Reddy, D.V., and A. Gunasekar. 2013. 'Chronic Kidney Disease in Two Coastal Districts of Andhra Pradesh, India: Role of Drinking Water', *Environmental Geochemistry and Health* 35(4): 439–54. doi:10.1007/s10653-012-9506-7.

Rigby, H., G. Gubitz, and S. Phillips. 2009. 'A Systematic Review of Caregiver Burden Following Stroke', *International Journal of Stroke: Official Journal of the International Stroke Society* 4(4): 285–92. doi:10.1111/j.1747-4949.2009.00289.x.

Sachdev, Harshpal S., Caroline H.D. Fall, Clive Osmond, Ramakrishnan Lakshmy, Sushant K. Dey Biswas, Samantha D. Leary, Kolli Srinath Reddy, David J.P. Barker, and Santosh K. Bhargava. 2005. 'Anthropometric Indicators of Body Composition in Young Adults: Relation to Size at Birth and Serial Measurements of Body Mass Index in Childhood in the New Delhi Birth Cohort', *The American Journal of Clinical Nutrition* 82(2): 456–66.

Salvi, Sundeep, Komalkirti Apte, Sapna Madas, Monica Barne, Sushmeeta Chhowala, Tavpritesh Sethi, Kunal Aggarwal, Anurag Agrawal, and Jaideep Gogtay. 2015. 'Symptoms and Medical Conditions in 204 912 Patients Visiting Primary Health-Care Practitioners in India: A 1-Day Point Prevalence Study (the POSEIDON Study)', *The Lancet Global Health* 3(12): e776–e784.

Sandhu, Gurprataap S., Sebhat Erqou, Heidi Patterson, and Aju Mathew. 2016. 'Prevalence of Triple-Negative Breast Cancer in India: Systematic Review and Meta-Analysis', *Journal of Global Oncology* 2(6): 412–21. doi:10.1200/JGO.2016.005397.

Saxena, Anita, Sivasubramanian Ramakrishnan, Ambuj Roy, Sandeep Seth, Anand Krishnan, Puneet Misra, Mani Kalaivani, Balram Bhargava, Marcus D. Flather, and Philip P.A. Poole-Wilson. 2011. 'Prevalence and Outcome of Subclinical Rheumatic Heart Disease in India: The RHEUMATIC(Rheumatic Heart Echo Utilisation and Monitoring Actuarial Trends in Indian Children) Study', *Heart* 97(24): 2018–22. doi:10.1136/heartjnl-2011-300792.

Shivashankar, Roopa, Sandeep Bhalla, Dimple Kondal, Mohammed K. Ali, Dorairaj Prabhakaran, K.M. Venkat Narayan, and Nikhil Tandon. 2016. 'Adherence to Diabetes Care Processes at General Practices in the National Capital Region-Delhi, India', *Indian Journal of Endocrinology and Metabolism* 20(3): 329–36. doi:10.4103/2230-8210.180000.

Siegel, Karen R., Mohammed K. Ali, Adithi Srinivasiah, Rachel A. Nugent, and K.M. Venkat Narayan. 2014. 'Do We Produce Enough Fruits and Vegetables to Meet Global Health Need?' *PLOS ONE* 9(8): e104059. doi:10.1371/journal.pone.0104059.

Singh, Ajay K., Youssef M.K. Farag, Bharati V. Mittal, Kuyilan Karai Subramanian, Sai Ram Keithi Reddy, Vidya N. Acharya, Alan F. Almeida, et al. 2013. 'Epidemiology and Risk Factors of Chronic Kidney Disease in India – Results from the SEEK(Screening and Early Evaluation of Kidney Disease) Study', *BMC Nephrology* 14(May): 114. doi:10.1186/1471-2369-14-114.

Singh, Ram B., Jan Fedacko, Daniel Pella, Zelmira Macejova, Saraswati Ghosh, K. de Amit, Raheena Begom, et al. 2011. 'Prevalence and Risk Factors for Prehypertension and Hypertension in Five Indian Cities', *Acta Cardiologica* 66(1): 29–37. doi:10.2143/AC.66.1.2064964.

Sridharan, Sapna E., J.P. Unnikrishnan, Sajith Sukumaran, P.N. Sylaja, S. Dinesh Nayak, P. Sankara Sarma, and Kurupath Radhakrishnan. 2009. 'Incidence, Types, Risk Factors, and Outcome of Stroke in a Developing Country: The Trivandrum Stroke Registry', *Stroke; a Journal of Cerebral Circulation* 40(4): 1212–18. doi:10.1161/STROKEAHA.108.531293.

Staimez, L.R., M.B. Weber, H. Ranjani, M.K. Ali, J.B. Echouffo-Tcheugui, L.S. Phillips, V. Mohan, and K.M. Narayan. 2013. 'Evidence of Reduced Beta-Cell Function in Asian Indians with Mild Dysglycemia', *Diabetes Care* 36(9): 2772–78. doi:10.2337/dc12-2290.

Tillin, Therese, Alun D. Hughes, Jamil Mayet, Peter Whincup, Naveed Sattar, Nita G. Forouhi, Paul M. McKeigue, and Nish Chaturvedi. 2013. 'The Relationship Between Metabolic Risk Factors and Incident Cardiovascular Disease in Europeans, South Asians, and African CaribbeansSABRE(Southall and Brent Revisited)—A Prospective Population-Based Study', *Journal of the American College of Cardiology* 61(17): 1777–86. doi:10.1016/j.jacc.2012.12.046.

Trivedi, Hargovind, Aruna Vanikar, Himanshu Patel, Kamal Kanodia, Vivek Kute, Lovelesh Nigam, Kamlesh Suthar, Umang Thakkar, Harsh Sutariya, and Shruti Gandhi. 2016. 'High Prevalence of Chronic Kidney Disease in a Semi-Urban Population of Western India', *Clinical Kidney Journal* 9(3): 438–43. doi:10.1093/ckj/sfw009.

Tuomilehto, J., N. Li, G. Dowse, H. Gareeboo, P. Chitson, D. Fareed, Z. Min, K.G.M.M. Alberti, and P. Zimmet. 1993. 'The Prevalence of Coronary Heart Disease in the Multiethnic and High Diabetes Prevalence Population of Mauritius', *Journal of Internal Medicine* 233(2): 187–94. doi:10.1111/j.1365-2796.1993.tb00672.x.

United Nations. 2011. 'Political Declaration of the High-Level Meeting of the General Assembly on the Prevention and Control of Non-Communicable Diseases'. Available at http://www.who.int.proxy.library.emory.edu/nmh/events/un_ncd_summit2011/political_declaration_en.pdf, last accessed on 31 August 2017.

Unnikrishnan, Ranjit, Ranjit Mohan Anjana, and Viswanathan Mohan. 2014. 'Diabetes in South Asians: Is the Phenotype Different?' *Diabetes* 63(1): 53–55. doi:10.2337/db13-1592.

Varma, P.P. 2015. 'Prevalence of Chronic Kidney Disease in India - Where Are We Heading?' *Indian Journal of Nephrology* 25(3): 133–5.

Vogelmeier, Claus F., Gerard J. Criner, Fernando J. Martinez, Antonio Anzueto, Peter J. Barnes, Jean Bourbeau, Bartolome R. Celli, et al. 2017. 'Global Strategy for the Diagnosis, Management, and Prevention of Chronic Obstructive Lung Disease 2017 Report. GOLD Executive Summary', *American Journal of Respiratory and Critical Care Medicine* 195(5): 557–82. doi:10.1164/rccm.201701-0218PP.

Vos, Theo, Ryan M. Barber, Brad Bell, Amelia Bertozzi-Villa, Stan Biryukov, Ian Bolliger, Fiona Charlson, et al. 2015. 'Global, Regional, and National Incidence, Prevalence, and Years Lived with Disability for 301 Acute and Chronic Diseases and Injuries in 188 Countries, 1990–2013: A Systematic Analysis for the Global Burden of Disease Study 2013', *The Lancet* 386(9995): 743–800. doi:10.1016/S0140-6736(15)60692-4.

Wadhwa, Pathik D., Claudia Buss, Sonja Entringer, and James M. Swanson. 2009. 'Developmental Origins of Health and Disease: Brief History of the Approach and Current Focus on Epigenetic Mechanisms', *Seminars in Reproductive Medicine* 27(5): 358–68. doi:10.1055/s-0029-1237424.

Wasay, Mohammad, Ismail A. Khatri, and Subhash Kaul. 2014. 'Stroke in South Asian Countries', *Nature Reviews. Neurology* 10(3): 135–43. doi:10.1038/nrneurol.2014.13.

Watkins, David A., Catherine O. Johnson, Samantha M. Colquhoun, Ganesan Karthikeyan, Andrea Beaton, Gene Bukhman, Mohammed H. Forouzanfar, et al.

2017. 'Global, Regional, and National Burden of Rheumatic Heart Disease, 1990–2015', *New England Journal of Medicine* 377(8): 713–22. doi:10.1056/NEJMoa1603693.

Weber, Mary Beth, Harish Ranjani, Lisa R. Staimez, Ranjit M. Anjana, Mohammed K. Ali, K.M. Venkat Narayan, and Viswanathan Mohan. 2016. 'The Stepwise Approach to Diabetes Prevention: Results From the D-CLIP Randomized Controlled Trial', *Diabetes Care* 39(10): 1760–67. doi:10.2337/dc16-1241.

Xavier, Denis, Prem Pais, P.J. Devereaux, Changchun Xie, D. Prabhakaran, K. Srinath Reddy, Rajeev Gupta, et al. 2008. 'Treatment and Outcomes of Acute Coronary Syndromes in India(CREATE): A Prospective Analysis of Registry Data', *The Lancet* 371(9622): 1435–42. doi:10.1016/S0140-6736(08)60623-6.

Yajnik, C.S. 2002. 'The Lifecycle Effects of Nutrition and Body Size on Adult Adiposity, Diabetes and Cardiovascular Disease', *Obesity Reviews* 3(3): 217–24. doi:10.1046/j.1467-789X.2002.00072.x.

———. 2004. 'Obesity Epidemic in India: Intrauterine Origins?' *Proceedings of the Nutrition Society* 63(03): 387–396. doi:10.1079/PNS2004365.

Yusuf, Salim, Sumathy Rangarajan, Koon Teo, Shofiqul Islam, Wei Li, Lisheng Liu, Jian Bo, et al. 2014. 'Cardiovascular Risk and Events in 17 Low-, Middle-, and High-Income Countries', *New England Journal of Medicine* 371(9): 818–27. doi:10.1056/NEJMoa1311890.

7

Unjust Social Differences

Health Inequalities in India

*Aditi Iyer and Gita Sen**

DRIVERS OF HEALTH INEQUALITY

Among the most powerful social determinants of health in different countries and contexts is inequality (CSDH 2008). Economic and social inequality not only affect the health of different subgroups in a population differently, but also drag down the averages for the country as a whole. Wilkinson and Pickett (2010) have argued persuasively that average income has much less effect on a country's social indicators than the extent of inequality. For each of a group of 21 high income countries, the composite index of a set of social indicators[1] including health was strongly correlated with the extent of income inequality in each country, but not with its level of per capita income. That is, the greater the income inequality, the worse the performance on health and other components. In reverse it can be shown, as we argue in the chapter, that health inequality itself works through multiple pathways to worsen people's economic and social status and overall well-being.

Health-related inequality manifests in three broad ways:

1. As health *outcomes* that range from differentials in health insults such as undernutrition within the womb and neonatal and infant mortality, through the burdens of specific diseases, injuries and violence, to death rates and life expectancy;
2. At the overall level of social and economic determinants that shape *vulnerability and exposure* to ill health through such factors as whether people live and work in safe, sanitary, and healthy conditions, whether they consume nutritious food, whether they get enough rest and leisure, whether their lives are free of discrimination and violence; and
3. In the form of inequality in *accessing and affording* appropriate preventive, promotive, curative, and restorative healthcare and services of decent quality.

Data availability for these three dimensions is uneven, and the data is fragmentary. For some health conditions, evidence is available for all three dimensions, while for

* We are grateful to our colleague, Baneen Karachiwala for her cheerful and efficient research assistance.

[1] The index is a composite of a set of health indicators (such as life expectancy, infant mortality, mental illness, teen pregnancy, and obesity) and other social indicators (such as literacy and mathematics proficiency, imprisonment, and homicides).

others the evidence is more limited. We have therefore integrated the data as best we could in the discussion in the next sections of the chapter. Some aspects of the three dimensions are also discussed in other parts of this chapter.

In addition to economic and social inequality, an important driver of health inequality is inadequate public spending on health. It is widely recognized that adequate public spending is essential to ensure that out-of-pocket expenses on health remain within control and don't become catastrophic, especially for poorer households that tend to be hit hardest by such expenses (World Bank 2018). In India, out-of-pocket expenses are between 60 and 70 per cent of total health expenditures and are responsible for large numbers falling below the poverty line each year (Karan et al. 2014).

Another key driver of health inequality is poorly regulated privatization of health services and medical education. A surge in privatization since the mid-1980s and the early 1990s has provided incentives to private corporate hospitals with little accountability, transferred government-run health facilities to registered trusts that are not very different from profit-making entities, and opened medical education to private players, eroding the incentives for doctors to work in poor and rural areas (Rao 2017; Sen and Iyer 2015). This has strengthened interests working against equitable access.

INDIA'S HEALTH INEQUALITY IN CONTEXT

It is no secret that, in comparison to a number of neighbours, India has underperformed significantly on the health front despite some notable achievements. Tables 7.1, 7.2 and 7.3 present India's performance on a set of key variables in the context of South Asian neighbours, Thailand,[2] China, and Japan. Annex 1 has the detailed definitions for the indicators in the three tables.

Table 7.1 compares basic health data for 2016 from the World Health Statistics for these countries (WHO

[2] An Asian country that is widely believed to have made significant progress towards universal health coverage (Tangcharoensathien et al. 2018).

Table 7.1 Indicators of India's health

Statistics for year 2015	India	Bangladesh	Pakistan	Sri Lanka	Thailand	China	Japan	India's Rank*
Life expectancy at birth: male (years)	66.9	70.6	65.5	71.6	71.9	74.6	**80.5**	6
Life expectancy at birth: female (years)	69.9	73.1	67.5	78.3	78.0	77.6	**86.8**	6
Healthy life expectancy at birth (years)	59.5	62.3	57.8	67.0	66.8	68.5	**74.9**	6
Maternal Mortality Ratio (per 100,000 live births)	174.0	176.0	178.0	30.0	20.0	27.0	**5.0**	5
Skilled births (%)	74.0	42.0	52.0	99.0	**100.0**	**100.0**	**100.0**	5
Under-five mortality rate (per 1,000 live births)	47.7	37.6	81.1	9.8	5.5	10.7	**2.7**	6
Neonatal mortality rate (per 1,000 live births)	27.7	23.3	45.5	5.4	3.5	5.5	**0.9**	6
Modern family planning (%)	63.9	72.5	47.0	69.4	**89.2**	NA	NA	4
Adolescent birth rate (per 1,000 women aged 15–19 years)	28.1	113.0	44.0	20.3	60.0	6.2	**4.4**	4
Stunting in children under 5 years (%)	38.7	36.1	45.0	14.7	16.3	9.4	**7.1**	6
Wasting in children under 5 years (%)	15.1	14.3	10.5	21.4	6.7	**2.3**	**2.3**	6
Overweight children under 5 years (%)	1.9	1.4	4.8	**0.6**	10.9	6.6	1.5	4
**Average of 13 International Health Regulations core capacity scores	94.0	88.0	43.0	71.0	98.0	99.0	**100.0**	4

* Rank 1 represents the best performance; the countries with the best performance have the values shown in bold.

** The 13 International Health Regulations core capacities include: Legislation, Coordination, Surveillance, Response, Preparedness, Risk Communication, Human Resources, Laboratory, Points of entry, Zoonosis, Food Safety, Chemical and Radionuclear. Country values are the average of 13 core capacity scores (%).

Source: WHO (2016).

2016). Although India ranks at the middle for core capacity on a set of 13 important health regulations, it is near the bottom on almost all other health indicators. Sri Lanka is the well-known outlier among the larger South Asian countries, performing significantly better on most. Thailand, China, and Japan, despite very different per capita income levels, are clustered together and are considerably better than the others, barring Sri Lanka.

How much of this differential health performance reflects socioeconomic inequality? Table 7.2 provides some clues based on the *Human Development Report, 2016*, which focused on inequality (UNDP 2016).

The Human Development Index (HDI), a composite of average income, health, and education, again clusters India, Bangladesh, and Pakistan at the low end (with country ranks above 130), with Sri Lanka, Thailand, and China significantly better, and Japan as is to be expected near the top of the global country ranks and performance. What is striking is that, when adjusted for inequality in the different components of the HDI, India loses more than a quarter of the value of its HDI, with Bangladesh and Pakistan faring a little worse. By contrast, HDI lowering on account of inequality is much less in Sri Lanka, Japan, and Thailand. The Gender Inequality Index shows how important gender inequality is for the poor performance of the South Asian countries barring Sri Lanka, and how closely it correlates with the inequality-adjusted HDI itself.

Table 7.3 uses the Multidimensional Poverty Index (MPI) to show how much health, education, and living standards contribute to poverty (UNDP 2016). Although the data are less uniformly available, health contributes almost one third to the MPI in India, significantly more than education.

Tables 7.1 to 7.3 provide a cross-country snapshot of the relationship between inequality, multidimensional poverty, and human development. They suggest that socioeconomic inequality is linked to poor performance in health and human development overall. The implications for India are concerning, since there is growing evidence that inequality has been increasing significantly in recent years. According to the Credit Suisse Research Institute's *Global Wealth Report 2016* (2016), the richest 1 per cent own 53 per cent of the country's wealth, the richest 5 per cent own 68.6 per cent, and the top 10 per cent have 76.3 per cent. The bottom 50 per cent of the population own 4.1 per cent of national wealth. This makes India one of the most unequal countries in the world today.

But inequality is not only a matter of the distribution of household income and wealth. Economic inequality

Table 7.2 India's Human Development

Statistics for the year 2015	India	Bangladesh	Pakistan	Sri Lanka	Thailand	China	Japan
Human Development Index	0.624	0.579	0.550	0.766	0.740	0.738	0.903
Rank*	131	139	147	73	87	90	17
Inequality Adjusted HDI	0.454	0.412	0.380	0.678	0.586	NA	0.791
Percentage (%) loss in HDI	27.2	28.9	30.9	11.6	20.8	NA	12.4
Gender Inequality Index	0.530	0.520	0.546	0.386	0.366	0.164	0.116
Rank*	125	119	130	87	79	37	21

* Rank 1 represents the best performance. This is based on data for 188 countries.
Source: UNDP (2016).

Table 7.3 Multi-Dimensional Poverty Index Statistics

Statistics	India	Bangladesh	Pakistan	Sri Lanka	Thailand	China	Japan
Applicable year	2005–6	2014	2012–13	NA	2005–6	2012	NA
Multi-dimensional poverty index	0.282	0.188	0.237	NA	0.004	0.023	NA
% contribution of education to MPI	22.7	28.4	36.2	NA	19.4	30.0	NA
% contribution of health to MPI	32.5	26.1	32.3	NA	51.3	36.6	NA
% contribution of living standards to MPI	44.8	45.5	31.6	NA	29.4	33.4	NA

Source: UNDP 2016.

is crosscut by long-standing social inequalities of gender, caste, and religion, to name a few of the most dominant sources of inequality. For example, compared to Hindus, poverty tends to be significantly higher among Muslims, especially those belonging to Other Backward Classes (OBC) (Government of India 2006).

Inequality in health status and outcomes, in access to services and affordability, and in exposures and vulnerability to ill health are deeply influenced by these intersecting economic and social forces (Iyer et al. 2007, 2010). The deep poverty (Sen and Iyer 2019) that besets those at the bottom of the multidimensional socioeconomic pyramid differentiates them in huge ways from those nearer the upper end when it comes to health inequality, as we show next. Although we experience good or poor health as individuals, this is not randomly distributed. Many of the causes and consequences of health status and outcomes are clustered in socioeconomic groups, with some groups more likely to suffer ill health while others are better off. In this chapter, we focus on health outcomes that are largely socially created and, therefore, are more amenable to policy solutions and public action.

DIMENSIONS OF HEALTH INEQUALITY

India's health can be judged by its life expectancy, mortality, morbidity, and nutritional status, and the distribution of these outcomes in the population. With death rates falling and life expectancy at birth rising from 59 years in 1990 to 68.5 years in 2016 (ISDBIC 2017), India's health can be said to be improving. Yet, mortality rates are uneven across regions and the socioeconomic divide (Po and Subramanian 2011). The levels and types of morbidity, and of undernutrition, are also differentiated by geography, gender, class, caste, and minority status.[3]

These inequalities contribute to an unevenly paced epidemiological transition.[4] By 2010, all states within India had entered stage three of the transition with non-communicable diseases becoming major contributors to the disease burden (ISDBIC 2017). States such as Kerala, Tamil Nadu, Goa, Punjab, and Himachal Pradesh are said to have made the transition in 1986, 24 years before Assam, Meghalaya, and all EAG states[5] (other than Uttarakhand) could get there.

Biological factors, socioeconomic power relations and geography interact to produce inequalities in health outcomes. In this section, we map these inequalities in the prevalence of deaths, ailments, and undernutrition from some key pieces of evidence.

One challenge is that much of the available evidence considers gender, economic class, caste, and minority status as separable axes of inequality, with little (if any) recognition of their intersections. But do these different inequalities work in synergy or against each other? We cannot really say on the basis of existing evidence. The result is that we do not know, for example, whether the burdens of economic disadvantage are equally shared across gender divides. We have limited evidence on whether and when gender, caste, or minority status become more important drivers of health inequity than economic class.[6] Questions such as these have implications for the design of policies and the effectiveness of programmes that aim to improve health outcomes (Sen and Iyer 2019).

UNFAIR DEATH

The fact that death rates overall in the country have been moving along a downward trajectory over time is well known.[7] Despite this, deaths that result from socioeconomic inequality—deprivation, discrimination, social exclusion, inaccessible/inappropriate/adversarial care—persist. In this section, we focus on deaths of children under the ages of one (infancy) and five (early childhood); deaths of childbearing women; and suicides,[8] many of which stem from inequality and injustice.

[3] Our discussion of minority status-based inequalities in health will be restricted to religious minorities, even though other bases for minority status (for example, alternative sexualities) are important.

[4] The epidemiological transition encapsulating the interaction between birth rates, death rates, medical innovations and development typically evolves from an age of 'pestilence and famine' characterized by high birth and death rates and low life expectancy, to the age of 'degenerative diseases' coinciding with declining mortality and fertility rates in ageing populations (Omran 1971).

[5] The empowered action group (EAG) states include Bihar, Jharkhand, Uttar Pradesh, Uttarakhand, Madhya Pradesh, Chhattisgarh, Rajasthan, and Odisha.

[6] Some relatively recent work has made advances on this front (Sen and Iyer 2012).

[7] The age-standardized death rates for the country fell from 1,653 per 100,000 population in 1990 to 1,139 in 2016 (ISDBIC 2017).

[8] Due to space constraints, we exclude from the discussion deaths occurring in situations of conflict.

Infant and Child Mortality

Deaths of children during infancy and early childhood have fallen sharply over time, albeit at different rates. Between 2000 and 2015, mortality among children aged 1–59 months fell at an average annual rate of 5.4 per cent, compared to 3.3 per cent among neonates (aged 0–1 month)[9] (Million Death Study Collaborators 2017). The relative obduracy of neonatal mortality stems from the intergenerational transfer of vulnerability: the phenomenon of full-term low birth weight babies[10] born to women who are undernourished and/or anaemic (James 2014; Million Death Study Collaborators 2017).

Infants of poor and economically weaker Indian homes are more vulnerable to untimely mortality than their more privileged counterparts (Jain et al. 2013; Subramanian et al. 2006). The extent of inequality in infant mortality across economic classes appears to have narrowed through the 1990s until the mid-2000s (1992–3, 1998–9, and 2005–6), but national estimates mask significant regional variations (Jain et al. 2013). While such inequality fell in the southern Indian states, which also had the lowest mortality rates; it actually rose in the northern Indian states, which had the highest mortality rates, and remained consistently high in the western Indian states (Jain et al. 2013).

Social inequality is also implicated in infant mortality. Mortality rates did not significantly differ between boys and girls in the late 1990s (Subramanian et al. 2006). Other data show small gender gaps against girls over the years (RGI, various years). Yet, these seemingly absent or small gender gaps point to the presence of significant gender bias against girls. Girls are endowed by nature with a significant biological advantage over boys, and normally ought to survive much better than infant boys. In addition to gender, being higher up the birth order or born within two years of a previous birth to a poorly educated mother are other factors that have made infants significantly more vulnerable to mortality (Jain et al. 2013).

Socioeconomic biases become even stronger during early childhood (13–59 months). Children who are disadvantaged or discriminated against (girls, scheduled tribes, children in poor and economically weaker households, children from mistimed or unwanted pregnancies) are significantly more likely to die than better-off children (Jain et al. 2013; Joe et al. 2010; Subramanian et al. 2006). Economic inequality, which widened between the 1990s (1992–3) and mid-2000s especially in south India, was a major contributor to inequality in child mortality (Chalasani 2012; Jain et al. 2013).[11]

Intra-household inequities in feeding, nurturing, and healthcare (including immunization) are also likely to contribute to socioeconomic inequalities in childhood mortality. Studies (Borooah 2004; Joe et al. 2010; Prusty and Kumar 2014; Singh 2012) have found significant inequalities in the uptake of the full immunization schedule: girls, the poor, and Muslims were less likely to be fully immunized, especially when their mothers were uneducated. Girls were also less likely to be fed nutritious food (Borooah 2004) or to receive treatment when sick with acute respiratory infection and diarrhoea (Singh and Patel 2017), especially when they were higher in the birth order and had no male siblings.

In addition to the inter-group and intra-household inequalities discussed so far, state boundaries and the rural–urban divide are conventional axes along which geographical inequalities are mapped. Yet, contiguous geographical regions cutting across state borders that share common developmental histories, ecologies, and cultures can have similar health outcomes. Singh et al. (2011) found stark intra-state and inter-regional disparities in infant and child mortality over the past two decades. Geographic regions across state boundaries that were underprivileged in terms of child nutrition, female literacy or wealth were also likely to be disadvantaged in terms of infant and child survival.

Maternal Mortality

Fertility rates in India have dropped by nearly 40 per cent over 35 years (1990–2015).[12] With women having fewer children, the risk of their succumbing to health problems that are caused or exacerbated by pregnancy and/or its management has reduced substantially. The maternal mortality ratio (MMR) fell from 556 per

[9] Most neonatal deaths tend to occur during the first week of life.

[10] Neonatal mortality rates linked to low birth weight rose from 12.3 per cent in 2000 to 14.3 per cent in 2015, especially in poorer states and in rural areas, whereas the rates linked to infections, birth asphyxia or trauma and tetanus fell substantially (Million Death Study Collaborators 2017).

[11] Since these studies treated economic and social inequality (gender, caste) as independent, rather than intersecting variables, we do not know what happened to the gender gap over time.

[12] The TFR was 2.3 in 2015 (ORGCCI 2016), down from 3.8 in 1990 (ORGI 2018).

100,000 live births in 1990 to 174 in 2015 (WHO et al. 2015). However, inter- and intra-state variations are enormous. According to 2014–16 estimates, MMR was much higher in the EAG states and Assam than in the south (188 versus 77) (ORGI 2018). The southern state with the highest MMR (Karnataka at 108) was much better off than the EAG state with the lowest MMR (undivided Bihar at 165).

These regional variations in MMR reflect differing childbearing trajectories of disempowered women from families that cannot be certain of child survival. In 2015, total fertility rates (TFRs) in the EAG states plus Assam ranged from 2.0 (Odisha) to 3.2 (Bihar), while the rates in the south were no more than 1.8 (ORGCCI 2016). These lowered fertility rates do not, however, tell the full story of pregnancy since they do not tell us about the extent of pregnancy wastage due to miscarriages or perinatal mortality. Indian data is weak in this regard, but evidence from Egypt (also a middle-income country) provides a few pointers. In a study of three teaching hospitals, Serour et al. (1981) found high rates of miscarriages among poor, anaemic and high parity women. It is plausible that similar rates may be found in India. This means that the toll that pregnancy takes on poor women's health may be higher than what may be predicted by fertility rates. With multiple pregnancies making women vulnerable, especially when they are already undernourished,[13] access to clinical care and services that assure maternal survival and health become critical.

Socioeconomic inequities, health system constraints, and geographical remoteness interact with policy decisions to determine the dynamics and consequence of care seeking, especially during obstetric emergencies. Even before the introduction of the National Rural Health Mission (NRHM)[14] in 2005, institutional intra-partum care was becoming increasingly popular in better-off states and districts, albeit in an unequal way. In a better-off district of south India, for instance, such care was more likely among the upper castes and non-poor (Adamson et al. 2012). For rural women in poorly developed regions of the country, institutional births were relatively uncommon, and their quality poor even when women sought help. The ability of women in a rural block of Uttar Pradesh to recognize and secure medical attention for excessive intra-/postpartum bleeding was low *regardless* of their socioeconomic and caste status (Sibley et al. 2005). Lack of acknowledgement of and accountability towards their need for care (George et al. 2005) could lead to women being denied services, shunted from one health institution to another, and being poorly treated during obstetric emergencies. This situation could be made much worse for poorer women due to financial barriers (Iyengar et al. 2009).

Since the NRHM, access to antenatal care and institutional deliveries have become less unequal across wealth and educational divides (Vellakkal et al. 2017). The incentives for health workers to take such work seriously are clearly in place.[15] However, limits to the readiness of health centres, the competence of healthcare providers, the quality of interpersonal communication, and of obstetric practices serve as major barriers to maternal safety. Health system weaknesses such as these are particularly burdensome for poor and disadvantaged women as shown by independent verbal autopsy investigations of maternal deaths in poor, semi-feudal, and gender-adverse regions across the country. Many actions can put women in harm's way. Inadequately recognized antenatal risks and intra-partum emergencies, harmful obstetric practices and/or brutal interpersonal care precipitating obstetric emergencies, and risk averse referrals, especially in the face of imminent death, are a few examples (Banerjee et al. 2013; Chattopadhyay et al. 2017; Iyer et al. 2012, 2013; Jithesh and Ravindran 2015; Subha Sri and Khanna 2014; Subha Sri et al. 2012). In the face of such evidence, some researchers have questioned whether and how much institutional deliveries have actually contributed to the observed reduction in maternal mortality (Ranadive et al. 2013).

Suicides

Suicides hold up a mirror to societal harshness in its inability to recognize and address the extreme distress that pushes individuals over the brink. Unjust social

[13] In 2015–16, 50.3 per cent of all pregnant women and 54 per cent of adolescent girls aged 15–19, who are often pushed into early marriages in disadvantaged regions, were anaemic (IIPS & ICF 2017).

[14] The NRHM actively promoted institutional deliveries via village health workers, a free ambulance service, conditional cash transfers and the opening of 24/7 primary and community health centres.

[15] Primary care facilities are assessed by their institutional delivery performance; the ASHAs (Accredited Social Health Activists) were paid by the number of women who received antenatal services and intra-partum care.

institutions and relationships form the bases for suicides. A study by Patel et al. (2012) recorded a geographical distribution that runs counter to the usual expectation that the southern regions of the country will be better off. Suicide rates were not higher in the EAG states but in the south, where human development indicators are significantly better than in many other parts of the country. We do not know how much of this may be due to differential reporting or recording. Questions about the role of gender and caste-based power relations may be important but have not been systematically studied thus far.

The study by Patel et al. (2012) systematically considers age-related differences and reports sex differences although it does not grapple sufficiently with questions about gender power. Even so, the study provides glimpses of findings that merit greater investigation. For instance, it found that suicide rates among women were clustered in the 15–29 age group (56 per cent of all suicides; 15 per cent of all deaths in the age group), a period corresponding to major milestones in the gender–power continuum. This is the period when girls find their already limited decision-making power and autonomy drastically curtailed. They are likely to be married, often while still in their teens, have to give up on educational attainment and employment aspirations, enter into involuntary marital relationships, early childbearing and increased burdens of unpaid work, and reduced leisure. Interestingly, the study also found that separated, divorced or widowed women were 1.5 times less likely to commit suicide relative to those who were married, a sad indicator of the pernicious nature of gender power within matrimony.

MORBIDITY: SOCIALLY PRODUCED, UNEQUALLY EXPERIENCED

Illnesses affect bodily functions, but are not purely biological events. Social forces play a role in shaping the way they emerge and are experienced by individuals and their caregivers. Depending on its severity and duration, an illness requiring resources, caregiving functions, and realigned work arrangements can be catastrophic for families.

In the past, communicable diseases like tuberculosis or leprosy were often the cause for such disruption. More recently, non-communicable diseases (NCDs) such as cerebrovascular and ischaemic heart disease with attendant risk factors (diabetes, hypertension, high cholesterol, and high body mass index [BMI]) have begun to test the resilience of families in ways that communicable diseases do not. NCDs have overtaken communicable diseases in terms of their relative contributions to deaths (61.8 per cent in 2016) and DALY lost (55.4 per cent in 2016) (ISDBIC 2017). These chronic ailments need to be managed lifelong with a combination of lifestyle changes and treatment that hinges critically on the ability to obtain and pay for healthcare.

NCDs emerge from a toxic interaction between biological and social and/or environmental factors, that is, nutrition/diet (WCRFI and The NCD Alliance 2014, WHO 2002), the stresses of daily living, lifestyle choices, and the physical and social environment with its share of environmental chemicals in the air, food, and water (Norman et al. 2013, WHO 2017). Differential exposure to these determining factors across the socio-economic spectrum gives rise to inequalities. Vineis et al. (2014) hypothesize that factors such as social adversity, diet, lack of physical activity, and pollution get 'embedded' in human biology through the epigenetic route, which make individuals susceptible to NCDs over time and across generations.

Studies indicate that although the incidence of NCDs has been growing among poor people, CVD and its risks are more prevalent among the rich than the poor (Subramanian et al. 2013). Risk factors such as hypertension increase with increasing BMI (Moser et al. 2014) and tend to be significantly more prevalent among the rich (Arokiasamy et al. 2016). In high-income countries, CVD was initially more prevalent among the rich before it became a disease of the poor. This crossover does not appear to have taken place in India. This may partly be a counting problem, since CVD can be undiagnosed and/or under-reported by the poor (Vellakkal et al. 2013). However, as Subramanian and others (2013) argue, it may also stem from the ironic fact that the undernourished poor in India continue to experience food insecurity and are, consequently, not highly at risk of developing diabetes or hypertension due to sudden increases in dietary intakes. Changing preferences for and access to calorific food offered by a globalized market may particularly affect those who are enough above the poverty line to be able to afford such food, but who have not yet graduated towards healthier foods. Such groups carry histories of undernutrition in their epigenetic makeup, making them more vulnerable to diabetes, obesity, elevated lipids, and hypertension. Hypertension was also found to be higher among women than men, especially if they were pushed into seclusion or had low decision-making power (Stroope 2015).

Apart from CVD, mental (ill)health is another by-product of the social transformations occurring in the country but is poorly recognized or counted. Depression is the most common problem due to mental, neurological, and substance use disorders accounting for 37 per cent (11·5 million DALYs) in 2013 in the country. The burden of depression rose by 67 per cent between 1990 and 2013 (WHO 2017). People with depression are 50 per cent more likely to die and have significantly higher risks of suicide (WHO 2017). A higher prevalence of depression for females across all age groups, among working age adults, among the elderly, and among those living in urban metros with causes including loneliness, terminal illness, and lack of autonomy among others, has been noted (WHO 2017). According to the National Mental Health Survey (2015–16) (NIMHANS 2016) depression was strongly associated with household income with the poorest quintile having almost double the prevalence of the richest.

Intimate partner violence, sexual assaults, and abuse in response to perceived threats to the system of unequal gender power relations have enormous mental health implications, including for depression. A study conducted in six states of India found that experiences of family violence and restrictions to independence made mental health problems more likely for both young men and women, but the latter also suffered from gender discriminatory practices (Ram et al. 2014). Young men belonging to a scheduled tribe (ST) or to poorer households were more likely to have mental health problems compared to their more privileged counterparts.

Chronic illnesses necessitate access to appropriate and affordable healthcare services. However, the care available for mental health problems can be thin on the ground in disadvantaged rural areas. Further, seeking outpatient care and buying drugs for chronic ailments can be impoverishing, even in major cities (Bhojani et al. 2012), since outpatient care is not covered by health insurance schemes but is financially burdensome (Berman et al. 2010, Shahrawat and Rao 2012).

The policy response to the problem of catastrophic out-of-pocket payments has taken the form of publicly-funded health insurance schemes for inpatient care for poor families. However, these schemes are not adequately set up to address the question of equity. Hamlets inhabited by the poor and lower castes, as well as remote regions inhabited by tribals and other disadvantaged groups tend to be poorly covered (Borooah et al. 2015; Rathi et al. 2012). Further, families without below poverty line (BPL) cards; those that have lost the 'household head' whose name appears on the government's list;[16] and migrants who cannot present themselves during enrolment drives (Jain 2013) also tend to get excluded. Within large households, the politics of leveraging (Sen and Iyer 2012) may also result in the exclusion of devalued members (Sen and Iyer 2019). Additionally, spiralling healthcare costs due to uncapped pricing of drugs, diagnostics, and treatment means that impoverishment can and does occur even if households are protected by health insurance (Fan et al. 2012; Selvaraj and Karan 2012).

CHILDHOOD UNDERNUTRITION: EMBODIED INEQUALITY

Wasting[17] (or low weight for height), stunting[18] (or low height for age) and anaemia are important dimensions of child health. In 2015–16, 21 per cent of the Indian population under the age of five were wasted and 38 per cent stunted (IIPS and ICF 2017). Around 31 per cent of the population aged 6–59 months were moderate-to-severely anaemic (IIPS and ICF 2017). These outcomes affect the cognitive development and well-being of children, their susceptibility to debilitating illness or death and ultimately results in reduced human capital during adulthood.

Wasting

Acute undernutrition, either due to insufficient intake of food or the presence of recurring infections, results in children being excessively underweight relative to their height. This phenomenon of wasting in a food surplus economy reveals the ill-effects of socioeconomic inequality. Its decadal rise from 19.8 per cent in 2005–6

[16] This list is based on population-based surveys of BPL households conducted by state governments across India in 2002. Each BPL family is identified by the member designated as the household's head (Ram et al. 2009). Households excluded in this way will also include female-headed households whose former male head may have either died recently or abandoned the household.

[17] A child is deemed to be wasted if his/her weight relative to height is two standard deviations lower than the median weight in the reference populations used to develop WHO's Child Growth Standards (WHO 2006).

[18] A child is deemed to be stunted if his/her height relative to age is two standard deviations lower than the median height in the reference populations used to develop WHO's Child Growth Standards (WHO 2006).

(IIPS and Macro International 2007) to 21 per cent (IIPS and ICF 2017) with even higher prevalence in states such as Jharkhand (at 29 per cent) and Chhattisgarh (at 25.8 per cent) point to the need for sustained action against the factors that drive acute undernutrition.

Two of the contributors to undernutrition, which are widely recognized, are oral: the *availability* of nutritious food and a child's *access* to it. These two factors are unequally experienced by children, depending on the amount of food their families are able to obtain, and the manner in which it gets distributed among different members. Dalit (scheduled caste; or SC) and adivasi (ST) children are more likely to be wasted than children from more privileged castes (Thorat and Sadana 2009). A study that decomposed the pan-India gap in average weight-for-height scores between the urban poor and non-poor also found that caste-based disadvantage was an important contributor, along with poor education and low BMI among mothers (Kumar and Singh 2013).

Three other factors—absorption, antibodies, and allopathogens which are linked to open defecation and faecally-transmitted infections (Chambers and von Medeazza 2014)—contribute to an inability to benefit from nutritious food, even if it were to become available and accessible to a child. These factors are more likely to affect the poor.

Stunting

Stunting reveals chronic undernutrition, the result of inadequate nutrition and of adverse environmental conditions and infections, both in vitro and for extended periods after birth. The prevalence of stunting in the under-5 population in the country was high in 2015–16 despite a reduction of 10 percentage points from 48 per cent in 2005–6 (IIPS and Macro International 2007). Regional variations in 2015–16 were wide: for instance, Bihar had more than twice the rate of Kerala (48.3 per cent versus 19.7 per cent) (IIPS and ICF 2017).

Studies show that Dalit and adivasi children are more likely to be stunted than their more privileged counterparts (Subramanyam et al. 2010; Thorat and Sadana 2009; van der Poel and Speybroeck 2009). However, caste interacts with and operates through other drivers of inequality. Its independent effect on the probability of stunting diminished after household wealth and maternal education had been accounted for (Subramanyam et al. 2010). Another study using NFHS-2 data (pertaining to 1998–9) found that the gap in stunting between SCs, STs and other castes was primarily due to differences in their levels of income, uptake of education, and of services (van der Poel and Speybroeck 2009).

Between 1992 and 2006, while the absolute levels of stunting among children under three fell steadily in India, economic disparities among them grew stronger, as improvements were more quickly achieved by the rich, especially in urban areas (Chalasani 2012; Subramanyam et al. 2010). Gender bias operated not at the level of children, but among their mothers. Maternal education was an important driver of inequality, even if it was less powerful than household wealth (Subramanyam et al. 2010).

Women who are stunted because of nutritional deprivation during childhood and adolescence are likely to give birth to stunted and underweight children, who are at greater risk of dying during childhood (Subramanian et al. 2009). Analysis of all-India data revealed that five out of 15 factors accounted for two-thirds (67.2 per cent) of the total population attributable risk of stunting in 2005–6 (Corsi et al. 2016). Three of these were linked to the deprivation and disempowerment experienced by mothers: short stature, underweight, and having no education. The fourth factor (household poverty) was economic in nature; the fifth (poor dietary diversity) stemmed from an interaction between poverty and maternal disempowerment. Clearly, poverty and maternal deprivation/disempowerment drive inequalities in stunting in India, as it does across South Asia (Krishna 2017).

Moderate to Severe Anaemia

Anaemia characterized by low levels of haemoglobin in the blood is mainly due to iron- or vitamin B-Complex deficiency. In 2015–16, 58.4 per cent of Indian children (6–59 months) were anaemic (IIPS and ICF 2017), 30.6 per cent being moderate-to-severely anaemic.[19] Although the prevalence rate of any anaemia is 11.1 percentage points lower than that in 2005–6 (IIPS and Macro International 2007), it continues to be an actionable public health problem.

The prevalence of childhood anaemia is not differentiated across geographical regions in any predictable manner. In 2015–16, the rates of moderate-to-severely anaemic children were higher in Chandigarh (45.6 per cent) and Haryana (43.5 per cent) than in the poor

[19] For children aged between 6 and 59 months, moderate and severe anaemia are indicated by haemoglobin levels between 9.9 and 7.0 g/l, and below 7 g/l respectively (WHO 2011).

states of Odisha (19.8 per cent) and Chhattisgarh (17.6 per cent) (IIPS and ICF 2017).

A cross-sectional study in two poor districts of Karnataka (Pasricha et al. 2010) found that three out of four children (12 to 23 months) were anaemic. The study found significant gender and wealth-based differences, with the average level of haemoglobin being lower among boys and in poor, food-insecure households. The study also identified maternal anaemia as a significant intergenerational gender effect, which was linked to the economic status of the household.

Another study found that household wealth and adult education were statistically non-significant in the presence of caste (Vart et al. 2015). However, abuses of gender power, typically in the form of maternal domestic violence, were strongly associated with childhood undernutrition. Children of women who experienced domestic violence more than once during one year prior to the NFHS-2 survey in 1998–9 were likely to be anaemic and wasted (Ackerson and Subramanian 2008).

POLICY DIRECTIONS

Our discussion so far shows that people suffering from social and economic disadvantages bear higher burdens of ill-health while having poorer access to affordable and quality services. Drivers of health inequality such as social and economic differentials, inadequate public spending on health, and poorly regulated privatization work through the availability, accessibility, acceptability, and quality (AAAQ) of healthcare and health promotion interventions (Hunt 2016). Directly, and indirectly through these intermediate factors, the drivers of health inequality affect behaviours such as healthcare seeking. Together they determine inequalities in health outcomes such as illness, disability, and death.

A potent mix of economic and social inequalities based on income/wealth, caste, religion, gender, and geography governs who is well and who is sick, and what they can do about it. The health of disadvantaged people is partly affected by factors such as where they live (more polluted environments with inadequate shelter), what and how much they eat (less nutritious food with insufficient calories, proteins, and micro-nutrients), the work they do (excessive, unsafe, unhealthy, and abusive conditions of work), and their entitlement to leisure to enable them to rest and recreate themselves. Poverty, caste, religion, and geography shape the health of households and their members. A first policy goal for better health for all must be to tackle these disadvantages and oppressions in a sustained way with a clear plan, funding, and effective monitoring of programmes.

Inequality and social subordination are also often the norm within their social and familial relationships, affecting how they are treated by others, their entitlements within homes and communities, and whether they have to contend with discrimination, disrespect, abuse or violence in these spaces. These factors work both from outside and within the home, particularly disadvantaging girls, women, disabled people, and the dependent elderly. A second policy goal is to recognize and tackle such power relations and their harmful effects in causing, illness, disability, injuries, and premature death.

Inequalities in the ability to access and afford care work both within and outside the home. They also affect the quality of care received, and whether it is free of discrimination and abuse. Explicitly tackling how such inequalities work goes beyond affirming a universal right to healthcare, which is a laudable goal but does not of itself guarantee equity or fairness on the pathways to that goal (Gwatkin and Ergo 2011). A third imperative is, therefore, to ensure that programmes such as social health insurance and others addressing healthcare services are designed in ways that ensure equitable pathways to primary, secondary, and tertiary care for all.

Taking such policy actions has two key co-requisites which are policies in themselves. Even if the health budget is increased, tracking and addressing health inequalities per se must be prioritized and protected or it is likely to fall victim to what may be called the politics of the squeaking wheel. This is the fourth policy imperative.

The fifth requirement is to make sure that policymakers and programme managers have enough data disaggregated not only by economic status of the household but also by social characteristics to enable effective focus and monitoring of what works or does not work to reduce health inequity. Such data should also be openly available to civil society organizations working to ensure accountability and fairness.

APPENDIX 7.1: DEFINITIONS

Table 7.1

(a) **Life expectancy at birth** is the number of years a newborn infant could expect to live if prevailing patterns of age-specific mortality rates at the time of birth stay the same throughout the infant's life.

(b) **Healthy life expectancy** provides an indication of overall health for a population, representing the average equivalent number of years of full health that a newborn could expect to live if they were to pass through life subject to the age-specific death rates and average age-specific levels of health states for a given period.

(c) **Maternal mortality ratio** is defined as the number of maternal deaths per 1,00, 000 live births.

(d) **Skilled births** are those births attended by skilled health personnel.

(e) **Under-five mortality rate** is the probability of a child born in a specific year or period dying before reaching the age of five, if subject to age-specific mortality rates of that period.

(f) **Neonatal mortality rate** is the number of deaths during the first 28 completed days of life per 1,000 live births in a given year or period.

(g) **Modern family planning** indicates the proportion of women of reproductive age (15–49 years) who have their need for family planning satisfied with modern methods.

(h) **Adolescent birth rate** is the number of births per 1,000 women aged 15 to 19 years.

(i) **Stunting** in children under five years is the prevalence of stunting (height for age <–2 standard deviation from the median of the WHO Child Growth Standards) among children under five years of age.

(j) **Wasting and over weight** in children under five years is the prevalence of malnutrition (weight for height >+2 or <–2 standard deviation from the median of the WHO Child growth standards) among children under five years of age, by type (wasting and overweight).

Table 7.2

(a) **Human Development Index** is a composite index measuring average achievement in three basic dimensions of human development—a long and healthy life, knowledge, and a decent standard of living.

(b) **HDI rank** Human Development Index and its components ranks countries by 2015 HDI value and details the values of the three HDI components: longevity, education (with two indicators), and income.

(c) **Inequality-adjusted Human Development Index** contains two related measures of inequality—the IHDI and the loss in HDI due to inequality. The IHDI looks beyond the average achievements of a country in longevity, education, and income to show how these achievements are distributed among its residents. An IHDI value can be interpreted as the level of human development when inequality is accounted for.

(d) **Percentage loss in HDI** is the relative difference between IHDI and HDI values is the loss due to inequality in distribution of the HDI within the country.

(e) **Gender Inequality Index** presents a composite measure of gender inequality using three dimensions: reproductive health, empowerment, and the labour market. Reproductive health is measured by two indicators: the maternal mortality ratio and the adolescent birth rate. Empowerment is measured by the share of parliamentary seats held by women and the shares of population with at least some secondary education by gender. And labour market is measured by participation in the labour force by gender. A low GII value indicates low inequality between women and men, and vice-versa.

Table 7.3

Multidimensional Poverty Index captures the multiple deprivations that people face in their education, health, and living standards. The MPI shows both the incidence of non-income multidimensional poverty (a headcount of those in multidimensional poverty) and its intensity (the average deprivation score experienced by poor people). Based on deprivation score thresholds, people are classified as multi-dimensionally poor, near multidimensional poverty or in severe poverty. The contributions of deprivations in each dimension to overall poverty are also presented.

REFERENCES

Ackerson, Leland K. and S.V. Subramanian. 2008. 'Domestic Violence and Chronic Malnutrition among Women and Children in India'. *American Journal of Epidemiology* 167(10): 1188–96. doi:10.1093/aje/kwn049.

Adamson, Paul C., Karl Krupp, Bhavana Niranjankumar, Alexandra H. Freeman, Mudassir Khan, and Purnima Madhivanan. 2012. 'Are Marginalized Women Being Left Behind? A Population-based Study of Institutional Deliveries in Karnataka, India'. *BMC Public Health* 12(1): 30. doi:10.1186/1471-2458-12-30.

Arokiasamy, Perianayagam, Uttamacharya, Paul Kowal, and Somnath Chatterji. 2016. 'Age and Socioeconomic

Gradients of Health of Indian Adults: An Assessment of Self-reported and Biological Measures of Health. *Journal of Cross-Cultural Gerontology* 31(2): 193–211. doi:10.1007/s10823-016-9283-3.

Banerjee, Soumik, Priya John, and Sanjeev Singh. 2013. 'Stairway to Death: Maternal Mortality Beyond Numbers'. *Economic and Political Weekly* 48(31): 123–30.

Berman, Peter, Rajeev Ahuja, and Laveesh Bhandari. 2010. 'The Impoverishing Effect of Healthcare Payments in India: New Methodology and Findings'. *Economic and Political Weekly* 45(16): 65–71.

Bhojani, Upendra, B.S. Thriveni, Roopa Devadasan, C.M. Munegowda, Narayanan Devadasan, Patrick Kolsteren, Bart Criel. 2012. 'Out-of-Pocket Healthcare Payments on Chronic Conditions Impoverish Urban Poor in Bangalore, India'. *BMC Public Health* 12(1): 990. doi:10.1186/1471-2458-12-990.

Borooah, Vani K. 2004. 'Gender Bias among Children in India in their Diet and Immunisation against Disease'. *Social Science & Medicine* 58(9): 1719–31. doi:10.1016/S0277-9536(03)00342-3.

Borooah, Vani K., Nidhi S. Sabharwal, Dilip G. Diwakar, Vinod K. Mishra, and Ajaya K. Naik. 2015. *Caste, Discrimination, and Exclusion in Modern India*. New Delhi: Sage Publications.

Chalasani, Satvika. 2012. 'Understanding Wealth-based Inequalities in Child Health in India: A Decomposition Approach'. *Social Science & Medicine* 75(1): 2160–9. doi:10.1016/j.socscimed.2012.08.012.

Chambers, Robert and Gregor von Medeazza. 2014. 'Reframing Undernutrition: Faecally-Transmitted Infections and the 5 As'. *IDS Working Paper* 45, Institute of Development Studies, Brighton, Sussex. Available at https://opendocs.ids.ac.uk/opendocs/bitstream/handle/20.500.12413/4941/Wp450rev.pdf, last accessed on 1 June 2016.

Chattopadhyay, Sreeparna, Arima Mishra, and Suraj Jacob. 2017. '"Safe", yet Violent? Women's Experiences with Obstetric Violence during Hospital Births in Rural Northeast India'. *Culture, Health & Sexuality* 20(7): 815–29. doi:10.1080/13691058.2017.1384572.

Corsi, Daniel J., Ivan Mejía-Guevara, and S.V. Subramanian. 2016. 'Risk Factors for Chronic Undernutrition among Children in India: Estimating Relative Importance, Population Attributable Risk and Fractions'. *Social Science & Medicine* 157: 165–85. doi:10.1016/j.socscimed.2015.11.014.

Credit Suisse Research Institute. 2016. *Global Wealth Report 2016*. Available at http://publications.credit-suisse.com/tasks/render/file/index.cfm?fileid=AD783798-ED07-E8C2-4405996B5B02A32E, last accessed on 20 October 2017.

CSDH (Commission on Social Determinants of Health). 2008. *Closing the Gap in a Generation: Health Equity through Action on the Social Determinants of Health*. Final Report of the Commission on Social Determinants of Health. Geneva: World Health Organization. Available at https://apps.who.int/iris/bitstream/handle/10665/43943/9789241563703_eng.pdf?sequence=1, last accessed on 5 August 2016.

Fan, Victoria, Anup Karan, and Ajay Mahal. 2012. 'State Health Insurance and Out-of-Pocket Health Expenditures in Andhra Pradesh, India', *International Journal of Health Care Finance and Economics* 12(3): 189–215. doi:10.1007/s10754-012-9110-5.

George, Asha, Aditi Iyer, and Gita Sen. 2005. 'Gendered Health Systems Biased against Maternal Survival: Preliminary Findings from Koppal, Karnataka, India'. *IDS Working Paper* 253, Institute of Development Studies, Brighton, Sussex. Available at https://opendocs.ids.ac.uk/opendocs/bitstream/handle/20.500.12413/4046/Wp253.pdf?sequence=1&isAllowed=y, last accessed on 24 November 2005.

Government of India. 2006. *Social, Economic and Educational Status of the Muslim Community of India: A Report*. Prime Minister's High Level Committee. New Delhi: Government of India.

Gwatkin, Davidson R. and Alex Ergo. 2011. 'Universal Health Coverage: Friend or Foe of Health Equity?' *The Lancet* 377(9784): 2160–1. doi:10.1016/S0140-6736(10)62058-2.

Hunt, Paul. 2016. 'Interpreting the International Right to Health in a Human Rights-based Approach to Health'. *Health and Human Rights* 18(2): 109–30.

IIPS (International Institute for Population Sciences) and ICF. 2017. *National Family Health Survey 4 (NFHS 4), 2015–16: India*. Mumbai: IIPS.

IIPS (International Institute for Population Sciences) and Macro International. 2007. *National Family Health Survey 3 (NFHS 3), 2005–06: India (Volume I)*, Mumbai: IIPS.

ISDBIC (India State-level Disease Burden Initiative Collaborators). 2017. 'Nations within a Nation: Variations in Epidemiological Transition across the States of India, 1990–2016 in the Global Burden of Disease Study'. *The Lancet* 390(10111): 2437–60. doi:10.1016/S0140-6736(17)32804-0.

Iyengar, Kirti, Sharad D. Iyengar, Virendra Suhalka, and Kalpana Dashora. 2009. 'Pregnancy-related Deaths in Rural Rajasthan, India: Exploring Causes, Context, and Care-seeking Through Verbal Autopsy'. *Journal of Health Population and Nutrition* 27(2): 293–302. doi:10.3329/jhpn.v27i2.3370.

Iyer, Aditi, Gita Sen, and Asha George. 2007. 'The Dynamics of Gender and Class in Access to Health Care: Evidence from Rural Karnataka, India', *International Journal of Health Services* 37(3): 537–54. doi:10.2190/1146-7828-5L5H-7757.

Iyer, Aditi, Gita Sen, and Piroska Ostlin. 2010. 'Inequalities and Intersections in Health: Review of the Evidence', in *Gender Equity in Health: The Shifting Frontiers of Evidence and Action*, edited by Gita Sen and Piroska Ostlin, pp. 70–95. New York: Routledge.

Iyer, Aditi, Gita Sen, and Anuradha Sreevathsa. 2013. 'Deciphering Rashomon: An Approach to Verbal Autopsies of Maternal Deaths', *Global Public Health: An International Journal for Research, Policy and Practice* 8(4): 389–404. doi:10.1080/17441692.2013.772219.

Iyer, Aditi, Gita Sen, Anuradha Sreevathsa, and Vasini Varadan. 2012. 'Verbal Autopsies of Maternal Deaths in Koppal, Karnataka: Lessons from the Grave', *BMC Proceedings* 6(Suppl. 1): P2.

Jain, Kalpana. 2013. 'Health Financing and Delivery in India: An Overview of Selected Schemes'. *WIEGO Working Paper (Social Protection)* No. 29, Women in Informal Employment: Globalizing and Organizing (WEIGO), Manchester. Available at https://www.wiego.org/sites/default/files/migrated/publications/files/Jain-Health-Financing-India-WIEGO-WP29.pdf, last accessed on 4 August 2016.

Jain, Nidhi, Abhishek Singh, and Praveen Pathak. 2013. 'Infant and Child Mortality in India: Trends in Inequalities across Economic Groups', *Journal of Population Research* 30(4): 347–65. doi:10.1007/s12546-013-9110-4.

James, K.S. 2014. 'Recent Shifts in Infant Mortality in India: An Exploration'. *Economic and Political Weekly* 49(3): 14–17.

Jithesh, Veetilakath, and T.K. Sundari Ravindran. 2015. 'Social and Health System Factors Contributing to Maternal Deaths in a Less Developed District of Kerala, India'. *Journal of Reproductive Health and Medicine* 2(1): 26–32. doi:10.1016/j.jrhm.2015.12.003.

Joe, William, Udaya S. Mishra, and K. Navaneetham. 2010. 'Socio-economic Inequalities in Child Health: Recent Evidence from India'. *Global Public Health* 5(5): 493–508. doi:10.1080/17441690903213774.

Karan, Anup, Sakthivel Selvaraj and Ajay Mahal. 2014. 'Moving to Universal Coverage? Trends in the Burden of Out-Of-Pocket Payments for Health Care across Social Groups in India, 1999–2000 to 2011–12'. *PLoS One* 9(8): e105162. doi:10.1371/journal.pone.0105162.

Krishna, Aditi, Iván Mejía-Guevara, Mark McGovern, Victor Aguayo, and S.V. Subramanian. 2017. 'Trends in Inequalities in Child Stunting in South Asia'. *Maternal and Child Nutrition* 14(suppl 4): e12517. doi:10.1111/mcn.12517.

Kumar, A., and A. Singh. 2013. 'Decomposing the Gap in Childhood Undernutrition between Poor and Non–poor in Urban India, 2005–06'. *PLoS ONE* 8(5): e64972. doi:10.1371/journal.pone.0064972.

Million Death Study Collaborators. 2017. 'Changes in Cause-specific Neonatal and 1–59-month Child Mortality in India from 2000 to 2015: A Nationally Representative Survey'. *The Lancet* 390(10106): 1972–80. doi:10.1016/S0140-6736(17)32162-1.

Moser, Kath A., Sutapa Agrawal, George Davey Smith, and Shah Ebrahim. 2014. 'Socio-Demographic Inequalities in the Prevalence, Diagnosis and Management of Hypertension in India: Analysis of Nationally-Representative Survey Data'. *PLoS ONE* 9(1): e86043. doi:10.1371/journal.pone.0086043.

NIMHANS (National Institute of Mental Health and Neuro Sciences). 2016. *National Mental Health Survey of India, 2015–16. Prevalence, Pattern and Outcomes*. Bengaluru: NIMHANS. Available at http://www.nimhans.ac.in/, last accessed on 14 May 2018.

Norman, Rosana E., David O. Carpenter, James Scott, Marie Noel Brunea, and Peter D. Sly. 2013. 'Environmental Exposures: An Underrecognized Contribution to Noncommunicable Diseases'. *Review of Environmental Health* 28(1): 59–65. doi:10.1515/reveh-2012-0033.

Omran, Abdel R. 1971. 'The Epidemiologic Transition. A Theory of the Epidemiology of Population Change'. *Milbank Memorial Fund Quarterly* 49(4): 509–38. doi:10.2307/3349375.

ORGCCI (Office of the Registrar General & Census Commissioner of India). 2016. *Sample Registration System Statistical Report 2015* (Field work period: 2016). New Delhi: Ministry of Home Affairs, Government of India. Available at http://www.censusindia.gov.in/vital_statistics/SRS_Report_2015/7.Chap%203-Fertility%20Indicators-2015.pdf, last accessed on 25 January 2018.

ORGI (Office of the Registrar General, India). 2018. *Special Bulletin on Maternal Mortality in India 2014–16*. New Delhi: Ministry of Home Affairs, Government of India. Available at http://www.censusindia.gov.in/vital_statistics/SRS_Bulletins/MMR%20Bulletin-2014-16.pdf, last accessed on 24 October 2019.

Pasricha, Sant-Rayn, James Black, Sumithra Muthayya, Anita Shet, Vijay Bhat, Savitha Nagaraj, N.S. Prashanth, H. Sudarshan, Beverley-Ann Biggs, Arun S. Shet. 2010. 'Determinants of Anemia among Young Children in Rural India'. *Pediatrics* 126(1): e140. doi:10.1542/peds.2009-3108.

Patel, Vikram, Chinthanie Ramasundarahettige, Lakshmi Vijayakumar, J.S. Thakur, Vendhan Gajalakshmi, Gopalkrishna Gururaj, Wilson Suraweera, and Prabhat Jha for the Million Death Study Collaborators. 2012. 'Suicide Mortality in India: A Nationally Representative Survey'. *The Lancet* 379(9834): 2343–51. doi:10.1016/S0140-6736(12)60606-0.

Po, June Y.T. and S.V. Subramanian. 2011. 'Mortality Burden and Socioeconomic Status in India'. *PLoS One* 6(2): e16844. doi:10.1371/journal.pone.0016844.

Prusty, Ranjan Kumar and Abhishek Kumar. 2014. 'Socioeconomic Dynamics of Gender Disparity in

Childhood Immunization in India, 1992–2006'. *PLoS ONE* 9(8): e104598. doi:10.1371/journal.pone.0104598.

Ram, F., S.K. Mohanty, and Usha Ram. 2009. 'Understanding the Distribution of BPL Cards: All-India and Selected States'. *Economic and Political Weekly* 46(7): 66–71.

Ram, Usha, Lisa Strohschein, and Kirti Gaur. 2014. 'Gender Socialization: Differences between Male and Female Youth in India and Associations with Mental Health'. *International Journal of Population Research* 2014, article ID 357145: 1–11. doi:10.1155/2014/357145.

Ranadive, Bharat, Vishal Diwan, and Ayesha De Costa. 2013. 'India's Conditional Cash Transfer Programme (the JSY) to Promote Institutional Birth: Is There an Association between Institutional Birth Proportion and Maternal Mortality?' *PLoS ONE* 8(6): e67452. doi:10.1371/journal.pone.0067452.

Rao, Sujatha K. 2017. *Do We Care? India's Health System*. New Delhi: Oxford University Press.

Rathi, Pradeep, Arnab Mukherji, and Gita Sen. 2012. 'Rashtriya Swasthya Bima Yojana: Evaluating Utilisation, Roll-out and Perceptions in Amaravati District, Maharashtra'. *Economic and Political Weekly* 47(39): 57–63.

RGI (Registrar General of India). n.d. *Compendium of India's Fertility and Mortality Indicators, 1971–2013, Based on The Sample Registration System*. New Delhi: Ministry of Home Affairs, Government of India. Available at http://www.censusindia.gov.in/vital_statistics/Compendium/Srs_data.html, last accessed on 18 April 2018.

———. n.d. *MMR Bulletin 2011–2013* New Delhi: Ministry of Home Affairs, Government of India. Available at http://www.censusindia.gov.in/vital_statistics/mmr_bulletin_2011-13.pdf, last accessed on 15 January 2018.

Selvaraj, Sakthivel and Anup K. Karan. 2012. 'Why Publicly-financed Health Insurance Schemes Are Ineffective in Providing Financial Risk Protection?' *Economic and Political Weekly* 47(11): 60–8.

Sen, Gita, and Aditi Iyer. 2012. 'Who Gains, Who Loses and How: Leveraging Gender and Class Intersections to Secure Health Entitlements', *Social Science & Medicine* 74(11): 1802–11.

———. 2015. 'Health policy in India: Some Critical Concerns', in *The Palgrave International Handbook of Healthcare Policy and Governance*, edited by Ellen Kuhlmann, Robert H. Blank, Ivy Lynn Bourgeault, and Claus Wendt, pp. 154–70. Hampshire: Palgrave Macmillan.

———. 2019. 'Beyond Economic Barriers: Intersectionality and Health Policy in Low- and Middle-income Countries', in *The Palgrave Handbook of Intersectionality in Public Policy*, edited by Olena Hankivsky and Julia Jordan-Zachery, pp. 245–61. Cham, Switzerland Palgrave Macmillan.

Serour, G., N. Younis, F. Hefnawi, H. Daghistani, M. El-bahy, M. Nawara, and S. Abdel-Razak. 1981. 'Pregnancy Wastage'. *Population Sciences* 2: 57–69.

Shahrawat, Renu and Krishna D. Rao. 2012. 'Insured yet Vulnerable: Out-of-Pocket Payments and India's Poor', *Health Policy and Planning* 27(3): 213–21. doi:10.1093/heapol/czr029.

Sibley, Lynn, Leila Caleb-Varkey, Jayant Upadhyay, Rajendra Prasad, Ekta Saroha, Neerja Bhatia, and Vinod Paul. 2005. 'Recognition of and Response to Postpartum Hemorrhage in Rural Northern India', *Journal of Midwifery & Women's Health* 50(4): 301–8.

Singh, Ashish. 2012. 'Gender-based within Household Inequality in Childhood Immunization in India: Changes Over Time and Across Regions'. *PLoS ONE* 7(4): e35045. doi:10.1371/journal.pone.0035045.

Singh, Abhishek and Sangram Kishor Patel. 2017. 'Gender Differentials in Feeding Practices, Health Care Utilization and Nutritional Status of Children in Northern India'. *International Journal of Human Rights in Healthcare* 10(5): 323–31. doi:10.1108/IJHRH-05-2017-0023.

Singh, Abhishek, Praveen K. Pathak, Rajesh K. Chauhan, and William Pan. 2011. 'Infant and Child Mortality in India in the Last Two Decades: A Geospatial Analysis'. *PLoS ONE* 6(11): e26856. doi:10.1371/journal.pone.0026856.

Stroope, Samuel. 2015. 'Seclusion, Decision-making Power, and Gender Disparities in Adult Health: Examining Hypertension in India'. *Social Science Research* 53: 288–99. doi:10.1016/j.ssresearch.2015.05.013.

Subha Sri, B. and Renu Khanna. 2014. *Dead Women Talking: A Civil Society Report on Maternal Deaths in India*. CommonHealth and Jan Swasthya Abhiyan.

Subha Sri, B., N. Sarojini, and Renu Khanna. 2012. 'An Investigation of Maternal Deaths following Public Protests in a Tribal District of Madhya Pradesh, Central India'. *Reproductive Health Matters* 20(39): 11–20. doi:10.1016/S0968-8080(12)39599-2.

Subramanian, S.V., Leland K. Ackerson, George Davey Smith, and Neetu A. John. 2009. 'Association of Maternal Height with Child Mortality, Anthropometric Failure, and Anemia in India', *JAMA* 301(16): 1691–701. doi:10.1001/jama.2009.548.

Subramanian, S.V., Daniel J. Corsi, Malavika A. Subramanyam, and George Davey Smith. 2013. 'Jumping the Gun: The Problematic Discourse on Socioeconomic Status and Cardiovascular Health in India', *International Journal of Epidemiology* 42(5): 1410–26. doi:10.1093/ije/dyt017.

Subramanian, S.V., Shailen Nandy, Michelle Irving, Dave Gordon, Helen Lambert, and George Davey Smith. 2006. 'The Mortality Divide in India: The Differential Contributions of Gender, Caste, and Standard of Living Across the Life Course', *American Journal of Public Health* 96(5): 818–25. doi:10.2105/AJPH.2004.060103.

Subramanyam, Malavika A., Ichiro Kawachi, Lisa F. Berkman, S.V. Subramanian. 2010. 'Socioeconomic Inequalities in Childhood Undernutrition in India: Analyzing Trends between 1992 and 2005'. *PLoS ONE* 5(6): e11392. doi:10.1371/journal.pone.0011392.

Tangcharoensathien, Viroj, Woranan Witthayapipopsakul, Warisa Panichkriangkrai, Walaiporn Patcharanarumol, and Anne Mills. 2018. 'Health Systems Development in Thailand: A Solid Platform for Successful Implementation of Universal Health Coverage', *The Lancet* 391(10126): 1205–23. doi:10.1016/S0140-6736(18)30198-3.

Thorat, Sukhadeo and Nidhi Sadana. 2009. 'Discrimination and Children's Nutritional Status in India', *IDS Bulletin* 40(4): 25–9.

UNDP (United Nations Development Programme). 2016. *Human Development Report, 2016*. Statistical Annex, Human Development Composite Indices, Table 1 (pp. 198–201), Table 3 (pp. 206–9), Table 5 (pp. 214–17), and Table 6 (pp. 218–19). New York: UNDP. Available at http://hdr.undp.org/sites/default/files/2016_human_development_report.pdf, last accessed on 30 October 2017.

van de Poel, Ellen and Niko Speybroeck. 2009. 'Decomposing Malnutrition Inequalities between Scheduled Castes and Tribes and the Remaining Indian Population', *Ethnicity & Health* 14(3): 271–87. doi:10.1080/13557850802609931.

Vart, Priya, Ajay Jaglan, and Kashif Shafique. 2015. 'Caste-based Social Inequalities and Childhood Anemia in India: Results from the National Family Health Survey 2005–2006', *BMC Public Health* 15(1): 537. doi:10.1186/s12889-015-1881-4.

Vellakkal, Sukumar, Adyya Gupta, Zaky Khan, David Stuckler, Aaron Reeves, Shah Ebrahim, Ann Bowling, and Pat Doyle. 2017. 'Has India's National Rural Health Mission Reduced Inequities in Maternal Health Services? A Pre-post Repeated Cross-sectional Study', *Health Policy and Planning* 32(1): 79–90.

Vellakkal, Sukumar, S.V. Subramanian, Christopher Millett, Sanjay Basu, David Stuckler, and Shah Ebrahim. 2013. 'Socioeconomic Inequalities in Non-Communicable Diseases Prevalence in India: Disparities between Self-Reported Diagnoses and Standardized Measures', *PLoS ONE* 8(7): e68219. doi:10.1371/journal.pone.0068219.

Vineis, Paolo, Silvia Stringhini, and Miquel Porta. 2014. 'The Environmental Roots of Non-Communicable Diseases and the Epigenetic Impacts of Globalization', *Environmental Research* 133: 424–30. doi:10.1016/j.envres.2014.02.002i.

WCRFI (World Cancer Research Fund International) and The NCD Alliance. 2014. *The Link between Food, Nutrition, Diet and Non-Communicable Diseases: Why NCDs Need to be Considered when Addressing Major Nutritional Challenges*. London: WCRFI. Available at https://www.wcrf.org/sites/default/files/PPA_NCD_Alliance_Nutrition.pdf, last accessed on 15 January 2018.

WHO (World Health Organization). 2002. Globalization, Diets and Non-Communicable Diseases. Geneva: World Health Organization. Available at https://apps.who.int/iris/bitstream/handle/10665/42609/9241590416.pdf?sequence=1&isAllowed=y, last accessed on 7 February 2018.

———. 2006. *WHO Child Growth Standards: Length/height-for-age, Weight-for-age, Weight-for-length, Weight-for-height and Body mass index-for-age. Methods and Development*. Geneva: Department of Nutrition for Health and Development, World Health Organization. Available at https://www.who.int/childgrowth/standards/Technical_report.pdf?ua=1, last accessed on 28 October 2019.

———. 2011. *Haemoglobin Concentrations for the Diagnosis of Anaemia and Assessment of Severity.* Vitamin and Mineral Nutrition Information System. Geneva: World Health Organization. Available at http://www.who.int/vmnis/indicators/haemoglobin.pdf, last accessed on 28 December 2017.

———. 2015. *Trends in Maternal Mortality 1990 to 2015: Estimates by WHO, UNICEF, UNFPA, World Bank Group and the United Nations Population Division*. Geneva: World Health Organization. Available at https://apps.who.int/iris/bitstream/handle/10665/194254/9789241565141_eng.pdf, last accessed on 18 April 2018.

———. 2016. *World Health Statistics 2016—Monitoring Health for the SDGs*. Annex B, Parts 1 and 2—Tables of Health Statistics by Country, WHO Region and Globally, pp. 103–19. Geneva: World Health Organization. Available at http://www.who.int/gho/publications/world_health_statistics/2016/EN_WHS2016_AnnexB.pdf?ua=1, last accessed on 30 October 2017.

———. 2017. *Preventing Non-Communicable Diseases (NCDs) by Reducing Environmental Risk Factors*. Geneva: World Health Organization. Available at http://apps.who.int/iris/bitstream/10665/258796/1/WHO-FWC-EPE-17.01-eng.pdf?ua=1, last accessed on 7 February 2018.

———. 2018. *Depression in India: Let's Talk*. Geneva: World Health Organization. Available at http://www.searo.who.int/india/depression_in_india.pdf, last accessed on 13 May 2018.

Wilkinson, Richard and Kate Pickett. 2010. *The Spirit Level: Why Equality is Better for Everyone*. London: Penguin Books.

World Bank. 2018. 'Equity on the Path to UHC Deliberate Decisions for Fair Financing'. Background Report (Conference Version) for the 3rd Annual UHC Financing Forum: Greater Equity for Better Health and Financial Protection Washington, D.C., April 19–20. Available at http://pubdocs.worldbank.org/en/588321524060370166/BGP-v-8-20180418-0930-FINAL.pdf, last accessed on 13 May 2018.

Part III
Structural Determinants of Health

8

A New Economics for Health

Smita Srinivas

THE INDUSTRIAL EVOLUTION OF HEALTHCARE

It is a transformative fact today that most countries and their citizens draw on essential medicines and vaccines designed and manufactured and then traded across hundreds and often, thousands of miles. Health technologies include both mature and innovative products, in some cases, entirely disrupting patient experiences, the medical profession, and the organization of industries. Several sub-sectors such as medicines, vaccines, diagnostic kits, medical devices, and surgical instruments are produced and governed within and across national boundaries. These technologies may be regulated for a range of health and safety reasons, and often through industrial policies. New economics for health focused on technological change and the evolutionary aspects of industrial organization in the health industry may therefore look different from health economics as we know it today.

One of the traditional ways of approaching the health sector is to see it understandably as something unique—a sector that deals with life, death, inequalities, and difficult philosophy questions. After all, the health sector is a moral dilemma all on its own, and health economists and other health policy specialists undertake inquiries traversing a complex terrain of theory, methods, and practicalities. A policymaker, regulator, medical practitioner, and certainly the patient, all face practical and more philosophical questions: what markets to create and support, is a dengue test or a biopsy necessary, how much to charge for it, is a medicine for an epidemic available at a reasonable cost or free, what types of public subsidies should be available for private firms, and what limits on data availability should exist as newer technologies and therapies come into being?

Yet there are several clues that the heath sector is not unique and has elements common with other industries: these are its industry dynamics and its technological aspects. These elements are practical and problematic because they cover a wide logistical and philosophical compass requiring closer scrutiny, often directly shaping clinical practice or field use: these features have to do with how industries change, how they overlap and converge with other industries, and the degree to which specific technological transformations result in new products, process, and knowledge. In turn, private, public, and hybrid organizations must be watchful and aware of these dynamic changes underway in their sphere: accommodating or embracing such change by bringing in new equipment, testing new treatment regimens, adapting skills and training streams for specialists with growing instrumentation requirements, finding funds for future investments, dynamic storage and stocking needs, and building relationships with a range of external actors—from trucking to pharmacies, patient advocacy organizations to regulators.

The health sector also shares attributes of connectedness: the wider health industry in one part of a world in which health policymaking is one facet but not the whole, and must respond to changes elsewhere. When an expensive magnetic resonance imaging (MRI) machine is produced and purchased in any country, the buyer (for example, a hospital) must recoup the costs, often by urging doctors to prescribe its use (or over-use) and where possible, charging as much for each use of the machine along with full-time costing of a qualified radiologist. When this MRI machine is produced in one place and imported to another part of the world, it can often sit unused for want of personnel, repair parts, and servicing, thereby running losses for the buyers and valuable time and energy for patients. The MRI machine is a part of a wider industrial dynamic through which it is designed, tested, manufactured, deployed, repaired, redesigned, and made obsolete. Therefore, sophistication in R&D or manufacture of these products and their spread into the wider health system of needs, diagnosis, and therapeutic care requires analysis in industrial context with make or buy decisions, skills and materials, logistics and testing.

We can go further whether we acknowledge or embrace the reality, the health industry comprises an increasingly dominant element of healthcare today, even in most lower-income countries. It has several moving parts and sub-sectors: generics, patented medicines, vaccines, and biotechnologies. Industrial policies, innovation, and new science and engineering knowledge, they all influence health regulations, and thus also the goals and direction of firms' product design and development and manufacturing priorities. Regulators in turn need to keep pace with medical and manufacturing advances, not merely with the finished products and processes they encounter, but to anticipate changes in the science, engineering, and health and social systems of knowledge that bring these into being. Industrial dynamics and its specific organization at a given time is thus vital to the analysis of healthcare today. These dynamics extend beyond R&D and manufacture into science-, technology-, and engineering-dependent and now industrially organized realms of demand (insurance, procurement, and so on), and delivery (diagnosis and tele-treatment, clinics and hospitals, logistics, trucking, cold storage, and so on) (Srinivas 2012).

A NON-EQUILIBRIUM, INSTITUTIONALLY DYNAMIC HEALTH ECONOMICS

The knowledge intensity of health sub-fields, and the technology intensity of the industry thus play vital roles in growing uncertainty, speed, information asymmetries, and competition among firms, and consequently rejects traditional health economics (Hodgson 2008). Dramatic differences in the health system concerning contingent technological advances open up across countries as well as in single countries across time. These are not explained by cost or efficiency considerations alone (Srinivas 2012). Consequently, as technological advances grow and equipment and methods increasingly specialist and narrow, economics ceases to be the simple cost calculus of cost–benefit analysis, neither a market-failure threshold for state intervention, nor indeed one that can rely on equilibrium analysis in fast-moving technological domains.

Several health success stories for India are therefore mixed technology and industrial successes: reductions in polio, improved childhood immunization rates for this and other vaccines, growing viability of genome-based oncology diagnostics, the use of machine learning in early stage detection and treatment regimens across diseases, the vast availability of generic medicines, and growing domestic alternatives for foreign on-patent drugs, vaccines, and medical diagnostics which help toward health security. This array of public and private firms, and rapidly increasing hybrid cooperation agreements between dispersed stakeholders, is opening up new realms of health technology advances that have dramatically expanded care options and organizational formats for Indian healthcare.

Consequently, the relationship and the emphasis on growth of the industrial and technological elements of healthcare deserves much more attention in claiming the economics to study it. While the options for Indian healthcare are often a function of their technology and industry attributes, health analysis in India has had a surprising and traditional over-reliance (despite varied ideology) on market vocabulary and market protagonists (Srinivas 2006, 2012). This over-reliance and yet imprecision in description of the markets under study, and contingent dependence of market design on technology evolution, make it clear that healthcare benefits do not automatically flow to the poorest or most susceptible. An alternate institutional and evolutionary approach must consider science and technology specifics. This is not to argue for a technological determinism; on the contrary, ironically without it, healthcare analysis and policy economics tend to attribute too much power to science and technology, which has resulted in a biomedically-centric policy environment.

The nation state is one way of drawing the system boundary for health analysis and most health economics preserves this traditional demarcation, focusing on national capabilities. Seen, however, from the vantage point of technology evolution, and the related capabilities of firms, the geographic and institutional ambit becomes much wider for 'Indian' health analysis. Grow at home it might, but the world is a firm's potential playground. Thus, the evolutionary and institutional discrepancies of 'Indian' healthcare and its domestic self-sufficiency rely on how well we can analyse the behaviour of firms (whether they be public, private, or hybrid), the nature of sub-sector investment and demonstration and process engineering challenges in their local environment. At the same time, the analysis depends on the globally traded industry and technology profile of 'Indian' firms which may have significant foreign investors. Firms which began as indigenous and entirely locally owned, have become increasingly international or entirely foreign in ownership. This financing pattern, ownership, and allegiances to shareholders undoubtedly affects priorities for domestic health and the expectations of the state's role in industrial and health policies. Gaps in equity and effectiveness at home require understanding the export profile of India's health industry, in which the domestic Indian consumer is one amongst a set of potential global users.

Industrial scholars are especially concerned with these systemic and boundary demarcation attributes of the innovation context. The Schumpeterian elements include uncertainty and non-equilibrium, cumulative convergence or divergence of firms, and wider institutional and organizational elements. These attributes of the system in local production contexts, are poorly served by a universal, homogenous approach to economic theory and methods. The arguments for a new economics are strongest when focused on technological and institutional change, and the uneven historic attributes of knowledge and theories of agency (including policy agency). Several potential economic theories inform the different historical threads that connect industry evolution; no single narrative or historical data arc undergirds a single economic model on positivist grounds (Hodgson 2008; Robert and Yoguel 2016). Once the technological dynamism of the sector is acknowledged, extant firms and product diversity in diverse geographies requires the use of multiple methods through comparative national analysis of the health industry's evolution. This context-specificity requires empirical strategy, is often case-focused, likely to push against universal explanations, and dependent on the non-equilibrium, open-endedness of different technology paths and specific institutional contexts. Health system studies are invariably inductive and mixed-methods approaches, iteratively building up plausible theoretical explanations for how products, processes, and technology platforms came into being in different societies and their varying degrees of success.

Newer disease threats, new approaches to health and well-being, and new citizenship and entitlement frameworks for care also evolve in a contingent technology context with social changes. An older economics approach, more narrowly seen in terms of an economics of market failure and public goods, provides us a conservative, overly narrow approach to leading institutions such as states and markets. This poorly fits those late industrializing nations that have sophisticated technological capabilities and where changing institutional influences prevail: intellectual property rights (IPR), technical standards, citizenship, insurance, or licensing arrangements. Demand patterns also emerge as distinctive in medical innovation history (for example, Lotz 1993) as do the organizational 'mission' structures for health (for example, Wilson et al. 2007 on vaccines), and a range of market varieties designed and legitimized at various times in supplier countries (Srinivas 2012). The global governance of diseases has extended these institutional and organizational arrangements: today HIV, AIDS, tuberculosis, malaria, and swine flu are increasingly arranged into cross-border science and engineering collaborations and funding patterns.

However, supplier countries are a special case of nations that have a robust local production structure and often manufacturing capabilities as well. Market failure provides a poor descriptor of their institutional dynamics; technological advance can boost economic growth and industrial plants, but the impact on health is less straightforward. Furthermore, a non-equilibrium and evolutionary approach to healthcare industrial dynamics results in a shift in policy analysis. 'Health policy' thus becomes a wider arena of methods and analysis: concerns of industrial, innovation, and science and technology (S&T) planning process, with technology-influenced policy design, and public administration. Health policy and the economics of health have tended to focus on delivery mechanisms and consumption.

Yet, as technological capabilities grow, a range of industrial and alternate institutional considerations grow alongside. Artificial intelligence, for example, may ease the viability of new point of care models. Technical standards, lab testing, STEM capabilities, technology transfer, and supply chain logistics for intermediate products and input reagents become critical. Financing and prototyping also become pivotal to access and affordability. Supplier countries therefore require an economics of industrial organization through which such technological capabilities are built, consumed, and delivered, a co-evolutionary process of at least 3 institutional domains as shown in Figure 8.1.

This heuristic represents a systemic linkage across production, demand, and delivery at any given time, where traditional health policy spheres are represented by Table 8.1 and Table 8.2, and industrial policy, and related innovation and S&T policy in Table 8.3. The heuristic represents the inter-linkage and changes across all three domains where these policy silos weaken

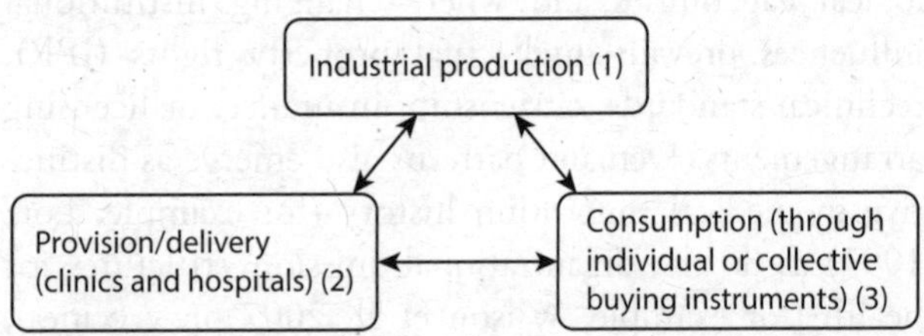

Figure 8.1 A Heuristic describing the Industrial Organization
Source: Srinivas (2012: 8).

Table 8.1 Specific Industrial Policy Instruments and Influences

Country	Institutional lasers (dominant institutions or policy instrument)
Zimbabwe	Procurement helps (3, 1)
Tanzania, Kenya, Mozambique	Global funds can weaken local producers (3, 1)
Tanzania	Industry-specific 'business-friendly' supports are absent (1)
India	Foreign welfare states have been pivotal ('the 3 Ws') (3, 2)
Brazil	Domestic welfare state pivotal (3,2)
Uruguay	Weak knowledge demand (3,2)

Source: Chataway et al. (2016) on Zimbabwe; Tibandebage et al. (2016) on Tanzania and Kenya; Russo and de Oliveira (2016) on Mozambique; Mackintosh et al. (2016, forth.) on Tanzania; Srinivas (2006, 2012) on India; Albuquerque (2007) on Brazil; Arocena and Sutz (2000) on Uruguay and other Latin American countries.

(for a fuller analysis, see Srinivas 2014, 2016). Another use is to study the heuristic as demonstrating evolution of single countries over time or within different forms of the national or localized governance. Table 8.1 considers how health systems will respond to democracy and to specific transformations in technology such as machine learning. Taken separately or together, policy and plans combine with technological change not in a single predictable way, but on the different politically amenable levers possible and the ways in which demand is identified and its delivery response.

Cuba, for example, is able to combine institutional design priorities in ways that are impossible or politically inadvisable in most democracies. Cuba's policies and health outcomes appear highly enviable: substantial biotechnology and scientific advances, simultaneous and extensive disease surveillance, registration of patients, free healthcare, or expansion of public research institutes. These reforms are difficult to replicate in most democratic supplier nations, but other permutations are possible and potentially health positive. Countries may draw on dynamic, privately owned firms, active NGOs, hybrid partnerships between public and private sectors, third-party accountability organizations, state–society experiments in process improvements in insurance or

Table 8.2 Policy Domains and Economic Activities of the Institutional Triad

Institutional vertex	Policy domain	Characteristic economic activities
1	Production (Industrial Policy, also Innovation, Science, R&D)	Manufacturing, R&D, prototyping, supply-driven 'catch-up' in medicines (generics and other), vaccines, diagnostics and devices
2	Provision/ Delivery (Health Policy, and some infrastructure and Industry policies)	Hospital services, primary and tertiary care, emergency services, diagnostics and devices, tele-medicine, radiology, logistics, trucking, and refrigeration, etc.
3	Consumption (Health policy, especially Insurance policies)	Individual or Collective buying instruments: Pay as you go, out of pocket cash payments, collective insurance-formal and informal.

Adapted from Srinivas (2012: 8).

Table 8.3 Late Industrial Development and Institutional Permutations

Iconic late industrial suppliers	Institutional bundles	Notable global exporting supply-side success	Health policy success
Democratic, or mostly democratic (if periods of authoritarianism)			
Brazil	1, 3	Only in some products, e.g. biologicals	Yes
Japan	1, 2, 3	Yes (across a wide range)	Yes
India	1, 2	Yes (across a wide range)	Only in some products
Costa Rica	2 (universal), 3	—	Yes
Egypt	1, 2	Mainly generics	—
Non-democratic and/or Maoist, other Communist)			
Cuba	1, 2 (universal), 3	In several products	Yes
China	1, 2 (universal or close), 3	Yes	Yes (data reliability is a caution)
Non-Suppliers (may have been suppliers at a time)			
Sri Lanka	2 (universal for a time), 3 (suffered from civil war loss of infrastructure)	-	Yes

Legend: 1: Industrial Production 2: Provision/Delivery 3: Demand/Consumption.
Adapted from Srinivas (2012: Figure 1.1, p. 8 and Table 8.2, p. 181).

delivery logistics, and the ability in principle to respond through financial or other incentives offered to firms, to reduce delays and shortfalls in supply chains and treatment options. A traditional economics focused as it is on market failure approaches and costing tends to underestimate the power of dynamic changes in the three co-evolving domains.

HEALTH AND TECHNOLOGICAL PRIORITIES OF THE NATION

As technological advances increase in India no sub-domain of healthcare will remain untouched, including different epistemic traditions of standardization whether in 'western' medicine or Ayurveda. These advances will also raise inevitable questions on the priorities and problem-solving capabilities of the state. Beyond several generations of chemical and drug advancement, newer dynamic and uncertain 'Industry 4.0' or the 'fourth Industrial Revolution' has had impact in Indian health-care too: rather than technological advances within R&D, prototyping, and manufacture, policymakers are additionally confronting technology transformations in other 'non-industrial' domains of healthcare—personnel skills, demand-signalling (including surveillance of needs, community feedback, monitoring of demand over time) as well as the evolution of demand (scale of governance and nature of demand). Moreover, technological advances are shaping delivery itself, to patients, hospitals, doctors, government, or other lead users. For example, refrigeration, mapping, tracking, and trucking technologies affect delivery of medicines, diagnostics, and vaccines from largely urban manufacturing and stocking centres to rural clinics. Similarly, technology platforms and large digital data advances are reshaping insurance coverage, privacy, and individual choice and policy autonomy. In other words, technological advances in any sphere of the triad lead (Figure 8.1) to (co-evolve with) multiple possible healthcare outcomes in other spheres as well.

One example of the complexities of conceptual and pragmatic framing is in the arena of non-communicable diseases (NCDs) surveillance. This is critically situated at the interface between demand and delivery dimensions of the triad (Figure 8.1) and is being fundamentally altered through several independent technology advances as well as some convergent industrial strategies on the production side. NCDs comprise heart diseases, stroke, cancer, diabetes, and chronic lung disease. NCDs exact an immense burden on Indian health, and NCD surveillance provides an important reminder of the need of systemic, institutional health capacity in all domains of the industrial triad.

Two large surveillance initiatives are underway in India—the WHO-ICMR NCD risk factor surveillance study and NCD risk factor survey under the Integrated Disease Surveillance Project (IDSP) (for example, Mishra et al. 2016). Both address India's NCD contributions of 14 per cent (5.2 million deaths) of the global total (WHO 2011). Technological advances in NCD surveillance are therefore pivotal to understanding whether and how the triad's dimensions are systemically functional or fragmented. For example, Nsubunga et al. (2006) refer to two hemispheres of surveillance itself: data generation and data use. Both aspects of surveillance have been transformed by digital technologies, telecommunications platforms, software and hardware advances. At the same time, they are also shaped by longstanding and newly forming industrial and innovation policy priorities, and by the independent strategies of businesses and nonprofits, patients, doctors, hospitals, and government programmes. Surveillance thus involves several actors using diverse technological advances (mobile phones, tablets, data analysis software) to interpret the data and disseminate them (again, by multiple means), including to decision-makers.

Therefore NCD surveillance requires considerable technical expertise and technology interventions on all three aspects of the WHO STEPS approach using behavioural, physical, and biochemical information (WHO 2003). Human resources and infrastructure needs alone in NCD surveillance include several technology-intensive requirements: use of information technology (IT) and data management, training and scaling up of training of community professionals, clinical tests and diagnostics of high-risk cases, and governance gaps across the jurisdiction of multiple ministries, for instance Ministry of Communications and Information Technology, Ministry of Skill Development and Entrepreneurship, and Ministry of AYUSH[1] (Mishra et al. 2016).

Just as with NCD surveillance, Indian microbial resistance also requires considerable convergence between the three domains of Figure 8.1 in order to bring together industrial and health policy-making efforts. Karnataka for instance, among India's more industrialized states, was the first to offer a biotechnology-specific policy map. It was one of the earliest to reap direct benefits of both public sector and private business investments in the cross-over domains of information technology and biotechnology development, and hosts a high concentration of scientific and engineering education and considerable private sector activity. It provides a strong health science and industrial production ecology, offering considerable 'bench to bedside' policy translation potential for the state government. Biotechnology advances and their considerable uncertainties shape the pace of growth and the nature of policy convergence in mature health sub-sectors.[2] For example, anti-microbial priorities which recognize the centrality of industry dynamics and healthcare potential within the state now comprise an important element of the biotechnology policy from 2017–22. Specific Karnataka state policy instruments focus technology on societal impact and offer policy inducements that push for closer ties between the science, engineering, technology, and demand and delivery concerns of social impact (for example, section 3.4).[3] An example of a social impact and policy convergence attempt is Karnataka state's Rare Diseases and Orphan Drugs (RDOD) policy. Drug-resistance strategies by the Karnataka state include several government departments, hospital networks, and other stakeholders; surveillance and informatics tools for human and animal diseases; identification of strains including genomics strategies to address rapid treatment; development of diagnostics technology to viral versus bacterial infections, as well as the production of new antimicrobials (discovery, development, manufacturing) (Karnataka government, 2017–22, p. 43).

Similarly, the Government of India has used financial incentives in policy steering of biotechnology initiatives towards reducing antimicrobial resistance thus orienting wider systemic reform between the Indian elements of Figure 8.1. These include the UK-funded Longitude Prize for seed funding to biotech startup firms and Finnish-funded (Tekes) to address competitiveness of Finnish and Indian firms in different biotechnology areas.

The reason to focus not only on market variety but markets at different scales of governance is influenced by India's quasi-federal system in which cities and rural areas, small towns, and state governments have to administer and manage a sizeable health system and determine its relevant moving parts. This subnational system offers additional permutations for institutional change such as an emphasis on economic development and local tax revenues, but also underscores complex economic incentives and regulatory pressures a state government may experience. As the policy thrust of the Karnataka government acknowledges, the capital city of Bengaluru is a hub for biotechnology and healthcare, and private firms in R&D, in manufacturing, and in hospitals, clinics, instrumentation, and IT-enabled healthcare services (ITeS healthcare). These have clustered for several reasons, but assisted through government incentives. While the incentives (fiscal, land, or other) operate at local levels, the regulatory levers on these firms (foreign

[1] AYUSH stands for Ayurvedic, Yoga and Naturopathy, Unani, Siddha and Homeopathy.

[2] Karnataka Industrial Policy 2014–19 (with Amendments)—G.O. no. CI 204 SPI 2015, Dated: 12 September 2016.

[3] 3.4. Invest in foundations of life sciences by creating technology platforms and encourage more effective multi-disciplinary collaborations to expand the scale and scope of biotechnology and its impact on the society and economy (Government of Karnataka, p. 27).

direct investment [FDI], technical standards, safety and quality, or pricing) are largely instituted at the national level. In times of health emergency, multiple subsystems begin to re-steer and come into conflict Repeated gaps in rabies vaccines, snake anti-venom, H1N1 flu (swine flu) treatments are industrial priorities: they require manufacturing capabilities, 'just-in-time', stocking and availability of the relevant drugs, and information and rapid testing and diagnosis. These are challenges not of market failure in the narrow sense but of the coordination of multiple market and non-market arrangements across the domains of production (from incubation to licensing), and of demand and delivery.

WHICH SYSTEM IS THE HEALTH INDUSTRY A PART OF?

It is no simple task therefore to determine the 'correct' economics for more complex ontological reasons, having to do with what a 'health system' is and in which wider economic system it is embedded. From an institutional perspective, and for pragmatic policy reasons, the health system includes jurisdictions of ministries and departments, budget allocations and transfers, specialization and discretion of personnel, and several 'hard' rules of technical standards, patents, and competition conditions. Until we know which 'system' we are referring to, we cannot correctly describe the appropriate 'rules of the game' to ensure that every Indian has access to the healthcare they need.

Rather than market failure and a single market for reference, multiple markets, the 'market menagerie' (Figure 8.1) permeate (at least) three interlinked contexts of production, demand, and delivery in which access to healthcare comes about. There are multiple markets operating at different geographic and organizational scales (Figure 8.1). The healthcare system itself is made up of several sub-systems that change and connect in ways that produce unpredictable outcomes for healthcare. Not only is the health industry and its technology components an essential part of any healthcare system, it is arguably the dominant element in it. This co-evolution is consistent with the combinatorial nature of institutions (Amable 2000). No single market for market failure exists in these three domains—rather these three institutional domains co-evolve. Even for countries with no indigenous production capability in product design, manufacturing, or industrial R&D labs, market concerns in the domains of delivery and demand are nevertheless still influenced by other institutions such as IPR, technical standards, clinics and hospital diagnostics and devices, pharmacy systems, and supply and stocking logistics.

For some time now, there has been a wider, growing articulation of how a historic institutionalism that informs political economy might benefit from an understanding of technological change. In my earlier work, I questioned the wisdom of advancing production capabilities in the absence of simultaneous exercising of the state's problem-solving muscle in demand and delivery. Poor signalling and systemic challenges pervade ministries and departments, which bear fewer responsibilities for healthcare and health outcomes. Cross-country evidence also demonstrates a range of social policy and industrial organization choices facing countries (Antonakis and Achilladelis 2001; Mackintosh et al. 2016; Srinivas 2012).

An evolutionary industrial analysis helps is because (a) it has been the area of economics with substantive empirical and theoretical breakthrough contributions on technological change and innovation analysis. Some originates in the Schumpeterian tradition, where dynamic attributes require non-equilibrium economics and open-ended outcomes; (b) it can also capture the evolutionary attributes of healthcare needs, and issues such as inclusion and demand (Hodgson 2008; Srinivas 2014, 2018); and (c) it has historic traditions that analyse social policy and industrial welfare. This is consistent with a wider political economy debate on structure, institutions, and economic transformation, identifying the autonomy and discretion that states and their bureaucracies retain in prioritizing their health interventions and reducing risks for ill-health. The evolutionary institutional approach in the realm of wider social policy has resonance not only in the industrial organization of Indian health, but also in the related domain of (largely socialist-driven but mixed-capitalist-enacted) aspirational 'European' industrial welfare entitlements. The division of labour between the ministries of health and labour, for instance, further exacerbates divisions in terms of entitlement structure which separates India's 'unorganized' sector (broadly, informal workers) from other citizens and residents, and at the same time, perpetuates tensions in place-based, work-based, and workplace-based (P, W, WP) entitlements for healthcare seekers and in which 'organized' factory labour still retains political influence, and industrial policy and fiscal importance (Srinivas 2010).

These tensions of political and programmatic entitlements keep India away from universal ambitions of healthcare. The cross-national perspective alerts us to the fact that a big differentiator among capable, and democratic, supplier nations such as India and Brazil are not supply side capabilities, considerable though those are, but policy approaches to healthcare demand. For this reason, the relationship between technological advances and structural inequalities is a core concern in innovation analyses, and has manifested in literature specifically focused on inclusion and studies on the demand side: the economics of wants, needs, effective demand, derived demand, and related concerns (see Srinivas 2014, 2018). However, the epistemological approach to this demand takes different routes in economics (Robert and Yoguel 2016). These paths may not have easy single or universal health measures of effective institutional change, for example, quality-adjusted life years (QALYs), disability-adjusted life year (DALYs), per capita income or number of hospital beds and doctors per 10,000 population. Instead, industry system concerns focus on alternative metrics and systems of product design, contexts in which access and affordability can be met, supply chain concentration and value extraction, input resources, market share and export revenue, manufacturing value addition, and so on.

Health, labour, S&T, industrial, finance, and trade ministries and line agencies are often disconnected on critical technology and healthcare outcomes. Uncoordinated outputs across government and public organizations emerge: from knowledge commissions, NITI Aayog, mission-mode elements of Indian technology plans, the new 2013 science, technology, and innovation (STI) planning documents for the country, and state-level planning departments, ministries of finance, labour, and industries and commerce, and a range of powerful and historically critical public sector companies in chemicals, vaccines, or electronics.

Healthcare and its economics are part of a wider set of phenomenological questions that can be asserted about India's longstanding but troubled romance with S&T in national development. Abrol (2004, 2014) for example, captures the specific and repeated tensions that have plagued Indian technological and scientific interventions from health to water, pointing to unresolved and perhaps irresolvable tensions between Gandhian, Nehruvian, and Left perspectives on how to expand socioeconomic inclusion and participation from technological advance and scientific knowledge. The prospects for resolution (and revolution) have often found outlets in the creation of pan-Indian, cross-technology institutes such as the Council for Scientific and Industrial Research (CSIR). Yet, because of a series of political and ideological compromises by ruling governments and advocates over time, no fundamental conceptual change emerged in policy design to better embed technology, engineering and science within the economy (Abrol 2004, 2014). As a consequence, India's flagship research and translation institutes: the Indian Institutes of Technology, Indian Institute of Science, CSIR, and others have struggled to offer a social alternative with consistency or political viability.

This national dependence on large-scale and mostly centralized ideals of industry and healthcare flies in the face of India's immense size and diversity. The diversity requires localized attention to technological innovation and the social context of demonstration and demand to which both policy design and a traditional economics of industrial change can be quite blind. Outside the scientific advances and engineering possibilities of formal health R&D and with considerable health impact are what can be termed 'scarcity-induced innovations' (Srinivas and Sutz 2008). These are idiosyncratic innovation outliers that are traditionally ignored by a cost and consumption calculus on the one hand, as well as the supply chains analysis. Examples include Cuba's Hib (Haemophilus influenzae type b) vaccine (high science), neonatal incubators from Uruguay (innovative engineering plus science), and India's Jaipur Foot (a rubber-based prosthetic leg; low-cost iterative experimentation and customization of materials and kinetics). These have a series of innovative attributes including scientific or process engineering breakthroughs. They are not simple process modifications of problems framed and solved elsewhere, but have local, customized, and cognitive dimensions of problem solving (Srinivas and Sutz 2008), and 'under the radar' policy challenges (Kaplinsky 2011) with weak demand (Arocena and Sutz 2000). Demand evolution and the management and coordination of supply is a policy challenge to theory and to the dynamic nature of divergence, feedback, and coordination of diverse actors (Hodgson 2008; Srinivas 2014, 2018).

THE DOUBLE-EDGED SWORD OF EXPORT SUCCESS: GLOBAL DIPLOMACY AND TRADE

Finally, every nation has, as its right, a broadly autonomous sphere in which to determine the degrees to which each of the three dimensions is an industrial, or health, priority as India becomes more globally relevant in geopolitics and foreign policy. Figure 8.1 provides a comparative, national viewpoint to view new partners and geographic leadership. In the previous century, extraordinary technological advances from fermentation and bioprocess engineering to genomics and diagnostics led to an enormous shift in supplier countries and firms. Brazil and India, both enormously successful in their industrial and innovation policies in boosting a domestic industry, have nevertheless chosen different balancing acts with Brazil spending far more to boost their demand institutions, with guaranteed social minimum wages and cash-transfer benefits toward education and health spending. Non-democratic Cuba tightly managed all three domains to extend access to medicines and vaccines through an extensive network of primary healthcare centres, and combined production and testing with extensive surveillance and registration of health users. Democratic experiments in Kenya have improved the production capabilities alongside delivery systems.

International exports from India are increasingly defining its diplomatic relationships. In 2012, Uganda led African countries with 57.6 per cent or USD 204 million of its pharmaceutical formulation imports coming from India, while South Africa at a lower 15.9 per cent, still imported USD 1,890 million (Chaudhari 2016: 110).

As we saw also in Table 8.1, Brazil, India, Cuba, and to some degree Kenya, have the degree of autonomy to link, extend, or deepen the ties between the three dimensions because of supply capabilities, including vertical integration and specialization in several technologies. This frees them up to greater degrees of make versus buy, relative to Sri Lanka, Tanzania, or Peru, which must depend on imports to ensure response to demand, and also coordinate delivery to clinics, hospitals, and pharmacies.

Co-evolution in Figure 8.1 of the three institutional domains is an idea centrally embedded in the economics of institutional analysis and Schumpeterian approaches to innovation. It is rarely used in orthodox cost–benefit economics where a zero-sum, winner–loser rhetoric has retained methodological narrowness and political sway in policymaking circles. Co-evolution reflects development complexity. It underscores a combinatorial notion of how multiple institutional effects may occur at once and change alongside. Co-evolution captures the fact that nations do not first technologically advance on the supply side, before attempting to ensure their citizens have access, and neither do they improve the delivery of essential vaccines or diagnostics without becoming aware of bottlenecks in refrigeration and electricity, trucking or storage, and of worrying gaps in personnel capabilities. Multiple spheres of state action make for higher thresholds to ensure coordinated and systemic responses: minimum sub-systems need to be in place with public capacities to plan, manage, tweak, and improve and distil necessary feedback and modifications.

Co-evolution makes more evident the opportunities and challenges of developing problem-framing and problem-solving capacity in simultaneous, coordinated fashion across state agencies and with non-state partners. 'Mission-mode' polio successes in India built extensive scope and reach through nodal agencies and established procedures for repeated, iterative coordination and sustained communication across multiple agencies and organizations from the government to Indian NGOs, to Rotary International. Deployment of actual immunization took place on a war footing, to bus stops, households, schools, and other everyday locations of people in their daily activity. Polio's mission-mode, however, technically required only partial co-evolution in the triad because polio production had been mostly accomplished—the oral polio vaccine was by then a mature technology and the response required was primarily of appropriate supply and stocking, and last-mile delivery successes. In contrast, Cuba's Hib vaccine was a breakthrough, emerging from intimate ties across the scientific, industrial, and health policy and delivery spheres.

Technology and supply leadership are not synonymous with national health self-sufficiency. Table 8.3 indicates dominant industrial policy instruments in India, Brazil, Tanzania, Kenya, and Mozambique.

India's new start-up ecosystem of genomics-based diagnostics for breast cancer, prostate, and others, reflects new plan and regulatory tensions between technological advances with better diagnosis and treatments. New India–Africa geopolitics is influenced by such new 'lasers' for policy use become available (as in Table 8.3). The incubation and growth of these diagnostics is predominantly private and fuelled by venture capital investing, while public sector research institutes have continued to play a role quite different from the US (VijayRaghavan and Saberwal 2017). This mixed ownership model has muddied a simpler economics that discussed costs and benefits divided between public and private owners. In such a model, the state bore the primary burden of the extraction of these public and windfall benefits.

As these new forms of ownership and responsibilities keep changing, so too do the expectations that the state can keep up with creating, shaping, or regulating the contexts in which these technologies emerge and advance. Nowhere is this interplay of relevant economics with changing technologies as visible as in the case of medical devices whose importance for development is now well-recognized and whose close ties to local production considered imperative (Mahal and Karan 2009; Miesen 2013; WHO 2010). The range of technical challenges and bottlenecks to formulate a viable medical devices policy is in sharp contrast to the strong supportive policy framework for Indian pharmaceutical generics and some vaccines (Srinivas 2004). There exist important details for why the medical devices industry has suffered this fate despite its enormous importance not only for healthcare but also for addressing inequality (Jaroslawski and Saberwal 2013; Kale and Wield 2018). Rather, medical devices require more closely crafted local production and testing (Miesen 2013), active industry associations with health policy advocacy closely linked to science–technological advances and industrial policy (Kale and Wield 2018), and ambitious public sector efforts (VijayRaghavan and Saberwal 2017).

Economics should be able to help us answer whether this supply dominance helps at home, helps others, and if so, how. In a localized analysis of health too, its technology attributes should be visible and dynamic. Here, trade analysis tied narrowly to export revenue provides little information. The complementarity or substitutability of India's (mostly) private firms exporting to, collaborating with, investing and physically establishing themselves in African sites, can be more systematically answered through a technology analysis using a framework that captures all three domains. For instance, the production growth of Indian cancer diagnostics is represented by significant advances in oncology product design and R&D, as well as manufacture. In addition, private Indian investments in cancer treatment is increasingly stretching to consumption-side interventions and to delivery logistics in India as well as Ghana, Kenya, and Tanzania. Collaborative ventures using a combination of incubation assistance through grants and other means can also eventually generate complex competition dynamics in Africa and the Indian subcontinent. India-based Villgro Innovations Foundation focuses on early-stage incubation of social enterprises in Kenyan healthcare.[4] Healthcare-related ITeS matches health providers such as Vaidam and PlanmyMedicalTrip.com with the patients across the public–private divide, using government links, a vast array of Indian and African referral partners (doctors, clinics, hospitals), and travel services providers such as Emirates and hotels.[5]

While the first market environment displays specific design and regulatory priorities, the second market environment for Indian firms raises other challenges (Srinivas 2004, 2006). The '3 Ws'—WHO, WTO, and the Wax–Hatchman Act—demonstrate the overseas regulatory pressures on Indian investment and response to overseas demand and delivery. Indian generic and vaccine firms successfully supplied large institutional buyers from the WHO to US and European healthcare regimes. Export success in this critical phase has since defined both the ability of private firms to expand further into new (and in some instances, technically simpler) markets of Africa; test Indian and African consumers alongside on a case-by-case basis for specific technology markets, while building out a large simultaneous services push into new demand and delivery segments.

Medical tourism and ITeS in diagnosis and logistics is a large part of the current Africa strategy with Nigerians (42.4 per cent), Tanzanians (18.5 per cent), and Kenyans (9.2 per cent) alone providing substantial historic and contemporary interest (India Tourism Statistics 2013; James et al. 2015, 2017). Indian FDI is growing in Africa, as are joint ventures with technology transfer (Chaudhuri 2016; Government of Kenya 2010; URT 2016). East Africa acts as a special hub today for IT-enabled search and rating in health-related e-commerce and logistics. The Indian government's overseas support include to tele-medicine and tele-education platforms via close connections to 12 specialty Indian hospitals launched in 53 African countries (KPMG and CII 2015; Ngangom and Aneja 2016). While the Indian private sector ventures and diplomatic initiatives are driven by commercial opportunities for Indian firms and feel-good diplomacy measures, only a more systematic future analysis of the specifics of technology transfer and local production outcomes will show whether Indian medicines and devices have acted as substitutes for local production in other nations or as an important complementary dynamic both at home and abroad.

***

An enormous healthcare transformation has been underway for decades, manifested in specific technological

[4] http://disrupt-africa.com/2017/02/indias-villgro-launches-healthcare-incubator-in-kenya/, last accessed on 14 December 2017.

[5] The medical tourism market in India is estimated at USD 3 billion as of 2015, with some estimates of a USD 8 billion valuation by 2020.

sub-revolutions in pharmaceuticals, vaccines, biotechnologies, new devices, and diagnostics, and vast new frontiers being broached with machine learning and wider artificial intelligence, genomics, materials, and devices.

The rapid evolution of the sector and specialized capital and knowledge accumulation with relatively low policy representation and others wielding enormous market and policy power, requires a new approach to economics—more attentive to an economics that moves well beyond market failure theory, focused on learning and technological change and explains sub-sector differences. Bottlenecks in financing, prototyping, commercialization, and feedback continue to plague health self-reliance. Consequently, technological analysis remains central to healthcare systems irrespective of their political contexts, but the 'why's, 'how's, and 'when's of policy design and public administration reform are contingent on how health policy and industrial aspirations come together.

REFERENCES

Abrol, D. 2004. 'Lessons from the Design of Innovation Systems for Rural Industrial Clusters in India', *Asian Journal of Technology Innovation* 12(2): 67–94.

———. 2014. 'Pro-poor Innovation Making, Knowledge Production, and Technology Implementation for Rural Areas: Lessons from the Indian Experience', in Innovation in India: Combining Economic Growth with Inclusive Development, edited by S. Ramani. New Delhi: Cambridge University Press.

Achilladelis, B. and N. Antonakis. 2001. 'The Dynamics of Technological Innovation: The case of the Pharmaceutical Industry', *Research Policy* 30(4): 535–88.

Chaudhuri, S. 2016. 'Can Foreign Firms Promote Local Production of Pharmaceuticals in Africa?' in *Making Medicines in Africa*, edited by M. Mackintosh, G. Banda, P. Tibandebage, and W. Wamae, pp. 103–21. London: Palgrave Macmillan.

Gehl-Sampath, P. 2008. 'India's Pharmaceutical Sector in 2008: Emerging Strategies and Global and Local Implications for Access to Medicines', report prepared by Department for International Development, UK.

Government of India. n.d.. National Biotechnology Development Strategy 2015–2020. Available at https://pib.gov.in/newsite/printrelease.aspx?relid=134035, last accessed on 15 March 2018.

Government of Karnataka. n.d. Karnataka Biotechnology Policy 2017–2022. Available at http://itbt.karnataka.gov.in, last accessed on 28 April 2018.

Harilal, M.S. 2009. 'Commercialising Traditional Medicine: Ayurvedic Manufacturing in Kerala', *Economic and Political Weekly* 44(16): 44–51.

Hodgson, G.M. 2008. 'An Institutional and Evolutionary Perspective on Health Economics', *Cambridge Journal of Economics* 32(2): 235–56.

James, T.C., Prativa Shaw, Payel Chatterjee, and Deepti Bhatia. 2015. 'India–Africa Partnership in Health Care: Accomplishments and Prospects', research report published by Research and Information System for Development Countries, New Delhi.

Jaroslawski, S. and G. Saberwal. 2013. 'Case Studies of Innovative Medical Device Companies from India: Barriers and Enablers to Development', *BMC Health Services Research* 13(1): 199–207.

Kale, D. and D. Wield. 2018. 'In Search of Missing Hand of Collaborative Action: Evidence from Medical Device Industry', *Innovation & Development* 9(1): 1–23.

KPMG and Confederation of Indian Industry. 2015. 'India and Africa—Collaboration for Growth'. Available at https://www.kpmg.com/IN/en/IssuesAndInsights/ArticlesPublications/Documents/India-Africa-Summit2015.pdf, last accessed on 12 December 2017.

Lotz, P. 1993. 'Demand as a Driving Force in Medical Innovation', *International Journal of Technology Assessment in Health Care* 9(2): 174–88.

Mackintosh, M., G. Banda, P. Tibandebage, and W. Wamae (eds). 2016. *Making Medicines in Africa*. London: Palgrave Macmillan.

Mackintosh, M., J. Mugwagwa, G. Banda, P. Tibandebage, J. Tunguhole, S. Wangwe, and M. Karimi Njeru. 2018. 'Health-Industry Linkages for Local Health: Reframing Policies for African Health System Strengthening'. *Health Policy and Planning* 33(4): 602–10.

Mahal, A. and A. Karan. 2009. 'Diffusion of Medical Technology: Medical Devices in India'. *Expert Review of Medical Devices* 6(2): 197–205.

Miesen, M. 2013. The Inadequacy of Donating Medical Devices to Africa', *The Atlantic*, 20 September. Available at http://www.theatlantic.com/international/archive/2013/09/the-inadequacy-of-donating-medicaldevices-to-africa/279855/, last accessed on 3 March 2018.

Mishra, U.S., S.I. Rajan, William Joe and Ali Mehdi. 2016. 'Health Surveillance of Chronic Diseases: Challenges and Strategies for India', Health Policy Initiative Policy Brief 4, Indian Council for Research on International Economic Relations (ICRIER), New Delhi.

Ngangom, T. and U. Aneja. 2016. 'Health is Wealth: Indian Private Sector Investments in African Healthcare', Issue Brief, no 145, Observer Research Foundation, New Delhi.

Nsubuga, P., M.E. White, S.B. Thacker, M.A. Anderson, S.B. Blount, C.V. Broome, T.M. Chiller, et al. 2006. 'Public Health Surveillance: A Tool for Targeting and Monitoring Interventions', in *Disease Control Priorities in Developing Countries*, edited by D.T. Jamison, J.G. Breman,

A.R. Measham, George Alleyne, Mariam Claeson, David B. Evans, Prabhat Jha, Anne Mills, and Philip Musgrov, second edition, pp. 997–1015. Washington, DC: World Bank.

Ramani, S. 2002. 'Who's interested in Biotechnology: R&D Strategies, Knowledge Base and Market Sales of Indian Biopharmaceutical Firms', *Research Policy* 31(3): 381–98.

Robert, V. and G. Yoguel. 2016. 'Complexity Paths in Neo-Schumpeterian Evolutionary Economics, Structural Change and Development Policies', *Structural Change and Economic Dynamics* 38: 3–14.

Srinivas, S. 2006. 'Industry and Innovation: Some Lessons from Vaccine Procurement', *World Development* 34(10): 1742–64.

———. 2010. 'Industrial Welfare and the State: Nation and City Reconsidered', *Theory and Society* 39(3–4): 451–70.

———. 2012. *Market Menagerie: Health and Development in Late Industrial States*. Palo Alto, CA: Stanford University Press, Economics and Finance imprint.

———. 2014. 'Demand and Innovation: Paths to Inclusive Development', in *Innovation in India: Combining Economic Growth with Inclusive Development*, edited by S. Ramani, pp. 78–104. New Delhi: Cambridge University Press.

———. 2016. 'Healthy Industries and Unhealthy Populations: Lessons from Indian Problem-Solving', in *Making Medicines in Africa*, edited by M. Mackintosh, G. Banda, P. Tibandebage, and W. Wamae, pp. 183–99. London: Palgrave Macmillan.

———. 2018. 'Evolutionary Demand, Innovation, Development', in *Development with Global Value Chains: Upgrading and Innovation in Asia*, edited by D. Nathan, S. Sarkar, and M. Tewari, pp. 349–73. New Delhi: Cambridge University Press.

VijayRaghavan, K. and G. Saberwal. 2017. 'Bio-business in Brief: The Case for Ambitious Action in the Public Sector', *Current Science* 113: 1841–5.

WHO (World Health Organization). 2003. 'Surveillance of Risk Factors for Noncommunicable Diseases: The WHO STEPwise Approach'. *Noncommunicable Diseases and Mental Health*. Geneva: World Health Organization.

———. 2010. 'Medical Devices: Managing the Mismatch', report of the Priority Medical devices project. Available at http://www.who.int/medical_devices/en/, last accessed on 3 March 2018.

———. 2011. *Global Status Report on NCDs: Description of the Global Burden of NCDs 2010, Their Risk Factors and Determinants*. Geneva: World Health Organization. Available at http://www.who.int/nmh/publications/ncd_report2010/en/, last accessed on 28 April 2018.

———. 2012. 'Local Production and Technology Transfer to Increase Access to Medical Devices: Addressing the Barriers and Challenges in Low- and Middle-Income Countries'. Available at http://www.who.int/medical_devices/1240EHT_final.pdf, last accessed on 3 March 2018.

Wilson, P., S. Post, and S. Srinivas. 2007. 'R&D Models: Lessons from Vaccine History', IAVI Policy Research Discussion Paper no. 14, International AIDS Vaccine Initiative, New York.

9

Health and Economy Linkage

Systems and Conditions in the Indian Context

Venkatanarayana Motkuri and Amir Ullah Khan

Conventional wisdom informs us that economic growth is a precondition for improvements in the domain of human health. Research studies and reports especially that of the World Health Organization (WHO) and the World Bank over the last few decades have made a turnaround in this regard. They established the impact of health investments in poverty reduction and economic growth (see Bloom and Canning 2008; Sachs 2001; Schultz 2005; World Bank 1993). The usual pathway is that better macroeconomic fundamentals such as high economic growth and stability are conditions enhancing the resources available for social spending including health and improves living standards of people by generating employment opportunities and improved income that in turn improves health conditions. Therefore, the two-way relationship established shows that human health condition affects the macroeconomic fundamentals which is affected by the macroeconomic policies and conditions/performance. It is very clear now that unless there is a lead priority for investment in health, the vicious circle of poor health condition affecting economic development, which in turn further depreciates the investment in health and health conditions of people continue.

Given the backdrop, this chapter explores conceptual and analytical macroeconomic framework for health and empirically analyses the linkages and two-way relationship between the health and economic growth.

IMPACT OF HEALTH ON ECONOMIC GROWTH AND VICE VERSA

The conventional indicator of development per capita income is, in fact, a manifestation of labour force participation rate, the sectoral composition or occupational distribution of workforce, and labour productivity in different sectors (Bhadhuri 2006). Structural change along with a rise in productivity (of factors of production) is considered as critical for economic growth (Kaldor 1957). Indeed, productivity of labour is critical for improving economic development at a macro level as well as the living standard of a household at a micro level. Labour productivity is influenced by the level of human capital consisting of education and health. Growth studies have been observing significant contribution of human capital to economic growth (see Becker 1964; Dennison 1967; Shultz 1961). Both education and health have intrinsic as well as instrumental values.

While they are fundamental in improving human welfare on their own right, they have economic values along with being considered as a means to enhance economic growth through labour productivity. There is a growing consensus that is emerging about health and education which considers them as not merely consumption goods but also critical investment goods. It is more or less clear on the effect of human capital involving education on productivity of labour and thereby on economic growth. In the same line, there is growing research interests in understanding the impact of health on economy.

Earlier studies that have examined the changes in demographic characteristics and health conditions in various societies broadly identified three factors in health improvements, particularly through declining mortality (see Preston 1980). They are: socioeconomic development, social policy measures, and technical changes (advancements in medicine and medical technology resulting in reduced cost of healthcare). The emphasis on the role of these three broad categories of factors varies across studies (Bloom and Canning 2008; Cutler, Deaton, and Lleras-Muney 2006; Preston 1975, 1980). Moreover, one of the points that emerged from the earlier studies was that the immediate fallout of decline in mortality is growth of population leading to Malthusian trap rather than leveraging any economic betterment. But later studies have shown that mortality decline followed by eventual decline in birth rate along with technological advancement in organization of production lead to betterment of human life (Boserup 1965).

Through earlier research it is known that socioeconomic development largely involved with income growth is one of the factors in improving health conditions. The Preston Curves has shown the changing relationship between life expectancy and income levels across countries (Bloom and Canning 2008; Preston 1975). Further, the Preston (1975) study observed that a significant portion of the improvement in life expectancy through the declining mortality rate was factors other than income growth. In the same line of thought, the Easterly (1999) study found a weak relationship between income and health in the sense that growth in income improving health conditions is not so great. It is also observed that there are instances (cross-country experiences) and phases (temporal) of health improvements without much corresponding economic growth and also income growth without corresponding health improvements (Preston 1980; Weil 2013). The other factors involved in health improvements were technological advancements in medicine and social institutions (Bloom and Canning 2008; Cutler, Deaton, and Lleras-Muney 2006; Preston 1975, 1980).

Moreover, with research emerging over the last two decades, there has been a turnaround in understanding the relationship between health and economic growth. Following the conventional wisdom of health depends on economic growth, and policy priority meant increasing income growth. But emerging research studies have been informing to change the policy priority investing in health, as they found impact of good health conditions on economic growth (Aghion, Howitt, and Murtin 2010; Bloom and Canning 2008; Bloom, Canning, and Fink 2009; Bloom, Canning, and Sevilla 2001; Murphy and Topel 2005; Schultz 2002, 2005, 2010; Weil 2005). With the advancement in methodologies estimating the aggregate production function, the improvements in health conditions are being accounted for as a source of economic growth (Bloom, Canning, and Sevilla 2001).

The growth accounting framework developed with the post-War development thinking was for identifying source of economic growth using the aggregate production function introduced by Solow. The exercise left a considerable residual part of economic growth accounting for factors other than labour and physical capital. The Solow residual, as it is referred, was considered as growth accounted for total factor productivity (TFP) which in turn comprises human capital and technological changes. Over a period, using evolving advanced methods, estimates are drawn for components of human capital separately from the pool of labour and TFP. In this regard, Bloom, Canning, and Sevilla (2001) study by constructing aggregate production that included health as a separate factor along with labour, capital, education, and experience found positive and statistically significant effect of health on economic growth. As their estimates show a one-year improvement in a population's life expectancy contributes to a 4 per cent increase in output. Behrman and Rosenzweig (2004) estimated certain returns to birth weights through schooling and better payoff in labour market. Murphy and Topel (2005) study estimated more than USD 1 trillion as the social value of increased longevity and progress against various diseases for the American economy.

Indeed, health is a multidimensional construct involving health inputs and various forms of outcomes and conditions. It consists of health outcomes or conditions such as mortality, ill-health, malnutrition, anaemia, low birthweights, and many more. Life expectancy is a one summary measure of the state of disease burden indicating probability of premature death (mortality) owing to any fatal disease. But life expectancy does not capture the impact of non-fatal diseases and disabilities on living humans restricting their potential physical and mental abilities and their participation in economic and non-economic activities. In this regard, the WHO in 1990 developed a metric for measuring disease burden through a construct referred to as disability-adjusted life years (DALYs). It consists of two components, that is years of life lost (YLLs) due to premature death (mortality) and years (of productive life) lost due to disease/disability or ill-health (or simply years lost due to disability [YLD]) of those living.

In fact, GDP growth discussions included the full income approach that adds value of life expectancy to the growth accounting calculations. This approach combines growth in national income, GDP, with the value people place on increased life expectancy—that is, the value of their additional life years (VLYs). Global Health 2035 report (Lancet 2013) estimates that 24 per cent of growth in full income in low- and middle-income countries between 2000 and 2011 resulted from health improvements. Hence, the initial health of a population is definitely a robust driver of economic growth. As Nordhaus (2002) has shown in the US, half of the growth in full income during the first half of the twentieth century had resulted from mortality declines, and slightly less than half during the second half of the twentieth century. Real income in the US went up six times and life expectancy went up by 25 years during this period. Clearly, the impact of health on GDP is substantial—an extra year of life expectancy is estimated to raise a country's per capita GDP by about 4 per cent, for example.[1]

The *World Development Report* (*WDR*) 1993 by the World Bank, which examined gains from investing in health nearly 25 years ago, had argued then that investing in health is one means of accelerating development (World Bank 1993). The *WDR* 1993 advocated then a threefold approach to health policy.[2] First, to foster an economic environment.[3] Second, redirect government spending away from specialized care and toward such low-cost and highly effective activities.[4] Third, encourage greater diversity and competition in the provision of health services by decentralization.[5] These reforms could translate into longer, healthier, and more productive lives for people around the world, and especially for the poor. The report of the Commission on Macroeconomics and Health that was set up by the WHO and headed by Jeffrey Sachs had addressed the impact of health investments in poverty reduction and economic growth (see WHO 2001). It is also observed that foreign direct investment is attracted to environments where labour is not vulnerable to heavy disease burdens (Alsan, Bloom, and Canning 2006).

Similarly, in 2004 the International Monetary Fund (IMF) asserted the following: first, improving health outcomes is linked not only to the provision of health services, but also to interventions outside the health sector.[6] Second, achieving sharp declines in maternal mortality requires behavioural changes in prenatal care and delivery and an improved road network, in addition to improved hospital care. Third, delivering health services effectively requires the coordination of policies across a number of fields.[7] In 2013, the European Commission stated that despite the improvement in average levels of health across the European Union (EU), the data is hiding major inequalities.[8] It observed that poorer and disadvantaged people die younger and suffer more often from disability and disease. The Commission argued that investing in sustainable health systems combines

[1] The intrinsic value of mortality changes, measured in terms of the value of a statistical life (VSL) is even more substantial.

[2] It is meant for governments in developing countries and in the formerly socialist countries.

[3] This will enable households to improve their own health. Policies for economic growth that ensure income gains for the poor are essential. So, too, is expanded investment in schooling, particularly for girls.

[4] Such as immunization, programmes to combat micronutrient deficiencies, and control and treatment of infectious diseases. By adopting the packages of public health measures and essential clinical care described in the report, developing countries could reduce their burden of disease by 25 per cent.

[5] Particularly decentralizing government services, promoting competitive procurement practices, fostering greater involvement by non-governmental and other private organizations, and regulating insurance markets.

[6] Access to clean water and education for mothers are both key determinants of infant and child mortality rates.

[7] These include public sector management policies that provide adequate incentives to health care providers; procurement and distribution policies for pharmaceuticals so that these are available in sufficient quantities in the right places; public health measures to protect the population; and suitable regulation and quality control for private providers, who often deliver more health services than public providers.

[8] The European Commission, in its document on 'Investing in Health', February 2013. Available at https://ec.europa.eu/health/sites/health/files/policies/docs/swd_investing_in_health.pdf, accessed on 11 August 2018.

innovative reforms aimed at improving cost-efficiency and reconciling fiscal consolidation targets with the continued provision of sufficient levels of public services.

An Opposite Argument and Consensus

However, the growing understanding of impact of health on economic growth has attracted criticism from certain sections of scholars. Some of the studies have come up with evidence that the degree of impact of health on economic growth is not so great as it has been estimated by some studies (Acemoglu and Johnson 2007; Acemoglu, Johnson, and Robinson 2003; Ashraf, Lester and Weil 2008; Weil 2013). They pointed out some methodological issues involved in estimating the impact of health on economic growth.

Some of the issues associated with estimating the value of health for economic growth is endogenity of health as a result of income growth or two-way causality between health and economic growth (Bloom, Canning, and Sevilla 2001). Secondly, the issue is the construct of a health input factor. In other words it is about what form of health involving health inputs or health outcomes (for instance, life expectancy, disease burden, illness, mortality rate, nutrition level and so on,) one can consider to place it in the aggregate production function for estimating the impact of health on economic growth (see Bloom and Canning 2008). Notwithstanding these issues, there is growing understanding and consensus that health has impact on economic growth but it is not a one-way street, there is a two-way casualty between the two.

Systems and Conditions of Health and Economy

The flowchart presented further (Figure 9.1) illustrates the linkages between economy and health through the systems and conditions in these domains. As Frenk (2004) observes growth, income, investment, and employment are functions of the performance and quality of the economic system including its regulatory frameworks, social and economic policies, social and human capital, and labour markets. The health conditions (morbidity, mortality, and disability) depend not only on economic conditions or standards of living but also on the actual performance of the health system (Frenk 2004).

The influence of health on the economy in general and per capita income in particular, is seen in terms of healthy workers being more productive than comparable others who suffer from poor health (Bloom and

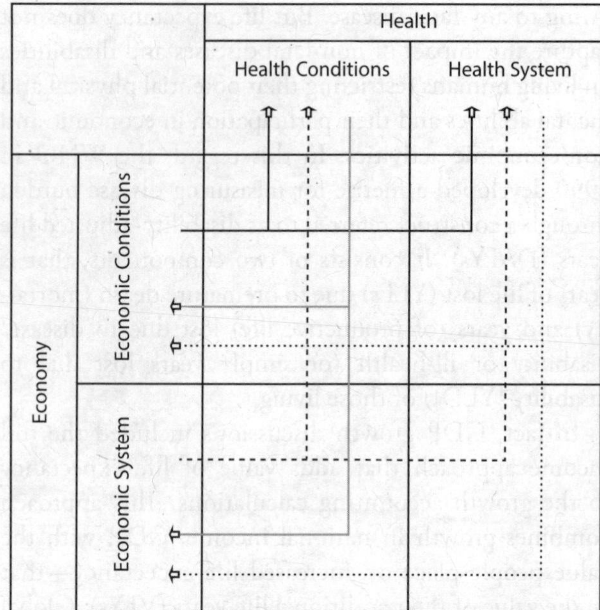

Figure 9.1 Relationship between Health and Economy
Adapted from Frenk (2004).

Canning 2008; Schultz 2002, 2005). The better health conditions improve the labourers' chances at productivity and thereby increasing their earnings. Better health also raises per capita incomes through investment, saving, and expenditure decisions[9] (Bloom, Canning, and Graham 2003). Health conditions of children improve their school attendance and learning that in turn improves their ability to earn more in their adult life (Aghion, Howitt, and Murtin 2010; Behrman and Rosenzweig 2004; Bloom and Canning 2008; Bloom, Canning, and Fink 2009; Bloom, Canning, and Sevilla 2001; Murphy and Topel 2005; Weil 2005).

On the other hand, better economic conditions enable people at the household level to afford healthcare and the state at the macro level to finance better health systems. Better macroeconomic fundamentals such as high economic growth and stability enhances the resources available for social spending and improves living standards of people by generating employment opportunities and improved income that in turn improves the health conditions by facilitating poor households to be able to afford the same (Aghion, Howitt and Murtin 2010; Behrman and Rosenzweig 2004; Bloom and Canning 2008; Bloom, Canning, and

[9] Retirement schemes and pension accounts raise large resources in countries with high life expectancy.

Fink 2009; Bloom, Canning, and Sevilla 2001; Frenk 2004; Murphy and Topel 2005; Weil 2005). Both health and economic growth each having its impact on the other, have other exogenous determinant factors working for each of them. Technology influences economic growth and plays a key role in improving health conditions.

Health as a Multi-Dimensional Concept

As mentioned earlier, health is by nature a multi-dimensional construct/concept (Weil 2013). Holistically, it is to reflect the person's mental (cognitive) and physical conditions. Usually it is considered that (a good) health is the state of being free from illness/diseases, infirmity and/or injury. It is also about psychomotor condition reflecting the coordination between cognitive functions and physical movements. The ideal life is that which involves living long and healthy. But certain conditions of diseases, disabilities, and disorders affect or restrict the cognitive functions and/or physical movements resulting in health conditions (morbidity) below normal healthy life. Fatal diseases and those otherwise if not attended would result in premature death (mortality).

In a person's lifecycle, life begins as a foetus in the uterus of the mother. External environment and health conditions of mothers facilitate or affect internal development of the foetuses. Depending on these and the delivery conditions, certain health conditions are acquired at birth (cognitive disorders, physical infirmities, low birthweight). Maternal health conditions such as women's body mass index, anaemia and malnutrition affects not only the foetus but also the growth of the child in the postnatal life. The postnatal life of infants and children is very sensitive and depends on delivery conditions, childhood diseases, anaemia, and nutritional status (stunting). Under-nutrition (stunting, underweight, and wasting) along with certain health conditions or diseases not only affect cognitive and physical development of children but also result in death (neonatal, infant or child mortality). The health status beyond childhood depends on the health conditions including cognitive and physical development during childhoods and conditions at each stage of life that one passes through. Of course, certain disease conditions vary across geographical regions such as tropical and humid, and within certain regions.

With this in the background, one can say that there is no single measure that can capture health status of population or individual comprehensively. The death probabilities captured through life expectancy and IMR as a summary measures of health do not reflect health status or conditions of those living (Weil 2013). Health conditions such as anaemia and malnutrition among women and children, low birthweight of children are different dimensions of health. Cognitive development captured through intelligent quotient (IQ) is another dimension of health. In this regard, along with DALY, the recent metric of health adjusted life expectancy (HALE) has combined the death probability and health status during the period of life lived. Still, it is very difficult to have a comprehensive measure of health status of population.

The studies that examined the impact of health on economic growth in fact varied in their construction of health variables (Weil 2013). For instance, the Preston Curves has shown the relationship between life expectancy and per capita income (Preston 1975). Behrman and Rosenzweig (2004) study examined the impact of low birthweight on the adult earnings in the labour market. The cross-country study by Shastry and Weil (2003) examined the relationship between income and women who are not anaemic. Some other studies have examined the impact of Flynn effect[10] of rising IQ on economic growth (Weil 2013). But all they did was establish the impact of health conditions on economic growth.

MACRO ECONOMY: PERFORMANCE OF THE INDIAN ECONOMY AND STATE POLICY

Macro Scenario

During the post-reform period, especially in the second phase, Indian economy has emerged as one of the fastest growing in the world.[11] In its growth trajectory the Indian economy has moved away (up) from the dubious feature of the 'Hindu rate of growth' (that is 3.5 per cent) since the 1980s and the rate of growth of Indian economy further accelerated to not less than 6 per cent (high growth trajectory) during the post-reform period. The Indian economy has waded through situations of poor agriculture growth with short supply of foodgrain that were unable to match population growth leading to severe food crisis in 1960s,[12] which resulted in importing

[10] It refers to the rise in measured IQ in developed countries over a period (see Flynn 1987).

[11] According to the World Economic Forum's valuation of 2017, of the 10 biggest economies in the world, India is placed at seventh with USD 2.1 trillion worth's economy.

[12] The first sign of severe food shortage was observed in 1965. The food production fell to an all-time low in 1966 and immediately foodgrain imports from USA had rescued India from an otherwise famine situation.

foodgrain; adverse impact of subsequent multiple wars with neighbouring countries (Pakistan and China) in 1960s and 1970s; oil crisis/shocks of 1970s;[13] and balance of payment problems of the late 1980s, leading to an economic crisis that culminated in 1991.[14] The economy was also able to withstand the global financial crisis (2007) as well. The policy initiative of the Green Revolution helped level up the Indian economy and turn it into a self-sufficient one in terms of food supply and economic reforms implemented since 1991 facilitated economic growth in the country. Foreign trade, exports, stock markets have been flourishing; large foreign direct investments have been attracted, current account deficit have been reached to manageable level and foreign exchange reserves are sufficient. Still, India holds a mere 2.83 per cent share in the world economy against the larger 17 per cent share in the world population. Consequently, one can find very low per capita income in the country when compared to some of the South Asian and developed countries all over the world.

The trend rate of GDP growth in the last 20-year period in India has been more than 6 per cent per annum (Dev 2013; Dev, Mishra, and Veeramani 2013; Panda 2013). The growth rate was touching even 9 per cent per annum between 2005–6 and 2007–8 (Dev 2013; Dev, Mishra, and Veeramani 2013; Panda 2013). There were certain macroeconomic challenges such as high inflation, high current account deficit, depreciation of rupee, high fiscal deficit, decline in exports, and so on that confronted the country (Dev 2013; Dev, Mishra, and Veeramani 2013; Panda 2013). The prospects for continuing on such a high growth trajectory tended to be high. The *Economic Survey* 2017–18 indicates that the Indian economy has grown at not less than 6 per cent during the last three years (GOI 2018). However, the recent slowdown in the light of Government of India's policy measures such as Demonetization and Goods and Services Tax (GST) has become a cause for concern.[15]

As mentioned before, one of the factors that are identified for substantially accounting for the economic growth of a country is its human capital (Becker 1964; Shultz 1961) and TFP (Dennison 1967; Griliches 1963). The new growth theory brings into focus the contribution of TFP involving the human capital in the growth accounting (Romer 1988). Empirical studies of growth accounting exercises across countries have been making efforts to estimate the TFP. In this line of research, studies have established the impact of health investments in poverty reduction and economic growth (WHO 2001; World Bank 1993).

In India as well there are such studies estimating the TFP of the country's economic growth and observed its contribution (Bosworth, Collins, and Virmani 2007; RBI 2014). The estimates in an RBI (2014) report on study of TFP including capital, labour, energy, material, and services (referred to as KLEMS—capital, labour, energy, materials, and services) shows that the Indian economy registered a TFP growth rate of 1.4 per cent during 1980–2008. The productivity growth during 2000–8 (2.3 per cent) has been improved over the period 1980–99 (1.1 per cent). In respect to labour productivity, it was observed to be 4.1 per cent[16] during 1980–2008.

There have not been many research studies in India on the individual impact of health and/or education on economic growth. However, one can imagine the level of human capital accumulation there has been in India under such circumstances of illiteracy, poor educational levels along with high disease burden and prevalence of undernourishment, and its impact on economic growth. A country like India can benefit from the impact of technological changes through import of technology or externality and spillover effects of changes at a global level. But the impact of human capital including

[13] Unprecedented rise in international price of petrol owing to oil embargo proclaimed by Organization of Petroleum Exporting Countries (OPEC) in October 1973 (referred to as first oil shock) and followed by drastic reduction in oil output in 1979. India was one among the oil importing countries which were affected with such price rises leading to inflation.

[14] The currency devaluation and current account deficits leading to balance of payments problem had begun since 1985 and culminated by the end of the decade and resulted in the meltdown of foreign exchange reserves below minimum level. Growing fiscal imbalances in the country were further precipitated by the steep rise in international oil prices owing to the Gulf War. Together, the country was virtually in economic and financial crisis in mid-1991.

[15] Growth has slumped. The recent *Economy Survey* shows that GDP growth declined from 8 per cent in 2015–16 to 7.1 per cent in 2016–17 (GOI 2017b). Further, the GDP growth slipped from 7.7 per cent in the first half of 2016–17 to 6.5 per cent in the second half of the same year. Projections for the financial year 2017–18 are volatile and uncertain ranging between 5 and 6 per cent. Job losses are mounting. Despite a very low international market prices, fuel prices in India are rising. Exports have slowed down while imports are going up. Gold imports have gone up recently too. The government has been celebrating the rise in the stock market but now that has also started crashing. The dollar is going back to nearly INR 65.

[16] That is of the median growth for the economy as a whole.

education and health condition on its economic growth is possible through the development of human capital within the country. Herein one can make a point that India has not reaped the potential contribution of human capital including health and education in its economic growth. It must be due to historical neglect of human capital components both on health and education in the drafting of important social and economic policies and underplayed the required measures for the same throughout the planning era. The policy focus for a long time has been on investing in industry, irrigation, energy, followed by resource allocations for short-run poverty alleviation programmes.

Employment, Poverty, and Inequality

Strangely, despite the high growth trajectory that Indian economy has been witnessing, the growth of employment has been decelerating over the 1990s and 2000s and hence is considered as jobless growth (Ghosh 2013; Himanshu 2011; Mehrotra et al. 2014; Thomas 2012). India's employment growth had been slowing down since 2004–5. It was about 2 per cent per annum between 1999–2000 and 2004–5. It declined to around 0.7 per cent per annum between 2004–5 and 2009–10. Subsequently, it further slowed down to around 0.4 per cent per annum between 2009–10 and 2011–12 (Mehrotra et al. 2014; Shaw 2013). It was observed that there was an absolute decline in size of employment in the rural agricultural sector.[17] Such a decline was estimated to be about 20 million between 2004–5 and 2009–10 (Himanshu 2011; Thomas 2012). Further a decline of about 13 million during 2009–10 and 2011–12 (Mehrotra et al. 2014). The growth of employment during the past few years further worsened and the economy witnessed a negative growth meaning an absolute decline in employment during the period 2013–14 to 2015–16 (Abraham 2017). Such a trend is occurring for the first time in independent India.[18]

The challenges with respect to labour and employment to be addressed in the country are of low productivity of labour, underemployment, and unemployment. We do not have much research in the Indian context that studied the relationship between health conditions and labour productivity and establishing significance of health conditions in this regard. But it is well examined in the global and developed countries context (Behrman and Rosenzweig 2004; Schultz 2002, 2005). Further, economic conditions such as underemployment and unemployment along with low wages and economic inequalities have an adverse impact on health conditions through access and affordability of healthcare.

India's experience seems to be remarkable in reducing percentage of poor. But the methodological issues in poverty estimates leave one to wonder about the performance of the country in this regard[19] (Mishra 2014; Subramanian 2012, 2014). The Rangarajan Committee has estimated that the percentage of poor in India was 38.2 per cent in 2009–10 and 29.5 per cent in 2011–12 indicating a sharp decline during the two years (Planning Commission, 2012). The latest estimate (2011–12) of population living in poverty (that is BPL) in India amounts to somewhere between 350 and 400 million. More worrisome is the rate of

[17] The deceleration in growth of employment in general and declined size of employment in agriculture in particular during this period was due to a decline in female employment and shifting of male employment to non-farm sectors (Abraham 2013; Mehrotra et al. 2014; Thomas 2012). In fact, the structural transformation theory of Lewis indicates decline in agricultural employment and rise in non-agricultural employment. Such a change is due to productivity and wage differences between the two sectors (see Lewis 1954). Again, such a transformation especially the transition from agriculture to industry is to be accompanied by the withdrawal of women from the labour force (see Goldin 1993). Most importantly, such transformation is expected to result in formalizing employment. But the structural transformation of workforce/labour force that the country has witnessed is nowhere of that kind. The decline in size of employment in agriculture has not been replaced with the corresponding compensatory growth of employment in non-agriculture sector (industry and/or services). Moreover, large portion (more than 90 per cent per cent) of the workforce in the country is engaged in unorganized and informal sector without any social protection/security measures (see NCEUS 2009).

[18] Moreover, it is worrisome to note that such a decline in size not only in the primary sector, but also in secondary (industry) sector particularly that in manufacturing and construction, and tertiary/services sector (Abraham 2017). Within the organized sector, along with a continuous sharp deceleration in information technology/business process outsourcing the other sub-sectors witnessed a decline in size of employment (Abraham 2017).

[19] The Planning Commission of India estimates, which are based on the Lakadawala methodology, shows that the poverty ratio in the country (rural and urban combined) was 54.93 per cent in 1973–4 and it declined to 27.5 per cent in 2004–5, whereas the estimates based on methodology of Tendulkar Committee show that it has declined from 45.3 per cent in 1993–4 to 21.9 per cent in 2011–12.

growing inequalities.[20] The Lucas Chancel and Thomas Piketty study (2017)[21] observed that income inequality in India is at its highest level since 1922. The study also observed that the increase in income inequality coincides with the sharp rise in Indian economic growth after 1980.[22] According to the IMF study (2015) which estimates the Gini coefficient, the inequality measure, the coefficient rose from 45 to 51 between 1990 and 2013.[23] The study based on NSSO's All India Debt and Investment Survey (AIDIS) also indicates growing wealth inequality in India[24] (Anand and Thampi 2016; Himanshu and Murgai 2016). Poverty and inequality have their impact on health conditions of the poor. Also, there are studies showing health expenditures especially the catastrophic ones, have adverse impact of pushing households into poverty.

[20] Oxfam's report shows that the gap between rich and poor all over the world in general is far greater now than before. Titled as 'An economy for the 99 percent', OXFAM, available at https://oi-files-d8-prod.s3.eu-west-2.amazonaws.com/s3fs-public/file_attachments/bp-economy-for-99-percent-160117-en.pdf, last accessed on 10 August 2018.

[21] The study observed that the year 1922 was the time when Income Tax Act was passed and the government began levying income tax since then. The study has calculated inequality from tax data, national income accounts, and sample surveys.

[22] The study observed that the top 1 per cent of earners captured less than 21 per cent of total income in the late 1930s, before dropping to 6 per cent in the early 1980s and rising to 22 per cent today. Over the 1951–80 period, the bottom 50 per cent group captured 28 per cent of total growth and incomes of this group grew faster than the average, while the top 0.1 per cent incomes decreased. Over the 1980–2014 period, the situation was reversed; the top 0.1 per cent of earners captured a higher share of total growth than the bottom 50 per cent (12 per cent v 11 per cent), while the top 1 per cent received a higher share of total growth than the middle 40 per cent (29 per cent v 23 per cent) (see Chancel and Piketty 2017).

[23] The estimates based on consumption expenditure using NSSO data of Consumer Expenditure Survey (CES) shows that the Gini coefficient has increased during the post-reform period (see Deaton and Drèze 2002; Himanshu 2015; Himanshu and Murgai 2016). The Gini coefficient based on NSSO-CES is usually observed to be an underestimation (Himanshu 2015). It is so because the coverage of NSSO–CES is little limited as it is based on only consumption expenditure of the sample households surveyed but does not cover the income and wealth of households and institutions.

[24] Indeed, the study observed that the rising levels of wealth inequality are deeply linked to the growth strategy being followed, by which the gains from growth have been redistributed among those who were already wealthy (see Anand and Thampi 2016).

State Policy and Course of Action: Performance in Correcting Mechanisms

The state policy in India has been inefficient and faltering on two important measures of redistributing mechanism such as taxation and social spending which are critical for reducing economic inequalities. The social sector spending is not only a policy measure of income redistribution mechanism, it has greater role in influencing macro fundamentals as well where it enhances growth and macro stability. In the circumstances of high inequality, considerably significant level of poverty and as most of the workforce engaged in unorganized and informal economy without any social security measures, the state policy of social spending on public services such as education, health, and social protection are important. But the reality has been showing that these appropriable measures have not been used for the purpose. The performance of the country particularly in respect of the measure of social spending correction mechanism has been consistently poor. The Centre and the states' budget allocations show that they have been not only inadequate but also misallocated. In fact, the recent *Economic Survey* 2017–18 admitted the fact that welfare spending in India suffers from misallocation (GOI 2017b). As the *Economic Survey* observed[25] that the expenditure on social services (both Centre and states) as a proportion of GDP was 7.0 per cent during 2016–17, while the education and health sectors accounted for 2.9 per cent and 1.4 per cent respectively. The average social sector spending in developed countries is to the tune of 14 per cent of their GDP (Goswami 2013). The *Economic Survey* has made a point that India has not been sufficiently invested in human capital such as education and health (GOI 2017b).

The fiscal policy of the Indian state especially that followed the initial phase of economic reforms initiated in early 1990s has compressed the social spending (Dev 2003; Joshi 2006). In the second phase of reforms, the social spending has been marginally improved and resulted in implementation of schemes such as the massive Mahatma Gandhi National Rural Employment Guarantee Act (MGNREGA) and other welfare schemes. However, competing populism in state social policy has been denting the social spending on productive investment that enhances the human capital.

[25] Based on the RBI data related to public expenditure in India.

Further, the governance structure in federal system of the country is such that most of social sector components such as education and health are 'state subjects'. Central government can make policy and initiate the Centrally Sponsored Schemes (CSS) while making certain contribution of financial resources. State governments are deciding factors in implementing the same while making their part of spending. As the state-specific policies and their priorities vary, one can observe the differences in social sector outcome including health condition across states. One can easily observe the uneven progress and inter-state variation in respect of success in implementing country-wide massive schemes like public distribution system (PDS) and MGNREGA. Similarly, there are considerable variations across states in respect of implementing central schemes related to health and progress in the healthcare sector, achievement in health outcome. Two extreme cases illustrating this are Kerala and Bihar.

HUMAN HEALTH CONDITIONS IN INDIA: HEALTH PARAMETERS

The performance of India in respect of many of the health parameters or indicators since independence has in fact improved but still lagging behind in terms of required outcomes when compared to many other countries. Twin dimensions of health, that is morbidity and mortality rates, are unacceptably high in India (Charan and Paramita 2016). India's performance when evaluated in respect of the MDGs indicates that though there have been improvements, none of the targets set for 2015 have been met (GOI 2015b; UN 2015b). Of the total of eight MDGs, the goals four, five, and six are directly connected to health—child mortality (goal 4), maternal health (goal 5), and combating diseases including HIV/AIDS (goal 6). Goal one—'eradicating extreme poverty and hunger'—is related to the nutrition aspect of health. Despite the remarkable progress, there remains a considerable gap between the achievement and the target on the health- and nutrition-related indicators in India (GOI 2015b; UN 2015b).

The new National Health Policy (NHP) 2017[26] was unveiled to deal with these issues. The policy seeks to reach everyone in a comprehensive integrated way to move towards wellness and aims at achieving universal health coverage and delivering quality healthcare services to all at an affordable cost.[27] How far it will succeed avoiding the fate that earlier policies witnessed is yet to be seen. Of the 17 SDGs, only one that focuses on 'to ensure healthy lives and promote well-being for all at all ages', goal three, is directly connected to the issue of health.

Taxing Burden of Disease

The most crucial parameter in health is life expectancy at birth.[28] It is an indicator that reflects the strength of the health system of a country throughout the lifecycle of a citizen or persons living in it. The life expectancy at birth in India as per the latest estimates is at nearly 68.78 years in 2016, and is one of the lowest in the world. Most of the developed countries including Japan have life expectancy of more than 80 years. When compared to China (75.19 years) on this indicator, India's performance is lagging behind. It is to be noted that in 1960 with an average life expectancy of 43 years, China's position was in fact close to that of India's but has improved to a great extent during the last four-and-a-half decades.

One of the disadvantages that the country has been witnessing in respect of human health is heavy disease burden. According to a 2017 GBD study published in the medical journal *The Lancet*,[29] India is ranked at a dismal 154 among 195 countries on the healthcare index.[30] In this study, India's performance is observed to be poor in tackling cases of tuberculosis, diabetes, chronic kidney diseases, and rheumatic heart diseases. The study identified India as one among the biggest underachievers in Asia in healthcare access. High disease burden brings down the DALYs and HALE of the country.

As is the case with most developing countries, India has been witnessing 'triple burden of diseases'—that is, along with still prevalent age-old communicable diseases, there are certain emerging infectious

[26] The Union Cabinet led by Prime Minister Narendra Modi approved the policy on 15 March 2017. The NHP 2002 preceeded it.

[27] For details see Press Note at http://pib.nic.in/newsite/PrintRelease.aspx?relid=159376, last accessed on 15 August 2018.

[28] It is the average number of years a person is expected to survive if existing patterns of mortality stayed the same throughout their life.

[29] See various entries in *The Lancet*, vol. 390, no. 10100, 12 September 2017.

[30] See at https://thewire.in/137902/india-rank-healthcare-index/, last accessed 20 May 2017.

diseases,[31] and chronic and NCDs where some of which are due to changing lifestyles (GOI 2015a). There is a growing burden of chronic NCDs[32] (Charan and Pramita 2016). The epidemiological transition of disease burden in India indicates that it is shifting from communicable, maternal, neonatal, and nutritional diseases (CMNNDs) to NCDs (ICMR/PHFI/IHME 2017; GOI 2018). According to the WHO's Country Profile 2014 for India, the NCDs contribute to 60 per cent of the mortality in the country (Charan and Paramita 2016). According to a scientific study by Roth, Murray, and Naghavi (2017), CVDs, including heart diseases and stroke, account for one-third of the deaths throughout the world.[33] India too experiences such high contribution, one-fourth of the total deaths in the country (Charan and Paramita 2016) are caused by CVDs. Along with the high mortality and morbidity owing to major diseases, injuries (accidental or otherwise) also become fatal and result in disability and/or mortality if not timely attended to.

The increasing life expectancy at birth along with a decline on the metric of DALYs over a period indicates the reduction in disease burden that jeopardized the potential and healthy human lives in India. Still such a disease burden (both the CMNNDs and NCDs) is very high when compared with any reference averages across the globe (GOI 2018). Such a high disease burden and epidemiological transition have far-reaching implications on the cost of healthcare[34] as it shifts from relatively less costly disease burden of CMNNDs to that of more costly NCDs (ICMR/PHFI/IHME 2017; GOI 2018).

[31] Although the epidemics and other fatal communicable and infectious diseases (plague, small pox, polio, cholera and others) have been controlled owing to the advancements in medical technology and public health systems, still there are some old and new variants of communicable and infectious diseases (swine flu, anthrax and so on) surfacing. Some of the vector-borne (malaria, dengue, kala-azar chikungunya) and water-borne (cholera, diarrhoea) communicable diseases and threatening infectious diseases (Ebola, SARS, H1N1 influenza virus) still continue to pose major challenges to public health in India.

[32] Besides, many forms/variants of NCDs (such as heart and pulmonary diseases, cancer, diabetes, hypertension, rheumatism) spread rapidly and some of them come close to becoming an epidemic.

[33] This study has examined the problem of CVD in every country over the past 25 years. It observed that in 2015, there were more than 400 million individuals living with CVD and nearly 18 million CVD deaths worldwide.

[34] The shift is relatively less costly over healthcare services attending the disease burden of CMNNDs nature to that of costlier NCDs (see ICMR/PHFI/IHME 2017; GOI 2018).

Moreover, it has been observed that while communicable diseases contribute to 24.4 per cent of the entire disease burden in India, over 75 per cent of communicable diseases are not part of existing national health programmes and universal coverage of these national health programmes covers only for less than 10 per cent of all mortalities and 15 per cent of all morbidities taking place in the country (Charan and Paramita 2016). In respect of tuberculosis, it has been observed that though a significant decline is observed from the MDGs baseline, India still contributes to 24 per cent of all the global new case detections (Charan and Paramita 2016). The prevalence of HIV/AIDS has become another challenge for disease control interventions and public health in India. Although intervention through various AIDS control programmes has brought down the prevalence rate in the general population over a period, it has still left millions of people living with HIV/AIDS (Charan and Paramita 2016). According to UNAIDS data, India has about 2.1 million people living with HIV/AIDS, of which 80,000 are new HIV infection cases indicating the continuing spread of the disease in the country (UNAIDS 2017).

Another challenge is that under-reporting of general ailments is quite prevalent in India. The estimates in the NSSO report based on its latest (seventy first) survey on health (2014) shows that about 9 per cent of rural population and 12 per cent of urban population reported ailments during a 15-day reference period. The reporting of ailments in the survey is not reflecting of the intensity of the health problems prevalent in the country. When we consider the prevalence of ailments based on reporting across states one can find that such a prevalence rate is higher in Kerala and lower in Bihar. The higher ailment prevalence rate in Kerala when compared to Bihar is due to higher incidence of reporting due to growing awareness, education, access, and affordability to healthcare.

Most of these diseases are preventable and loss of lives can be averted. Prevention is the cost-effective strategy of public health. But the performance of the country in this regard is poor. The NHP 2017 seeks to establish a system for regular tracking of DALYs index as a measure of burden of disease and trend in its major categories. How far the new health policy will succeed in controlling and minimizing the disease is a million dollar question given its wherewithal, inadequate resources, and capacities.

Maternal and Child Health and Nutrition

The most important component of human health is maternal and child health. The performance of India over a period in this regard in fact has been improving but still lagging behind in terms of required outcomes and the situation at the global level. India has a considerably high infant mortality rate (IMR) and maternal mortality ratio (MMR). There is huge gap in its achievements in respect antenatal care, institutional delivery, and nutritional levels.

According to the Sample Registration System (SRS) of India estimates, IMR in the country has come down from 57 (per 1,000 live births) in 2006 to 34 in 2016, indicating remarkable decline of 23 infant deaths over the last 10-year period. The SRS estimate of under-five mortality rate in 2015 was 43. These mortality rates are still considerably at high level above the MDG target of 28. Similarly, the World Bank estimate shows that the MMR[35] for India in 2015 is 174 whereas the MDG target for the same year was 109, indicating huge gap between target and achievement. Most of the mothers succumb to heavy blood loss (that is postpartum haemorrhage).[36] Although the trend indicates a significant decline over a period (MMR in the year 2000 was 374), the latest estimate of MMR is still very high wherein it shows about five women die every hour in India due to complications during childbirth. It amounts to nearly 45,000 deaths and accounts for 17 per cent of maternal deaths globally. The maternal mortality is fallout for lack of adequate health facilities attending to prenatal and postnatal care.

In the WHO's guidelines to reduce MMR in India an emphasis is placed on antenatal care. As of now, the most critical antenatal care is yet to be universalized. The recent NFHS-4 of 2015–16 estimates show that mothers who had antenatal check-up in the first trimester in India was 58.6 per cent and mothers who had at least four antenatal care visits was further low at 51.2 per cent. It is staggering to note that the mothers who had full antenatal care in the country was very low at 21 per cent. Also, the country is still lagging behind in respect of institutional deliveries—the percentage of live births where the mothers received medical attention at delivery either at government-run hospitals or at private hospitals. As per the SRS estimates only little more than one-third (34.9 per cent) of live births in the country were attended to by institutional skilled health personnel in 2006 and it increased to little more than three-fourths of live births (79.3 per cent) by 2015. The NFHS-4 of 2015–16 as well indicates the same, the percentage of institutional deliveries in India was 78.9 per cent. Although it indicates a remarkable performance over a period, still more than one-fifths of child births are not attended to by proper skilled health personnel and have not taken place at health institutions.

Malnutrition, especially undernutrition and anaemia, among children and women is another severe problem in India. Undernutrition is due to insufficient intake of energy and nutrients to meet an individual's needs to maintain good health. The WHO says that when individuals are undernourished, they can no longer maintain natural bodily capacities, such as growth, resisting infections, recovering from diseases, learning, and physical work, as well as pregnancy and lactation in women. Such malnourishment, when it comes to children, results in disorders such as stunting (proportionately short height as per age), underweight (proportionately low weight in terms of age), and wasting (dangerously thin body). The NFHS-4 of 2015–16 estimates show that nearly 38.4 per cent of children below five years of age are stunted, 21 per cent of them are wasted, and 35.7 per cent of them are underweight. Anaemia is another condition that reflects the problem of undernutrition. In this regard, the NFHS-4 of 2015–16 shows about 58.6 per cent of children aged between 6 and 59 months were found to be anaemic. Such a problem of anaemia is prevalent among adults as well especially among women. The estimates of the same NFHS shows that about 53 per cent of all women aged 15–49 years are found to be anaemic.

Sanitation, Hygiene, and Drinking Water

One of the factors affecting nutrition and other issues related to maternal and child health are sanitation, hygiene, and drinking water. In this regard, UNICEF makes a point that access to safe water and sanitation is children's right and not a privilege. Access to safe water and sanitation, and practices of hygiene is considered to be most cost-effective preventive strategy for controlling certain communicable and infectious diseases. The state policy initiatives such as Total Sanitation Campaign (TSC) and the Swachh Bharat Abhiyan (SBA) have seen attempts to raise the common understanding of cleanliness and universal sanitation, but much needs to be done before India catches up with the rest of the world. Protected tap water for drinking has remained a mirage for millions of households in India. In respect

[35] The MMR is the number of mothers dying per 100,000 live births. See Kaul (2017).

[36] Postpartum haemorrhage is defined as the loss of more than 500–1,000 ml of blood within the first 24 hours following childbirth.

of universalizing access to drinking water, the country's performance is falling behind. According to the 2011 Census, only 43.3 per cent of households in India had access to tap water. But access to the tap water from any treated source was even lower at 32 per cent. In rural India the access to tap water and especially from treated source was lower (30.8 per cent and 17.9 per cent, respectively).

As per the 2011 Census, only 48.9 per cent of households have latrine facility within the premises of the house. The NFHS-4 of 2015–16 estimates also show 48.4 per cent of households are using improved sanitation facility. In other words, more than half of the households are deprived of such facilities. According to the 2011 Census, on the matter of bathing facility, only 42 per cent of households in India have bathrooms. About 48.9 per cent of households in India have no drainage (open or closed) system. Rural areas bear the burden wherein the percentage of rural households in India having latrines and bathrooms was very low (30.7 per cent and 25.4 per cent, respectively) and for those with no drainage systems, the percentage was very high (63.2 per cent). Herein the pointer is that although it seems to be largely lack of facility owing to affordability at household level and apathy of state policy initiatives in providing such basic facilities and the lacunae in required behavioural change and awareness are also factors that affect the situation in India.

HEALTH SYSTEMS AND POLICY MEASURES

Health Infrastructure and Human Resources for Health

Preventive and curative care involving hospital care, public health measures, and emergency medical services are critical for the healthcare system. The country has to deal with the challenge of inadequate infrastructure required for healthcare on all these fronts. Public sector is nowhere matching the requirement and needs of the people in the country. Mounting pressure owing to growing demand on public health system without adequate infrastructure has been resulting in healthcare tragedies such as children's mass death in Uttar Pradesh[37] and that of female sterilization deaths in Chhattisgarh.[38] Private sector is highly concentrated in urban areas (towns and cities) and the cost of healthcare in the private sector is at an unaffordable level, especially for the poor, hence a cause of concern. Together, access to healthcare for certain sections of population remained far from universalized coverage. As we have seen above, there have been deficiencies in institutional deliveries, and child and maternal care. Similarly, the percentage of deaths that received medical attention at healthcare institutions (either at government or private hospitals) is very low. The SRS estimates show that only 28.1 per cent of the total deaths recorded in 2006 received medical attention and it increased 44.4 per cent in 2015.

Rural Healthcare Facilities

Healthcare needs of people in rural areas are attended to a large extent by unqualified and unlicensed private medical practitioners (J.P. Narayan 2004; K.V. Narayana 2006). Under the minimum needs programme/basic minimum services programme, certain health facilities have to be established and maintained by the state, mostly the provincial or state governments in a federal structure (GOI 2015a). As per the Indian Public Health Standards (IPHS), there should be one health sub-centre facility for every 5,000 population in plains and 3,000 population in the hills. Similarly, there should be one primary health centre (PHC) for every 30,000 (plains)/20,000 (hills) population, one community health centre (CHC) for every 120,000 (plains)/80,000 (hills) population. When the rural population is estimated to be at 891.6 million in 2016, as per the IPHS norms rural India requires a minimum of 0.178 million health sub-centres, around 30,000 PHCs, and more than 7,000 CHCs to serve the rural population of the country. If taken into account the norm referred for tribal areas along with the population in Census towns, the requirement of health centres would be even higher (see Table 9.1).

Against the requirement considered earlier, the rural health statistics information related to existing number of centres, however, shows that there are 153,000 health sub-centres, 25,000 PHCs, and little more than

[37] Referring to the tragedy of more than 85 children and newborns who died in Gorakhpur, Uttar Pradesh, in August 2017. It was Gorakhpur's Baba Raghav Das Medical College that witnessed the tragedy. Following that 49 babies died in a month at a government hospital in Farrukhabad in Uttar Pradesh. For details see Laxminarayan (2017) and Ghosh (2017).

[38] Referring to sterilization deaths, a doctor performed tubectomy on 83 women in 90 minutes without proper care in the district government hospital in Chhattisgarh where 18 of these women had died because of such careless action in February 2017. For details see Ananya (2017).

Table 9.1 An Estimate of Required Number of Rural Health Centres in India, 2015

S. no.	Details	HSCs	PHCs	CHCs
1	**Norm***: Population per Centre (Plain/Hilly area)	5,000/3,000	30,000/20,000	120,000/80,000
2	Total Number of Rural Health Centres required for usual rural population (*a minimum*)	178,322	29,720	7,430
3	Total Number of Rural Health Centres required for non-ST Rural & ST Rural population (*a medium*)	191,740	31,398	7,849
4	Total Number of Rural Health Centres required for non-ST Rural, ST Rural population and Population of Census Towns (*a maximum*)	203,925	66,428	8,357
5	**Existing (actual) Centres (as on 31st March 2015)**	**153,655**	**25,308**	**5,396**
Minimum Shortage: Difference (2–5)		*24,667*	*4,412*	*2,034*
Medium Shortage: Difference (3–5)		*38,085*	*6,090*	*2,453*
Maximum Shortage: Difference (4–5)		*50,270*	*8,120*	*2,961*

Source: Authors' calculations; also see Khan and Motkuri (2017); and Motkuri, Vardhan, and Ahmed (2017).
Note: 1. * Indian Public Health Standards (IPHS).
2. Based on projected population.

5,000 CHCs in India in 2015 (GOI 2015a). When we compare the requirement as per the population norms of IPHS and the existing number of health centres in India, it indicates a considerable shortage in terms of availability of health facilities in rural areas.

Severe Shortage of Human Resources for Healthcare Services

Inadequate availability of human resources for providing healthcare is most prevalent in the country. The WHO's standardized threshold indicates 4.45 skilled health professionals per 1,000 people (WHO 2016). In this regard India needs about 5.9 million health professionals and workers given its population as 1326.8 million in 2016. As per the Government of India report,[39] the total number of health professionals and workers registered in India is about 5.49 million in 2016. It indicates the shortage of more than 0.4 million (or about 4.1 lakh) health professionals and workers in the country. The shortage would shoot up depending on the size (or proportion) of those who are not actively rendering their service among the registered health professionals and workers.[40]

The Census information[41] on workers by industrial classification or occupational classification covers both the public and private sectors, it does not even

[39] In the Government of India's National Health Profile 2017 report, one would find that India has one million doctors possessing recognized medical qualifications (under Indian Medical Council Act 1956) and registered with any of the state medical councils in India and/or with Medical Council of India (as of 2016). Also about 0.2 million are the dental surgeons registered with either any of the state dental councils or Dental Council of India (as of 2016). Besides, 0.8 million is the number of doctors registered as AYUSH practitioners in the country. In respect of the paramedics in India, the registered number of auxiliary nurse midwives (ANMs) in 2015 was 0.82 million, number of nurses and midwives was 1.9 million, and the other female health assistants (that is lady health visitors or LHVs) was at 0.06 million. Together, there was 5.49 million health professionals and workers registered in India in 2015.

[40] One has to note that the registration records-based number of any category of health professionals or workers does not indicate that they are all alive and actively rendering their services in the Indian healthcare system, for different reasons such as mortality, migrations and so on (see Motkuri, Vardhan, and Ahmed 2017; Motkuri and Naik 2010; Rao, Shahrawat, and Bhatnagar 2016). It is an accumulated number over a period ever since the concerned authorities have been set up for the purpose.

[41] While the Census 1991 had followed the National Industrial Classification of 1987 (NIC-87), the Census 2001 had followed that of 1998 (NIC-98) for classification of workers by the industry or activity that they engaged in. In the NIC-87, the Group 930 of Division 93 in Section 9 and that in the NIC-98, Group 851 in Division 85 represents the activities related to human health. The activities in human health group is further categorized into five (930.1, 930.2, 930.3, 930.4, and 930.9) classes of workers in NIC-87 and three (8511, 8512, and 8519) classes of workers in NIC-98. And Census 2011 adopted the NIC-2009.

differentiate workers between these sectors.[42] A caveat is that the Census information on workers by industrial classification is so comprehensive that it includes all workers in the healthcare sector.[43] According to the Census,[44] the total number of workers engaged in the activities related to human healthcare (main and marginal category together) was nearly 1.89 million in 1991, it increased to 2.35 million in 2001, and further to 4.60 million in 2011. The population of India was 838.6 million in 1991, 1028.7 million in 2001, and 1210.9 million in 2011. If considered only the number of actual skilled health personnel such as doctors and nurses/midwives, it would be even fewer (Anand and Fan 2016; Rao, Shahrawat, and Bhatnagar 2016). Given the size of India's population and WHO's threshold (of 4.45 health workers per 1,000 people), it could have required nearly 3.73, 4.58, and 5.39 million skilled workforce for its healthcare services respectively for the years 1991, 2001, and 2011. It shows that even if we set aside the caveat on the Census information mentioned above, the obvious shortage of skilled health professionals and workers in 1991 was 1.85 million, 2.23 million in 2001, and 0.79 million in 2011. It would shoot up if we take into account the caveat on Census information. Hence, it can be safely deduced that the Indian healthcare system is suffering from a major shortage of human resources particularly of skilled health professionals (i.e. doctors and nurses) and other workers (including paramedics and supporting staff).

The foremost issue is that as availability of human resources for health has impact on health outcomes (Motkuri and Mishra 2018; Motkuri and Naik 2010), the shortage of the same has severe implications. Secondly, the fundamentals of economic theory, principles, and its laws in a market economy indicate that work for the labour market as well apply here. The phenomenon of inadequate human resources particularly that of various cadres/categories of skilled personnel available in healthcare sector when in short supply would drive up wages. Due to imbalance between demand and supply the cost of healthcare gets augmented as well, which would in turn enhance the financial burden for the state and household budget. Ultimately, it would result in unaffordable healthcare services for the poor. On the other hand, mounting pressure on short supply of human resources may result in tragedies such as the deaths of children in Gorakhpur and death of sterilized case of women in Chhattisgarh discussed earlier.

Expenditure on Health

The Government of India (both central and state) spends around one per cent of its GDP on health, though some estimates put it at 2 per cent (Rajagopal and Mohan 2015). The NHP 2017 wants to improve this to 2.5 per cent of GDP by 2020 while the global average is 6 per cent. As the *Economic Survey* 2016–17 pointed out, the public spending on health was unusually low at below 1 per cent for a long time. It was 0.22 per cent of the GDP in 1950–1 and increased to little above 1 per cent in the recent past (GOI 2017b). As public expenditure on health has been very low, it has a corresponding burden on private out-of-pocket expenditure. For the year 2014, the estimates[45] of WHO and National Health Accounts (NHA) have shown that the private health expenditure in India forms more than 3 per cent of its GDP. It is thrice that of public expenditure on health.[46] Both private and public expenditure on health forms little less than 5 per cent of GDP. As the estimates for the year 2014–15 have shown of the total expenditure on health, the out-of-pocket expenditure accounts for more than three-fifths of it and the government expenditure contributes little above one-fourth of it (see Table 9.2). Government expenditure on health as a per cent of total expenditure on health (including both the public and private sources of expenditure on health) has increased, but it is still very low.

[42] If we explore the Census of India information, some of the B series Tables of the Census of India provide numbers of workers by industrial classification as well as by classification of occupations. Research studies such as Anand and Bärnighausen (2004), Anand and Far (2016), Rao et al. (2011), and Rao et al. (2013) have explored earlier the Census information in this respect.

[43] Along with skilled healthcare professionals (allopathy), paramedics, and other workers, practitioners of various forms of Indian medicine, it also consists of laboratory technicians, pharmacists, even the unqualified private medical practitioners who have been predominant in rural areas, and other personnel of administration and management in healthcare institutes (that is hospitals and nursing homes).

[44] The Census 2011 data of B Series Tables has just been released and we have information of Census 1991 and 2001.

[45] Based on the WHO's Global Health Expenditure Database. The WHO has maintained the database for the past 10 years. It provides internationally comparable numbers on national health expenditures.

[46] It also means that private per capita expenditure on health is thrice that of public expenditure.

Table 9.2 Expenditure on Health in India—National Health Accounts

S. no.	Details	2004–5	2014–15
1	Total Health Expenditure (THE) as a % of GDP	4.2	3.9
2	Per Capita THE (INR)	1201	3826
3	% of Government Health Expr. in THE (% of Government in GDP)	22.5 (0.95)	29.0 (1.1)
4	% of Private (Out-of-Pocket) Health Expr. in THE	69.4	62.6
5	% of Other Stakeholders health Expr. in THE	8.1	8.4

Source: National Health Accounts 2014–15, Government of India.

Notes: 1. THE includes current and capital as well both public and private including out-of-pock expenditure.
2. Other Stakeholder are: Insurance companies, external or donor funding, and social security expenditure.

Such a high private (out-of-pocket) expenditure has been a burden and denting the household budgets especially that of the poor due to lack public health facilities and insufficient public spending on health. Insurance market in general and that of health insurance in particular is not that prevalent in India. The NSSO's health survey report shows that as high as 86 per cent of rural population and 82 per cent of urban population in India was not covered under any scheme of health expenditure support (NSSO 2016). It is scanty although some of the southern states have come up with innovative health insurance schemes successfully implementing it, particularly two Telugu states (Andhra Pradesh and Telangana) have been implementing the Rajiv Arogyasri Scheme that provides a coverage of up to INR 200,000 worth of hospital care expenses per year for poor families[47] (below poverty line, or BPL). At the national level Rashtriya Swasthya Bima Yojana (RSBY) is an important scheme that serves to help the poor in financial distress.

In response to felt need to improve access to and utilization of healthcare services particularly in developing countries and among the poor there emerged the concept of Demand Side Financing (DSF) (Gupta, Joe, and Rudra 2010). When financial barrier in terms of cost of healthcare, including transportation and transaction costs, causes the lack of access to and lower utilization of healthcare services, the DSF is implemented to address such challenges. It has been observed that although the concept has certain merits, its long-term sustainability is a cause of concern (Gupta, Joe, and Rudra 2010). It has been implemented in certain countries and regions largely with donor funds on which a country or region cannot depend on for long (Gupta, Joe, and Rudra 2010). Similarly, in India, although it has been implemented by some of the civil society organizations[48] as a pilot, so far it has not been scaled up.

The estimates of Centre for Integrated Health (CIH) of the Department of Health, University of Mississippi, USA, indicate that India would need to invest an average of about USD 24 billion annually over the next 20 years. It suggests that roughly half of India's health investments will need to be targeted towards health system strengthening to develop a health sector capable of scaling up priority interventions. It is considered that as India's health system becomes stronger, more investments should then be targeted towards programmatic scale-up. The largest investments in India would be for maternal and newborn health, malaria, and child health. These health areas would require an average annual investment of USD 2.2 billion, USD 2.6 billion, and USD 2 billion respectively, annually for the next 20 years.

Drug Policy, Prices and Out-of-Pocket Expenditure

The drugs industry while contributing to employment generation and economic growth, supplies essential drugs for improving health conditions of patients. In this regard, economic or industrial, health and social policies are intertwined. Drug prices have strong impact on both the public and private out-of-pocket expenditure. As India's NHAs of 2014–15 have shown more than one-fourth (29 per cent) of total health expenditure (private and public together) is spent on pharmacies/medicines. A large part of the out-patient medical expenses is associated with medicines. As observed in the NSSO report, out of the total private medical expenditure, around 72 per cent in rural and 68 per cent in urban areas was made for purchasing 'medicine' for non-hospitalized treatment (NSSO 2016). One of the problems in healthcare sector is high prices of drugs/medicines and

[47] For details see http://www.aarogyasri.telangana.gov.in/aarogyasri-scheme.

[48] Such as many non-governmental organizations (NGOs) like Centre for Enquiry into Health and Allied Themes (CEHAT).

prescribing high valued non-generic medicine along with spurious/counterfeit/substandard drugs.

In this regard India lacks a comprehensive drug regulatory mechanism.[49] The Mashelkar Committee noted that although the Drugs and Cosmetics Act 1947 has been in force for the past 56 years,[50] the level of enforcement in many states has been far from satisfactory[51] (GOI 2003). The drugs price control orders have been issued from time to time on a need basis since 1962. Thenceforth they have been at the centre of debate. The Drug Price Control Order (DPCO) of 2013 involved issues of not only the span of control (that is list of drugs under price control) but also the method of price fixing (Motkuri and Mishra 2018). Instead of the Active Pharmaceutical Ingredients (APIs) which were earlier used for price control, drug formulations are now considered for price control in the new order (that is DPCO 2013). Also, the method of price fixation changed from cost-based price which was in practice since 1979 to market-based price.

When it was observed that the prices of certain drugs fixed based on market-based price were higher than average market price or the alternative procurement prices paid by different organizations, the Supreme Court of India had to intervene and ordered the concerned authorities to take appropriate action in this regard (DPCO 2013). Along with drugs the prices of medical devices such as coronary stents and knee implants drew policy attention. There are many other ways in which the cost of medicines and equipment can come down. Tamil Nadu's and Rajasthan's success with respect to procurement and inventory management is indeed a great example (Sharma and Chaudhury 2015).

Innovation is the key to the reduction of drug prices. The increasing demand for healthcare along with the goal of universal healthcare (UHC) provision requires affordable and easily available life-saving drugs. In this regard it needs a policy environment providing the best incentive to pharmaceutical research by way of encouraging higher outlays in research and development. Patent protection for drug companies that invested large sums of money in research and development of new medicines, their molecules, and formulations act as an incentive. On the other hand, it also needs a proper regulating mechanism in place.

***

This chapter explored a conceptual and analytical macroeconomic framework for health and empirically analysed the linkages and two-way relationship between the health and economic growth. It is to bring in a perspective of health as an investment good beyond the perspective of it as a human well-being in itself. The conditions of economy and health in India are examined and discussed in this conceptual and analytical framework.

In this macroeconomic framework discussion it has been exhibited that investing in health is critical not only for the well-being of people but also important for economic growth. However, Indian policymakers have not been drawn up required policy attention and priority for health. The Indian economy could not realize the beneficial effect of better health conditions in its economic growth and development process due to poor health outcomes. On the other hand, its improved performance in economic growth particularly in the post-reform period has not led it to prioritize the investment in human capital in general and that of healthcare in particular. As a result, as observed, the health outcomes in the country are still far from the required and UHC remains a distant dream.

The policy experts must understand the full income approach and the argument that health investments impact economic growth. Health and education have suffered in respect of investment priority of the state and hence illiteracy and poor health outcomes and low life expectancy have prevailed in the country. Health expenditure otherwise viewed in terms of consumption

[49] Such concerns are expressed by the Supreme Court of India, the National Human Rights Commission, and members of Parliament and suggested improving the drug regulatory system in the country (GOI 2003).

[50] The first Drugs Act 1940 was enacted in British India is a central legislation for the present Drugs and Cosmetics Act 1940. The Drugs Act was enacted in pursuance of the recommendations of the Chopra Committee, which was constituted in 1930 by the British Government of India. The act was to regulate the import, manufacture, distribution, and sale of drugs and cosmetics in the country. The main objective of the act is to ensure that the drugs available to the people are safe and efficacious and conform to prescribed quality standards, and the cosmetics marketed are safe for use. Following that the Drugs Rules were promulgated in December 1945 and the enforcement of these Rules had begun only in 1947. The first Drugs Act 1940 and following Rules had been amended several times. The Drugs & Cosmetics Act covers a wide variety of therapeutic substances, diagnostics, and medical devices (see GOI 2003).

[51] The Committee had observed the idea of setting up of National Drug Authority (NDA) as suggested in Hathi Committee report (1975) and it was reiterated in Drug Policy (1986 and 1994) has not been implemented (GOI 2003).

needs to be considered as an investment. Health requires priority as a sector that enables fast-paced growth through decreased mortality, higher life expectancy, and increased productivity. A critical factor is that it requires a commitment towards enhancing the required financial resources for improving the healthcare sector in India. The bottom line is that no country can proceed in providing universal healthcare without providing good healthcare infrastructure and larger public investments in health.

REFERENCES

Abraham, Vinoj. 2017. 'Stagnant Employment Growth: Last Three Years May Have Been the Worst'. *Economic and Political Weekly* 51(38).

Acemoglu, D., S. Johnson, and J. Robinson. 2003. 'Disease and Development in Historical Perspective'. *Journal of the European Economic Association, Papers and Proceedings*, vol. 1: 397–405.

Acemoglu, Daren, and Simon Johnson. 2007. 'Disease and Development: The Effect of Life Expectancy on Economic Growth'. *Journal of Political Economy* 115(6): 925–85.

Aghion, Philippe, Peter Howitt, and Fabrice Murtin. 2010. 'The Relationship between Health and Growth: When Lucas Meets Nelson-Phelps'. NBER Working Paper No. 15813, National Bureau of Economic Research, New York. Available at http://www.nber.org/papers/w15813.

Alsan, M., D.E. Bloom, and D. Canning. 2006. 'The Effect of Population Health on Foreign Direct Investment Inflows to Low- and Middle-Income Countries'. *World Development*, vol. 34: 613–30.

Anand, S. and T. Bärnighausen. 2004. 'Human Resources and Health Outcomes: Cross-Country Econometric Study', *Lancet* 364(9445): 1603–9.

Anand, S., and V. Fan. 2016. *The Health Workforce in India*. Human Resources for Health Observer Series No. 16, Geneva: World Health Organization. Available at http://www.who.int/hrh/resources/16058health_workforce_India.pdf?ua=1, accessed on 6 October 2017.

Anand, Ishan, *and Anjana Thampi*. 2016. 'Recent Trends in Wealth Inequality in India'. *Economic and Political Weekly* 51(50):.

Ananya, I. 2017. 'Chhattisgarh Sterilisation Deaths: Thanks to Our Ministers, the Lives of Women Continue to Remain Cheap', *FirstPost*, 28 February. Available at http://www.firstpost.com/india/chhattisgarh-deaths-thanks-to-our-ministers-the-lives-of-women-continue-to-remain-cheap-3307762.html, last accessed on 14 April 2018.

Ashraf, Qamurul, Ashley Lester, and David Weil. 2008. 'When Does Improving Health Raise GDP?' NBER Working Paper No. 14449, http://www.nber.org/papers/w14449. Also in *NBER Macroeconomics Annual*, vol. 23(1): 157–204.

Becker, Gary S. 1964. *Human Capital: A Theoretical and Empirical Analysis with Special Reference to Education*. New York, NY: National Bureau of Economic Research.

Behrman, J.R., and M.R. Rosenzweig. 2004. 'The Returns to Birthweight'. *Review of Economics and Statistics* 86: 586–601.

Bhaduri, Amit. 2006. *Development with Dignity*. National Book Trust, New Delhi.

Bloom, D.E., and D. Canning. 2008. 'Population Health and Economic Growth', Working Paper 24, Commission on Growth and Development, The World Bank.

Bloom, D.E., D. Canning, and B. Graham. 2003. 'Longevity and Life-Cycle Savings'. *Scandinavian Journal of Economics* 105: 319–38.

Bloom, D.E., D. Canning, and J. Sevilla. 2001. 'The Effect of Health on Economic Growth: Theory and Evidence'. NBER Working Paper No. 8587, National Bureau of Economic Research, New York. Available at http://www.nber.org/papers/w8587, accessed on 5 August 2018.

———. 2004. 'The Effect of Health on Economic Growth: A Production Function Approach'. *World Development* 32: 1–13.

Bloom, D.E., D. Canning, D.T. Jamison. 2004. 'Health, Wealth and Welfare', *Finance and Development*, March, pp 10–15. Available at http://web.worldbank.org/archive/website01055/WEB/IMAGES/BLOOM.PDF, accessed on 2 August 2018.

Bloom, David E., David Canning, Günther Fink. 2009. 'Disease and Development Revisited'. NBER Working Paper No. 15137, National Bureau of Economic Research, New York. Available at http://www.nber.org/papers/w15137, accessed on 5 August 2018.

Boserup, Ester. 1965. *The Conditions of Agricultural Growth: The Economics of Agrarian Change Under Population Pressure*. London: Allen & Unwin.

Bosworth, Barry, Susan M. Collins, Arvind Virmani. 2007. 'Sources of Growth in the Indian Economy'. NBER Working Paper No. 12901, National Bureau of Economic Research, New York. Available at Issued in February 2007.

Chancel, Lucas, and Thomas Piketty. 2017. 'Indian Income Inequality 1922–2014: From British Raj to Billionaire Raj?', WID.world Working Paper Series No. 2017/11, July, World Wealth and Income Database, World Inequality Lab. Available at https://wid.world/document/chancelpiketty2017widworld/, accessed on 6 August 2018.

Charan M.S., Sengupta Paramita. 2016. 'Health Programs in a Developing Country: Why do we Fail?', *Health System Policy Research* 3(3). doi:10.21767/2254-9137.100046.

Chaudhury, N., J. Hammer, M. Kremer, K. Muralidharan, and F.H. Rogers. 2006. 'Missing in Action: Teacher and

Health Workers' Absence in Developing Countries', *Journal of Economic Perspective* 20(1): 91–116.

Cutler, D.M., A.S. Deaton, and A. Lleras-Muney. 2006. 'The Determinants of Mortality'. *Journal of Economic Perspectives* 20(3): 71–96.

Deaton, Angus, and Jean Drèze. 2002. 'Poverty and Inequality in India'. *Economic and Political Weekly* 37(36).

Dennison, Edward F. 1967. *Why Growth Rates Differs.* Washington, DC: The Brookings Institution.

Dev, S. Mahendra. 2003. 'Social Sector Expenditures in India: Trends and Patterns', in *India Infrastructure Report.* New Delhi: Infrastructure Development Finance Corporation (IDFC).

——— (ed.). 2013. *India Development Report 2012–13.* New Delhi: Oxford University Press.

Dev, S. Mahendra, Srijit Mishra, and C. Veeramani. 2013. 'Overview—India's Experience with Reforms: What Next?', in *India Development Report 2012–13* edited by S. Mahendra Dev. New Delhi: Oxford University Press,.

Drèze, Jean, and Amartya Sen. 2013. *An Uncertain Glory: India and Its Contradictions.* New Delhi: Oxford University Press.

Easterly, W. 1999. 'Life During Growth'. *Journal of Economic Growth* 4, pp. 239–76.

European Commission. 2013. Investing in Health. Available at www.ec.europa.eu/health/strategy/docs/swd_investing_in_health.pdf, last accessed on 8 June 2018.

Flynn, J.R. 1987. 'Massive IQ gains in 14 Nations: What IQ Tests Really Measure'. *Psychological Bulletin* 101: 171–91.

Frenk, Julio. 2004. 'Health and Economy: A Vital Relationship'. *OECD Observer*, no. 243. Available at http://oecdobserver.org/news/archivestory.php/aid/1241/Health_and_the_economy:_A_vital_relationship_.html, last accessed on 25 July 2018.

Ghose, Jayati. 2013. 'The Strange Case of the Jobs that did not Appear: Structural Change, Employment and Social Patterns in India', Presidential Address, 55th Annual Conference, The Indian Society of Labour Economics, 16–18 December, Centre for Economic Studies and Planning, Jawaharlal Nehru University, New Delhi.

Ghosh, D. 2017. 'In UP Again, 49 Children Die In Hospital Allegedly Due To Oxygen Shortage', NDTV.com, 4 September. Available at https://www.ndtv.com/india-news/in-up-again-49-children-die-in-hospital-allegedly-due-to-oxygen-shortage-in-farukhabad-1745751, last accessed on 18 March 2018.

Government of India (GOI). 2003. *Report of The Expert Committee on A Comprehensive Examination of Drug Regulatory Issues, Including the Problem of Spurious Drugs* (Mashelkar Committee Report). New Delhi: Ministry of Health and Family Welfare.

———. 2015a. *Rural Health Statistics 2014–15.* New Delhi: Statistics Division, Ministry of Health and Family Welfare.

———. 2015b. *Millennium Development Goals: The India Country Report 2015.* New Delhi: Social Statistics Division Central Statistics Office, Ministry of Statistics and Programme Implementation.

———. 2017a. National Health Profile 2017. Central Bureau of Health Intelligence, Directorate General of Health Services, Ministry of Health and Family Welfare, Government of India, New Delhi.

———. 2017b. *Economic Survey 2016–17*, Volumes I and II. New Delhi: Economic Division, Department of Economic Affairs, Ministry of Finance. January (vol. I) and August (vol. II).

———. 2017c. National Health Policy 2017. Ministry of Health and Family Welfare, Government of India, New Delhi.

———. 2018. *Economic Survey 2017–18.* New Delhi: Economic Division, Department of Economic Affairs, Ministry of Finance.

Goldin, Claudia. 1993. 'The Quiet Revolution That Transformed Women's Employment, Education, and Family'. Richard T. Ely Lecture and NBER Paper. Available at https://www.nber.org/papers/w11953.pdf, last accessed on 2 August 2013.

Goswami, Urmi. 2013. 'Social Sector Outlays: An Assessment'. *Yojana*, vol. 57, March.

Griliches, Zvi. 1963. 'The Sources of Measured Productivity Growth: United States Agriculture, 1940–60', *Journal of Political Economy* 71: 331.

Gupta, Indrani, William Joe, and Shalini Rudra. 2010. 'Demand Side Financing in Health: How Far Can it Address the Issue of Low Utilization in Developing Countries?' Background Paper 27 of World Health Report, World Health Organization, Geneva.

Himanshu. 2011. 'Employment Trends in India: A Re-examination'. *Economic and Political Weekly* 43(59): 43–59.

———. 2015. 'Inequality in India'. *Seminar*, Issue 672. Available at https://www.india-seminar.com/semframe.html, last accessed on 30 July 2018.

Himanshu, and Rinku Murgai. 2016. 'Inequality in India: Dimensions and Trends'. Presentation at UN-WIDER Conference on Inequality, 22 January, UN-WIDER and ICRIER, New Delhi. Available at https://www.wider.unu.edu/sites/default/files/Events/PDF/Slides/Himanshu_seminar_inequality.pdf, last accessed on 30 May 2018.

ICMR/PHFI/IHME. 2017. *India: Health of the Nation's States—Disease Burden Trends in the States of India 1990 to 2016.* New Delhi: Indian Council of Medical Research (ICMR), Public Health Foundation of India (PHFI) and Institute of Health Metrics and Evaluation (IHME), New Delhi. Available at https://icmr.nic.in/sites/default/files/reports/2017_India_State_Level_Disease_Burden_Initiative_Full_Report.pdf, last accessed on 5 August 2018.

IMF (International Monetary Fund). 2015. 'Causes and Consequences of Income Inequality: A Global Perspective', June, Strategy, Policy, and Review Department, International Monetary Fund. Available at https://www.imf.org/external/pubs/ft/sdn/2015/sdn1513.pdf, last accessed on 20 May 2018.

Joshi, Seema. 2006. 'Impact of Economic Reforms on Social Sector Expenditure in India'. *Economic and Political Weekly* 41(4): 358–65.

Kaul, Rhythma. 2017. 'India's Maternal Mortality Rate on a Decline', *Hindustan Times*, 27 May.

Khan, Amir Ullah, and Venkatanarayana Motkuri. 2017. 'Health Policy Concerns: Where are we Going Wrong?', in *Paths for Sustainable Economic Development* edited by R. Lensink, S. Sjögren, and C. Wihlborg. Gothenburg, Sweden: Lensink, Sjögren & Wihlborg.

Lancet. 2013. 'Global Health 2013: A World Converging within a Generation', The Lancet Commissions. Available at http://www.globalhealth2035.org/sites/default/files/report/global-health-2035.pdf, last accessed on 10 August 2018.

Laxminarayan, R. 2017. 'Uttar Pradesh's Child Death Crisis', Livemint, 29 August. Available at http://www.livemint.com/Opinion/c92nu3gIscxEHmuA2BdlyH/Uttar-Pradeshs-child-death-crisis.html, last accessed on 14 March 2018.

Lewis, W. Arthur. 1954. 'Economic Development with Unlimited Supplies of Labor', *The Manchester School* 22(2): 139–91. doi:10.1111/j.1467-9957.1954.tb00021.x.

López-Casasnovas, Guillem, Berta Rivera and Luis Currais (eds). 2007. *Health and Economic Growth: Findings and Policy Implications*. Cambridge, USA: The MIT Press.

Mehra, P. 2014. 'Only 17% have health insurance cover'. *The Hindu*, 22 December. Available at https://www.thehindu.com/news/national/only-17-have-health-insurance-cover/article6713952.ece, last accessed on 4 August 2017.

Mehrotra, Santosh, Jajati Parida, Sharmistha Sinha, and Ankita Gandhi. 2014. 'Explaining Employment Trends in the Indian Economy: 1993–94 to 2011–12'. *Economic & Political Weekly* 49(32): 49–57.

Ministry of Statistics and Program Implementation, India (MOSPI). 2004. *National Sample Survey 60th Round Report on Morbidity, Health Care and the Condition of the Aged*. New Delhi: National Sample Survey Organization, MOSPI,.

Mishra, Srijit. 2014. 'Reading between the Poverty Lines'. *Economic & Political Weekly* 49(39):123–7.

Misra, Rajiv, Rachel Chatterjee, and Sujatha Rao. 2003. *India Health Report*. New Delhi: Oxford University Press.

Motkuri, Venkatanarayana. 2011. 'Access to Health Care in Andhra Pradesh: Availability of Manpower'. MPRA Paper No. 47932, Munich Personal RePEc Archive, Germany. Available at https://mpra.ub.uni-muenchen.de/47932/1/MPRA_paper_47932.pdf, accessed on 15 June 2018.

Motkuri, Venkatanarayana, and Uday S. Mishra. 2018. 'Human Resources in Health and Health Outcomes'. MPRA Paper 85217, Munich Personal RePEc Archive, Germany. Available at https://mpra.ub.uni-muenchen.de/85217/1/MPRA_paper_85217.pdf, accessed on 15 June 2018.

Motkuri, Venkatanarayana, and Suresh V. Naik. 2010. 'Workforce in Indian Health Care Sector'. *The Asian Economic Review* 52(2): 377–88.

Motkuri, Venkatanarayana, T. Sundara Vardhan, and Shakeel Ahmed. 2017. 'Quantity and Quality of Human Resources for Health: A Note on Shortage of Health Workers in India'. MPRA Paper No. 84332, Munich Personal RePEc Archive, Germany. Available at https://mpra.ub.uni-muenchen.de/84332/1/MPRA_paper_84332.pdf, last accessed on 10 June 2018.

Motkuri, Venkatnarayana, and Rudra Narayana Mishra. 2018. 'Pharamaceuticals Industry and Regulations in India: A Note', Working Paper No. 250, Gujarat Institute of Development Research (GIDR), Ahmadabad.

Murphy, Kevin M., and Robert H. Topel. 2005. 'The Value of Health and Longevity'. NBER Working Paper No. 11405, National Bureau of Economic Research, New York. Available at http://www.nber.org/papers/w11405, last accessed on 6 March 2018.

Narayan, J.P. 2004. 'Ensuring a Healthy Future', *Loksutta*, Hyderabad. Available at www.loksutta.org, last accessed on 12 August 2009.

Narayana, K.V. 2006. 'The Unqualified Medical Practitioners: Methods of Practice and Nexus with the Qualified Doctors'. Working Paper No. 70, Centre for Economic and Social Studies, Hyderabad.

National AIDS Control Organization (NACO). 2007. People Infected with HIV, Press Release. Available at http://www.naco.gov.in/pressrelease/25-million-people-india-living-hiv-according-new-estimates, last accessed on 8 August 2018.

National Commission on Macroeconomics and Health. 2005. *Financing and Delivery of Health Care Services in India*. New Delhi: Government of India.

National Health Systems Resource Centre. 2016. National Health Accounts Estimates for India (2013–14). New Delhi: Ministry of Health and Family Welfare, Government of India.

Nordhaus, W.D. 2002. 'The Health of Nations: The Contribution of Improved Health to Living Standards', NBER Working Paper No. w8818, National Bureau of Economic Research, New York.

National Sample Survey Office (NSSO). 2016. *Health in India*. Report No. 574 (71/25.0), New Delhi: Ministry of Statistics and Programme Implementation, Government of India.

NCEUS (National Commission on Enterprises in Unorganised Sector). 2009. 'The Challenges of Employement in India: An Informal Economy Perspective', Main Report, Volume I. New Delhi: NCEUS. Available at http://dcmsme.gov.in/The_Challenge_of_Employment_in_India.pdf, last accessed on 11 May 2017.

Panda, Manoj. 2013. 'Macroeconomic Overview: The Growth Story', in *India Development Report 2012–13*, edited by S. Mahendra Dev. New Delhi: Oxford University Press.

Planning Commission. 2007. *Tenth Five Year Plan (2002–07): India*, Volume III. New Delhi: Government of India.

———. 2011. *High Level Expert Group Report on Universal Health Coverage for India*, Report No. 4646. New Delhi: Government of India.

Preston, Samuel H. 1980. 'Causes and Consequences of Mortality Declines in Less Developed Countries during the Twentieth Century', in *Population and Economic Change in Developing Countries*, edited by Richard A. Easterlin. Chicago, IL: University of Chicago Press. Available at http://www.nber.org/books/east80-1, last accessed on 10 August 2018.

———. 1975. 'The Changing Relation between Mortality and Level of Economic Development'. *Population Studies* 29(2): 231–48.

Rajagopal, D. and R. Mohan. 2015. 'India's disproportionately tiny health budget: A national security concern?', *Economic Times*, 31 October. Available at http://economictimes.indiatimes.com/industry/healthcare/biotech/healthcare/indias-disproportionately-tiny-health-budget-a-national-security-concern/articleshow/49603121.cms, last accessed on 18 March 2018.

Rao, Krishna D. 2013. 'Situation Analysis of the Health Workforce in India'. Human Resources Background Paper 1, Public Health Foundation of India (PHFI), New Delhi.

Rao, Krishna D., A. Bhatnagar, and P. Berman. 2009. 'India's Health Workforce: Size, Composition and Distribution', in *India Health Beat*, edited by J. la Forgia and Krishna D. Rao. New Delhi: World Bank and Public Health Foundation of India. Rao, Krishna D., Renu Shahrawat, and Aarushi Bhatnagar. 2016. 'Composition and Distribution of the Health Workforce in India: Estimates Based on Data from the National Sample Survey', *WHO South-East Asia Journal of Public Health* 5(2): 133–40.

Rao, M., Krishna D. Rao, A. Shiva Kumar, M. Chatterjee, and T. Sundararaman. 2011. 'Human Resources for Health in India', *The Lancet* 377(9765): 587–98. Available at https://www.thelancet.com/journals/lancet/article/PIIS0140-6736(10)61888-0/fulltext, last accessed on 30 May 2016.

Reserve Bank of India (RBI). 2014. *Estimates of Productivity Growth for the Indian Economy*, by B.N. Goldar; Deb Kusum Das; Suresh Aggarwal; Abdul Azeez Erumban; Sreerupa Sengupta; Kuhelika De, and Pilu Chandra Das. Mumbai: Reserve Bank of India.

Roth, Gregory, Catherine Johnson, Amanuel Abajobir, Foad Abd-Allah, Semaw Ferede Abera, Gebre Abyu, Muktar Ahmed, et al. 2017. 'Global and National Cardiovascular Disease Prevalence, Mortality, and Disability-Adjusted Life-Years for 10 Causes, 1990 to 2015', *Journal of the American College of Cardiology* 70(1): 1–25.

Sachs, J.D. (ed.). 2001. *Macroeconomics and Health: Investing in Health for Economic Development*. Geneva, Switzerland: World Health Organization.

Schultz, T.P. 2002. 'Wage Gains Associated with Height as a Form of Health, Human Capital'. *American Economic Review* 92(2): 349–53.

———. 2005. 'Productive Benefits of Health: Evidence from Low-Income Countries', Centre Discussion Paper No. 903, Economic Growth Centre, Yale University, New Haven, CT.

———. 2010. 'Health, Human Capital and Economic Development'. *Journal of African Economies* 19(3 Suppl): 12–80.

Schultz, Theodore W. 1961. 'Investment in Human Capital'. *American Economic Review* 51(1): 1–17.

Selvaraj, Sakthivel, and Anup K. Karan. 2009. 'Deepening Health Insecurity in India: Evidence from National Sample Surveys since 1980s', *Economic & Political Weekly* 44(40): 55–60.

Sharma, S., and R.R. Chaudhury. 2015. 'Improving Availability and Accessibility of Medicines: A Tool for Increasing Healthcare Coverage'. Archives of Medicine. Available at https://www.archivesofmedicine.com/medicine/improving-availability-and-accessibility-of-medicines-atool-for-increasing-healthcare-coverage.php?aid=7046, last accessed on 27 April 2018.

Shastry, G.K., and D.N. Weil. 2003. 'How Much of Cross-Country Income Variation is Explained by Health?', *Journal of the European Economic Association* 1(2–3): 387–96.

Shaw, Abhishek. 2013. 'Employment Trends in India: An Overview of NSSO's 68th Round'. *Economic & Political Weekly* 48(42): 23–5.

Sheehan, P., B. Rasmussen, and K. Sweeny. 2014. 'The Impact of Health on Worker Attendance and Productivity in the APEC Region', Report to the APEC Business Advisory Council, VISES, Melbourne, July. Available at http://www.vises.org.au/documents/2014_VISES_Impact_of_Health_on_Productivity.pdf, last accessed on 5 May 2018.

Subramanian, S. 2012. *The Poverty Line*. Oxford India Short Introductions Series. New Delhi: Oxford University Press.

———. 2014. 'Getting it Wrong Again… and Again: The Poverty Line', *Economic & Political Weekly* 49(47): 66–70.

Thomas, Jayan Jose. 2012. 'India's Labour Market during the 2000s: Surveying the Changes'. *Economic & Political Weekly* 48(51): 39–51.

United Nations. 2015a. 'World Population Prospects: The 2015 Revision (Medium Fertility Variant)', Population Division, Department of Economic and Social Affairs, United Nations (UN), Geneva.

———. 2015b. 'The Millennium Goals Report 2015'. United Nations (UN), New York.

UNAIDS. 2017. 'UNAIDS Data 2017'. United Nations AIDS (UNAIDS) Programme, Geneva. Available at https://www.unaids.org/sites/default/files/media_asset/20170720_Data_book_2017_en.pdf, last accessed on 3 July 2018.

Weil, David N. 2013. 'Health and Economic Growth', in *Handbook of Economic Growth*, edited by Philippe Aghion and Steven N. Durlauf, vol 2. Available at https://www.brown.edu/Departments/Economics/Faculty/David_Weil/Health_and_Economic_Growth_Handbook_Article.pdf, last accessed on 10 August 2018.

———. 2005. 'Accounting for the Effect of Health on Economic Growth', NBER Working Paper No. 11455, National Bureau of Economic Research, New York. Available at http://www.nber.org/papers/w11455, last accessed on 8 August 2018.

World Health Organization (WHO). 2001. *Macroeconomics and Health: Investing in Health for Economic Development*, Report of the Commission of Macroeconomics and Health (headed by Jeffrey Sachs), World Health Organization, Geneva.

———. 2006. *The World Health Report 2006: Working Together for Health*. Geneva: World Health Organization.

———. 2012. 'World Health Statistics 2012', World Health Organization, Geneva.

———. 2016a. 'Global Strategy on Human Resources for Health: Workforce 2030', World Health Organization, Geneva.

———. 2016b. 'The WHO Health Systems Framework', World Health Organization, Geneva. http://www.wpro.who.int/health_services/health_systems_framework/en, last accessed on 5 September 2018.

———. 2011. Global Health Observatory, select data. Available at http://apps.who.int/ghodata/, accessed 13 January 2011.

World Bank. 1993. *World Development Report 1993: Investing in Health*. New York: Oxford University Press.

———. 2001. *India: Raising the Sight—Better Health Systems for India's Poor*, Report No. 22304, 28 May, Health, Nutrition and Population Sector Unit, India, South Asia Region, New Delhi. Available at http://web.worldbank.org/archive/website00811/WEB/PDF/HOVR.PDF, last accessed on 3 March 2017.

———. 2014. 'Health and Nutrition Population Statistics', World Bank, Washington, DC.

10

Unravelling the 'Social' in Social Determinants and Health

Rama V. Baru

The relationship between socioeconomic factors and health is well recognized and has a long history. Its roots go back to the eighteenth and nineteenth centuries where there were a number of empirical observations between socioeconomic conditions and ill health. There were several surveys that were conducted by social scientists on poverty among the working classes in the rapidly industrializing cities in England and several European countries. Booth and Rowntree's surveys in England challenged the traditional view of poverty that placed the onus on individual failing. Both of them undertook a house-to-house survey and provided the evidence of poor wages, disease, and lack of food security among the working classes. Following these two important studies, in the late nineteenth and early twentieth centuries, there was active engagement with the poverty question. Several surveys were conducted in the towns and cities of Britain (Glennerster 2004). These surveys provided the evidence to push for State responsibility for social and health welfare measures.

More specifically relating to health, the work of Farr, Villerme, and Engels highlighted the relationship between poor working and living conditions to high levels of mortality and morbidity (see Susser and Susser 1996). These studies were able to demonstrate how inadequate wages, long hours of work, poor housing, water supply and sanitation, hunger and undernutrition resulted in high mortality due to communicable diseases like tuberculosis, fevers, and enteric infections. The improvement in wages, living conditions, and welfare measures were largely responsible for the decline in mortality due to communicable diseases (McKeown 1979). With the rise of germ theory the causal links of disease was primarily reduced to a single causative agent. With the discovery of sulphanomides, and later antibiotics, in the first half of the twentieth century the focus of mainstream public health was concentrated on curing the diseases. Increasingly, in public health, the responsibility of individuals for their health gained importance and the broad understanding was that behavioural change could result in better compliance to access health services and accept the treatment. Allopathy was seen as a modern scientific project that could not only treat disease but by doing so would also address poverty. Considerable funds were allocated for information, education, and communication for affecting behavioural change at the individual and community levels in the major public health programmes. The behavioural approach in public health placed excessive emphasis on individual responsibility and does not adequately address the structural determinants of behaviour.

In a highly stratified country like India there is much variation in health outcomes and access to health services, which broadly corresponds to multiple axes of inequalities. These include region, class, religion, caste, and gender that are not discreet but intersect and interact with one another. These inequalities have an impact on both health outcomes and access to health services across the axes mentioned above (Baru et al. 2010). From a normative perspective, it is unfair and unjust that some social groups are denied what is rightfully due to them as Indian citizens.

It is indeed a paradox that a country that has performed fairly well in terms of economic growth does poorly in terms of social indicators. As per the ranking of countries by the Human Development Index (HDI) and Gender Development Index (GDI), the ranking for India has not improved in any significant way over the last three decades. The HDI value for India was 0.428 in 1990 and this increased to 0.624 in 2016. However, when adjusted for inequality this value fell to 0.454. The HDI is a composite index that is a measure for the quality of life of the population in a given country. These are average measures and in the Indian case the HDI value had increased over a 15-year period. However, averages mask inequalities and this was evident when the increase in the value was adjusted for inequality. The UNDP report estimates that 55.3 per cent of India's population is living under multidimensional poverty. This highlights the extent of inequality and lack of adequate public investment in health services and other welfare enhancing programmes that impact health.

This is due to underfunding and a fragmented approach to welfare policies that lacks a comprehensive view of health. Health outcomes are a result of investments that promote social equity and justice. The reciprocal relationship between health and development which was well articulated in the Alma Ata declaration on Primary Health Care Approach in 1978 (WHO 1978). This declaration emphasized the reciprocal relationship between development and health that went beyond medical care and technology. The values of equity, universality and comprehensiveness were the three pillars of the declaration. This approach to public health reclaimed the importance of health service and social determinants for health improvements. The tussle between technological determinism and a holistic approach to health improvement started soon after the signing of the declaration. The primary healthcare approach was seen as too radical and not practical enough for implementation. The lobby for maintaining a selective, technologically driven approach replaced the comprehensive healthcare with selective healthcare.

However, the comprehensive approach was shelved by the dominant trend within public health that privileged technological solutions to health problems. This was derived from an understanding that technology and science could solve the problem of disease and poverty. The comprehensive approach was seen as radical that would require far reaching structural changes, which would challenge the existing power relations at the global, national, and local levels. Through the 1980s and the 1990s, the emphasis was on delivery of technology and medical care for public health programmes in both low- and middle-income countries. The Health Sector Reform agenda of the 1980s and the 1990s, continued the selective approach and also encouraged commercialization of healthcare. This resulted in a commercialized public sector through the introduction of user fees, contracting in and out of nonclinical services and health workers and so on. There was a conscious move on the part of government to encourage private sector to provide curative services at the secondary and tertiary levels of care. The private sector has grown in a haphazard and unregulated manner over the last three decades and is a major provider of medical care in urban and rural areas. Today, the for-profit sector is the major provider of health services leading to high out-of-pocket expenditure and indebtedness. The nonprofit sector has also been transformed under the influence of the market. Several trust hospitals that were set up before and after Independence have adopted market principles to remain viable. Many others were forced to shut down due to paucity of revenues as was seen in the case of several small and medium missionary hospitals (Baru 1999). Nundy's study of charitable hospitals (Nundy 2010) established soon after Independence have entered into partnerships with 'for-profit' entities resulted in the undermining of normative values that defined them.

Thus one can argue that spaces for the 'public' and normative values are no longer a core concern for health policy. With growing inequities in access to health services and the global concern for universal coverage, the focus is on extending insurance coverage that is targeted for the poor. Many of the welfare schemes today target the poor, which has a history in addressing absolute poverty. Poverty alleviation programmes were conceptualized and designed soon after Independence and came up with an income cut-off for defining the poverty line. India had one of the largest poverty alleviation programmes in the world that was based on the idea of absolute poverty, which was measured in terms of income and consumption. These calculations helped to determine the poverty line that determined access to welfare programmes. One could argue that welfare provisioning was not informed by the principle of universality but rather used instrumentally for the larger goal of industrialization. The Nehruvian vision of welfarism was to improve the skill base and productivity of labour for a modern, industrial nation. Therefore, one would agree with Jayal's argument that it would probably be more apt to characterize the Nehruvian period as an interventionist state rather than a welfare state (Jayal 2001).

In a country with an extremely fragmented public insurance coverage meant that not only the poor but also the differentiated middle class has to pay for medical care. The differentiated middle class is comprised of persons with insecure employment in the services sector, which has been a growth area for the Indian economy. As a result, one observes a social gradient in the burden of household expenditure on medical care in both rural and urban areas (Baru et al. 2010). The role of private insurance is still small and is purchased mostly by white collar workers. It would therefore not be an exaggeration to say that India is facing a serious crisis both in terms of health and access to affordable health services. The lack of adequate resources results in untreated morbidities. The poor are the worst affected but a substantial section of the middle class is burdened due to high out-of-pocket expenditures on medical care.

The consequence of this was seen in rising inequities in access to health services, poor coverage of preventive programmes, high out-of-pocket expenditures for outpatient and inpatient care. The rise in out-of-pocket expenditure led to working class households being driven into poverty, untreated morbidities due to inability to pay, and indebtedness for medical care expenses.

The change in welfare and health policies has also meant an erosion of social solidarity and normative values. Commercialization has emphasized individual choice and responsibility with regard to welfare provisioning. Therefore, even when it comes to public programmes, there is a shift to targeted programmes across lines of income, caste, gender, age, religion, and other vulnerabilities. Increasingly, the emphasis is on targeted cash transfer welfare programmes that provides a notional support to the poor. One observes that this has resulted in the growth of welfare schemes across states in India. There is too much variation in scope, breadth, and depth of these schemes and they are managed vertically. This essentially means that the imagination and space for intersectoral coverage is minimal. The welfare schemes are populist and seen as a useful strategy to garner votes. In that sense their lifespan maybe short if there is a change in political parties. This fundamental shift in the perception of welfare schemes by all major political parties means that the idea of a comprehensive and universal welfare provisioning is a thing of the past.

WHAT IS THE 'SOCIAL' IN SOCIAL DETERMINANTS AND HEALTH?

As discussed earlier, until the discovery of the germ, social factors were associated with health outcomes. With the discovery of medicines, social factors were only seen as contributory factors. Once again the social factors get attention with the negative consequences of undue emphasis on growth over development. In most countries high economic growth did not translate into an equitable distribution of wealth and assets. Therefore, there was a growing concern with socioeconomic inequalities that was detrimental to social justice and for market interests. It has been observed that there is a substantial proportion of persons who are unable to engage with global markets because of poor purchasing power. Therefore, several corporations have started engaging with NGOs to enhance interaction with markets among the poor. The government has also focused their welfare schemes on those who fall below the poverty line. So, today the dominant discourse in welfare provisioning is on targeted, cash transfer schemes that have replaced a state-financed and administered services.

The growing inequalities have led to the exclusion of social groups from participating in globally integrated markets. This was seen as detrimental to political stability and therefore various targeted welfare measures were introduced globally. The Millenium Development Goals (MDGs) highlighted the need for nation states to improve a number of social, economic, and health goals. Several countries, including India, were unable to meet some of the MDGs. There was considerable variation in the MDGs across states in India. One does not have data to analyse the economic and social variations of the outcomes. Across countries, there were a few achievements of the MDGs but it was well recognized that more work was required to address social and health inequities. The Sustainable Development Goals (SDGs) are an indication of the seriousness of inequities and includes a number of social, economic, infrastructural, institutional, and environmental concerns. As a signatory to the SDGs, Indian policymakers and the political class have to engage with the questions of poverty, hunger, and growing inequities more seriously.

Here, we need to distinguish between inequalities and inequities in health outcomes. While inequalities in health can be measured and quantified, inequities are informed by moral values that recognize that these are due to flouting of the principle of fairness and social justice. There are two broad approaches to explain health inequities. The dominant perspective within public health sees health inequalities as an outcome of individual responsibility and choices that people make with respect to the determinants of ill health. For example, smoking and unhealthy lifestyles at an individual level is seen as risk factors for non-communicable diseases. Therefore, the emphasis is on individual behavioural change and empowerment as means to influence choices to promote healthy behaviour. There is sufficient evidence to show that there are limits to improving personal health due to the complex interaction of biology and socioeconomic circumstances of an individual. Here it is important to recognize that social class, caste and gender, region and religion intersect to determine life chances and opportunities for individuals that shape health outcomes and health-seeking behaviour. Intersection and interaction of the multiple axes of inequalities is critical for addressing the complex interaction of human life and health.

Several studies have also demonstrated how these inequalities get reflected in the 'place' of the habitat of different classes. It shows that poorer neighbourhoods are exposed to environmental risks that are detrimental for health as compared to middle and upper class areas. The continued exposure to the risks of poor housing, nutrition, water supply, and sanitation through the life course of the individual within and across generations has an effect on health outcomes. The availability, accessibility, affordability, and quality of health services are also determined by geographical and socioeconomic factors. Clearly, the determinants of health and health services are rooted in the question of development.

INEQUALITIES IN HEALTH OUTCOMES AND ACCESS TO HEALTH SERVICES

Health inequalities can be seen as a mirror to the failure of development policies. Economic growth without redistributive justice does not seem to have the desired effect to reduce socioeconomic and health inequalities. The persistence and widening of inequalities is a collective concern that requires a comprehensive and universal approach to development.

As discussed earlier, inequalities in health outcomes have been measured and a body of analysis has emerged over the 1990s and the 2000s. Macro data sets like the National Sample Survey Office (NSSO) and National Family Health Surveys (NFHS) have shown that inequalities exist across income quintiles, caste, region, and gender. Figures 10.1 to 10.5 demonstrate these

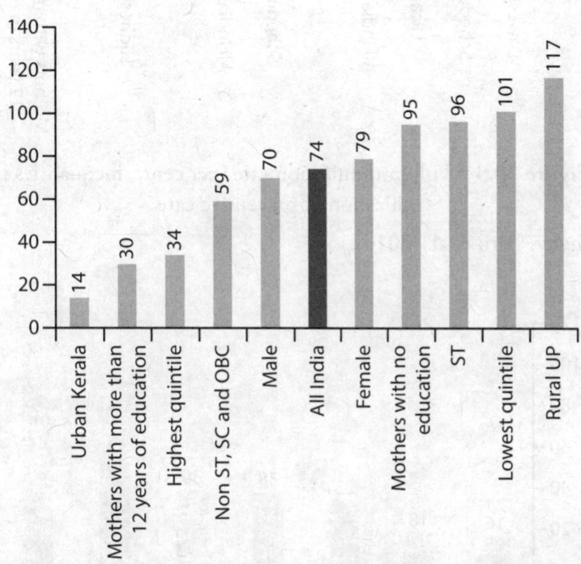

Figure 10.1 Inequalities in Under-Five Mortality in India, 2006

Source: Baru et al. (2010).

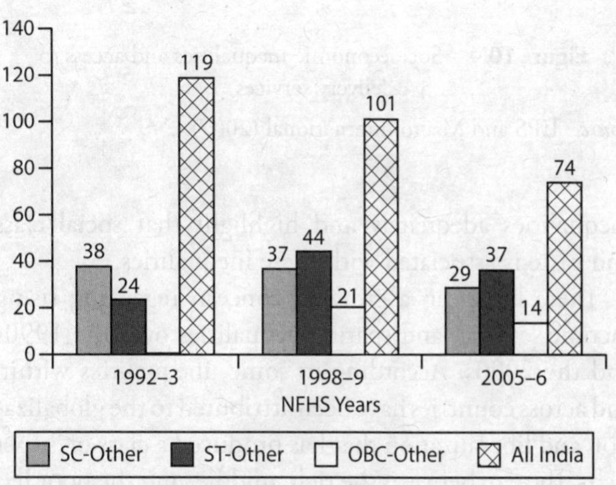

Figure 10.2 Social Gap in Under-Five Mortality for three periods 1992–3, 1998–9 and 2005–6

Source: Baru et al. (2010).

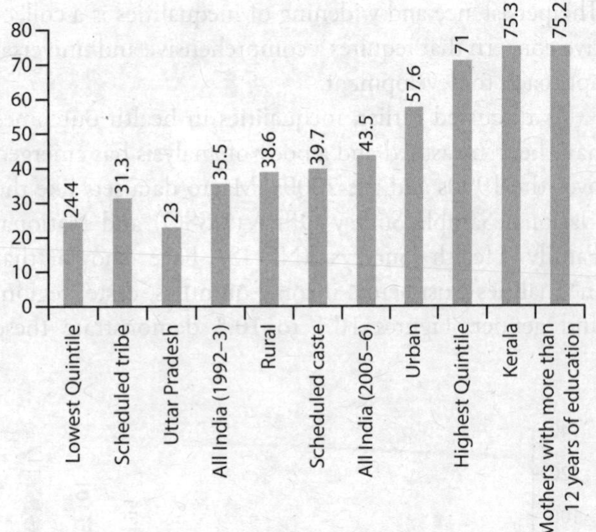

Figure 10.3 Full immunization rate (per cent), inequalities in utilization of preventive care

Source: Baru et al. (2010).

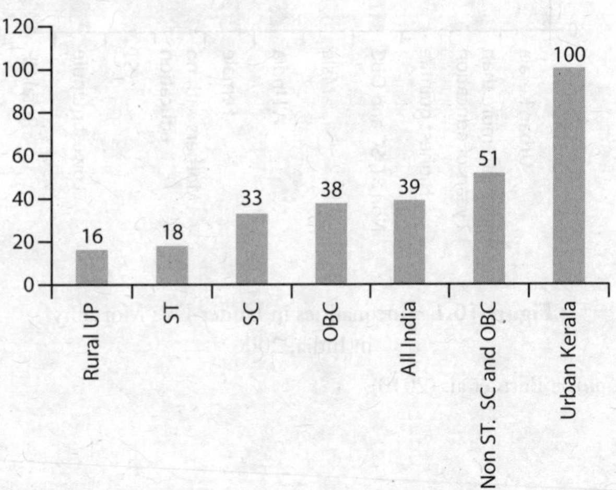

Figure 10.4 Socioeconomic inequalities and access to delivery services

Source: IIPS and Macro International (2007).

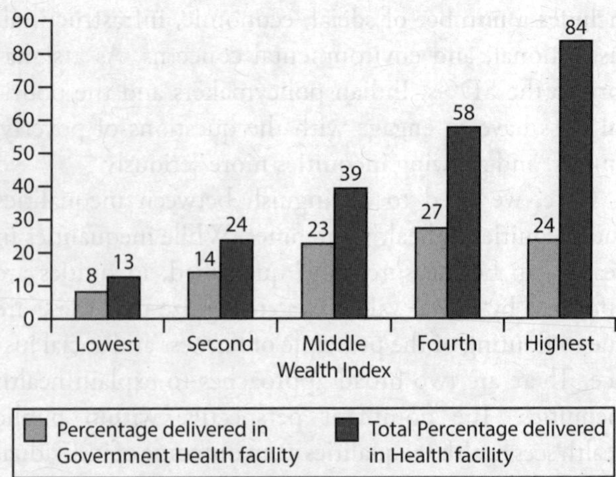

Figure 10.5 Delivery in health facility across wealth index

Source: IIPS and Macro International (2007).

inequalities adequately and highlight that social class and caste is associated with these inequalities.

There has been a growing concern regarding rising income, ethnic, and spatial inequalities over the 1990s and the 2000s. According to some, inequalities within and across countries have been attributed to the globalization and liberalization that has produced a class of 'super rich'. The gap between the rich, middle, and the poor has widened resulting in tension and discontentment across societies. The inequalities in health outcomes have been well recognized and cited as an important reason for the underachievement of the health related MDGs. The large data sets like the District Level Household Surveys (DLHS), NFHS, NSSO can be analysed for variation across states, income quintiles, religion, caste, and gender. In order to analyse the complex intersections between the multiple axes of inequality, one needs to access the raw data of these surveys. Mohanty and Ram's analysis (2010) of the intersection between caste and economic condition on life expectancy at birth shows an interesting trend. They show that life expectancy at birth is similar among the poor across caste groups.

INEQUALITIES IN ACCESS TO HEALTH SERVICES

Several studies have examined the multiple axes of inequality in access to health services. Analysis of the various rounds of the National Sample Surveys (42nd to 61st) on utilization of medical care shows a greater reliance on the private sector for both outpatient and inpatient services. This has resulted in high out-of-pocket and catastrophic expenditures. Baru et al. (2010) analysed the burden of expenditure incurred on medical care across income quintiles for outpatient and inpatient care. They observed a social gradient in the burden of expenditure across income quintiles. The lower-income quintiles have the highest burden followed by the middle-income quintiles and the least burden is among the highest-income quintiles. The important point to note is that the middle-income quintiles have a high burden and it is only a very small upper quintile that has a lower burden. Therefore, what one observes is a social gradient in the burden of expenditure for both outpatient and inpatient care (Baru et al. 2010). These trends reaffirm the Hart (1971) law that states:

> The availability of good medical care tends to vary inversely with the need for it in the population served. This inverse care law operates more completely where medical care is most exposed to market forces, and less so where such exposure is reduced. The market distribution of medical care is a primitive and historically outdated social form, and any return to it would further exaggerate the maldistribution of medical resources.

The important learning from this analysis is that the excessive focus on the poor does not acknowledge the social gradient of the burden of medical expenditure resulting in a significant proportion of the population in rural and urban India having unmet needs for treatment. If we superimpose the intersections between gender, caste, class, disability, and age, then the patterns of inequities get very complex. Iyer, Sen, and George (2007) studied the dynamics of gender and class in treatment-seeking patterns in rural Karnataka. When the two variables are studied independently it does not capture the complexity of the interactions between the two. These intersections play out differently in access to treatment and also on the postponement and rationing of healthcare.

SOCIAL DETERMINANTS OR SOCIAL DETERMINATION OF HEALTH?

It is not adequate to map health inequalities because it does not lend itself to answer why they occur and how they are to be redressed. There are two broad approaches to explain these inequalities. One approach places importance on individual responsibility for reducing inequalities, while the other goes beyond the individual to the role of social groups. In the more recent debates, there is a recognition that there are different ways in which social determinants are conceptualized. The WHO Commission on Social Determinants and Health (2008) sought to take a layered view of the interaction between society and health. The individual characteristics represents the micro level that moves to the meso layer which consists of social networks, community relations and the macro layer includes the socioeconomic and political context. This model is used to capture the interaction between the three levels and is most popularly used in analysis on health inequalities. The drawback of this model is that it adopts a factor analysis to explain health inequalities at a point in time. It tends to be informed by a positivist understanding of inequalities especially by making a distinction between downstream and upstream determinants. Here, the solutions derive from empowering individuals and communities to take greater responsibility to reduce inequalities, while the upstream determinants that include the role of the State and corporations are not analysed through the lens of power.

In all human interactions the role of power and its circulation is important for understanding how income, religion, caste, and gender intersect and impact health outcomes and access to health services. This kind of a conceptual framework does not find much currency in the health inequalities literature today. There is greater emphasis on placing the onus on individuals and social networks to assume responsibility for health improvements. Several government and NGO initiated programmes have focused on giving agency and voice to marginalized groups. As a result, self-help groups for women, Adivasis, and disabled persons have started gaining attention. These initiatives are seen as a means to redress poverty in society. While improving the agency of these groups has value in itself, it does not question the unequal power relations between the privileged and the less privileged in society. Thus the structural limit to agency is not questioned by this approach. From the late 1980s, the role of social capital has gained currency as a means to reduce inequalities in health.

Several scholars have studied social capital and social cohesiveness as an important source of support (Kawachi and Kennedy 1997). These networks of social support act as a means to find local solutions through individual and collective action. In the creation of these networks, civil society organizations are seen to play an important role in mobilizing and giving voice and agency to marginalized groups. These networks could also put pressure on the State and its institutions to respond to a diverse set of local needs.

SOCIAL CAPITAL IN ADDRESSING INEQUALITIES AND SOCIAL JUSTICE

The concept of social capital has been used in various ways to address inequalities in health. As Szreter and Woolcock (2004: 650) have pointed out, there are distinct ways in which this concept has been used. These include a 'social support' perspective that argues that informal networks are central to objective and subjective welfare; an 'inequality' thesis posits that widening economic disparities have eroded citizens' sense of social justice and inclusion, which in turn has led to heightened anxiety and compromised rising life expectancies; a 'political economy' approach sees the primary determinant of poor health outcomes as the socially and politically mediated exclusion from material resources.

While the social support perspective has gained a great deal of attention by epidemiologists, policymakers and the neoliberal state, it has been contested and criticized by those who see material inequalities as important for health. The access to the nature and extent of social capital is itself determined by one's position in the social hierarchy. It is well known that socially supportive networks through the family, community, and state provided services play an important role for individuals to cope and recover from illness. Poorer communities who are stressed economically may not have equal access to these resources that would have an impact on their health outcomes. Therefore, one needs to go beyond social support and include the idea of bridging and linking social capital. Szreter and Woolcock argue that material deprivation produces disruption in social relationships and has serious psychological consequences. The role of the State as an arbiter of the interests of citizens and the creation of democratic spaces and institutions that allow representation of the needs of different sections of the population is also a critical aspect of social capital.

If we apply some of these ideas to the Indian context, the bonding and bridging aspects of social capital is still fairly strong. Also, in some regions the State has played a proactive role in strengthening this aspect through its programmes. Civil society organizations have also contributed to strengthening this in various ways in some parts of the country. The weak link has been the role of the State in improving the material conditions by reducing structural inequalities. The gradual fragmentation of welfare provisioning that often lacks depth in its breadth and height of entitlements cannot contribute significantly to reducing inequities. Also a means tested targeted provisioning of these services does not address the graded social inequalities in a rapidly transforming society.

***

Indian society has been undergoing rapid socioeconomic transitions over the past three decades. This has created many challenges for social life and quality of human relationships that have consequences for health. There are multiple axes of intersecting inequities—region, caste, class, and gender in health and access to health services. In order to address this an intersectoral and comprehensive policy is needed rather than programmes that operate in silos. For example, child undernutrition needs to be addressed through the lens of chronic poverty, intergenerational transfer of poverty, intra-household inequity in distribution of food, undernutrition among women, transfer of undernutrition from mother to child, nutritional adequacy of the child along with safe water supply and sanitation, preventive strategies for infection and its treatment. This is to illustrate how a comprehensive approach is needed across sectors. This is unfortunately not the case today because the policy establishment has opted for a silo approach to welfare services.

This chapter argued that the relationship between society and health needs to go beyond medical care as the important determinant. Public policy needs to ensure that there is intersectoral coordination to address the basic needs are available to all sections of the population that impact on health. As a signatory to the sustainable development goals, India needs to address all the goals that have health consequences by ensuring that there is convergence across sectors. This can be effected through inter-ministerial coordination and the forging of relevant alliances and partnerships for effective outcomes. Health impacts need to be spelt out in the economic and social sectors with a special focus on reducing inequities. The government needs to take a lead role by increasing public funding for health services, regulate the quality and ensure accountability of the for-profit and non-profit sectors in health.

REFERENCES

Baru, R. 1999. 'Missionaries in Medical Care'. *Economic and Political Weekly* 34(9).

Baru, R., A. Acharya, S. Acharya, A.K. Shivakumar, and K. Nagaraj. 2010. 'Inequities in Access to Health Care: Caste, Class and Region'. *Economic and Political Weekly* 45(38): 51–8.

Glennerster, H. 2004. 'The Context for Rowntree's Contribution in Glennerster H.', in *One Hundred Years of Poverty and Policy*, edited by J. Hills, D. Pichaud and J. Webb. York, UK: Joseph Rowntree Foundation.

Hart, J. Tudor. 1971. 'The Inverse Care Law'. *The Lancet* 297(7696): 405–12.

IIPS (International Institute for Population Sciences) and Macro International. 2007. National Health and Family

Survey 2005–06 (NFHS 3). Mumbai: IIPS and Macro International.

Iyer, A., G. Sen, and A. George. 2007. 'The Dynamics of Gender and Class in Access to Health Care: Evidence from Rural Karnataka, India'. *International Journal of Health Services*, 37(3): 537–54.

Jayal, Niraja G. 2001. 'The Gentle Leviathan: Welfare and the Indian State', in *Disinvesting in Health: The World Bank's Prescriptions for Health*, edited by Mohan Rao, pp. 39–47. New Delhi: Sage.

Kawachi, I., and B.P. Kennedy. 1997 'Socioeconomic Determinants of Health: Health and Social Cohesion: Why Care about Income Inequality?', *British Medical Journal* 314: 1037. doi:10.1136/bmj.314.7086.1037.

McKeown, T. 1979. *The Role of Medicine: Dream, Mirage or Nemesis?* Oxford: Blackwell.

Mohanty, S.K., and F. Ram. 2010. 'Life Expectancy at Birth among Social and Economic Groups in India', Research Brief Number 13, International Institute for Population Sciences.

Nundy, M. 2010. 'Social Transformation of "Not for Profit" Hospitals in Delhi', Unpublished PhD thesis submitted to the Centre of Social Medicine and Community Health, Jawaharlal Nehru University, New Delhi.

Susser, M and E. Susser (1996) Choosing a future for epidemology: I. Eras and Paradigms. American Journal of Public Health. Volume 86. No.5

Szreter, S., and M. Woolcock. 2004. 'Health by Association? Social Capital, Social Theory, and the Political Economy of Public Health', *International Journal of Epidemiology* 33(4): 650–67. doi:10.1093/ije/dyh013.

WHO (World Health Organization). 1978. *Health for All by 2000: The Alma Ata Declaration on Primary Health Care Approach*. Geneva: WHO.

———. 2008. *Closing the Gap in a Generation: Health Equity through Action on the Social Determinants of Health*, Final Report of the Commission on Social Determinants of Health. Geneva: WHO. Available at https://apps.who.int/iris/handle/10665/43943, last accessed on 15 March 2019.

11

Spatial Determinants of Urban Health

V.S. Saravanan

Diseases are rapidly urbanizing in India. Ageing infrastructures, high inequality, poor environmental quality, poor urban governance, rapidly growing economies, changing lifestyles, and the highly dense and mobile populations that occupy urban spaces all create an environment conducive to communicable and NCDs. Urban space can be conceptualized to influence human health through the way people/society interact with its built environment. The quality of built environment, the mobility of people across this environment, and the attitudes and behavioural patterns of such people influence the way the urban environment is imagined and designed. Urban space has its own semiotics that reveal the policies, cultures, societies, securities, and economies of urban regions. These semiotics shape the way we plan, design, and manage our urban spaces, which impact our health. This chapter examines the determinants of health from a sociospatial perspective in urban India. A sociospatial perspective recognizes the social, economic, ecological, and political institutions that shape urban inequalities and result in differential health implications in India. In particular, it examines the six sociospatial determinants—segregation of settlements, housing patterns, facilities in the household, environmental hygiene, changing lifestyles, and access to healthcare facilities—that shape urban health.

Existing data on urban health is scarce, as such data is largely confined to a few conventional (infectious) diseases, ignoring a large set of NCDs. Furthermore, these data are often not aggregated according to cities or intra-urban populations unless the information is manually collected and documented from each city. Correlating these data with socioeconomic and demographic information according to built environment is even more challenging because the data are confined to administrative units. Given these limitations, this chapter is based on a systematic review of the literature (Web of Science, PubMed, and Google's searchable products), and reports from government and private institutions in India and multilateral/intergovernmental agencies. In Web of Science, the search term included '"urban health" AND India' (returning 2,583 articles), with the additional search strings 'spatial' (returning 93 articles), '"communicable diseases" AND India' (295 articles), and '"non-communicable diseases" AND India' (123 articles). A similar search term in PubMed resulted in 1,048, 170, 1,838, and 223 articles, respectively. A Google Scholar search resulted in a few reports from the Government of India and some international agencies. Despite these searches, many articles were excluded as they cited the search terms in their keywords, were clinically-focused articles, and were part of the systematic international reviews. Finally, about 30 articles were relevant, which were complemented with reports to address the two main questions posed by this chapter, namely, how should we approach the understanding of health in relation to the urban built environment, and which of these urban components dominates in terms of its impact on health? These are addressed in six sections following sociospatial determinants of urban space. The last section draws policy recommendations for a secure urban health.

SPATIALITY OF URBAN SEGREGATION

Urbanization in India is marked by rapid economic growth, a natural increase in the urban population, and in-migration, rather than systematic planning and regulation of urban regions. Although the urban planning process has produced several master plans in urban India, many of these plans have led to chaos in urban development. One of the visible consequences of these is an unequal settlement pattern—slums and non-slums. Slums are densely packed settlements with inadequate provision of services and infrastructure, including poor access to sanitation, water, electricity, waste management, and security. These conditions expose residents to the spread of disease and poor health outcomes, which are also fuelled by their intimately shared environments. Official statistics (Government of India 2015) claim that about 17 per cent of the total urban Indian population lived in slums as of 2011. However, such estimates do not account for squatter settlements, unrecognized slums, and pavement dwellers. The proportion of the population living in these clusters is estimated to be about 50 per cent to 60 per cent of the urban population (see, for instance, Agarwal 2011). Most of those living in official slums and unrecognized settlements are among the highest concentration of urban poor in the lowest quartile (poorest 20 per cent of the urban population) and are often suffering the worst living conditions. The mechanisms through which densely packed environments affect slum residents' health are termed 'neighbourhood effects'. Neighbourhood effects may result in poor health outcomes for slum inhabitants in comparison to non-slum dwellers.

There are differences in the health status among residences in slum and non-slum settlements, which are analysed in the National Family Household Survey round 2005–6 (referred to as the NFHS-3). Ghosh and Bose (2012) reveal that children living in slums are more susceptible to diarrhoea, acute respiratory infection (ARI), anaemia, and stunted growth than those living in non-slums. Furthermore, of the various socioeconomic variables, location (slums or non-slums) and household income were found to exert the greatest degree of influence on the health of children in urban areas (Ghosh and Bose 2012; Hatekar and Rode 2003). Women in slums receive poorer maternity care than those among non-slum populations (Agarwal 2011). Drawing on the NFHS-3 data set, Agarwal reveals that only 54 per cent of pregnant women from slums had access to antenatal care visits, compared to 83 per cent for the rest of the urban population. The slums also reported a low number of births assisted by health personnel in the poorest quartile. Poor maternity care is significantly associated with age, level of education, and knowledge of contraceptive methods (Hazarika 2010). Overall, slums are under-served by government facilities. It has historically been synonymous with urban poverty and poor urban health. An analysis of Ahmedabad revealed a significant correlation between slum population and disease prevalence, especially the prevalence of water-borne infectious diseases, such as gastroenteritis, jaundice, and cholera (Saravanan 2013). Interestingly, vector-borne diseases do not appear to have any significant relationship with the density of slum populations (see Table 11.1), which suggests that vector-borne diseases are widespread in urban regions as well.

Although slums and non-slums are officially designated categories, Indian cities are residentially segregated

Table 11.1 Correlations between Slums and Density of Population—2011–12

Diseases	Slum Population		Density of Population	
	2011	2012	2011	2012
Gastroenteritis	0.460**	0.508**	0.429**	0.424**
Jaundice (Indoor)	0.430**	0.465**	0.508**	0.389**
Jaundice (Outdoor)	0.155	0.162	0.253	0.216
Typhoid	0.356**	0.435**	0.376**	0.389**
Cholera	0.309*	0.394**	0.062	0.302*
Malaria (Positive cases of PV and PF)	0.259	0.323*	−0.021	−0.015
Dengue	0.294*	−0.153	0.029	0.031

Spearman's Correlation Coefficient. ** 2-tailed significance; * 1-tailed significance
Source: Saravanan (2013: 879).

according to caste, religious, and socioeconomic status. Using longitudinal data, Mehta (1968, 1969) displayed residential segregation in Pune along caste, religion, education, and occupational lines. Vithayathil and Singh (2012) conducted a study across seven major cities (Ahmedabad, Bengaluru, Chennai, Delhi, Hyderabad, Kolkata, and Mumbai) from the 2001 Census, revealing that Kolkata and Ahmedabad reported the highest level of residential segregation along caste lines, followed by Chennai and Bengaluru. The lowest level of residential segregation along caste lines was reported in Hyderabad. The authors also found that residential segregation along caste lines was greater than segregation according to socioeconomic status. Sidhwani (2015) draws on a similar approach using 2011 Census data for the 10 most densely populated Indian cities. Sidhwani finds that there is significant residential segregation by caste and by access to in-house drinking water and latrines. Chaplin (2011) argues that spatial inequality over access to water and sanitation are a result of the colonial legacy of segmented planning and inadequate land tenure, which is exploited by contemporary actors (international agencies, politicians, private companies, citizens, and government bureaucrats) using public goods to benefit private interests. These, coupled with neoliberal reforms, have reduced the role of the State to the execution of mere crisis-driven interventions that are either technocentric or overly focused on social solutions to address growing health insecurities (Saravanan 2013).

HOUSING CHARACTERISTICS

Housing is essential to urban health. A housing unit is characterized by a set of physical conditions that shield individuals from adverse socio-environmental exposures. Every house has a unique set of hygiene-related attributes, such as those related to indoor pollution, dampness, lighting, adequate space for movement, water, sanitation, waste disposal, storage, and consumption of food. With about 80 per cent of an individual's time is spent in houses, these characteristics heavily influence their everyday activities (Leech et al. 2002). These household activities carry inherent health risks that are mitigated or enhanced by the configuration of a house's internal and external spaces. Information on ownership, quality of housing, overcrowding, adequate ventilation, and number of rooms among urban households facilitates understanding of the magnitude of the health problems in urban India.

A detailed analysis from the NFHS-3 in select cities revealed that about 73 per cent of residents in Mumbai owned the house they lived in, compared to only 55 per cent of residents in Kolkata (Gupta, Arnold, and Lhungdim 2009). In slum areas of these cities, slightly more than half of poor households in Mumbai and 38 per cent of the poor households in Kolkata owned houses, with the rest living in unsecured tenure housing. Unsecured tenure housing is characterized by poor quality, which is of great concern. In every city, the percentage of households living in poor quality housing—such as in *kutcha* or semi-*pucca*—is much higher among the poor. In Meerut, Indore, and Nagpur more than 60 per cent of the poor live in poor-quality houses. The poor quality of housing results in overcrowding and poor ventilation.

Overcrowding is associated with lack of privacy, which contribute to both physical and mental illness and increased risk of infectious disease. Residential crowding is assessed based on the average number of rooms available within a dwelling and the average number of persons per sleeping room. The 2011 Census (Government of India 2011) revealed that about 62 per cent of urban households lived in one- or two-room houses. Interestingly, about 66 per cent of the households had four to eight members. Living in a crowded house contributes to the spread of infectious diseases. The NFHS-3 (Gupta, Arnold, and Lhungdim 2009) revealed that in all cities (sampled for study) the average number of persons per room used for sleeping ranged from 1.8 in Indore and Chennai to 2.3 in Mumbai. In all the cities covered by the NFHS-3, on average, less than two rooms per household were used for sleeping (Gupta, Arnold, and Lhungdim 2009). The slums revealed more crowding than the non-slum neighbourhoods, with more than five persons per room reported in over 30 per cent of the slum population, and in Delhi, Kolkata, and Mumbai, this rate was over 40 per cent. Overcrowding, along with high density of houses, results in suffocation and exposure to indoor pollutants if houses are not adequately ventilated.

The NFHS-3 collected information on the presence and type of windows in residences (Gupta, Arnold, and Lhungdim 2009). In the eight cities examined, 84 per cent to 91 per cent of the households inhabited spaces with at least one window, but windows were a lot less common in slum areas than in non-slum areas. The percentage of households with a window was particularly low for poor households in every city, ranging from only 26 per cent in Delhi to 56 per cent in Hyderabad.

Hyderabad, Chennai, and Nagpur were the only cities in which more than half of poor households had a window in their house.

Overcrowding also results in poor ventilation, which is exacerbated by the presence of in-house kitchen facilities in urban households. The 2011 Household Amenities Census (Government of India 2011) reported that the majority (about 70 per cent) of urban households have separate kitchen facilities inside their houses, and most of them (about 65 per cent) use clean-burning fuel (such as liquid petroleum gas). However, differences exist within urban regions. The NFHS-3 (Gupta, Arnold, and Lhungdim 2009) reports that about one-third of the slum population has a separate kitchen, and the majority of poor households use kerosene, coal, or charcoal for cooking. Use of kerosene and solid fuels is very high among poor households, which could cause health hazards.

Overcrowding has long been associated with higher premature mortality rates and enhanced risk of both infectious and non-infectious diseases. Tuberculosis and asthma are widely reported among overcrowded households with poor ventilation (NFHS-3). The incidence of tuberculosis showed marked coincidence with slum living and was significantly higher among the poorest quartile of the urban population (Gupta, Arnold, and Lhungdim 2009). An independent study (Firdaus and Ahmad 2011) revealed that overcrowding was reported among one in two households in Delhi, although higher overcrowding was reported in the city zone than in the Najafgarh and Shahdara zones. Overcrowded households reported a higher incidence of tuberculosis, asthma, and other common ailments (such as nausea, fever, and headache). However, asthma showed a significant relationship with indoor air pollution and damp and mouldy housing conditions. In addition, ARIs were found to be significantly correlated with overcrowding, poor ventilation, and poor structural conditions in homes. A similar study by Bansal and Saxena (2002) revealed that 92 per cent of individuals living in overcrowded conditions were susceptible to communicable, infectious, and parasitic diseases.

Overcrowding and dense settlements have a significant impact on the urban micro-climatic conditions that influence urban health. Unfortunately, meteorological stations cannot adequately assess the role of heat variability and humidity in diverse urban morphological settings because there are not many weather stations to capture the differences within a city, and thus do not reflect the true climatic conditions in urban areas. Climate change is likely to exacerbate variability in urban micro-climatic conditions. Dholakia, Mishra, and Garg (2015) reveal that India is likely to witness a predicted increase in heat-related mortality due to climate change in the near future. Cities like Delhi, Ahmedabad, Bangalore, and Mumbai are likely to witness the highest absolute increases in heat-related mortality. Azhar et al. (2014) reveal that a heat wave in Ahmedabad in May 2010 resulted in a 43 per cent higher rate of all-cause mortality than that of the same period in May 2009 and May 2011. Tran et al. (2013) reveal that age, pre-existing medical conditions, occupational heat exposure, access to resources, and access to health information are associated with self-reported heat illness among slum residents in Ahmedabad.

Water and Sanitation Facilities

Quality of housing has huge impacts on the availability of basic amenities, such as drinking water, sanitation, and hygiene amenities. Most urban households (70 per cent) were found to have access to tap water (treated and untreated) (Government of India 2011). However, the NFHS-3 reported that this access was strikingly low among the poorest quartile of the urban population (Agarwal 2011). About 81.5 per cent of the poorest quartile did not have access to piped water at home. Even in the best performing states, only half the population in the poorest quartile had piped water in their homes. For all of India, this figure was less than 20 per cent, and in Delhi—India's capital and one of its wealthiest cities—it was only 30 per cent. In Bihar, just 2 per cent of the poorest quartile had access to a piped water supply at home; in Uttar Pradesh, the state with the largest urban population, it was just 12 per cent. What is also noticeable is that more than one-third of urban households in the rest of the urban population did not have piped water supplied to their home. Just having a piped connection does not guarantee adequate quantity or quality of water.

Shaban and Sharma (2007) conducted a study in select cities (Delhi, Mumbai, Kolkata, Hyderabad, Kanpur, Ahmedabad, and Madurai) and revealed that only about 71 per cent of the households in these cities considered their water supply adequate. Furthermore, the per capita consumption of water in all the cities was much lower (that is, 92 litres per capita per day [lpcd]) than the recommended standard by the Bureau of Indian Standard, IS:1722–1993 of 135 lpcd, and consumption was much lower among poorer members of society, although the per capita consumption varied from 77 litres in Kanpur to 115 in Kolkata. The consumption also varied within these cities. Only 35 per cent of the total population in these cities consumed more than 100 lpcd of water. There were variations among cities, with one in two households in Kolkata and one in four households in Kanpur receiving more than 100 lpcd. Furthermore, water supply in most cities was intermittent. Such intermittent and insecure quantity and quality of water creates hygiene and sanitation problems.

Given the intermittent supply of water, households tend to gain more access to water using various strategies. Households living in bungalows and housing complexes use pumps to draw more water and use storage tanks within their house to store excess water for their daily needs. These settlements have concrete structures and enough money to install pumps and construct storage tanks inside their houses and apartments. The poor urban households, most of whom reside in the tail-end of the urban water network, cannot afford storage tanks or pumps, so they tend to lower their pipelines below ground level to gain access to a higher quantity of water. Thus, the poorest live at the mercy of the rich- and middle-class households. Although these strategies may enable poorer households to obtain a little more water, they also run the risk of having their water supply contaminated with rainwater, overflowing sewage water, and run-off from roadside waters. The intermittent supply also results in unhygienic water storage practices. A study by Brick et al. (2004) revealed that treated municipal water sources in Vellore town were all contaminated when freshly pumped. The contamination increases with household storage practices. In Vellore, about 67 per cent of households surveyed showed increased contamination during storage periods from one to nine days (Brick et al. 2004). Poor household facilities are significantly correlated with the spread of disease, especially water-borne illnesses. A sociospatial understanding not only reveals how the urban poor are pushed toward the margins but also cautions that poor housing could be a ticking time bomb for the emergence and re-emergence of infectious diseases in cities.

Poor Environmental Hygiene

Poor environmental hygiene is a major cause of the spread of infectious diseases in urban India. Poor toilet facilities aggravate the problem of sanitization, even though the official statistics claim over 80 per cent of urban households have latrine facilities. In the four metropolitan cities—Mumbai, Delhi, Chennai, and Kolkata—less than 25 per cent of the urban population uses improved, non-shared latrines. In a few smaller cities like Meerut, Indore, Nagpur, and Hyderabad, the usage of such facilities is higher than in the four metros. Urban households using improved toilet facilities that are not shared with other households is rare in slums and among the poorest quartile of the urban population (Gupta, Arnold, and Lhungdim 2009). Even more unfortunately, many households are not connected with city sewage networks to dispose of their wastewater. In India, only about 35 per cent of the wastewater from Tier I cities (more than 100,000 inhabitants) and Tier II towns (between 50,000 and 100,000 inhabitants) is treated, posing potential hazards to human health (Bhardwaj 2005). The Household Amenities Survey (Government of India 2011) revealed that only 44.5 per cent of urban households had a closed drainage facility, and about 37 per cent had open drainage. An official survey indicated that about 20 per cent of the urban households did not have any drainage facilities. However, this coverage in urban areas does not reflect the quality of service provided. Poor infrastructure is an obstacle, including unaccounted for water, poor metering, poor cost recovery, poor drainage, and ageing infrastructure. Poor disposal and treatment of wastewater remains a problem.[1]

The parliamentary panel in its report expressed 'distress' over an overwhelming number of sanitation and drainage projects (Sood 2012). It reports that almost 50 per cent of households in cities do not have sewerage connections and that 4,861 of the 5,161 cities in the country do not even have a partial sewage network. Even those receiving treated water are at the mercy of the erratic power supply and uncertain availability of water. Whereas the metropolitan cities treat about two-fifths of their wastewater, the smaller urban centres treat less than one-fourth of their wastewater. With a rapidly growing urban population, these smaller urban centers are likely to emerge as urbanizing sewage wetlands.

Water stagnation and contamination is one of the major causes of various infectious diseases in urban India. Technically speaking, poor water quality in urban regions could result from a combination of poor water treatment and contamination during distribution, especially between the distribution point of the treated water and

[1] See Narain (2012) for an extensive survey on the status of wastewater treatment in India.

the receiving end in the household. Chaotic alignment of water and sewage pipelines caused by encroachment, ageing pipelines, and illegal water connections remain the main cause (Saravanan et al. 2015). Contrary to engineering specifications, many piped networks (especially the tertiary pipelines) adjoin one another, with one pipe above or below the other. The close spacing of these pipelines has consequences on public health (Saravanan et al. 2015). As the drinking water flows under the force of gravity and is supplied only for a few hours in a day, it has low or no pressure throughout the day, except during peak hours of water supply. By contrast, the sewage lines are always full and have high pressure throughout the day, as these pipes are at least 50 years old and are not able to accommodate the current demand. All these pipelines (sewage and drinking water networks) have rubber joints, which expand and contract due to high diurnal temperature variations, creating space for leakage. Because of the close proximity of these pipelines, the high-pressure water from the sewage pipelines easily enters drinking water pipes when there is no water flowing during much of the day. This unhealthy mixing increases when the pipes are old, when rainfall causes waterlogging, when pipelines are tampered with during illegal connections, during periods of higher water intake in the summer, and when domestic or industrial wastewater is disposed of in an open area. Waterlogging is common in slums and informal settlements and it is especially common in low-lying areas, thereby encouraging the breeding of pathogens. Drawing on two years (2012–13) of spatial data in two administrative wards in Ahmedabad city revealed that leaky pipelines, mixing of drinking and sewage water, and different pressure systems in the Ahmedabad water network spatially coincided with the prevalence of jaundice, gastroenteritis, and malaria in an administrative ward in Ahmedabad (Saravanan et al. 2015).

Without the provision of adequate sewage treatment, wastewater is therefore becoming a serious health threat. On the other hand, wastewater is perceived as a saviour for the water starved peri-urban and rural hinterlands. Buechler, Devi, and Keraita (2006) estimate in their case study on the Musi River in Hyderabad that about 16,000 hectares of land generates INR 1 million from wastewater irrigation. In Vadadora in Gujarat, wastewater irrigation generates annual production equivalent to about INR 266 million. However, although wastewater reuse may generate benefits, it is not without medium or long-term costs, particularly in terms of public health risks.

The variability in climatic conditions also has a significant impact on water quality and the incidence of infectious diseases in India. Kulinkina et al. (2016) revealed that seasonality in water quality and diarrhoeal disease rates is affected by overcrowding and exacerbated by high temperatures associated with lower water availability for hygiene and sanitation. Drawing from their study in the south Indian town of Vellore, they revealed that potential of hydrogen (pH) value may be lower in seasons with the highest amount of rainfall and higher during hot and dry seasons. Peak nitrate concentrations were observed during seasons characterized by high amounts of rainfall, and total coliform was more pronounced during relatively wet seasons. Diarrhoeal peaks were observed under two seasonal conditions: during periods of high temperature and moderate rainfall and during periods of lowest rainfall and lowest average temperature.

Poor environmental hygiene poses serious health threats to urban residents. The re-emergence of malaria and new dimensions of the dengue epidemic are also linked to the morphology of urban environments. Construction activities, green belts, open drainage, and high levels of sealing off land provide ideal conditions for the breeding of disease vectors. A brainstorming session at the WHO New Delhi office in November 2006 (WHO 2006) revealed dengue spreading rapidly to newer areas, with outbreaks occurring more frequently and explosively; Chikungunya re-emerging in India after a gap of more than three decades; and a Japanese Encephalitis endemic in 135 districts and 15 states and union territories of India. The 2017 outbreak of dengue and chikungunya across the country should raise concern for rapidly urbanizing areas in India.

URBAN LIFESTYLES—A TICKING TIME BOMB

Urban life encourages consumption of goods with less nutritious value, increased pace of life, and sedentary lifestyle—one of the major drivers for the spread of non-communicable diseases (NCDs) in urban India. In India, NCDs contributed to an estimated 61 per cent of all deaths in 2014, and this is expected to increase to 67 per cent by 2030 (Mohan, Reddy, and Prabhakaran 2011). The most common NCDs in India are diabetes, cardiovascular diseases, cancers, and chronic respiratory diseases. Although these diseases are highly prevalent across the country, the rate of NCDs is reported to be two to three times higher in urban areas than in rural ones (Gupta and Ahuja 2010). The prevalence of coronary heart disease (CHD) is estimated to be much higher (6.5 per cent to 13.2 per cent) in urban areas than in rural ones (1.6 per cent to 7.4 per cent). The prevalence was projected to increase from 47.6 per 1,000 people in 2000 to 93.1 per 1,000 people in 2015. The geographic distribution of cardiovascular diseases (CVD) spatially coincides with states in southern and western regions of the country that have high urbanization (Gupta, Mohan, and Narula 2016). Rajan and Prabhakaran (2012) indicate that these diseases are prevalent among affluent members of society. However, Gupta, Mohan, and Narula (2016) caution that these diseases are also spreading among the urban poor.

India reports one of the highest rates of diabetes in the world. It is estimated that about 51 million Indians are currently diabetic, and 87 million may have diabetes by 2025 (Mohan, Reddy, and Prabhakaran 2011). Although more cases are reported in urban areas than in rural ones, this could be due to poor surveillance and reporting in rural areas. Among different urban areas, the incidence of diabetes is higher among the southern cities (Chennai and Hyderabad) and eastern cities (Kolkata) with more than 2,000 cases reported per 100,000 people (Gupta and Ahuja 2010). Within urban areas, diabetes rates are higher among the non-slum population than among the slum population. The prevalence of diabetes is higher among both women and men in the non-slum population, and diabetes rates among non-slum populations are more than three times higher than in slum areas, probably because people living in slums are less likely to have sedentary lifestyles or to be overweight or obese. Diabetes substantially increases the risk for macro and micro vascular complications. It is reported that a third of heart attack patients in India have diabetes (Rajan and Prabhakaran 2012). There are several barriers to reducing the burden from diabetes; these include sociocultural barriers (such as dietary patterns), inadequate awareness of diabetic risk factors, and poor monitoring and treatment. Unless these barriers are addressed, the number of diabetes cases in India is expected to increase to 101.2 million by 2030 from its current prevalence of 61.3 million (Gupta, Singh, and Lehl 2015).

Asthma, a chronic respiratory disease, is strongly correlated with increasing use of automobiles, industrial emissions, and increased population density in urban regions (Gupta Arnold, and Lhungdim 2009). The prevalence of asthma varies significantly across cities and between genders. Drawing on the NFHS-3 study, Gupta Arnold, and Lhungdim (2009) reveal that asthma prevalence varied from 591 per 100,000 people in Delhi to 3,133 per 100,000 people in Kolkata. Among men, the prevalence varied from 3,269 and 3,275 cases per 100,000 in Kolkata and Nagpur to as low as 593 and 243 cases per 100,000 in Chennai and Indore, respectively. Within the cities, the prevalence of asthma was higher among men and women in non-slum areas, whereas a reversal held true in Mumbai, Hyderabad, and Chennai.

URBAN HEALTH COVERAGE

The private medical sector is the primary source of healthcare among urban residences in both slums and non-slums. The NFHS-3 survey reveals that in most of the cities surveyed, public health facilities are used by few residents, except in Chennai, where more than 40 per cent of them access these facilities (Gupta Arnold, and Lhungdim 2009). Among the slum population, less than 20 per cent access these facilities in Meerut, Indore, and Hyderabad. In three of the four major metros, over 25 per cent of residents reported accessing these services, except in Chennai, where about 50 per cent of residents reported accessing public health services. Among the poorer cities of the urban population—Kolkata, Mumbai, and Hyderabad—more than 40 per cent of residents were able to access public health services, with Chennai leading at 63 per cent. Public health facilities are obviously not the ideal choice due to poor quality of care and excessive waiting times (Gupta Arnold, and Lhungdim 2009). In addition, the opening hours of these facilities, which coincide with daytime working hours, make it inconvenient for the working population to make use of them, since they have to take time off work.

POLICY RECOMMENDATIONS

Urban India is facing a complex burden of disease from urban poverty, poor governance, changing lifestyle, diverse micro-climatic conditions and widening inequalities. Although they affect the urban poor the most, diseases—such as malaria, dengue, and chikungunya—are increasingly spreading to rich neighborhoods, whereas NCDs—such as obesity, diabetes, and cardiovascular diseases—are catching up with the urban poor as well. To complicate things further, demographic changes and poor healthcare are affecting the aging population with the rise of chronic and degenerative diseases (such as arteriosclerosis, diabetes mellitus, hypertension, and osteoarthritis) and socio-psychological disorders. In addition, poor spatial planning and inadequate healthcare services foster vulnerability to floods, heat waves, and droughts among urban households.

There is a vicious cycle of exploiting poor governance at the cost of unequal urban health. Densification, segregation, and hierarchy of settlements; micro-climatic conditions; changing lifestyles; growing inequality; poor infrastructure; environmental pollution; and changing family structures characterize the urban economy. In these economies, inequalities are widening. Continuation of the colonial legacy of urban planning, limited investment, rapid economic growth, increasing rural–urban migration, and governance failures have created a foundation for growing inequalities (Chaplin 2011; Saravanan et al. 2016). In this unequal society, individuals compete, negotiate, and exchange goods with actors (individuals and organizations) by exploiting the vacuum created by poor policies, programmes, and socio-institutional regulations and shaping and reshaping urban space, resulting in poor and highly unequal urban health (Saravanan et al. 2016). It is, therefore, important for urban institutions to strengthen their structures, mechanisms and capacities for a secure urban health regime.

Strategically focusing on environmental hygiene (housing, integrated water supply and sanitation, food quality regulation, and solid waste management) may be more effective than the contemporary approach of healthcare delivery and the conventional approach to addressing material poverty.

Recent interest in urban health has mainly focused on improving coverage and expanding service delivery. An assessment of healthcare reforms across India's rapidly growing economy reinforces this interest and calls for improvement of healthcare quality by taking a comprehensive approach to urban health (Government of India 2014), increasing public spending, stewarding mixed public–private systems, ensuring equity, meeting growing resource demands, and addressing the social determinants of health (Marten et al. 2014). However, these measures are focused on health as a sector in facilitating preventive and curative care, rather than an overarching theme of urban health. In the urban governance of cities with rapidly growing economies, health remains a non-priority that only receives attention during disease outbreaks. Rarely are health and environmental hygiene on the agenda of other departments involved in planning, housing, and water infrastructure. It is strategically important to focus on improving environmental hygiene in urban regions, which might be more effective than the contemporary approach.

Harmonizing and geo-referencing urban health-related parameters is of the utmost importance to tailor risk management strategies and monitor progress for the betterment of urban health.

One of the biggest challenges facing urban regions is inadequate surveillance and monitoring of urban health-related information. According to the Household Amenities and Assets Survey (Government of India 2011), in recent years, from the national to the city level, the country has managed to strengthen its socioeconomic and demographic information up to the lowest administrative unit in the country. In 2011, the country also managed to collect information on the same parameters from a slum survey. However, this information has yet to be harmonized with corresponding health statistics. Further complicating the situation is the fact that information on health statistics is collected from different agencies for different purposes. The Office of the Registrar General and Census Commissioner (Government of India) collects vital statistics, which primarily cover death rates, birth rates, infant mortality rates, and other vital information. This information is aggregated at the state and national scale. The city corporations have their own mechanism for recording health information at various public and private clinics and hospitals, but they are again scaled up to the ward and city scale. Such health information recording efforts have recently become involved with the WHO supported Integrated Disease Surveillance Project (IDSP), launched by the government of India in November 2004 under the National Health Mission for all states. To facilitate this project, surveillance units were established at the central, state, and district levels. Most of these surveillance units focus on conventional health information and are managed by national and international agencies. Information on NCDs is rarely scaled up, and even when it is, it is not in the public domain. Furthermore, it is still not clear how such information is harmonized for decision-making, let alone the skills and knowledge involved in collecting health statistics. Given the size and diversity of urban settings, such aggregated statistics on India considerably ignore the diversity of health statuses within urban India.

REFERENCES

Agarwal, S. 2011. 'The State of Urban Health in India: Comparing the Poorest Quartile to the Rest of the Urban Population in Selected States and Cities. *Environment and Urbanization*, vol. 23(1): 13–28. doi:10.1177/0956247811398589.

Azhar, G.S., D. Mavalankar, A. Nori-Sarma, A. Rajiva, P. Dutta, A. Jaiswal, P. Sheffield, K. Knowlton, and J.J. Hess. 2014. 'Heat-related Mortality in India: Excess All-cause Mortality Associated with the 2010 Ahmedabad Heat Wave', *PLOS ONE* 9(3). doi:10.1371/journal.pone.0091831.

Badwe, R.A., R. Dikshit, M. Laversanne, and F. Bray. 2014. 'Cancer Incidence Trends in India'. *Japanese Journal of Clinical Oncology* 44(5): 401–7. doi:10.1093/jjco/hyu040.

Bansal, R. and D. Saxena. 2002. 'Overcrowding and Health'. *Indian Journal of Medical Sciences* 56(4): 177–9.

Bhardwaj, R. 2005. 'Status of Wastewater Generation and Treatment in India', International Work Session on Water Statistics, Vienna, 20–22 June. Available at https://unstats.un.org/unsd/environment/envpdf/pap_wasess3b6india.pdf, last accessed on 18 March 2020.

Brick, T., B. Primrose, R. Chandrasekhar, S. Roy, J. Muliyil, and G. Kang. 2004. 'Water Contamination in Urban South India: Household Storage Practices and their Implications for Water Safety and Enteric Infections', *International Journal of Hygiene and Environmental Health* 207(5): 473–80. doi:10.1078/1438-4639-00318.

Buechler, S., G. Devi, and B. Keraita. 2006. 'Wastewater Use for Urban and Peri-urban Agriculture', in *Cities Farming for the Future: Urban Agriculture for Green and Productive cities*, edited by R. van Veenhuizen, pp. 243–73. Den Haag and Ottawa: Resource Centre for Urban Agriculture and Food Security (RUAF) and International Development Research Centre (IDRC).

Chaplin, S.E. 2011. 'Indian Cities, Sanitation and the State: The Politics of the Failure to Provide', *Environment and Urbanization* 23(1): 57–70. doi:10.1177/0956247810396277.

Dholakia, H.H., V. Mishra, and A. Garg. 2015. 'Predicted Increases in Heat-related Mortality Under Climate Change in Urban India', Working Paper No. 2015-05-02, Indian Institute of Management, Ahmedabad. Available at https://web.iima.ac.in/assets/snippets/workingpaperpdf/15605627532015-05-02.pdf, last accessed on 18 March 2020.

Firdaus, G. and A. Ahmad. 2011. 'Indoor Air Pollution and Self-reported Diseases: A Case Study of NCT of Delhi', *Indoor Air* 21(5): 210–11. doi.org/10.1111/j.1600-0668.2011.00715.x.

Ghosh, S., and S. Bose. 2012. 'Morbidity among Urban Children in India: Distinctions between Slum and Non-slum Areas', International Quarterly for Asian Studies 43(1–2): 47–59.

Government of India. 2011. *Housing, Household Amenities and Assets 2011*. Available at http://censusindia.gov.in/2011census/hlo/HLO_Tables.html, last accessed on 18 March 2020.

———. 2014. 'Executive Summary—Reaching Health Care to the Unreached: Making the Urban Health Mission Work for the Urban Poor', *Report of the Technical Resource Group, Urban Health Mission*, New Delhi: National Health Systems Resource Centre. Available at http://nhsrcindia.org/sites/default/files/Executive%20Summary%20-%20Report%20of%20TRG%20for%20NUHM.pdf, last accessed 18 March 2020.

———. 2015. *Slums in India: A Statistical Compendium 2015*. New Delhi. doi:10.1017/CBO9781107415324.004.

———. 2016. *Elderly in India*. New Delhi: Ministry of Statistics and Programme Implementation. Available at http://mospi.nic.in/sites/default/files/publication_reports/ElderlyinIndia_2016.pdf, last accessed on 18 March 2020.

Gupta, A. and R. Ahuja. 2010. 'Disease Burden in Urban India', *India Health Beat-Supporting Evidence Based Policies and Implementation* 4(9): 4.

Gupta, K., F. Arnold, and H. Lhungdim. 2009. *Health and Living Conditions in Eight Indian Cities*. National Family Health Survey 3 (NFHS-3) 2005–06. Mumbai: International Institute for Population Sciences. Available at https://dhsprogram.com/pubs/pdf/od58/od58.pdf, last accessed on 18 March 2020.

Gupta, M., R. Singh, and S.S. Lehl. 2015. 'Diabetes in India: A Long Way to Go', *International Journal of Scientific Reports* 1(1): 1–2. doi:10.18203/issn.2454-2156.IntJSciRep20150194.

Gupta, R., I. Mohan, and J. Narula. 2016. 'Trends in Coronary Heart Disease Epidemiology in India', *Annals of Global Health* 82(2): 307–15. doi:10.1016/j.aogh.2016.04.002.

Hatekar, N., and S. Rode. 2003. 'Truth about Hunger and Disease in Mumbai: Malnourishment among Slum Children', *Economic and Political Weekly* 38(43): 4604–10. doi:10.2307/4414196.

Hazarika, I. 2010. 'Women's Reproductive Health in Slum Populations in India: Evidence from NFHS-3', *Journal of Urban Health* 87(2): 264–77. doi:10.1007/s11524-009-9421-0.

NFHS-3. 2007. National Family Health Survey (NFHS-3), 2005–06, India: Volume I. Mumbai: International Institute for Population Sciences and Macro International.

Kulinkina, A.V., V.R. Mohan, M.R. Francis, D. Kattula, R. Sarkar, J.D. Plummer, H. Ward, G. Kang, V. Balraj, and E.N. Naumova. 2016. 'Seasonality of Water Quality and Diarrheal Disease Counts in Urban and Rural Settings in South India', *Scientific Reports* 6(1): 1–12. doi:10.1038/srep20521.

Leech, J.A., W.C. Nelson, R.T. Burnett, S. Aaron, and M.E. Raizenne. 2002. 'It's About Time: A Comparison of Canadian and American Time–Activity Patterns', *Journal of Exposure Analysis and Environmental Epidemiology* 12(6): 427–32. doi:10.1038/sj.jea.7500244.

Mallath, M.K., D.G. Taylor, R.A. Badwe, G.K. Rath, V. Shanta, C.S. Pramesh, R. Digumarti, et al. 2014.

The Growing Burden of Cancer in India: Epidemiology and Social Context', *The Lancet Oncology* 15(6): e205–e212. doi:10.1016/S1470-2045(14)70115-9.

Marten, R., D. McIntyre, C. Travassos, S. Shishkin, W. Longde, S. Reddy, and J. Vega. 2014. 'An Assessment of Progress Towards Universal Health Coverage in Brazil, Russia, India, China, and South Africa (BRICS)', *The Lancet* 384(9960): 2164–71. doi:10.1016/S0140-6736(14)60075-1.

Mehta, S. 1968. 'Patterns of Residence in Poona (India) by Income, Education, and Occupation (1937–65)', *American Journal of Sociology* 73(4): 496–508.

———. 1969. 'Patterns of Residence in Poona, India', *Demography* 6(4): 473–91.

Mohan, S., K.S. Reddy, and D. Prabhakaran. 2011. *Chronic Non-Communicable Diseases in India Reversing the Tide*. New Delhi: Public Health Foundation of India.

Narain, S. 2012. *Excreta Matters—Vol 1 & Vol 2*. New Delhi: Centre for Science and Environment.

Rajan, V. and D. Prabhakaran. 2012. 'Non-Communicable Diseases in India: Transitions, Burden of Disease and Risk Factors—A Short Story', *India Health Beat: Supporting Evidence Based Policies and Implementation* 6(1): 1–8.

Saravanan, V.S. 2013. 'Urbanizing Diseases: Contested Institutional Terrain of Water- and Vector-borne Diseases in Ahmedabad, India', *Water International* 38(7): 875–87. doi:10.1080/02508060.2013.851363.

Saravanan, V.S., M. Ayessa Idenal, S. Saiyed, D. Saxena, and S. Gerke, S. 2016. 'Urbanization and Human Health in Urban India: Institutional Analysis of Water-borne Diseases in Ahmedabad', *Health Policy and Planning* 31(8): 1089–99. doi:10.1093/heapol/czw039.

Saravanan, V.S., D. Mavalankar, S.P. Kulkarni, S. Nussbaum, and M. Weigelt. 2015. 'Metabolized-Water Breeding Diseases in Urban India: Socio-spatiality of Water Problems and Health Burden in Ahmedabad City', *Journal of Industrial Ecology* 19(1): 93–103. doi:10.1111/jiec.12172.

Scommegna, P. 2012. 'India's Aging Population'. Available at https://www.prb.org/india-older-population/, last accessed 18 March 2020.

Shaban, A. and R.N. Sharma. 2007. 'Water Consumption Patterns in Domestic Households in Major Cities', *Economic and Political Weekly* 42(23): 2190–97.

Sidhwani, P. 2015. 'Spatial Inequalities in Big Indian Cities', *Economic and Political Weekly* 50(22): 55–62.

Sood, P. 2012. 'Urban Sanitation Hopelessly Inadequate: Parliament Panel', *DNA*. Available at https://www.dnaindia.com/india/report-urban-sanitation-hopelessly-inadequate-parliament-panel-1682592, last accessed on 18 March 2020.

Tran, K.V., G.S. Azhar, R. Nair, K. Knowlton, A. Jaiswal, P. Sheffield, D. Mavalankar, and J. Hess. 2013. 'A Cross-sectional, Randomized Cluster Sample Survey of Household Vulnerability to Extreme Heat among Slum Dwellers in Ahmedabad, India', *International Journal of Environmental Research and Public Health* 10(6): 2515–43. doi:10.3390/ijerph10062515.

Vithayathil, T. and G. Singh. 2012. 'Spaces of Discrimination', *Economic and Political Weekly* 47(37): 60–6.

World Health Organization (WHO). 2006. *Vector-borne Diseases in India: Report of a Brainstorming Session*. New Delhi: Regional Office for South Asia, World Health Organization.

12

Environmental Health Risks in India

Modern Plus Remaining Traditional Hazards

Kalpana Balakrishnan, Anoop Jain, and Kirk R. Smith

Environmental pollution creates major health hazards in India today with both significant traditional and modern sources at levels rarely experienced historically in any population. Recent studies enable an understanding of the scale of the health problems overall. Figure 12.1, for example, from the India Burden of Disease study (ICMR 2017) shows that ambient air pollution (AAP), household pollution from solid fuel use, poor water and sanitation, lead exposures, and occupational pollution exposure are all within the top 15 risk factors in the country. On an age-adjusted per capita basis, their impacts rival those anywhere in the world for these factors.[1]

Here we focus on the two major categories of air pollution, ambient and household, as well as sanitation, a major part of the total burden from poor water, sanitation, and hygiene (WASH), but note that these do not make up for all pollution risks by any means. Others, including those compromising food safety, leading to climate change, causing pesticide exposures, and leading to occupational diseases, are not yet evaluated on a sufficiently systematic basis to allow overall national health impact analysis, but are likely large or, in the case of climate change, becoming so. Systematic studies of the other factors are clearly needed to put them into perspective with known risks to health.

Table 12.1 shows the trends in the burden of disease from these major air and water contaminants over time in India, here divided into traditional forms highly associated with poverty (household air pollution, poor water/sanitation) and modern forms (ambient particle and ozone pollution, occupational exposures, and lead exposure).[2] In this table, we have included a portion of the impacts from the ambient pollution created by household fuel use into the traditional category since it would be reduced by the same actions to clean up household fuels. Thus, 26 per cent of the ambient particle pollution impacts here are found in both the household and ambient particulate matter (PM) categories,

[1] Per capita age-adjusted values are the accepted way to compare impacts across populations.

[2] The data come from the database for 2016 of the Institute of Health Metrics and Evaluation (IHME), one of the two sources of burden of disease information, the other from WHO. Details of and issues with these assessments are presented in the further sections of the chapter.

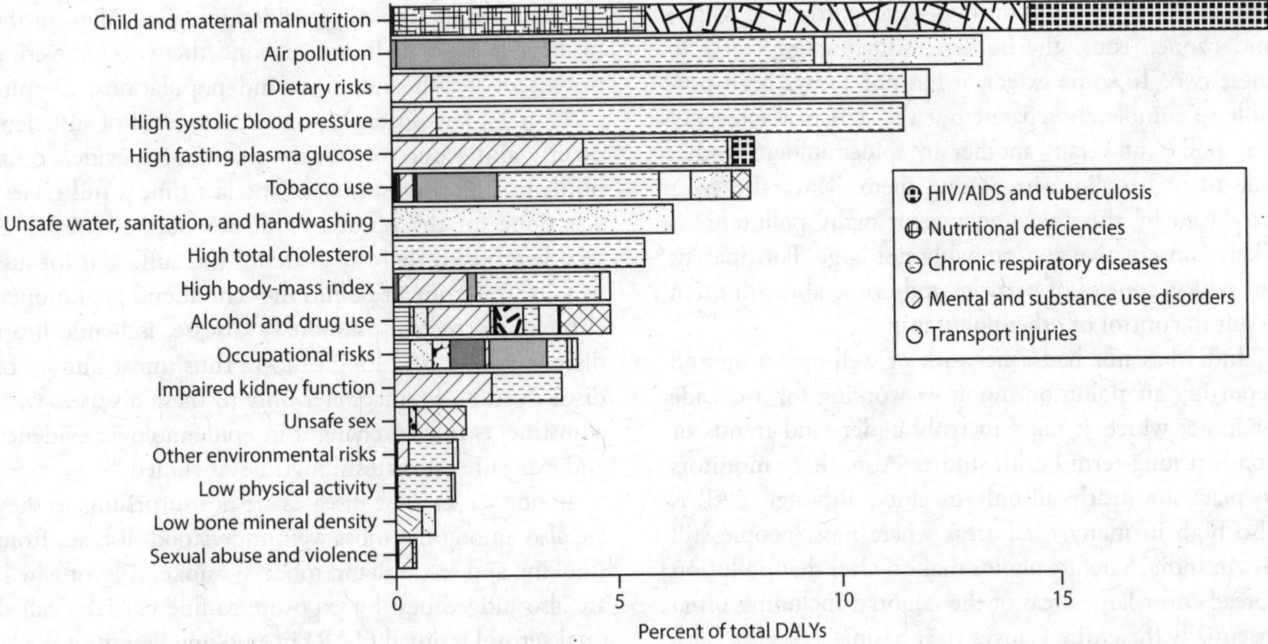

Figure 12.1 The risk factors affecting the burden of disease in India in 2016, which have been evaluated in Burden of Disease studies. Although not shown here, the uncertainty ranges in these estimates are large and not all risk factors have been evaluated. In addition, numbers change regularly due to new data and methods and thus should be considered indicative only.

Source: Dandona 2017.

which is one of the lower estimates available (Chafe 2014) although there are higher ones (for example, see Lelieveld 2015). Chowdhury et al. (2019) provide a comparison across seven such estimates. It shows that, as a group, although declining sharply this set of traditional pollution exposures still causes somewhat more ill health than the modern ones, recognizing the many gaps and uncertainties in all such estimates.

Table 12.1 Trends in health impacts of major traditional and modern environmental risks in India in units of percentage of total DALYs each year. Here, 26% of ambient PM is thought to be due to household fuel use and thus overlaps between the two categories

	1990	2000	2016	Trend
WASH	11.8	9.5	5.2	
HAP-total	10.7	9.7	7.2	
Total Traditional	22.5	19.2	12.4	
Ambient PM	6.4	6.4	7.1	
Ambient Ozone	0.3	0.4	0.5	
Pb Exposure	0.8	0.9	1.1	
Occup Exposures	1.5	1.6	1.9	
Total Modern	9	9.3	10.6	

Source: IHME 2017.

In the next few sections, we review the evidence base for the burden of disease in each category and discuss major issues for each.

AMBIENT AIR POLLUTION

The burden of disease estimates for environmental risks in India, as for other countries, rely on three separate lines of evidence:[3]

1. An estimate of the relevant exposures of the pollutant of interest in the population based on measurements, surveys, and modeling;
2. An estimate of the disease specific exposure–response relationships based on epidemiologic studies, systematic reviews, and meta-analysis/modelling;
3. An estimate of the actual national burden for each relevant disease, usually taken from burden of disease statistics available from IHME or WHO.

Although there are many ambient air pollutants with some health impact, exposure–response information is

[3] http://www.healthdata.org/gbd/about/protocol.

only available in detail for two—fine particles (PM2.5) and ozone. Thus, the burden estimates only refer to these two. To some extent, it has not always been possible to completely separate out the statistical effects of one pollutant versus another in epidemiologic studies due to high colinearity among them. Thus, the error produced by this focus on two of many pollutants is likely conservative and probably not large. Fortunately, for policy, control of particles and ozone also will often result in control of other pollutants.

India has not had a network of well-operating and reporting air pollution monitors working for a decade or more, which it takes to truly understand trends or conduct long-term health studies. Also, those monitors in place are nearly all only in cities, although AAP is also high in many rural areas where most people still live in India. Satellite photos make it clear that pollution spreads over large areas of the country, including often essentially the entire Ganges river basin.

Consequently, national exposure estimates for burden of disease studies must rely heavily on satellite data, bolstered by emission inventories of varying quality, completeness, and date, and what local measurements exist. Basically, the models triangulate on the best estimate in each place based on these three types of inputs combined with atmospheric chemistry and dispersion models. The conversion of satellite imagery, which of course examines the entire air column, to a ground-level value of use for health assessment, is of particular difficulty as it changes by season, time of day, location, and such other factors. As more ground-level measurements become available, however, these conversions are improving. In general, however, as new models are applied and new data become available, the estimates change, even if there are just incremental changes actually occurring on the ground. It is a work in progress.

UrbanEmissions.info[4] maps the ambient fine particle concentrations estimated in a triangulation fashion, combining ground measurements, satellite measurements, and source inventories. It represents a national population-weighted concentration of about 77 μg/m^3, but with major populations, such as that in the entire Gangetic river basin, experiencing annual levels greater than 100 μg/m^3.[5]

There are thousands of epidemiologic studies on the health effects of AAP done around the world, covering dozens of health endpoints and populations. Despite this, only a few dozen or so are considered of sufficient quality and scope to provide quantitative evidence for burden of disease estimates. The last time a full review was done for the burden of disease studies (2011), it was determined that the evidence was sufficient for just five diseases from air pollution—childhood pneumonia, chronic obstructive pulmonary disease, ischemic heart disease, stroke, and lung cancer. Thus, most burden of disease estimates since refer only to these diseases, with adjustments due to changes in epidemiologic evidence and exposure estimates sometimes included.[6]

In one sense, these diseases are not surprising, as they are also among the most well understood diseases from smoking and secondhand tobacco smoke, risks of which are also judged best by exposure to fine particles called total aerosol residual (TAR) in smoking literature. Risks are higher of course when putting the burning material in one's mouth, but the same set of diseases occur, albeit at different relative risks.

Posing higher risks, having been studied longer with more resources, and with easier exposure metrics, however, smoking has a much greater range of other diseases associated with it. The evidence base for many of these same diseases, however, is also rising for AAP. In particular, there is growing evidence of other cancers, adverse pregnancy outcomes of several kinds, flus, adult pneumonia, and diabetes, among others.[7] Some of these will undoubtedly be upgraded to be part of the official burden of AAP the next time the Global Burden of Diseases (GBD) is formally revised. As these diseases represent large background burdens in India and elsewhere, the total burden associated with AAP is likely to rise as a result.

Perhaps the most contentious aspect of applying the methods in the burden of disease studies to India is the

[4] See http://www.urbanemissions.info/india-air-quality/india-satpm25-maps/, last accessed on 28 December 2019. Readers are advised to compare the maps for 1998 and 2016.

[5] Indian long-term standard is 40 ug/m^3 and the WHO guideline is 10 ug/m^3.

[6] It is important to recognize that the absolute burden estimates are revised over time according to the newest data, and thus may be somewhat different in years beyond 2018 in the online database (https://vizhub.healthdata.org/gbd-compare/) than the precise estimates in this chapter. The general relationships described in this chapter, however, should remain fairly stable.

[7] By 2019, impacts on diabetes and adult pneumonia had been included, although these do not add much to the total mortality burden in India from AAP (~110,000). It has been planned for 2020 to add adverse pregnancy outcomes due to exposures to pregnant women.

lack of studies used to derive the risk estimates from India itself. Some government observers have cast doubt on the whole exercise as a result.

It is of course natural to prefer local evidence, but the question is whether excellent evidence from other places is insufficient for action in India. There are several ways to consider this problem. One argument is that people living in India are somehow immune or less susceptible to pollution due to genetics or generations having lived with pollution. Actually, available evidence on factors that change vulnerability to pollution exposures, particularly poor nutrition/growth and access to healthcare, would indicate that, on average, Indians ought to be more susceptible than the largely North American and European populations where the studies were done. Furthermore, the few studies that pick out ethnicity show no special resistance to pollution effects on Indians who moved to those areas after being born in India. In addition, new cohort studies (such as Yin et al. [2017]) being published from the other major polluted middle-income country, China, show if anything more vulnerability not less than in 'western' populations.

Second, although there are as yet no long-term prospective cohort studies done in India that can be included in the group used to derive global risks for AAP, there are other categories of studies done in India that do show effects. In particular, time series studies, which are quicker, cheaper, and less data-intensive to conduct, show effects in India that are within the range of what is found in other countries (for instance, Atkinson 2012; Balakrishnan 2012). These do not provide sufficient evidence of long-term risks needed for the burden assessments, but raise the question of why Indian populations would show the same short-term effects as others and not show similar long-term ones. In addition, as noted in the following section, much of the world literature on the health effects of household air pollution is derived from South Asia. Indians show no special resistance.

Finally, to wait for long-term studies to be completed in India in order to put air quality actions in motion would pose ethical challenges. Environmental guidelines for public health have always been uniformly applicable across all populations with virtually no precedence for differential exposure standards for individual countries. Indeed, that has been the basis for the adoption of WHO air quality guidelines as the framing for the revised Indian National Ambient Air Quality Standards.

It is therefore be very important to acknowledge the available scientific evidence for action and not defer the implementation of required programmes and policies to reduce population exposures. As new studies from India generate additional evidence, they will inform future updates to the guidelines but holding back the momentum on actions now can have serious consequences for public health.

One uncertainty about AAP risk estimates in general, and for India in particular, is whether dust (blown from the ground) should be treated the same as combustion particles. High-level reviews to date have concluded that there is insufficient evidence to treat the particles differently in policy and thus in those countries with rigorous regulation of air pollution, cities and other jurisdictions are required to conduct dust control measures equally to those for combustion sources (WHO 2006). There is, however, toxicological evidence of lesser effect, which leads some to suggest that ought to be treated differently. On the other hand, there is also evidence that dust particles are often associated with combustion material that has been deposited and resuspended. Finally, of course, there are issues of practicality in that it would add considerable cost and complexity to try to monitor and regulate the two types of sources separately, which also varies seasonally. More work would be justified to examine this issue in India.

Recommendations on Ambient Air Pollution

There is little space here to discuss control measures required in India to reduce its large burden from AAP, but three points could be considered as high priority:

1. India has many air pollution laws and regulations in place already. Much greater efforts are however needed for enforcement. Doing better at it could have a major benefit with little additional regulation.
2. India needs to recognize that the problem of household air pollution (HAP) is also an ambient problem, indeed perhaps the largest single contributor to AAP. A recent study found, for example, that household fuels contribute more than vehicles, power plants, or industries in India (GBD MAPS 2018). Although many sources need to be controlled to completely tackle ambient pollution, it may be impossible to achieve clean outdoor air when two-thirds of the population continues to burn solid cooking fuels every day (Chowdhury et al. 2019).
3. India needs to consider development of regional air quality management entities, since pollution

concentrations in any one place is only partly due to sources in that place. As in other countries, these bodies must have clear enforcement authority and operate at roughly the system of the problem (that is the air shed), which are much broader than single municipalities, but rather range across the entire air basin in which the city lies. China has done this for the Beijing region, covering more than 1,000 km, because, like India, much of the pollution derives from outside the city itself.

HOUSEHOLD AIR POLLUTION

Household air pollution resulting from the use of solid cooking fuels is now understood to be a major risk factor for health. According to the GBD 2016 study, diseases caused by HAP pollution were responsible for an estimated 2.5 million premature deaths in 2016 (4.7 per cent of all deaths worldwide) and 77 million disability-adjusted life years (DALYs) (3.2 per cent of all DALYs worldwide) with low-and middle-income countries (LMICs) bearing the largest share of this burden (GBD 2016: Risk Factors Collaborators 2017). While other slightly varying estimates for this burden have been available, all overwhelmingly point to the large and significant burden continuing to be borne by poor and vulnerable populations that currently rely on solid fuels for meeting their household energy needs (Landrigan et al. 2017).

Estimates of the HAP disease burden from exposure to PM2.5 is based on cause-specific integrated exposure–response functions that use the relative risk of mortality from ischemic heart disease, stroke, chronic obstructive pulmonary disease, lung cancer, and acute lower respiratory infections (ALRI), (Burnett et al. 2014; Smith 2014) together with estimates of household PM2.5 concentrations and exposures for men, women, and children (derived from spatio-temporal Gaussian process modelling [GBD 2016 Cause of Death Collaborators 2017]).

Nearly 70 per cent of the HAP burden is attributable to non-communicable diseases (NCDs) affecting both men and women (GBD 2016 Risk Factors Collaborators 2017). The burden for children continues to be high despite the decline in attributable burden. Further, with an expanding base of evidence for associations with health end-points such as adverse pregnancy outcomes and neuro cognition (Smith 2014), this burden is likely to be even larger for children, who can be at risk for extremely low-dose exposures to pollutants during windows of vulnerability in utero.

In 2013 exposure to ambient and HAP cost the world's economy some USD 5.11 trillion in welfare losses (World Bank 2015), with countries in South Asia experiencing HAP attributable welfare losses of the order of USD 1.52 trillion and up to 5 per cent of their GDP.

The Health Burden of HAP in India

The India State-level Disease Burden Initiative (India State-level Disease Burden Initiative Collaborators 2017) produced as part of the GBD 2016 study provides some of the most comprehensive state-level estimates for disease burden in India. The leading risk factors in India in 2016 have been shown in Figure 12.2.

Together, outdoor and HAP accounted for a substantial proportion of cardiovascular disease (4.4 per cent), chronic respiratory disease (2.5 per cent) and lower respiratory infection (2.5 per cent) burden in India. HAP accounted for about 780,000 premature deaths and 22 million DALYs in India (India State-level Disease Burden Initiative Collaborators 2017) with more than half the deaths and DALYs attributable to deaths from chronic respiratory and cardiovascular diseases.

The summary exposure value or the relative risk-weighted prevalence of exposure to HAP from solid fuels has dropped by 52 per cent (with the raw proportion of solid fuel users declining from 85 per cent to around 42 per cent) in India since 1991. This decrease has been largely offset by a simultaneous increase in population with essentially no change in the total number of people relying on solid-cook fuels over this period (Bonjour 2013; IHME 2017).

The HAP attributable burden in India has, however, decreased from around 42 million DALYs in 1990 to around 22 million DALYs in 2016. Given the relatively constant number of people exposed across the years, the reduction is largely on account of the steep decrease in the baseline incidence of childhood pneumonia (due to better nutrition, healthcare, and vaccines) resulting in a proportional reduction attributable to HAP.

There is considerable variation in the DALY rates as well as the total HAP burden across states (IHME 2017). DALYs rates and the burden were amongst the highest in the states of Rajasthan, Bihar, Uttar Pradesh, Madhya Pradesh, and Assam. The DALYs rates were among the lowest in the southern states of Tamil Nadu, Kerala, and union territories. However, with increasing contributions from NCDs (in particular cardiovascular

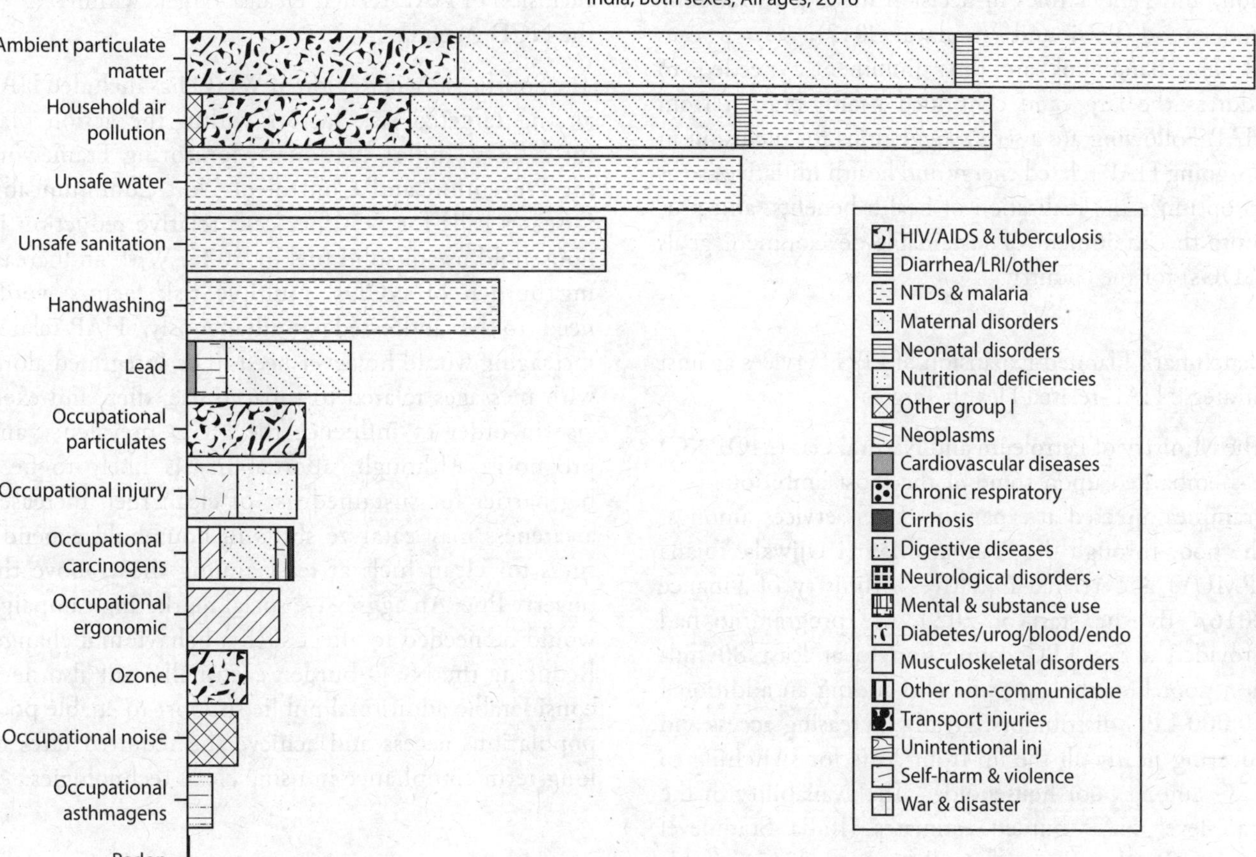

Figure 12.2 Burden of disease in India from major environment and occupational risk factors

Source: IHME 2017.

diseases) in the states of Punjab, Tamil Nadu, Kerala to the disease burden, future reductions in HAP exposures may not result in similar gains with the overall HAP attributable burden (as was the case since 1990 on account of decreasing ALRI incidence).

THE WAY FORWARD

There is currently an overwhelming body of scientific evidence (Smith 2014) that has pointed to the increased risks from HAP for various adverse health outcomes, only a portion of which are even currently addressed in available disease burden estimates. Merely viewing this as a poverty-related issue and waiting for development to catch up is unlikely to reduce the burden in the foreseeable future (Smith and Pillarisetti 2017).

Furthermore, an increasing body of literature points to the inability to achieve health-relevant exposure reductions through the use of 'improved' or even 'advanced combustion' cookstoves, both on account of insufficient emission reductions and stove stacking (Balakrishnan 2015; Bruce 2014; Pillariseti 2014; Sambandam 2014; WHO 2014). Clean fuels such as liquefied petroleum gas (LPG) meet the International Organization for Standardization (ISO 2012) and WHO recommendations (WHO 2014), for potentially achieving WHO air quality standards within homes but are contingent upon adoption and sustained use of clean fuels by households. Income, education, and urban location have been shown to promote adoption of cleaner stoves and fuels but the role of uninterrupted fuel availability and prices, household size and composition, and gender roles in decision making is not fully understood (Lewis and Pattanayak 2012).

New paradigms are thus imminently needed to address the large and continued health burden from HAP. Following are a series suggestions for inclusion in on-going HAP related energy and health initiatives so as to optimize the realization of health benefits, and promote the attainment of sustainable development goals (SDGs) for the country.

Benchmark Planned Expansion of LPG Services against Strategic HAP-related Health Targets

The Ministry of Petroleum and Natural Gas (MOPNG) has embarked upon some of the most ambitious programmes directed at expanding LPG services amongst the poor through the Pradhan Mantri Ujjwala Yojana (PMUY) and related initiatives (Ministry of Finance 2016). By the start of 2020, the programme had provided a free LPG connection to at least 80 million poor households, while also adding an additional 10,000 LPG distributors, greatly increasing access and covering nearly all the up-front costs for switching to LPG among poor households.[8] The availability of the state-level HAP burden estimates (India State-level Disease Burden Initiative Collaborators 2017) affords an unprecedented opportunity to prioritize and target LPG expansion across states by benchmarking against specific health targets. Expanding LPG access in states with highest ALRI burdens and covering entire districts for example, may allow a quick and easy ecological assessment of the benefits of HAP reduction on children's health. Further, adverse pregnancy outcomes are not currently included in HAP disease burden estimates but, available evidence suggests significant impacts from solid fuel use on birthweight (Amegah 2015). Providing subsidies to cover costs of LPG use among BPL pregnant women for the duration of the pregnancy and the first year of the child has the potential to achieve and document health benefits of LPG provision, while serving to also reduce the overall HAP attributable burden. Strategic alignment with health targets would greatly increase the ability of the ministry to market and promote the use of LPG thereby increasing the effectiveness of their programmes while also addressing the HAP attributable burden.

Inclusion of HAP-related Health Targets within the NCD Agenda

The Southeast Asia Region of WHO has included HAP among targeted risk factors within the action plan for NCDs. India's National Monitoring Framework for Prevention and Control of Non-Communicable Diseases calls for a 50 per cent relative reduction in household use of solid fuel by 2025. With an increasing burden of NCDs, multiple risk factors would need to be addressed simultaneously. HAP-related messaging would however need to be integrated along with messages related to tobacco use, diet, and exercise in order to influence the NCD prevalence and prognosis. Although, affordability is likely to be a big barrier for sustained use of clean fuel, increased awareness may catalyze shifts in household expenditures for clean fuels at least among those above the poverty line. An aggressive social marketing campaign would be needed to affect such a behavioural change. Reducing the NCD burden eventually will also need considerable additional public support to enable poor populations access and achieve the required rates of long-term compliance in using clean technologies.

Expansion of AAP Monitoring in Rural Areas to Aid Surveillance for HAP-related Exposure Reductions

As noted earlier, HAP contributes substantially to AAP in India. In densely populated communities, health relevant reductions in exposures cannot be accomplished without entire habitations transitioning to clean fuels (Desai 2016). As the PMUY enters its next phase of expansion and other initiatives such as 'smokeless villages' are launched, it will be critical to see the signal in HAP exposure reductions to aid surveillance. Currently, any information on HAP exposure reductions is generated only via research studies, which presently is too resource intensive to scale. Further, the current hybrid models (that use a combination of satellite and chemical transport-based methods) to provide gridded AAP concentrations for estimation of associated burden of disease (Cohen 2017) lack information from rural monitors to ground-truth the estimates. AAP monitoring in rural areas would thus allow an efficient modality to monitor both AAP and HAP associated exposure trends across both rural and urban areas of India.

[8] In February 2018, it was announced in the annual budget speech that the target was being raised to 80 million.

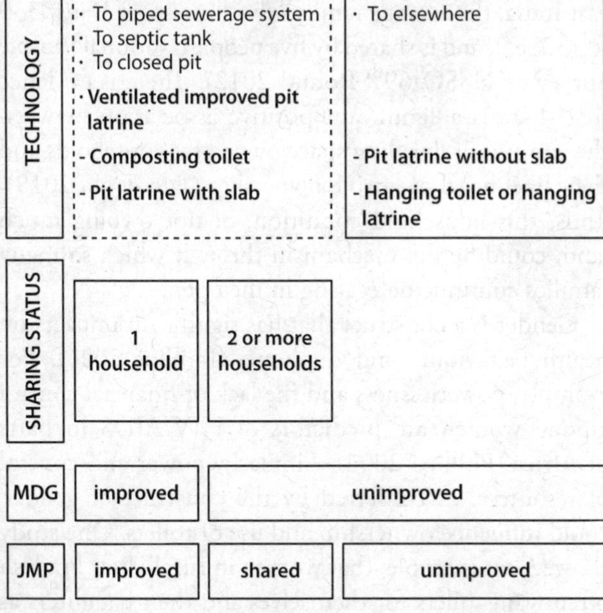

Figure 12.3 Joint Monitoring Programme and Millennium Development Goal classifications of improved, shared, and unimproved sanitation technologies

Source: Exley 2014.

SANITATION

Globally, more than half the burden from the combination of poor WASH is due to poor sanitation, and this amounts to about one-third in India (see Figure 12.3). Sanitation has long been considered to be the bedrock of public health. Indeed, readers of the *British Medical Journal* voted sanitation the single most important medical milestone since 1840 (Ferriman 2007). Yet globally, billions of people continue living without access to improved sanitation, which the Joint Monitoring Programme (JMP) for Water Supply and Sanitation defines as sanitation facilities that are not shared with other households, and that hygienically separate excreta from human contact (JMP 2017). Approximately 2.3 billion people (32 per cent of the world's population) still rely on some form of unimproved sanitation (JMP 2017). This includes shared sanitation facilities and pit latrines without a slab, or bucket latrines. Unimproved sanitation also includes open defecation, the practice of defecating in fields, forests, open bodies of water, and other open spaces. Globally, 892 million people still defecate in the open (JMP 2017).

Epidemiological studies have drawn inextricable causal links between unimproved sanitation—which often leads to fecal contamination—and disease. One gram of faeces can contain 10^6 viral pathogens, $10^{6\text{-}8}$ bacterial pathogens, 10^4 protozoan cysts, and $10\text{-}10^4$ helminth eggs (Mara 2010). This contamination is the cause of diarrhoeal disease, which is the second leading cause of deaths in children under the age of five globally (Hammer and Spears 2016), and can cause other diseases such as urinary tract infections, soil-transmitted helminth infections, trachoma, schistosomiasis, and cholera (Coffey 2014).

India is home to the largest share of people that defecate in the open. Over 520 million people in India (40 per cent of India's total population as of 2017) defecate in the open. Additionally, 16 per cent of India's population uses some other form of unimproved sanitation. Thus, only 44 per cent of Indians have access to improved sanitation (JMP 2017).

Estimates show that over 2.5 per cent of all DALYs in India are attributable to unimproved sanitation (IHME 2017). This is almost one percentage point higher than global DALYs attributable to the same risk factor (IHME 2017). Open defecation costs India nearly USD 54 billion annually, of which over USD 38 billion is the health-related economic impact (WSP 2011), and poses a significant threat to children under the age of five. Studies in India reveal that a 10 per cent increase in open defecation leads to a 0.7 per cent increase in stunting and severe stunting (Spears 2013a), both of which are proxy indicators for long-term social and economic outcomes (Spears 2013b).

Current Efforts to Improve Sanitation Outcomes

Although there is little doubt that unimproved sanitation causes disease, there remains uncertainty vis-à-vis the etiology of why so many people in India continue resorting to some form of unimproved sanitation. Researchers have posited a variety of theories, many of which converge towards a central theme: flawed attitudes and poor knowledge, at the individual level, about the benefits of toilet use lead to high rates of open defecation throughout India.

This belief, that India's sanitation crisis persists due to individual-level determinants, has spurred the creation of several interventions. For example:

1. The Government of India's Swachh Bharat Abhiyan (Clean India Mission or SBA) tries to convince households to build toilets by providing

families with up to INR 12,000 (USD 168) for toilet construction. This assistance comes in the form of a reimbursement after a family has completed construction of a toilet at their house.[9]

2. Community-Led Total Sanitation (CLTS) is a sanitation behaviour change curriculum that seeks to raise awareness about the benefits of toilet use by promoting the idea that disease can spread through an entire community even if just one person defecates in the open (Kar 2008). Families living in communities exposed to CLTS thus have the awareness to put pressure on one another to construct and use toilets. CLTS workers also lead communities on 'walks of shame' through the fields they commonly use to openly defecate. These walks attempt to shame communities to demand toilets (Kar 2008). This curriculum also recommends toilet construction not be subsidized, citing evidence that suggests financial assistance often undermines 'ownership' of goods or services, which can lead to non-use (WSP 2007).

Possible Social Determinants of Sanitation Outcomes

Despite the efforts, hundreds of millions of people throughout India continue defecating in the open. This could be because SBA and CLTS both ignore the possible social determinants of open defecation in India. Social determinants can be broadly defined as the economic, social, political conditions, and systems (Krieger 1994). This section elucidates how some of these determinants such as housing conditions, occupation, gender, caste, and educational attainment, along with prevailing economic, social, and political structures/relationships, might influence sanitation outcomes throughout India.

Household conditions are primarily used to indicate the material circumstances of a family. For example, the materials used to build a home can be indicative of the family's wealth. But housing conditions can also be the mechanism that dictates certain health behaviours or outcomes (Galobardes 2006). In rural Bihar, a state in east India, the average family's dwelling space is just 330 ft^2 (30 m^2), and is shared by five people (National Sample Survey or NSSO 69th Round 2012). There is evidence that there is a significant positive association between the amount of dwelling space owned by households and their likelihood of latrine ownership (Jain et al., 2019). Thus, this household condition, of not owning much land, could be the mechanism through which so many families continue defecating in the open.

Gender is a construct that has significant impacts on health behaviours and outcomes (Phillips 2004). For example, powerlessness and the lack of financial control among women are predictors of HIV/AIDS in parts of Africa (Phillips 2004). Similarly, power and control of resources, as conferred by the construct of gender, could influence ownership and use of toilets. One study showed, for example, that women in rural Uttar Pradesh often want toilets for themselves and their daughters as they help protect privacy (Khanna and Das 2016). Yet this is not a priority for their husbands, who spend the money on other things. Thus, segments of the population—in this case women—might already demand toilets, but do not control the resources needed to construct them (Khanna and Das 2016). Therefore, policies and programmes should be designed to address power imbalances stemming from gender norms to actually meet the demand for toilets.

India's ancient caste system has always been a mechanism that distributes social advantage or disadvantage. As a result, caste could influence education outcomes and occupation, which are both predictors of economic outcomes. These economic outcomes, in turn, predict a household's ability to own, maintain, or use a toilet. It is necessary, then, to examine the pathways through which caste-based discrimination influences sanitation outcomes.

Occupation is often considered a predictor of health insofar as it is indicative of a person's socioeconomic position (wealth, income) (Galobardes 2006). But occupation can predict health in other ways, too. For example, protections offered to workers often vary by occupation. One study showed that construction workers in India were far less likely to have access to a toilet at the workplace than factory workers (Rajaraman 2013). Similarly, farmers might have a toilet at home. Yet they defecate in the open if they are in the fields far from home during the day (Rajaraman 2013). Thus, improving sanitation related outcomes depends not only on ensuring that households have access to a safe, hygienic,

[9] It should be noted that the Prime Minister of India, Narendra Modi, declared India open defecation free thanks to SBA on October 2, 2019. The Indian government's data suggests that 110 million toilets were installed for 600 million people between 2014 and 2019. Yet the reliability of these data and the government data source, the National Annual Rural Sanitation Survey, has been questioned. (ref)

and functional toilet but policies are needed to ensure that this vital infrastructure is made available at all places of employment.

Education is similar to occupation in that it is typically used as an indicator of socioeconomic position, and thus a predictor of income and wealth. But education can be indicative of more. For example, educational attainment and literacy influence how individuals are able to access and engage with health services (Galobardes 2006). For example, India's literacy rate of 74 per cent remains below the global average (Census 2011). In states such as Bihar, the literacy rate is still only 64 per cent (Census 2011). Individuals are required to fill out necessary paperwork in order to receive the government reimbursement after toilet construction. Low literacy rates could deter families from even engaging with this process as they might not know how to receive the services they are entitled to, which could contribute to poor sanitation outcomes. Therefore, any policy should be designed so that it can be accessed even by those who are illiterate.

International guidelines, set by the JMP, limit what kinds of infrastructure constitute improved sanitation. As noted above, sanitation facilities must not be shared with other households and must hygienically separate excreta from human contact in order to be considered improved (JMP 2017). The emphasis on ensuring that sanitation facilities not be shared is motivated in part by the belief that shared sanitation might be harder to maintain. As a result, people might revert to defecating in the open if this infrastructure is not kept clean. However, shared sanitation might be the best option in densely populated urban areas, or in rural areas where people do not own enough land to construct their own toilet. More thought needs to be put into how shared sanitation could be maintained in both urban and rural settings. Diversifying the type of sanitation infrastructure that constitutes improved sanitation could help improve access to this vital infrastructure.

HEALTH AND SANITATION

Numerous studies have attempted to quantify the health improvements associated with increased sanitation coverage and use. The results from even the most robust and thoroughly planned studies have been mixed, however. For example, Clasen et al. conducted a cluster-randomized trial to assess the health impact of India's Total Sanitation Campaign in the state of Odisha. While this study did find significant improvements in self-reported latrine coverage (9 per cent to 63 per cent in treatment villages versus 8 per cent to 12 per cent in control villages), the intervention was not found to protect against diarrhoea in children under the age of five (Clasen et al. 2014).

The results of the WASH benefits trial from 2018 paint a somewhat similar picture, albeit in Bangladesh, India's eastern neighbour. Luby et al. found no significant improvements in linear growth for children in neither the individual water, sanitation, and hand washing groups of the study, nor when these interventions were combined (Luby et al. 2018). The study did find, however, significant reductions in diarrhoea in all treatment groups, except for the water treatment group (Luby et al. 2018). Similarly, The SHINE study, a cluster-randomized control trial conducted in Zimbabwe, found no impact of WASH on stunting or anemia (Humphrey et al., 2019).

There are various explanations for these mixed, and often times disappointing, results. For instance, Patil et al. note that a significant viral load might remain in the environment well after increased toilet coverage and use (Patil 2013). Thus, studies might have to last longer in order to notice improved health. Furthermore, there are countless other exposure pathways to disease, particularly in places such as rural India. Dirt floors inside the home, along with living in close proximity to farm animals, can also increase the risk of disease despite high toilet ownership and use.

Yet, the externalities associated with toilet ownership and use extend beyond the realm of 'traditional' health indicators. Access to sanitation affords people safety and privacy, which is particularly important for women and girls. Furthermore, access to sanitation, especially in schools, helps girls manage their menstrual hygiene needs. Additionally, the Water and Sanitation Programme (WSP) found that open defecation costs India nearly USD 54 billion, of which USD 10 billion is lost productivity (from illness or searching for a safe place to defecate) (WSP 2011).

Therefore, while sanitation is a fundamental mechanism through which improvements to public health can be made, there still remains some ambiguity vis-à-vis the quantifiable impact sanitation has on health outcomes in places such as India. This evidence, or the lack thereof, should not be taken to undermine the need for sanitation. Rather, continued efforts should be made to promote coverage and use of toilets, along with improving all-around living conditions, in order to not only improve health, but social and economic outcomes as well.

***

Air pollution in the form of AAP and HAP has emerged as the single largest environmental risk factor contributing significantly to the burden of disease in India. Interventions directed at AAP are already part of a regulatory framework that seek to constrain emissions but are plagued by the diversity and the volume of emissions that do not translate into exposure reduction. Despite the large attributable burden, reducing HAP exposures has not been explicitly a part of the regulatory requirement within the ambient air quality programmes. Increasing access and promoting sustained use of clean fuels provide the single most important opportunity to achieve the required exposure reductions with accompanying massive reductions in the health burden, while being in alignment with existing programmatic objectives and societal preferences. It is imperative that such an opportunity not be missed and that evidence from HAP interventions be used to spur the larger discourse on health burden from air pollution in India.

India's Ministry of Health and Family Welfare, however, has initiated a pioneering effort to evaluate how air pollution can be viewed as part of its health mandate (Sagar 2015). In addition, in examining air pollution as a health hazard, it did not pick out urban or rural, indoor or outdoor, but took an exposure approach, that is assessing those sources that lead to human exposures, not organizing to clean up particular parts of the environment. Few if any health ministries have taken up air pollution around the world, as nearly all countries place it within ministries of environment. In addition, to our knowledge, no jurisdiction has taken an exposure approach to its control (Sagar 2016). This bodes well for India to set up the mechanism to effectively control this large health hazard for its population.

Hundreds of millions of people throughout India continue relying on some form of unimproved sanitation. The most common form, open defecation, causes the spread of untreated and disease-spreading human faeces, which leads to high rates of morbidity and mortality. Current efforts aim to improve access to improved sanitation. They focus, however, on a very narrow set of etiological factors that might cause risky sanitation behaviours, such as open defecation. There is a need to examine a broader set of social determinants that might also lead to this behaviour. Doing so might lead to population-level changes in health outcomes. Lastly, efforts to quantify the health impacts of sanitation have yielded mixed results. Nevertheless, these should not undermine the need for sanitation, as toilets provide benefits beyond the realm of 'traditional' health indicators. Clearly, studies need to be done that better capture these extended benefits.

India has big challenges remaining in all three of these areas. Through the SBA, for example, it is beginning to address those for sanitation and through the PMUY LPG programme, those for HAP, although these need continued monitoring, re-adjustment, and expansion to promote usage as well as access. The large-scale AAP episodes in the Delhi region that are becoming a regular feature of the October/November period on top of its persistent high levels of AAP should have stimulated plans for more stringent controls. It remains to be seen how much impact they will have.

REFERENCES

Amegah, A.K., R. Quansah, and J.K. Jaakkola. 2014. 'Household Air Pollution from Solid Fuel Use and Risk of Adverse Pregnancy Outcomes: A Systematic Review and Meta-analysis of the Empirical Evidence', *PLOS One* 9(12): e113920.

Atkinson R.W., A. Cohen et al. 2012. 'Systematic Review and Meta-analysis of Epidemiological Time-series Studies on Outdoor Air Pollution and Health in Asia', *Air Qual Atmos Health* 5: 383–91.

Balakrishnan K., B. Ganguli et al. 2012. 'A Spatially Disaggregated Time-series Analysis of the Short-term Effects of Particulate Matter Exposure on Mortality in Chennai, India', *Air Qual Atmos Health.* doi:10.1007/s11869-011-0151-6.

Balakrishnan, K., S. Sambandam et al. 2015. 'Household Air Pollution Exposures of Pregnant Women Receiving Advanced Combustion Cookstoves in India: Implications for Intervention'. *Annals of Global Health* 81(3): 375–85. doi:10.1016/j.aogh.2015.08.009.

Bonjour S., H. Adair-Rohani et al. 'Solid Fuel Use for Household Cooking: Country and Regional Estimates for 1980–2010'. *Environmental Health Perspectives.* doi:10.1289/ehp.1205987.

Bruce, N., D. Pope et al. 2015. 'WHO Indoor Air Quality Guidelines on Household Fuel Combustion: Strategy Implications of New Evidence on Interventions and Exposure-risk Functions'. *Atmospheric Environment* 106: 451–57. doi:10.1016/j.atmosenv.2014.08.064

Burnett, R.T., Pope III et al. 2014. 'An Integrated Risk Function for Estimating the Global Burden of Disease Attributable to Ambient Fine Particulate Matter Exposure'. *Environmental Health Perspectives.* doi:10.1289/ehp.1307049.

Chafe, Z., M. Brauer et al. 2014. 'Household Cooking with Solid Fuels Contributes to Ambient PM2.5 Air Pollution and the Burden of Disease'. *Environmental Health Perspectives* 122(12): 1314–20. doi:10.1289/ehp.1206340.

Chowdhury, S., Z.A. Chafe, A. Pillarisetti, J. Lelieveld, S. Guttikunda, and S. Dey. 2019. 'The Contribution of Household Fuels to Ambient Air Pollution in India: A Comparison of Recent Estimates', Policy Brief, May, CCAPC/2019/01, Collaborative Clean Air Policy Centre, New Delhi.

Chowdhury, S., S. Dey, S. Guttikunda, A. Pillarisetti, K.R. Smith, and L.D. Girolama. 2019. 'Indian Annual Ambient Air Quality Standard is Achievable by Completely Mitigating Emissions from Household Sources', *Proc. US Nat Acad Sciences* 116: 10711–16.

Clasen, T., S. Boisson, P. Routray, B. Torondel, M. Bell, O. Cumming, ... W.P. Schmidt. 2014. 'Effectiveness of a Rural Sanitation Programme on Diarrhoea, Soil-transmitted Helminth Infection, and Child Malnutrition in Odisha, India: A Cluster-randomised Trial', *The Lancet Global Health* 2(11): e645–e653. doi:10.1016/S2214-109X(14)70307-9.

Coffey, D. 2014. *Revealed Preference For Open Defecation: Evidence From A New Survey In Rural North India.* First edition.

Cohen, A.J., M. Brauer et al. 2017. Estimates and 25-year Trends of the Global Burden of Disease Attributable to Ambient Air Pollution: An Analysis of Data from the Global Burden of Diseases Study 2015. *Lancet* 389: 1907–18.

Dandona, L., R. Dandona et al. 2017. 'Nations within a Nation: Variations in Epidemiological Transition across the States of India, 1990–2016 in the Global Burden of Disease Study', *Lancet.* doi:10.1016/S0140-6736(17)32804-0.

Desai, M.A. 2016. 'Model of Postulated Coverage Effect from Clean Cooking Interventions in Multiscale Drivers of Global Environmental Health', doctoral dissertation, Environmental Health Sciences Graduate Group, University of California, Berkeley.

Exley, J.L.R., B. Liseka et al. 2015. 'The Sanitation Ladder: What Constitutes an Improved Form of Sanitation?', *Environmental Science & Technology* 49(2): 1086–94. doi:10.1021/es503945x.Ferriman, A. 2007. 'BMJ Readers Choose the "Sanitary Revolution" as Greatest Medical Advance since 1840', *BMJ* 334:111.

Galobardes, B. 2006. 'Indicators of Socioeconomic Position (Part 1)'. *Journal of Epidemiology & Community Health* 60(1): 7–12. doi:10.1136/jech.2004.023531.

GBD 2016 Causes of Death Collaborators. 2017. 'Global, Regional, and National Age–Sex Specific Mortality for 264 Causes of Death, 1980–2016: A Systematic Analysis for the Global Burden of Disease Study 2016'. *Lancet* 390: 1151–210.

GBD 2016 Risk Factors Collaborators. 2017. 'Global, Regional, and National Comparative Risk Assessment of 84 Behavioural, Environmental and Occupational, and Metabolic Risks or Clusters of Risks, 1990–2016: A Systematic Analysis for the Global Burden of Disease Study 2016', *Lancet* 390: 1345–422.

GBD MAPS Working Group. 2018. *Burden of Disease Attributable to Major Sources of Air Pollution in India*, Special Report #21. Boston: Health Effects Institute.

Hammer, J. and D. Spears. 2016. 'Village Sanitation and Child Health: Effects and External Validity in a Randomized Field Experiment in Rural India', *Journal of Health Economics* 48: 135–148. doi:10.1016/j.jhealeco.2016.03.003.

Indian Council of Medical Research (ICMR), Public Health Foundation of India (PHFI), Institute for Health Metrics and Evaluation (IHME). 2017. *India: Health of the Nation's States—The India State Level Burden Initiative.* ICMR, PHFI, and IHME.

Institute for Health Metrics and Evaluation (IHME). 2016. GBD Compare Data Visualization. Seattle, WA: IHME, University of Washington. Available at http://vizhub.healthdata.org/gbd-compare, last accessed on 20 November 2017.

International Organization for Standardization (ISO). 2012. Guidelines for Evaluating Cookstove Performance. Available at https://www.iso.org/standard/61975.html, last accessed 20 November 2017.

Kar, K., R. Chambers, and Plan UK. 2008. *Handbook on Community-led Total Sanitation.* London: Plan UK.

Khanna, Tina and Madhumita Das. 2016. 'Why gender matters in the solution towards safe sanitation? Reflections from rural India', *Global Public Health,* 11(10): 1185–201. doi:10.1080/17441692.2015.1062905.

Krieger, N. 1994. 'Epidemiology and the Web of Causation: Has Anyone Seen the Spider?', *Social Science & Medicine* (1982), 39(7): 887–903.

Landrigan P.J., R.J. Fuller et al. 2017. 'The *Lancet* Commission on Pollution and Health', *The Lancet.* doi:10.1016/S0140-6736(17)32345-0.

Lelieveld, J., J.S. Evans et al. 2015. 'The Contribution of Outdoor Air Pollution Sources to Premature Mortality on a Global Scale', *Nature* 525: 367–74.

Lewis, J.J. and S.K. Pattanayak. 2012. 'Who Adopts Improved Fuels and Cookstoves? A Systematic Review', *Environmental Health Perspectives.* doi:10.1289/ehp.1104194.

Luby, S.P., M. Rahman, B.F. Arnold, L. Unicomb, S. Ashraf, P.J. Winch, ... J.M. Colford. 2018. 'Effects of Water Quality, Sanitation, Handwashing, and Nutritional Interventions on Diarrhoea and Child Growth in Rural Bangladesh: A Cluster Randomised Controlled Trial',

The Lancet Global Health 6(3): e302–e315. doi:10.1016/S2214-109X(17)30490-4.

Ministry of Home Affairs. 2011. Census of India 2011. Available at http://censusindia.gov.in/2011-Common/CensusData2011.html, last accessed on 18 November 2019.

NSSO (National Sample Survey Office). 2012. *Key Indicators of Drinking Water, Sanitation, Hygiene, and Housing Conditions in India*, 69th Round National Sample Survey. New Delhi: NSSO.

Patil, S.R., B.F. Arnold, A. Salvatore, B. Briceno, J.M. Colford, and P.J. Gertler. 2013. *A Randomized, Controlled Study of a Rural Sanitation Behavior Change Program in Madhya Pradesh, India*. The World Bank. doi:10.1596/1813-9450-6702.

Phillips, S.P. 2005. 'Defining and Measuring Gender: A Social Determinant of Health Whose Time has Come', *International Journal for Equity in Health* 4(1). doi:10.1186/1475-9276-4-11.Pillarisetti, A., M. Vaswani et al. 2014. 'Patterns of Stove Usage after Introduction of an Advanced Cookstove: The Long-term Application of Household Sensors', *Environmental Science and Technology* 48(24): 14525–33. doi:10.1021/es504624c.

Rajaraman, D., S.M. Travasso, and S.J. Heymann. 2013. 'A Qualitative Study of Access to Sanitation amongst Low-income Working Women in Bangalore, India', *Journal of Water, Sanitation and Hygiene for Development* 3(3): 432. doi:10.2166/washdev.2013.114.

Sambandam, S., K. Balakrishnan, et al. 2015. 'Can Currently Available Advanced Combustion Biomass Cook-Stoves Provide Health Relevant Exposure Reductions? Results from Initial Assessment of Select Commercial Models in India', *Ecohealth* 12(1): 25–41. doi:10.1007/s10393-014-0976-1.

Sagar, A., S. Reddy et al. 2015. *Report of the Steering Committee on Air Pollution and Health-Related Issues.* New Delhi: Ministry of Health and Family Welfare, Government of India, New Delhi. http://www.mohfw.nic.in/showfile.php?lid=3650.

Sagar, A.D., K. Balakrishnan, et al. 2016. 'India Leads the Way: A Health-centered Strategy for Air Pollution', *Environmental Health Perspective* 124(7): A116–17.

Scott, B. and D. Trouba. 2010. 'Sanitation and Health', *PLOS Medicine* 7(11): e1000363. doi:10.1371/journal.pmed.1000363.

Shaddick, S., M.L. Thomas, et al. 2017. 'Data Integration Model for Air Quality: A Hierarchical Approach to the Global Estimation of Exposures to Ambient Air Pollution', *Applied Statistics*. doi:10.1111/rssc.12227.

Smith, K.R., N. Bruce, et al. 2014. 'Millions Dead: How Do We Know and What Does it Mean? Methods Used in the Comparative Risk Assessment of Household Air Pollution', *Annual Review of Public Health* 35: 185–206.

Smith and Pillariseti. 2017. in *Injury Prevention and Environmental Health: Key Messages from Disease Control Priorities* edited by C.N. Mock, K.R. Smith, O. Kobusingye, R. Nugent, and authors of , Third Edition, volume 7. Washington, DC: World Bank.

Spears, D., A. Ghosh, and O. Cumming, O. 2013. 'Open Defecation and Childhood Stunting in India: An Ecological Analysis of New Data from 112 Districts', *PLOS One* 8(9): e73784. doi:10.1371/journal.pone.0073784.Spears, D., and S. Lamba. 2013. *Effects of Early-Life Exposure to Sanitation on Childhood Cognitive Skills: Evidence from India's Total Sanitation Campaign*. The World Bank. Retrieved from http://elibrary.worldbank.org/doi/book/10.1596/1813-9450-6659.

Water and Sanitation Programme. 2011. *Economic Impacts of Inadequate Sanitation in India.* New Delhi: Write Media.

World Health Organization (WHO). 2006. *WHO Air Quality Guidelines for Particulate Matter, Nitrogen Dioxide, and Sulfur Dioxide: Global Update for 2005.* Copenhagen, Denmark: WHO Regional Office for Europe, pp. 484.

———. 2014. *WHO Indoor Air Quality Guidelines: Household Fuel Combustion.* Geneva: World Health Organization.

World Sanitation Programme. 2007. *Community-Led Total Sanitation in Rural Areas: An Approach that Works.* New Delhi.

Yin, Peng, Michael Brauer, Aaron Cohen., Richard T. Burnett, Jiangmei Liu, Yunning Liu, Ruiming Liang, et al. 2017. 'Long-term Fine Particulate Matter Exposure and Nonaccidental and Cause-specific Mortality in a Large National Cohort of Chinese Men', *Environmental Health Perspectives* 125(11): 117002-1 – 117002-11.

Part IV
Health Sector Determinants and Resources

13

The Policy Framework
A Critical Assessment

K. Sujatha Rao

The health sector has two objectives that drive public policy: (a) improving population health; and (b) ensuring no one gets financially impoverished while seeking health services.

All countries have formulated policies to achieve the above mentioned objectives. India is no exception. Over the past 70 years, India came up with three NHPs—1983, 2002, and 2017—over 25 expert committees and various working group reports as well as sections on health in various Five Year Plans of the erstwhile Planning Commission. This chapter provides a critical overview of national health policies from the perspective of these twin objectives, starting out with a brief overview of the historical context.

HISTORICAL CONTEXT

A year prior to India's Independence, Sir Joseph Bhore submitted the comprehensive *Health Survey and Development Report* to the Government of India in 1946. The report made detailed recommendations for establishing a decentralized architecture for the delivery of services and laid down a dictum that continues to elude us 70 years on—'nobody should be denied access to health services for his inability to pay'—and emphasized the need to focus on rural areas.

Within available resources, the post-colonial India centred its attention on eliminating and reducing the burden of infectious diseases and promoting maternal care. The Mudaliar Committee, set up in 1959 to review the implementation of the Bhore Committee recommendations, highlighted the achievements made by India post-Independence.

By the late 1970s, some significant gains were achieved with the eradication of small pox and reduction of malaria from an estimated 75 million cases to less than 2 million. Plague was no longer a threat and mortality due to cholera reduced appreciably. Attention shifted to family planning as population growth seemed to outstrip resources. Promotional campaigns of small family and the red triangle gave way to forced sterilizations, generating huge public dissatisfaction and prompting the formulation of India's first health policy in 1983.

THE NATIONAL HEALTH POLICY OF 1983

The NHP 1983 came in the wake of two significant developments: the centralization of health policy implementation such as the family planning sterilization drive, and the international resolve at Alma-Ata (now Almaty) in 1978 to ensure everyone has access to comprehensive primary care. For achieving the lofty vision of Health For All (HFA) by 2000 (as proposed at the Alma Ata Conference), a set of quantifiable targets were also listed.

Achieving the goal of HFA required a thorough revamp of existing approaches to health manpower policies as well as the reorganization of the delivery structure to enable greater community participation and intersectoral convergence of health and its social determinants such as safe water, public hygiene, and nutrition. Accordingly, the NHP 1983 envisioned a three-tier structure for service delivery, consisting of community health workers, a network of primary health centres, and district hospitals at the top. The NHP 1983 also proposed establishing at the sub-regional levels sanitary and epidemiological stations for providing preventive, promotive, and mental health services under the regular supervision of the epidemiological unit at the district level. To attract private investment for setting up facilities and widen access, the policy recommended provisioning of logistical, financial, and technological support. It proposed a standing mechanism at the central and state levels to monitor policies related to disease-causation, malnutrition, lack of access to safe water, sanitation and so on.

The NHP 1983 was comprehensive in its approach, and had it been implemented, the long-term impact on the trajectory of the health sector in India would have been significant. However, primarily due to low public spending, its implementation remained tardy.

Low funding was due to a rapidly deteriorating economy that shortly later resulted in India resorting to International Monetary Fund (IMF) borrowings and binding itself to reducing fiscal deficit by restraining public spending. Public health budgets were slashed and funds available primarily through loans that the World Bank was willing to provide for a few selected national health programmes. Given the adverse resource position, the goal of attaining HFA receded, replaced by the more pragmatic vision of focusing on diseases that affected the poorest, had low-cost proven technologies and wide externalities, such as malaria, tuberculosis (TB), leprosy, and reproductive child health (RCH). The adverse fiscal situation of states increased dependence on the centre and for a decade and a half, health interventions were largely those for which central grants were available under the centrally sponsored schemes.

Chronic underfunding and the increasing proportion of operational costs and salaries meant squeezing out capital investment. While new facilities as per national guidelines could not come up, existing ones crumbled due to lack of maintenance. Obsolescent equipment and non-availability of drugs further eroded the credibility of these facilities and hospitals. To bridge this gap, in the late 1990s, the World Bank provided loans to a few states such as Andhra Pradesh, Tamil Nadu, Karnataka, West Bengal, Uttar Pradesh, and Rajasthan, for undertaking the construction of facilities at sub-district levels.

To bridge the mounting investment deficit, incentives were extended to the private sector such as land- and custom-duty waivers. By the end of the century, the situation reversed, with the private sector gaining dominance in all aspects of healthcare—manufacturing of drugs, technology, medical, and paramedical education and service delivery. In the meanwhile, government hospitals also began to charge user fees for mobilizing resources for operational expenses based on the World Bank-funded willingness-to-pay studies. Household data from the National Sample Survey Office (NSSO) surveys brought into the open evidence of an increasing trend of people getting impoverished on account of medical bills and, worse, one in five not availing health services on grounds of unaffordability.[1]

THE NATIONAL HEALTH POLICY OF 2002

The non-realization of HFA by the year 2000 and the new global resolve in the form of Millennium Development Goals (MDGs), containing quantified, measurable goals for disease control (malaria, TB, and leprosy) and maternal and child health to be achieved by 2015, the emergence of non-communicable diseases (NCDs), shifting aspirations of people and the deteriorating public health delivery system contributed to the articulation of the second National Health Policy of 2002 (NHP 2002).

Another ineluctable compulsion was the unabated prevalence of preventable infections. Malaria persisted in a more drug resistant form alongside TB and water-borne diseases. New infections (such as HIV/AIDS), lifestyle diseases, and geriatric illnesses were added. Evidence showed growing differentials—spatial, interstate,

[1] NSSO Survey, 60th Round.

gender, economic, and social—calling for a more equitable and just system. Given this backdrop, the NHP 2002 mapped out a comprehensive vision, laying down quantified goals to be achieved by 2010.

The design for realizing the vision consisted of a large number of strategies such as reviving the near-collapsing and dysfunctional public health delivery infrastructure, converging vertically driven disease-control programmes with an integrated approach to patient care, establishing autonomous health societies at the state (for monitoring) and district levels, engaging the community, revamping the medical curriculum, task-shifting to paramedics, intensifying the promotion of generic drugs, and establishing a two-tier public health infrastructure in urban areas. It proposed the establishment of a medical grants commission for funding medical and dental colleges to come up to standard and stepping up disease surveillance for building a baseline for disease prevalence.

The policy called for raising public health spending to 2 per cent of the gross domestic product (GDP), with 25 per cent of it provided by the central government and stimulate state spending to increase from an average of 4.5 per cent of revenue expenditure to the desired level of 8 per cent. The policy recommended encouraging private investment, particularly in the primary and tertiary care sectors of the service delivery chain and supported using insurance as an alternate means of health financing.[2]

THE NATIONAL RURAL HEALTH MISSION, 2005

The new UPA I government, that took charge in 2004, accorded high priority to health. Taking up the NHP 2002, the government formulated the NRHM, India's first serious effort to address fundamental biases in the health sector. Within the broad contours provided in the NHP 2002, the design of NRHM focused on reviving the primary health system in rural areas that accounted for 70 per cent of the country's population. It co-opted most of the policies stated in NHP 2002 such as providing integrated care by converging vertical programmes, creation of autonomous societies at the state and district levels alongside management structures such as the village health and nutrition societies and the facility level committees at the block level and district hospitals. At the community level, a system of community health workers, the Accredited Social Health Activists (ASHAs), was established per 1,000 population. Health budgets trebled and new concepts such as conditional-cash transfers and performance-based incentives introduced.

Achievements in the initial years (2005 to 2012) were positive as, under the revamped RCH programmes, maternal and infant mortality levels dropped by half, as did the incidence of HIV/AIDS. Over a million trained workers were brought into the health system and close to 175,000 personnel recruited, mostly on contractual basis. Refurbishment of facilities and provisioning of improved quality of care in accordance with the Indian Public health Standards (IPHS) significantly increased footfall, while the cash incentives combined with improved quality of care motivated pregnant women to deliver in public hospitals, substantially increasing the utilization of these facilities.

The momentum was, however, not sustained. As aspirations and activities expanded, the funding failed to keep pace. With a lower priority to disease control programmes, the policy failed to effectively integrate all health interventions. In the meanwhile, within five years of the launch of the NRHM, new goalposts were introduced, with the 12th Five Year Plan focusing attention on Universal Health Coverage (UHC) as the new vision to aspire for.

With the centrally-driven NRHM focused on rural primary healthcare, states shifted their policy attention to cope with the rising clamour for providing cashless treatment for inpatient hospital care and surgeries. Starting with the Yeshasvini model in Karnataka in 2004, several states are currently implementing health insurance programmes for the poor under which the state governments pay/subsidize the premium. Institutional mechanisms such as autonomous trusts have been established for purchasing, accrediting, and reimbursing costs to hospitals. The central government also introduced a nation-wide Rashtriya Swasthya Bima Yojana (RSBY) in 2009 for workers in the informal sector.

Such initiatives got a further boost with the emergence of UHC as the new global focus area for the health sector around 2010. Its importance is underscored by its inclusion under the Sustainable Development Goal (SDG) 3 to be achieved by 2030. Its direct policy implication for a country like India has been threefold—enhancing policy attention on NCDs, co-opting the private sector with the State shifting its role as a facilitator and

[2] See Annexure I to the NHP on the website of the Ministry of Health and Family Welfare, http://mohfw.nic.in/.

financier, and stepping up insurance as an important financial instrument for boosting demand and incentivizing providers.

The Ministry of Health and Family Welfare (MoHFW) was, however, reluctant to adopt UHC as the core policy since it seemed to imply shifting resources and policy attention towards contracting private sector for surgeries and NCDs. Instead, it recommended enhancing resources for accelerating the existing momentum for achieving the last mile on RCH goals and communicable disease control, alongside building capacity in public facilities to screen, diagnose, counsel lifestyle modifications, stabilize, and refer to higher facilities for the treatment of NCDs, particularly diabetes, hypertension, and old-age diseases. The stand-off of the MoHFW with the Planning Commission resulted in reduced budgets to the health sector. With the coming of the National Democratic Alliance (NDA) government in 2014, the Planning Commission got rechristened as the NITI Aayog. At the end of the 12th Plan period, total releases against allocated amounts in the plan remained about half.

Stagnant funding stymied the momentum of the NRHM, now rechristened as National Health Mission (NHM), with the inclusion of urban health. The practice of releasing central grants directly to state and district health societies was also discontinued with, dealing a further death blow to NRHM, since in several states release of funds was unpredictable, delayed, denied, or provided in instalments, severely affecting implementation and credibility. For want of capacity, not much headway was made on partnering with the private sector either. Initiatives for community-based tackling of NCDs by way of screening, diagnosis, and referral of patients suffering from hypertension and diabetes did not take-off at the desired pace. As a means of overcoming the pervasive sense of stagnation and inject fresh energy, the new government introduced the third NHP in 2017.[3]

NATIONAL HEALTH POLICY OF 2017

The NHP 2017 came about to fulfil a commitment made in the election manifesto of the new government to announce a new health policy and provide the framework for implementing universal health assurance through a public–private partnership (PPP) mode. This approach was driven in no small measure by two considerations. One pertained to the private sector that had invested heavily in building an infrastructure that had little effective demand, creating a financial crisis of sorts. And second was the good economic growth rates providing enhanced fiscal capacity for a new NHP. Accordingly, the new NHP aimed at widening access, lowering costs of care, and improving quality.

The NHP 2017 is an eclectic document, covering the wide expanse of the health sector, full of good intentions and some strategies. Its merit lies in the fact that, for the first time, a policy document spelt out the approach to the private sector within the overarching umbrella of a health system. The policy also has an exhaustive list of time-bound targets.[4]

The NHP indicates the future policy direction consisting of focusing on comprehensive care, monitoring outputs, providing free and universal access to drugs, diagnostics and emergency care to all in all public facilities, building primary care in urban areas on a partnership mode with existing providers, focusing on the underserved and backward regions and sub-population groups for higher public investments in order to build the infrastructure bottom-up in accordance with IPHS norms, and clearly committed to providing assured universal access to all health services with a combination of tax-based funding and insurance for services delivered on a cashless basis by public and private care providers.

The policy has several new ideas and approaches for revamping the architecture of service delivery and makes the following impressive commitments:

1. Declaring primary care as the fundamental obligation of the State that 'must be assured', the policy proposes to upgrade all sub-centres as health and wellness centres, responsible for every family under its jurisdiction, along with not-for-profit, charitable organizations working in this space. Smart health cards with portable medical information are proposed to be provided to each family to enable access to a package of free primary healthcare services anywhere in the country.

[3] See Annexure III to the NHP on the website of the Ministry of Health and Family Welfare, http://mohfw.nic.in/.

[4] See Annexure II to the NHP on the website of the Ministry of Health and Family Welfare, http://mohfw.nic.in/.

2. All district hospitals are to be strengthened to provide all secondary care services that are currently being provided in tertiary hospitals, alongside upgrading those in underserved areas to medical colleges.
3. To ensure access to emergency care within the golden hour rule, the policy commits to providing two emergency beds per 1,000 population along with transport services, besides ensuring the availability of 10 categories of specialists at district level and four or five at sub district level.
4. Establish more medical colleges and institutions similar to the All India Institute of Medical Sciences (AIIMS) to deal with the challenge of shortage of human resources;
5. As a short-term measure, the policy recommends to 'strategically' purchase services from private hospitals in order to expand access to secondary and tertiary care services in deficit areas and for diseases that have limited capacity in the government.
6. It also spells out interventions related to human resources, ranging from providing incentives to attract and retain doctors and paramedical personnel to work in government facilities, increasing availability of personnel in proposed wellness centres by paramedicalizing primary care, revisiting curricula to ensure training is relevant, need-based, appropriate, and so on.
7. Finally, the policy also commits to introducing the much delayed institutional reform by proposing the establishment of bodies and institutions to cope with the complexities of the health system and smoothen the transition process from welfarism to markets such as the National Institute for Chronic Diseases, the National Health Standards Organization, Medical Tribunals, National Digital Health Authority, and so on.

The NHP 2017 indicates increase in public spending to 2.5 per cent of GDP by 2025, but falls short of making any specific recommendations regarding the share of central government, and instead proposes to take steps to incentivize states to spend more than 8 per cent of its revenue expenditures on health. It further makes two important recommendations: government grants to be based on the fiscal backwardness of the districts and states and funding provided to primary health providers on a per capita basis.

A CRITIQUE OF THE THREE NHPS

The following section offers a critique of the NHPs within a broader analytical framework consisting of four pillars: clarity of vision, clarity of design, clarity of financing, and finally, clarity in incentive structures.

Clarity of Vision

It is remarkable that all three NHPs had a grand, all-inclusive, comprehensive vision of achieving the twin principal goals of improved population health and reduced impoverishment on account of healthcare.

Equally remarkable is that all the policies provided a list of targets to be achieved within a certain time frame. As can be seen from the accompanying Table 13A.1, such listing was whimsical, arbitrary, and not based on acceptable methodologies, resulting in shifting the goal posts and adding new indicators, without explaining the reasons for dropping the old or why governments failed to achieve the targets laid down earlier. Besides, many targets, particularly under NHP 2017, had no baselines, making accountability problematic.

Clarity of Design

If the vision provides the direction of what is to be done by when, the policy design reflects the 'how' part of the equation—how to achieve the vision and by whom? Designing policy must then involve a rigorous examination of the evidence, undertaking a detailed gap analysis and a critical assessment of the strengths and weaknesses of the various stakeholders in order to determine the policy levers that need to be activated for optimizing strengths, building capacity in weak areas, finding opportunities, and assessing the threats that normally follow any action to change the existing status quo.

Unfortunately, none of the policies reflect any such processes and, to that extent, were missed opportunities to usher change and make the system more reflective of the dynamic shifts in the external environment and context.

While all policies were enabling, there was no prioritization. Such prioritizing would have required sound, credible, and reliable data on all aspects of the health system, starting from the disease burden to the inadequacies in the organization of the delivery system in the public and private sector.

For assessing the epidemiological status, countries rely on the vital registration system, cause of death studies, and periodic household surveys for estimating the incidence of disease. India reneged in this regard despite NHP 1983 flagging the immediate necessity to build a robust disease surveillance architecture. For example, incidence assessments of TB were last done in 1956. While researchers estimate nearly 50,000–100,000 deaths due to vector-borne diseases (Dhingra et al. 2010), which a government committee of experts revised to approximately 30,000, the government continues to plan on programme data that is a gross underestimation. Likewise, there is no longitudinal surveillance data of childhood diseases nor any rigorously collected incidence data on vascular or other diseases such as mental health. Most estimates are extrapolations of small surveys or programme data that are often unreliable due to lack of in-built processes of concurrent validation.

However, in the case of infant, under-five, and maternal mortality rates, district-level estimations for three years (2011–13) are available for high-priority districts through the Annual Health Surveys (AHS), while the National Family Health Surveys (NHFS) provide valuable longitudinal data on several family welfare indicators. But such collection of district data needs to be routinized and expanded to cover all districts in the country. Hopefully, starting with the recent NFHS-4 (2015–16), this would be possible data related to incidence and prevalence of disease, populations most affected, direct and indirect causal factors, and so on is critical for ensuring better designing of implementation plans and efficient resource utilization.

While the facility surveys carried out by the IIPS[5] provide information on the current status of the public health infrastructure at district level and below, there is hardly any information on the private sector—its spread, character, financing, location, service mix, human resources employed, and so on. The rigorous implementation of the Clinical Establishment Act of 2010 would have enabled building up the required database. The question which then arises in hindsight is, whether the cavalier manner in which all the three NHPs dealt with the critical issue of private provisioning of health services was due to the absence of such vital data, or was it on account of an inadequate understanding of the complex nature of health markets and its characteristics.

Though policy articulation on the role of the private sector has been non explicit and vague, and despite the absence of vital data, every policy only strengthened and promoted the private sector, be it the provisioning of land and custom duty exemptions, opening up the pharma industry or medical education to private investment, concessional credit, income tax exemptions, handing over public assets and functions or a lax regulatory environment—untrammelled by laws and rules that most countries enforce to ensure that privatization does not degenerate to crass profiteering at the cost of patients' health or achieving the larger welfare goals. Such extensive concessions and subsidies were all given piecemeal and not as an integral component of a well-thought-out policy architecture.

Though PPPs have been a feature of policy design, they have hitherto been essentially in the nature of outsourcing routine tasks such as cleaning, laundry, and transport. Privatization in the form of handing over fixed assets for mobilizing additional investment is a recent trend and is confined to a few cases such as the handing over of land and hospital to a corporate entity (Adani Group) in Bhuj, Gujarat and, more recently, in Chittoor, Andhra Pradesh (Apollo Hospitals). It is significant that none of these initiatives have been evaluated till date.

PPP in a more extensive form is, however, being implemented under the government-sponsored health insurance programmes. Under these programmes, budgets are earmarked, hospitals empanelled, and cost of treatment reimbursed to the hospital as per rates agreed to prior to entering into a contract. These programmes, too, have not been evaluated rigorously by a third party. There are, however, a few studies on the impact of the RSBY by making a difference to difference comparative analysis of the data available in the NSSO surveys (Karan, Yip, and Mahal 2017). Likewise, an impact assessment on household expenditures was done for the Rajiv Arogya Shri based on household surveys (Rao et al. 2014), while the World Bank reviewed the impact of the Vajpayee Health Insurance programme in Karnataka (Sood et al. 2014). Almost all these studies showed increased utilization of services and reduced household expenditures for inpatient treatment. However, the overall impact on either catastrophic expenditures or household spending was found to be negligible. The

[5] The International Institute for Population Studies (IIPS) has conducted three rounds (1998–9, 2004–5 and 2010–11) of the District Level Household and Facility Surveys.

studies also showed that the middle classes benefitted disproportionately over the last two quintiles.

A major issue being faced in the further expansion of such programmes to reach the poorest is the non-availability of human resources and health facilities. A key infirmity in the design of most PPPs is the unequal spread of risk between the public and private partners and ineffective remedies in the event of non-compliance to any part of the agreement. In short, in promoting a dual system of care without adequate study or data for assessing the long-term implications, the NHPs have been responsible for the continued lack of clarity resulting in diffused policy attention over a wide canvas with meagre financial resources.

The NHPs were equally ambivalent about community engagement, the role of civil society, and patient/user groups for whom the health system is designed for. While the NHP 2017 is silent on this issue, the first two NHPs provided a strong thrust towards engaging civil society and communities for building a sustainable health system. The NHP 1983 even suggested earmarking 10 per cent of the total resource envelope for NGOs, which was enhanced to 25 per cent under the NRHM. But the policy vision remained only on paper as the policy design failed to spell out with any clarity as to how and in what manner and on what terms they are to be engaged. Similar confusion prevails on policies regarding human resources where much is said, but little done—not for want of ideas, but the forces of political economy, where private sector and doctor lobbies have a vice-like grip on all professional education and HR policies in the health sector. Until this dynamic changes, the issue of shortages in the availability of adequately qualified doctors will continue to elude India. The initiatives of NHP 2017 for ensuring availability of specialists at the district level—establishing more institutions, revamping the regulatory architectural and education policies—continue to be mere aspirations.

Such wide discrepancies between policy vision and policy design dot all health policy documents. Planning and monitoring on aggregate data does not help in identifying the areas, the population groups or the causal factors that need bulleted attention.

Clarity of Financing

Most discussions on health tend to start and end with lamenting on low public investment. It is true that India has the abysmal record of providing about 1.1 per cent of GDP on health, making it one of the few countries with the lowest public health spending in the world. Low public investment is the reason for over 62 million people getting pushed below the poverty line, of whom roughly 15 per cent face catastrophic expenditures. Indian households spend nearly 6 per cent of their household incomes on healthcare that shrinks their spending choices on goods that could improve their health and well-being. Private hospitals charge several times more than government hospitals, yet social security to buffer these shocks barely cover a third of the population.

Of serious concern is the chronic underfunding of national health programmes that deal with infectious disease control. India is perhaps one of the few countries that has failed to make the epidemiological transition, resulting in being saddled with the dual burden of disease—burden that has high levels of prevalence of both communicable and infectrious diseases that normally are prevalent in poor/developing countries alongside non-communicable diseases that are also known as lifestyle diseases and are more prevalent among better-off sections of society. A third of the disease burden is on account of communicable diseases that are not showing any signs of abatement, with TB re-emerging in a more virulent multidrug resistant form and malaria being overtaken by other vector-borne diseases such as dengue, Japanese encephalitis (JE) and chikungunya. Declines in HIV incidence have also stagnated for want of funds and policy attention.

Infectious diseases know no boundaries, but they strike the poorest who live in abysmal conditions that are conducive for such diseases to thrive. Minimal access to clean water, sanitation, hygiene, and good nutrition are reasons for the persistence of water-borne diseases such as cholera and diarrhoea that have claimed the lives of millions of under-five children in the country.

In view of the above, the NHP 1983 underscored the fact that financing was a critical determinant for achieving the stated goals and targets. The NHP 2017 also reiterated the need for public health spending of 2.5 per cent of GDP by 2025. While seeking to promote procurement of services from the private sector at market rates, the 2017 policy also seeks to simultaneously strengthen the full range of public sector facilities from the sub-centres to medical colleges. Clearly, there is no serious intention to implement the policy as the mismatch between resources required and policy strategies cannot be starker.

Additionally, private sector services are not free. Purchasing services throughout the three sub-markets of primary, secondary, and tertiary healthcare exposes the sector to market forces and leaves little room for containing costs. In UK, primary care is provided by private general practitioners, but then not only is there a single buyer of these services, the National Health Service (NHS) also owns and controls the more expensive cost-centres of secondary and tertiary care. Likewise, in Japan, all provisioning of health services is by private doctors, but at administered prices set by the government which has a monopoly.

The NHP 2017 proposes a mixed system where public and private healthcare sectors will co-exist and compete in a multi-payer environment, entailing serious problems for the fiscal sustainability of the policy. The proposal to forge symbiotic partnerships with the private sector through a system of 'strategic purchasing' for 'gap'-filling (where the gap is a huge hole, with the private sector providing 80 per cent of outpatient and 60 per cent of inpatient care, with a disproportionately higher share in the two sub-markets of tertiary and secondary care), is a sure way of further undermining the public sector.

In multi-payer systems, the public and private are in direct competition for patients. Besides, salary streams, motivation levels, working methods, prescription practices, monitoring and accountability systems, work expectations—all vary. While financing compulsions drive the private sector towards profit maximization by resorting to irrational care and unnecessary procedures in a manner that standard treatment protocols cannot address, it also results in price escalations.

Notwithstanding these, the options for India are limited and providing tertiary services requires partnering with the private sector. Till such time demand does not outstrip supply, prices will remain competitive. Once utilization increases with no commensurate increase in supply—shortage of beds and doctors—prices will rise, impacting sustainability.

In proposing strategic purchasing of services from the private and commercial sector of service providers without assessing its long-term fiscal implications for the government, the NHP 2017 is suggesting a course of action that will entail costs that it may not be able to afford, particularly at times when the economy is not doing well. The fact that this issue has not been seriously drilled down and thought through is clear from the recent policy interventions to contain costs of care by capping prices of drug and medical devices. For example, prices of stents have been capped at a third of the cost being charged. Within six months, the hospitals shifted the 'loss' under the stents to surgeon fees. In other words, knee-jerk responses to cost-containment are of little value as they can be gamed when done in a piecemeal manner without changing the fundamentals of the current system.

The financing provided under NHP 2017 is not in sync with its vision. Low spending has meant that India provides barely 15 per cent of the primary care services that ought to be available. Ensuring IPHS in high-priority districts will requires over INR 700 billion. Considering these districts are backward with high levels of poverty, the NHP 2017 skirts around this key issue instead of assessing the availability of required fiscal space. Such an approach would have forced a strict prioritization of those activities that, if left unattended, could entail substantial costs to growth and development.

Clarity of Incentives

Behavioural responses of stakeholders depend on incentive structures. Culture, intangible factors such as trust borne of personal experience, and values and notions of quality and dignity determine human behaviour to a large extent. It is for this reason that cash transfers have gained policy attention and examples of Mexico have convincingly demonstrated how demand for services did change on account of cash vouchers. Likewise, in India, cash transfers under the Janani Suraksha Yojana (JSY), combined with improved infrastructure, helped double institutional deliveries from 47 to 65 per cent between 2005 and 2015.

Incentives profoundly impact on behavioural responses and are an integral part of the design to enhance output and maximize gain or minimize harm. For example, general practitioners in UK double their base income from achieving quality targets. Rewards and incentives can also come in other forms. The Christian Medical College at Vellore (Tamil Nadu) has low attrition levels despite reportedly paying lower remuneration to its doctors than corporates. The explanation to such counterintuitive behaviour is a bundle of factors starting with the incredibly low amount charged for education, an excellent work environment, excellent housing and schools for their children and, in addition, permission to work abroad on lien.

Unlike NHPs of 1983 and 2002, NHP 2017 does mention the issue of incentives, providing some broad approaches. The policy, however, does not touch the politically sensitive issue of permitting private practice in lieu of a non-practicing allowance. The inability of government to stop doctors doing private practice is a principal reason for sub-optimal functioning of the public delivery system. A clear understanding of the drivers of human behaviour is central to managing human resources in highly competitive environments and imperfect markets.

Governance

Finally, the NHPs' weak commitment towards governance in general and regulations in particular has been a serious issue. While the policy stance towards private sector collaboration is aggressive, the need to strengthen the weak regulatory environment is perfunctory. The existing regulatory authorities such as the Professional Councils, the Food Safety and Standards Authority of India (FSSAI) and the Central Drugs Standard Control Organization (CDSCO) are all functioning suboptimally on account of understaffing, inadequate budgets, corruption, conflicts of interest, and virtual capture of the regulatory bodies by sectional interests. Weak supervision of pharmacies due to inadequate and poor-quality staff is responsible for the rampant misuse of antibiotics, endangering public health in the form of antimicrobial resistance (AMR), which has recently emerged as an issue of major global concern, and on which India has now formulated a national policy.

Weak enforcement of regulations has played havoc, making it cheaper to break a rule than abide by one. Enforcement of regulations is not cheap and calls for substantial recurring expenditures necessitating full assessment of the fiscal implications of building and sustaining the required institutional capacity to enforce laws at all levels of governance.

Going Ahead

One can put forth five recommendations to address some of the major challenges discussed here:

1. Focus on building a sound surveillance system and datasets as required for planning interventions.
2. Based on a realistic assessment of the availability of financial resources, prioritize and formulate micro plans[6] that clearly indicate what is to be done by when and by whom and construct monitoring systems to build in accountability.
3. Since the health sector is knowledge-driven, embed research into policymaking by providing dedicated budgets to incentivize a dozen Indian research institutions to take up operational research and concurrent evaluations of major policy initiatives.
4. Build clarity on the role of the State to stay focused on public goods and ensuring that choices are consistent with welfare goals.
5. Move away from rhetorical assertions to reasoned debate in policy formulation and design by widening the consultative process and including those that are most affected by the policy.

***

India's health policies have been unfocused, lacked prioritization, and reflected the desire to be a please-all document than a tool for designing and planning in detail the strategies in a sequential and systematic manner to achieve national health goals. This has contributed to the current crisis of a health system that was seen to often work at cross-purposes.

More than seven decades have gone by since Independence. Several countries that were on the same level as India in 1947 have moved far ahead. While not paying enough attention to health is one aspect of India's problem, having distorted priorities is the other, compounding the problem further. Ultimately, bureaucracies and political systems design systems exactly for their purposes and as convenient to them. Change if any will then have to be fought for and demanded. Being silent is not an option. People, doctors, academicians, and all other stakeholders need to mobilize themselves to ensure health policies that reflect societal aspirations of good health and well-being without impoverishing citizens in the process. India's finance minister announced an ambitious National Health Protection Scheme (NHPS) in his Union Budget 2018–19, in which the actual allocational increase to the health sector has been minuscule. Only time will tell how far will it go to protect the health and wealth of the citizens of this nation.

[6] In Malaysia such microplanning is referred to bringing plans from 3000 ft to 300 ft, that is, making them more manageable. Such processes have been instrumental in helping Malaysia achieve goals laid down and is now being attempted in the new state of Andhra Pradesh for some sectors.

APPENDIX

Table 13A.1 Comparison of Key Targets and Current Achievement through the Three NHPs

S. No.	Goal	Achievement by 2000 (NHP 1983)	Achievement by 2010 (NHP 2002)	Achievement by 2025/30 (NHP 2017)	Status as of 2019
1.	Increase Life Expectancy at birth	64		70 (2025)	68.56
2.	IMR/1000	60	30	28 by 2020	32
3.	MMR/1 Lakh Live Births	200	100	100 (2020)	130
4.	Reduction of TFR at national and sub-national level	2.3		2.1 (2025)	2.3
5.	Reduce Under Five Mortality	10		23 (2025)	39 (2018)
6.	Reduce neo-natal mortality	10		16 (2025)	24 (2017)
7.	Polio Eradication		2005		Achieved in 2014
8.	Eliminate Kala Azar		2010	2017	Not achieved
9.	Reduce Mortality TB /Vector borne disease	90%	50%	85% cure rate Elimination by 2025	>80% cure rate bit incidence is 19.9/10 lakh. Elimination requires <1/10lakh
10.	Blindness Incidence	0.3	0.5	0.25	1
11.	Zero HIV Incidence	—	2007	2020	84,000 new cases in 2017
12.	Increase utilization of public health facilities from current Level of <20% to >75%		2010	—	Not measured
13.	Establish an integrated system of surveillance	—	2005	2020	No information
14.	Increase health expenditure by Government as a percentage of GDP from the existing 0.9% to 2.0%	—	2010	2.5% by 2025	1.18% (2018 NHA)
15.	Increase State Sector Health spending from 5.5% to 7% of the budget 2005 and Further increase to 8%	—	2010	2020	Lesser than 5%

Source: Relevant NHP documents from the Government of India.

REFERENCES

Dhingra, Neeraj, Prabhat Jha, Vinod P. Sharma, Alan A. Cohen, Raju M. Jotkar, Peter S. Rodriguez, Diego G. Bassani et al. 2010. 'Adult and Child Malaria Mortality in India: A Nationally Representative Mortality Survey', The Million Death Study Collaborators, *The Lancet* 9754(1774):1768–74. doi:S0140-6736(10)60831-8.

Karan, Anup, Winnie Yip, and Ajay Mahal 2017. 'Extending Health Insurance for the Poor in India: An Impact Evaluation of the Rashtriya Swasthya Bima Yojana on Out of Pocket Spending for Health Care'. *Social Science & Medicine*, 181: 83–92.

Rao, M., A. Katyal, P.V. Singh, et al. 2014. 'Changes in Addressing Inequalities in Access to Hospital Care in Andhra Pradesh and Maharashtra States of India: A Difference-in-Differences Study Using Repeated Cross-Sectional Surveys'. *BMJ Open*, 4: e004471. doi:10.1136/bmjopen-2013-004471.

Sood, Neeraj, Eran Bendavid, Arnab Mukherji, Zachary Wagner, Somil Nagpal, Patrick Mullen, et al. 2014. 'Government Health Insurance for People Below Poverty Line in India: Quasi-Experimental Evaluation of Insurance and Health Outcomes'. *BMJ*, 349: g5114.

14

Major Actors Influencing Health Policy in India

A Historical Perspective*

Roger Jeffery

Public health and medical services in India have undergone dramatic changes since the early 1980s. At that time, public health was clearly seen to be the responsibility of the various levels of government, marshalled (if only in general terms) by the then Planning Commission (Jeffery 1986). Most health and medical expenditures were privately financed. Insurance schemes were limited to government employees, a few of the largest employers and some other protected industries (railways and tea estates, for example). Private hospitals, medical colleges, and clinics were dwarfed by state provision, with only a few large philanthropic trust hospitals. Although the Indian pharmaceuticals industry had already benefited from the protections offered by the Patents Act of 1970, drug companies were still relatively small, focused on the domestic market. International assistance to the health sector was welcomed, and it supported public health initiatives and family planning (Jeffery 1982).

In the 2010s, India's health and medical services look very different. The share of the public sector in health provision has continued to decline. Public–private initiatives in health insurance have been tried out since 2010. 'Corporate' hospitals and private medical colleges are increasingly visible in all the metropolitan and Tier 1 cities. The promoters of these colleges—politicians, capitalists, philanthropists—have used their political muscle to secure corruption at the heart of the Medical Council of India. Since 2003, international development assistance to India's public healthcare sector has been restricted to a few donors (Bijoy 2009), but large multinational lenders have invested in India's 'health industry'. International commitments made by the Government of India—such as to the Millennium and Sustainable Development Goals (MDGs and SDGs

* I am grateful to many people with whom I have worked on issues of public health in India since the 1980s for some of the ideas that underpin this chapter: Rama Baru, Ian Harper, Patricia Jeffery, Anuj Kapilashrami, Salla Sariola, and Jeevan Sharma. Special thanks to Amar Jesani, Bertrand Lefebvre, and Mohan Rao for commenting on an earlier draft. Errors, omissions, and responsibility for the arguments advanced here remain, of course, mine.

respectively), have, however, been written into plan documents. Progress towards meeting the goals now receives regular attention in the Indian media.

The dominant ideas that underpin or justify health policies have also changed. In the 1970s, ideas about 'Health for All' with community health overseen by local health committees exemplified a quasi-socialist goal of moving towards a full welfare state. Such an emphasis was Janus-faced: in supporting community activities, they disparaged state health services, and failed to notice the growth of private interests in health. They also showed little interest in doctors. At one point, the ideas of Ivan Illich (1976) advocating fewer doctors, and less medical intervention, held sway. They were unable to offer much resistance when, starting in the 1980s, but accelerating in the 1990s, the ideal of free medical care at the point of contact between patient and practitioner or institution was progressively abandoned.

This chapter reviews these changes in the health policy environment. It asks particularly how and why different levels of government, different kinds of non-governmental actors, and international advisors, have played greater or smaller roles. It will point to the inadequacy of existing regulatory frameworks, particularly with respect to public–private partnerships (PPP) and the increasing salience of philanthro-capitalism. The basic framework for this chapter is that India's 'new' health policy advocates have taken little or no notice of Gandhi's injunction to 'recall the face of the poorest and the weakest' and to how they will benefit from what is being proposed, leaving the country poorly prepared for key public health challenges.

CONTEXT

Whatever date is preferred for India's decisive turn towards a neoliberal economic development strategy (Corbridge, Harriss, and Jeffrey 2013; Kohli 1989), for India's 'health' economy, a significant shift towards greater commercialization and the opening of the health sector to more private sector investment is visible in the early 1980s (Baru 1998), when government encouragement of corporate hospitals first became visible (Hodges 2013) and private medical colleges became the norm. Of the 108 medical colleges opened by 1976, 91 per cent (98 colleges) were in the public sector; between 1977 and 2006, only 25 per cent (37 out of 150) were.[1]

The causes of these changes are often ascribed to politicians or government officials, or to pressures from the international economy such as the World Bank or donor countries (Qadeer 2013). Others argue, however, that the impetus came from a new breed of Indian entrepreneurs (Pedersen 2000) who acquired deep roots in the health sector from 1980 onwards and developed positions of influence in some states. Pedersen argues that they used these positions to weaken the public sector through assertive actions, starting with PPPs. Such policies are seen by radical critics to have eroded India's healthcare system: '… a clear attempt to undermine public health systems and to privilege the role of private medical care' (Sengupta and Prasad 2011: 72). This chapter reviews these changes and identifies some of the key actors—individual and institutional—who contributed to these policy changes.

Why and how do substantive changes in public policy take place? Major policy shifts occur when three independent streams—problems, policies, and politics—come together (Kingdon 1984; Shiffman and Ved 2007). 'Conditions,' such as poor health indicators, need to become 'problems' before they affect a public discourse involving collective action; 'policies' depend on the availability of sets of possible solutions; and 'politics' matters because elections, protests, pressure groups, and/or international attention prompt politicians to focus their attention on 'problem' issues. Michael Reich (2002: 1669) sees the state being reshaped by multiple forces (from above, within, and below) acting simultaneously. It is constrained by agreements with international agencies and by multinational corporations, by increasing trends toward marketization, and by problems of corruption, by the expansion of decentralization and by the rising influence of non-governmental organizations (NGOs).

Health reform depends on the strategies and actions of specific policy entrepreneurs, particularly leaders who can change the distribution of power to facilitate reform. The focus here is on the period since 1980, considering: the changing roles of international influences on policymaking; the shifting balance in central, state, and other levels of government; the significance of commercial interests; and finally, the roles of civil society organizations (CSOs).

[1] https://mciindia.org/ActivitiWebClient/informationdesk/listofCollegesTeachingMBBS, last accessed on 6 October 2017. Eight medical colleges identified in 2007–16 as 'Government/Society' have been included in the government totals. Colleges debarred from admission, not permitted for renewal of permission, or with conditional recognition, have been excluded.

INTERNATIONAL INFLUENCES ON INDIAN HEALTH POLICYMAKING

Bilateral and multilateral donors provided ideological support to the shifts identified above. The total contributions to government health expenditures from international agencies have never been substantial in the overall context of India's public-sector health expenditures, but their funding has helped with new initiatives, from family planning in the 1960s and the 1970s to HIV/AIDS control programmes in the 2000s (Sridhar and Gomez 2010: 13). From the early 1990s, the World Bank offered advice and financial support to an appreciative audience:

> Until that time, the government funded primary care on its own and did not seek policy advice from the Bank in the health sector. Financial difficulties in the early 1990s and new leadership in the Ministry of Health and Family Welfare, however, provided an opening for the Bank to fund two types of projects: disease-specific interventions and broader, state-level health system reforms. (Ridker and Musgrove 1999)

Ridker summarizes how Bank staff pushed for an increased role for the private sector in health and medicine. The World Bank funded four health reform projects between 1995 and 1999, in Andhra Pradesh (USD 159 million); an extension to three other states (USD 350 million); an Orissa (Odisha) project (USD 57 million); and a Maharashtra project (USD 98 million). These gave the Bank a chance to influence 'how the public health system works at the state level' from

> increasing access to primary care in remote areas, to establishing a new institution to manage the hospital system, to improving service quality at community health centers, focusing on maternity cases.
>
> Another cross-cutting issue is the need to better integrate NGOs and the private sector, which provide the vast majority of health services into health sector programming.... A strategy needs to be developed to involve the private sector that considers the division of labor, pricing and subsidy policies, licensing and regulation of private providers and health insurers, and appropriate training programs. The Bank ... can help by examining experience in other countries and in other sectors in India; encouraging the private provision of services, where appropriate; and encouraging and evaluating experimental programs. (Ridker and Musgrove 1999)

The Bank's approach can be seen in the publications of Peter Berman. In the early 1990s, he worked for the Ford Foundation in India; from 2004 to 2008 he was in the World Bank's New Delhi office as lead economist for health, nutrition, and population, overseeing a portfolio of almost USD 2 billion; and from 2008–11 he was a lead health economist for the Bank in Washington.[2] In 1998 he argued forcefully that the

> long-term strategy to develop a 'national health service'-type model of health care provision is misguided and wasteful. The current and potential role of nongovernment health care providers in achieving high levels of access to basic services is highlighted.... India and many other countries need to rethink their health care system development strategies to acknowledge and build upon the opportunities offered by the already extensive non-government health care sector. (Berman 1998: 1463)

The International Finance Corporation (IFC), an arm of the World Bank Group, has also become a significant source of funding for the private healthcare sector since the 1990s (see the next section as well). Where the Bank led, other large donors—notably the EU and the UK—tended to follow.

For the 2000s, the source of influential international advice has shifted and is now backed by the financial clout of the Gates Foundation. Some NGOs—such as international ones operating in India—have maintained a quiet but influential position, especially with some state governments. As the National Rural Health Mission (NRHM) was being established during 2004–5, a group of mostly US-based public health experts was called in to help shape it. Jeffrey Sachs, of the Earth Institute at Columbia University, chaired an International Advisory Panel (IAP) that met at least annually from 2005–13. Other members of the IAP included Sonia Ehrlich Sachs at the Centre for Sustainable Development at the Earth Institute and representatives of the Bill and Melinda Gates Foundation. The IAP pressed regularly for a role for the private sector. Sachs himself argued that 'other health policy issues like health insurance and public–private partnership' were important, 'but maintained that for poor, there was no substitute to a well-functioning public system' (IAP 2007: 2). With such mixed messages, it is not surprising that the NRHM lost a clear sense of direction (see also the next section).

[2] https://www.hsph.harvard.edu/peter-berman/, last accessed on 26 September 2017.

In a more general sense, international connections clearly influence statements of health policy in India, even if these do not always turn into actions with identifiable effects. Through various international forums—such as those that generated the SDGs, UN agencies, the G20, and a variety of bilateral relationships, international influences are brought to bear on India's health policies, so that issues such as antimicrobial resistance (AMR) have been incorporated into national action plans.

CHANGE AND CONTINUITY IN CENTRE–STATE RELATIONSHIPS

Medical and health issues are constitutionally mostly reserved for the states, but the central government tries to influence state health policies through advice and financial support. In the 1980s, the centre provided about 20 per cent of public health spending, and tried to set health priorities, especially in public health, family welfare and significant communicable disease control programmes such as those for HIV/AIDS, tuberculosis (TB), and malaria (Berman and Ahuja 2008; Deolalikar et al. 2008; Sridhar and Gomez 2010).

During the 1990s, central government expenditures stagnated. Poorer states failed to replace central funds. As the influence of the Planning Commission weakened, state health ministers preferred to support large-scale hospitals and medical colleges, and programmes that offered large construction contracts. State bureaucracies rarely developed coherent ideas about public health issues. Public health doctors are rarely appointed as a director-general of health services—these posts go to the most senior doctor in government service, usually someone with a clinical career, often spent mostly in medical colleges. Similarly, senior bureaucrats in the various state health ministries spend only a few years in post before moving elsewhere. Between 1991 and 2001, there was 'no systematic effort at the state level to plan, and monitor the delivery of health services (which) continue to be supply pushed (rather) than demand driven' (Ramani and Mavalankar 2006: 4).

In the early 2000s, the NRHM was seen by many Indian health planners as a means to meet the MDG health goals that India had signed up to in 2000, against which India's progress would be judged. India's healthcare indicators were lagging well behind those of other resource-constrained countries such as Sri Lanka, and very far from those of middle-income countries. But whatever the other benefits of the MDGs, they did lead to a narrow focus on a limited set of indicators in maternal and child health and the control of infectious diseases—TB, malaria, and HIV/AIDS in particular. The United Progressive Alliance (UPA) government in 2004 brought in new health policymakers to address these issues. Although never as much a matter for public debate as other innovations, health became one of the priorities in the coalition's 'common minimum programme' (CMP), which was the basis on which smaller parties supported the minority Congress-led Government. The CMP stated that India's poverty reduction must be built on both rapid economic growth and targeted investments aimed at the poorest of the poor (Bajpai and Sachs 2004: 3). Outside Parliament, the UPA had support from increasingly well-organized CSOs, as well as from Amartya Sen, Jean Drèze, and Aruna Roy. Drèze and Roy served briefly on UPA Chairperson Sonia Gandhi's National Advisory Council (NAC), which successfully lobbied for innovative social welfare programmes—education, food, and employment—and the Right to Information Act (2005). The UPA worked within the framework of the National Health Policy (NHP, 2002) to address issues of health equity involving analyses based on the social determinants of health. It attempted to integrate existing health programmes into a single administrative programme and to implement principles of equity, decentralization, empowerment of local institutions, and to strengthen the primary health system (Das and Cottler 2017: 155).

The main channel for central government funding was the NRHM (for details see Dhingra and Dutta 2011; Hota 2006; Husain 2011). Shiffman and Ved (2007) use Kingdon's framework to show how maternal mortality came to prominence within the NRHM. A similar story can be told for the PPP health insurance scheme, the Rashtriya Swasthya Bima Yojana (RSBY):

> By creating the NAC and the NCEUS [National Commission for Enterprises in the Unorganised Sector], Sonia Gandhi increased the salience of social security issues and empowered selected advocacy groups. Manmohan Singh's decision to disregard the NCEUS report except for health insurance made it clear within the bureaucracy which initiative was a priority. Similarly, Sudha Pillai and Anil Swarup's creation of the task force both enabled the design of this program to happen swiftly and quietly and provided a role for technocrats from the international agencies influencing what was produced. (Shroff, Roberts, and Reich 2015: 114)

Key to being able to implement any of these ideas was the massive increase in central government revenues, which rose by 15 per cent or more per year through the Eleventh Plan (2007–8 to 2012–13). By 2012–13, the central government was spending INR 184 billion through the NRHM, specifically designed to benefit differentially 18 'focus' states with relatively poor health indicators, the Empowered Action Group (EAG) states of the central north Indian belt and the northeast region of the country.[3]

There was a shift between the first UPA government (2004–9) and the second (2009–14). In the first phase, there was a clear emphasis on strengthening the public health sector, but, by the second phase, the NRHM emphasized links to NGOs and the private sector, decentralization, and a search for alternate sources of finances and insurance schemes (Dhingra and Dutta 2011: 1521). It claimed to provide flexible financial opportunities for innovations at the state level, alongside district-level planning and management, but the criteria for expenditure were very tightly drawn (Gill 2009: 11–12). The central government promised steady increases in its funding, while demanding that the states increase their contributions as well. Crucially, however, central government transfers were made directly to state-level 'societies', bypassing state budget mechanisms (Rao and Choudhury 2012: 16; see also Narwal 2015: 126).

These massive changes in NHP involved relatively little input from the states (Rao and Choudhury 2012: 17). In only a few fields, such as drug procurement, health insurance, or maternal and child health services, did states provide examples of innovative schemes that could be scaled up to the national level. The confluence of problems, policies, and politics rarely came together in the states: the NRHM was a semi-integrated mix of central government concerns, international perspectives, and CSO pressures. Despite the evidence that health outcomes in the EAG states are much worse than elsewhere, their state policymakers have never identified this as a 'problem' that needs to be addressed urgently, nor have policy entrepreneurs emerged in these states. Even after the expansion in health resources, most of India's states had '(i) insufficient state funding for health; (ii) a regulatory environment that enables the private sector to deliver social services without an appropriate regulatory framework; and (iii) lack of transparency in governance' (Nishtar 2010: 74).

The minister and the IAP wanted to exclude state politicians and administrators. There was disdain for state politics: 'there is a management challenge' and in states the 'view is narrow and segmented'. There was a desire to find out how to 'institutionalize a 10-year perspective, insulated from politics at state and union level sufficient to ensure vision reaches the end point' (Sachs comments, IAP 2006: 2). Or as the minister put it, a need to have the 'district as a unit not a state' (IAP 2006: 5).

Many EAG states did not make matching and additional contributions; the large allocations in central funding could not be spent, and unspent sums were reallocated to those states that could spend the money appropriately (Rao and Choudhury 2012: 17). Most EAG states spent their construction funds, with greater opportunities for corruption, rather than the other elements (Fan et al. 2014: x, 9, 11).

Interstate differences are well-established, depending on their evolving political economies, the nature of political leadership, the capacity and autonomy of the bureaucracy, along with the strength of CSOs and other organized interest groups, and their relationship with the state (Tillin, Deshpande, and Kailash 2015: 17). (See Table 14.1 and also Tillin and Duckett 2017.)

This model has some heuristic benefits, though not everything fits. While some states have followed a fairly consistent path towards a welfare state (Kerala, and for a while, West Bengal) on the basis of social democracy,

[3] Bihar, Jharkhand, Madhya Pradesh, Chhattisgarh, Uttar Pradesh, Uttaranchal, Odisha, and Rajasthan were the EAG states; Assam, Arunachal Pradesh, Manipur, Meghalaya, Mizoram, Nagaland, Sikkim, and Tripura were the eight northeast states. Himachal Pradesh and Jammu & Kashmir (the erstwhile state of Jammu & Kashmir, which is now split into two union territories—Jammu & Kashmir and Ladakh) also had special status.

Table 14.1 State Welfare Regimes in India

Cluster	Sub-Cluster A	Sub-Cluster B	Sub-Cluster C
Welfare regimes	'Social Democratic' e.g. Kerala, West Bengal (in the past)	'Competitive populist' e.g. Andhra Pradesh, Tamil Nadu	'Incorporationist' e.g. Chhattisgarh, Odisha
Inconsistent welfare regimes	'Pro-business' e.g. Gujarat	'Competitive clientelist' e.g. Uttar Pradesh, Bihar	'Predatory states' e.g. Jharkhand

Source: Tillin, Deshpande, and Kailash (2015: 16–20).

others (like Andhra Pradesh and Tamil Nadu) have moved in this direction as part of competitive populism. Odisha and Chhattisgarh (since 2000) are 'incorporationist': a top-down set of policies have achieved some measure of welfare state achievements. Elsewhere, welfarist policies have emerged only occasionally. In Gujarat, welfare has been tied to business interests and initiatives; in Uttar Pradesh and Bihar, identity politics has left little space for collective agreement to address common social welfare challenges (Jeffery, Jeffrey, and Lerche 2013; Singh 2014). Yet in Tamil Nadu—also often seen as hostage to identity politics—social development programmes have been implemented quite widely. In Jharkhand (and other states, sometimes) resources are skimmed off by a small political and business elite. In the 2000s, Kerala and Odisha saw steady growth in human development indicators (HDI), whereas Gujarat and Uttar Pradesh were nearly stagnant. The outliers here are Andhra Pradesh (before the division)—also stagnant—and Jharkhand, which improved considerably, albeit from a very low starting point (Drèze and Khera 2012).

Efforts to induce the states to follow a welfare-oriented route, therefore, succeed only where the state is already welfare-oriented. The Thirteenth Finance Commission has shifted more resources directly to the states. The NITI Aayog (or National Institution for Transforming India), which replaced the Planning Commission in 2015, avoids directly influencing state policies,[4] so the central government now has fewer levers at its disposal (Fan et al. 2014: 6). According to Prime Minister Narendra Modi's office, 'The centre-to-state one-way flow of policy, that was the hallmark of the Planning Commission era, is now sought to be replaced by a genuine and continuing partnership of states.'[5] In this emerging framework, it is not clear what if anything can or will be done to redress interstate disparities or address the particular problems of poorer states, or whether this policy claim remains merely rhetorical.

THE RISE OF THE HEALTH CORPORATES

Corporate hospital chains begin to take off in the 1990s. The Manipal group, which T.M. Pai (1898–1979) had started with a medical college and associated hospital in the early 1950s, began to expand its hospital chain at that time.[6] Prathap Chandra Reddy (b. 1933), the founder of the Apollo Hospital chain, was the first of the new breed of corporate hospital entrepreneurs. He propagated a justification for how this would benefit the country that was largely mythical (Gupte 2013; Hodges 2013). Prathap Reddy was connected to Chandraswami, an influential guru in the 1980s, and a leader of Youth Wing of the Congress Party in Andhra Pradesh in the 1970s. P.V. Narasimha Rao and R. Venkatraman, the Indian finance ministers in the 1980s, helped with Reddy's loans, land acquisition, and imports of medical equipment (Lefebvre 2008). Apollo and other chains have increasingly marketed their services abroad, targeting European and North American as well as Asian markets such as the Persian Gulf and Southeast Asia, with Chennai, Bengaluru, and Hyderabad as key centres of corporate efforts to attract overseas patients. Apollo Hospitals group claims over 7,000 doctors working in over 56 different specialities in August 2016.[7]

Reddy's initiative attracted many others who have transformed the medical cityscapes across India (see Table 14.2). Fortis represents a different trajectory, one in which profits from the pharmaceuticals sector were used to expand into hospitals. Fortis was founded in 1996 by the sons of Parvinder Singh (1943–1999) from the Ranbaxy pharmaceuticals company. They opened their first hospital in the suburbs of Chandigarh in 2001 but expanded rapidly by acquiring the Escorts Heart Institute in Delhi and hospitals from the Wockhardt chain in Mumbai, Bengaluru, and Kolkata. Fortis also began a rapid expansion abroad, only to sell off many of its overseas assets by 2015. In 2018, the group was bought out by a Malaysia-based group, IHH Healthcare.[8]

The establishment of these mostly family-run businesses depended heavily on government support. Like other private hospitals, Apollo was supported by government providing, among other things, land and tax

[4] http://niti.gov.in/, last accessed on 30 August 2017.

[5] ENS Economic Bureau, 'NITI Aayog replaces Planning Commission, Prime Minister Modi bids farewell to "one size fits all" approach', 2 January 2015, http://indianexpress.com/article/business/business-others/niti-aayog-to-replace-plan-panel/, last accessed on 2 January 2015.

[6] See https://www.manipalhospitals.com/about-us/; see also Pai (1982).

[7] https://www.apollohospitals.com/patient-care/find-a-doctor, last accessed on 15 August 2016.

[8] Shabana Hussain, 'Fortis tames debt burden, but at a cost', Forbes.com, 10 September 2015, http://forbesindia.com/article/big-bet/fortis-tames-debt-burden-but-at-a-cost/41045/1#ixzz3pJMOIsU4, last accessed on 20 April 2016.

Table 14.2 Private Hospital Chains in India in 2017

Hospital Chain	Year of Creation	Base	Number of Hospitals	Number of Beds
Manipal	1953	Bangalore (Kar)	11	2,333
Apollo	1983	Chennai (TN)	36	7,778
RG Stone	1987	Delhi	14	349
Kuval	1987	Coimbatore (TN)	3	857
Wockhardt	1989	Mumbai (Mah)	9	1330
Seven Hills	1992	Visakhapatnam (AP)	2	556
Sahyadri	1993	Pune (Mah)	10	900
Vrundavan Shalby	1994	Ahmedabad (Guj)	7	640
CARE	1997	Hyderabad (AP)	17	2,400
Metro Heart	1997	Delhi	12	1,814
Global	1998	Hyderabad (AP)	5	1,950
Vikram	2000	Mysore (Kar)	7	329
Sterling	2001	Ahmedabad (Guj)	7	1,006
Fortis	2001	Delhi	27	4,564
HealthCare Global	2001	Bangalore (Kar)	13	550
Narayana Hrudayalaya	2001	Bangalore (Kar)	13	6,650
Max	2002	Delhi	9	1,840
Rockland	2004	Delhi	5	1,315
Vaatsalya	2005	Bangalore (Kar)	17	1,143
Columbia	2005	Bangalore (Kar)	11	1,181
All			230	38,909

Source: Lefebvre (2013: 233) and respective company websites as accessed on 21 September 2017.

incentives in what was described as a PPP. The 'private' included the corporate hospitals, who were understood to be prepared to act as charitable institutions by providing free beds and outpatient services for the poor, as had been the case for the voluntary hospitals that preceded the corporate phase. Land was allotted to 42 hospitals and dispensaries in irregular ways, and there was no attempt to enforce the terms under which the land had been provided (Public Accounts Committee 2005: 26).

A public interest litigation filed by the All India Lawyers' Union in 1997 asked the Delhi high court to ensure free medical treatment in terms of the lease agreement between the Delhi Administration and Apollo Hospitals of March 1994. The case was settled in 2009, and it required the Delhi Administration to demand that Apollo (and others similarly placed) must provide free care in at least one third of their beds and up to 40 per cent of those seeking outpatient care, as had been agreed when land was allocated to them, some 15 years previously (Thomas and Krishnan 2010: 1).[9] Even since then, it has been hard—if not impossible—to enforce this rule, especially given the pressures on hospital consultants to 'meet targets for generating revenue by overprescribing diagnostic tests and avoidable surgeries' (Kay 2015). Anecdotal evidence suggests that, in line with many other practices followed by large private hospitals (Nundy, Desiraju and Nagral 2018) 'free patients' are pressured to leave (for example, by giving them access to facilities only at inconvenient hours).

Through procedures such as this, returns in the commercial hospital sector have sometimes been considerable.

[9] For full details of the judgment see http://lobis.nic.in/ddir/dhc/APS/judgement/05-10-2009/APS22092009CW54101997.pdf, accessed on 15 August 2016. Delhi government's order of 13 October 2009 is available at http://www.delhi.gov.in/wps/wcm/connect/3f4f14004ffe7cb580969bd9d1b46642/APOLLO.pdf?MOD=AJPERES&CACHEID=3f4f14004ffe7cb580969bd9d1b46642, last accessed on 15 August 2016.

Table 14.3 Indian Billionaires with Wealth from Healthcare or Pharmaceuticals, as of 2017

Global Rank	Name	Wealth (billion USD)	Age	Company	Rank in Indian List
84	Dilip Shanghvi	13.7	61	Sun Pharmaceuticals	4
159	Cyrus Poonawalla	8.1	76	Serum Institute of India	7
303	Pankaj Patel	5.2	64	Cadila Pharmaceuticals	13
348	Desh Bandhu Gupta	4.7	79	Lupin Pharmaceuticals	15
501	Ajay Piramal	3.7	62	Piramal	21
660	B.R. Shetty	3	75	NMC Healthcare	31
782	P.V. Ramprasad Reddy	2.6	59	Aurobindo Pharma	34=
867	Hasmukh Chudgar	2.4	83	Intas Pharmaceuticals	44=
1030	Leena Tewari	2	59	USV	49
1290	Murali Divi	1.6	66	Divi's Pharmaceuticals	62=
1376	Yusuf Hamied	1.5	81	Cipla	68=
1567	Habil Khorakiwala	1.3	74	Wockhardts	80=
1567	Shamsheer Vayalil	1.3	40	VPS Healthcare	80=
1678	Mahendra Prasad	1.2	77	Aristo Pharmaceuticals	89=
1678	Analjit Singh	1.2	63	Max Healthcare	89=
1795	Satish Mehta	1.1	66	Emcure Pharmaceuticals	93=
1795	Samprada Singh	1.1	91	Alkem Laboratories	93=
1940	Chirayu Amin	1	70	Alembic pharmaceuticals	97=
1940	Azad Moopen	1	64	Aster DM Healthcare	97=

Source: https://www.forbes.com/billionaires/list/2/#version:static_country:India, last accessed on 21 August 2017.

Corporate hospitals have been 'a new growth opportunity for business families. In what used to be a cottage industry with small family-run facilities, these groups are bringing unmatched financial strength and managerial skills' (Lefebvre 2010, 2013: 11).

The healthcare sector has proved sufficiently profitable that 19 of India's 100 billionaires found their initial success in either pharmaceuticals or healthcare (see Table 14.3). There are strong financial links between the two sectors, with many of the corporate hospital chains founded by business families involved in the pharmaceutical sector: Wockhardt, Fortis, and Max are the most obvious examples where the pharmaceuticals interest came first; in the case of Apollo, its retail network of pharmacies was built on the back of its hospital chain.

At the same time as the public sector attempted to increase its role in healthcare in India, 'The Indian hospital and diagnostic centres attracted foreign direct investment worth $2,793.72 million between April 2000 and January 2015.... [T]he market ... is witnessing a compound annual growth rate of around 13 per cent as affluent Indians get willing to pay a premium for better-equipped facilities.'[10]

Apollo Hospitals has also taken four substantial loans from the IFC (see Table 14.4). Max India, which created Max Healthcare in 2000 and operated its first hospitals in 2002, has also turned to the IFC for support, as have smaller groups such as Portea (Healthvista India), a home-based healthcare provider, and Regency (a hospital group based in Kanpur). This is one indicator of the extent to which these hospitals increasingly operate outwith the control of the government, whether central or state. Another indicator is the efforts being made by the corporate hospitals to acquire recognition by Joint Commission International (JCI), to enhance their attraction to overseas patients, which put the country's own hospital standards, National Accreditation Board

[10] Pramughda Mamgain, 'Global hospital chains, PE majors in race to buy India's CARE Hospitals: Report', 7 September 2015, https://www.dealstreetasia.com/stories/global-hospital-chains-pe-majors-in-the-race-to-buy-hyderabad-based-care-hospitals-report-11674/, last accessed on 25 August 2017.

Table 14.4 Indian Corporate Hospitals' Projects Funded by the International Finance Corporation, 1997–2017

Corporation	Project Cost (million USD)	IFC Loan/Investment (million USD)	IFC Input as Percentage of Total Project Cost	Year of Signing
Duncan-Gleneagles	29	7	24%	1997
Max Healthcare	84	18	21%	2002
Apollo Hospitals	70	20	29%	2005
Artemis	40	10	25%	2006
Max Healthcare	90	67	74%	2007
Rockland	76	22	29%	2008
Max Healthcare	93	30	32%	2009
Apollo Hospitals	200	50	25%	2009
Apollo Hospitals	n.s.	60	n.a.	2012
Global Hospitals	60	25	42%	2013
Fortis	n.s.	100	n.a.	2013
Portea	37	7	19%	2015
Eye-Q	10	5.7	57%	2015
Regency	25	9	36%	2016
Apollo Hospitals	135	68	50%	2016
Glenmark	200	75	38%	2016
Granules	84	48	57%	2016
HealthCare Global	n.s.	15	n.a.	2016
Max Healthcare	325	75	23%	2017
Biological E	n.s.	60	n.a.	2017

Source: www.ifc.org and Lefebvre (2010: 12).
Notes: n.s. = not stated; n.a. = not available. The loan to Eye-Q was denominated in Indian rupees; the exchange rate applied was INR 60 = USD 1.

for Hospitals and Healthcare Providers (NABH), in the shade.

Other corporate interests also attempt to intervene in their own spheres of interest, most notably in attempts to limit programmes of tobacco control, leading to India's premier public health institute losing, for a while, its ability to receive foreign funding for any research. The influence wielded in this way, whether by internationally-oriented hospitals, pharmaceutical companies, and wealthy individuals and their companies is hard to identify—it tends to happen behind closed doors. Not so the efforts of CSOs, whose noisy objections to the commercialization of health services often reflect their weakness in decision-making.

CIVIL SOCIETY ORGANIZATIONS

CSOs have actively tried to redraft health priorities in different ways and with different levels of success according to the prevailing political atmosphere. CSO leaders have often been invited to serve on health committees established by the central government, to provide 'blue-skies' thinking. In 1978, a joint panel of the Indian Councils of Social Science (ICSSR) and Medical Research (ICMR) operated outside the normal departmental setup and produced a visionary report that aimed to bring 'health for all' to India (Antia 2009; Nayar 2012; Ramalingaswami et al. 1981). Despite the report providing the basis of the 1983 NHP, few of its recommendations were taken forward in practice, and some of those involved in the original report such as Nosher Antia (1922–2007) and Rajnikant Arole (1934–2011) tried to take the insights forward in their advice to the NRHM, 25 years later. Other health activist groups, also established in the late 1970s and the early 1980s, include the Medico Friend Circle, founded in 1974 and with 'over 350 members who represent a wide spectrum of civil societal interest in the health of the people of

Table 14.5 Membership of the High Level Expert Group for Universal Health Coverage, 2010–11

Abhay Bang	Community physician: Society for Education, Action and Research in Community Health' (SEARCH); Gadchiroli, Maharashtra
Mirai Chatterjee	Director of Social Security: Self-Employed Women's Association; Ahmedabad, Gujarat
Jashodha Dasgupta	Community advocate: SAHAYOG, Lucknow, Uttar Pradesh
Anu Garg	Administrator: Principal Secretary-cum-Commissioner (Health and Family Welfare department, Odisha
Yogesh Jain	Community physician: member of Jan Swasthya Sahyog (JSS), Bilaspur, Chhattisgarh
A.K. Shiva Kumar	Development economist: member, National Advisory Council and advisor to UNICEF–India; Harvard and Hyderabad, Andhra Pradesh
Nachiket Mor	Economist: ex-ICICI Foundation for Inclusive Growth to rural development, Sugha Vazhvu Healthcare, Thanjavur, Tamil Nadu
Vinod Paul	Doctor: Head of AIIMS's paediatrics department, New Delhi
P.K. Pradhan	Administrator: Secretary, Health and Family Welfare, Government of India, New Delhi
M. Govinda Rao	Economist: Director, National Institute of Public Finance and Policy, New Delhi
K. Srinath Reddy (Chair)	Cardiologist and public health doctor: Director, Public Health Foundation of India, New Delhi
Gita Sen	Economist and global health expert: Centre for Public Policy, IIM Bangalore; Karnataka
N.K. Sethi (Convenor)	Senior Advisor (Health), Planning Commission, Government of India, New Delhi
Amarjeet Sinha	Administrator: Joint Secretary, Health and Family Welfare, Government of India; New Delhi
Leila Caleb Varkey	Midwife: member of the White Ribbon Alliance India; New Delhi

Source: Reddy et al. (2011).

India'.[11] Eighteen such organizations came together in 2001 to form the Jan Swasthya Abhiyan (JSA), the national regional circle of the global People's Health Movement.[12] Members of the JSA have been particularly active organizing around women's reproductive health issues, HIV/AIDS, and clinical trials, as well as campaigning in support of the public sector in health. They have also deepened their links with parallel organizations working in other resource-constrained countries. Their direct influence on policymaking has somewhat evaporated since 2014, but even before then, when they contributed strongly to discussions on the 2009 NHP, they were unable to influence how far its major commitments were implemented.

Under the UPA Government, CSOs changed their nature (Goswami and Tandon 2013) and grew rapidly in number. A few were able to exercise some influence directly, as members of important (though not necessarily, key) committees. Eighteen health activists joined the Advisory Group on Community Action of the NRHM in 2005, set up at the urging of Nosher Antia. Mirai Chatterjee, and Abhay Bang (husband of Rani Bang) were also members of the High Level Expert Group for Universal Health Coverage, 2010–11 (Table 14.5). Significantly, under the UPA government, CSOs were well represented, whereas under the 2014–19 BJP government, the Mission Steering Group—the highest-level committee—had 10 public health professionals, outweighed by 10 ministers, 16 secretaries in ministries in the Government of India, as well as four representatives of 'high focus' states and two representatives of the NITI Aayog. Membership of the Empowered Committee was entirely of administrators, barring two 'health professionals', one of whom was also in government service as director-general of the ICMR.[13]

Some CSOs have campaigned through the media and through direct approaches to parliamentary committees and the courts. One of the most successful campaigns concerned the ethics of clinical trials. CSOs such as Swasthya Adhikar Manch from Indore campaigned over irregularities in trials carried out in Bhopal. Delhi-based SAMA resource group for women and health, Drug Action Forum, and Delhi Science Forum campaigned vigorously over the ethical issues raised by the introduction of the HPV vaccine. Swasthya Adhikar Manch and

[11] http://www.mfcindia.org/, last accessed on 6 October 2017.

[12] http://phmindia.org/about-us/, last accessed on 6 October 2017.

[13] http://nhm.gov.in/monitoring/empowered-programme-committee.html, last accessed on 2 October 2017.

SAMA raised public interest litigation petitions in the Supreme Court, and gave evidence to the joint parliamentary committee which considered the roles played by the Drug Controller-General India and the Central Drugs Standards Control Organization (for more details see Divan 2016; Terwindt 2014). Civil society organizations thus helped to induce regulatory changes that tightened the regulation of those clinical trials that need to be registered with the central government, implementing those changes is an even harder task.

CSOs are unevenly distributed across states. In Kerala, West Bengal, Andhra Pradesh, and Tamil Nadu, CSOs can press state governments to implement welfare measures. Gujarat has a strong history of CSOs, and some notable pilot projects in health and education, but business interests in the state are even more strongly entrenched. Most of the other states have CSOs that struggle to get their voices heard by state governments, for example in EAG states such as Uttar Pradesh (Dasgupta 2016).

An alternative set of actors has always been part of the CSO health sector, involving philanthropists and those pursuing religious agendas. Their work, often focusing on medical treatment, for example through free clinics and eye camps, expanded and has become more closely linked to right-wing Hindu interests (sometimes including efforts to close down Christian-run activities). This part of the health sector is being increasingly affected by the requirement for larger Indian companies to set up corporate social responsibility schemes, for which two of the priority areas are reducing child mortality and improving maternal health, and combating HIV, AIDS, malaria and other diseases.[14] Some of these schemes are little more than off-shoots of their funders; rarely are there mechanisms in place that make them accountable to the community being served, nor can they offer independent advice to government on how its health policies might be implemented.

***

This chapter has shown the relevance of the analyses of both Kingdon and Reich. Centre–state relationships in health are of diminishing relevance for three main reasons: the shrinking role of public health provisions in large parts of India; the shift of resources to state governments; and the increasing role of global pressures that reduce the options for both levels of government. There has been a continuing failure over much of the country to invest in social welfare programmes even when increasing state revenues made this possible (Drèze and Sen 2013: 177). Although the examples of Tamil Nadu and Kerala, and to a lesser extent, Andhra Pradesh and West Bengal, show what is possible, mechanisms to extend those lessons to other states are weak and getting weaker.

Interstate and other inequalities are no longer seen to be important (Bhagwati and Panagariya 2013: 45–6). A host of health indicators, and evidence of differential access to and use of central government funds, show that southern India is a world apart from the EAG states. Gujarat has experienced a model of social and economic development that is primarily growth- and private-entrepreneurship-driven. The post-2014 BJP government sees this model as superior to the Kerala model of primarily redistribution and state-driven development championed by Drèze and Sen.

In Kingdon's terms, the preconditions for policy changes are not present in the poorer states, and (in most cases) the situation shows little sign of change. Indian health policymaking is characterized by a massive gulf between the impressive national policy statements and strong (if unevenly distributed) activist CSOs on the one hand, and the reality of day-to-day public health provisions that are increasingly commodified.

In conclusion I would like to raise five questions as a contribution to public policy and debate:

1. How can health politics and policymaking become more salient, particularly in the poorer states?
2. Are governance issues being adequately addressed in the new corporate social responsibility arrangements?
3. How can the corporate hospitals be properly regulated, and their statutory obligations enforced?
4. What is the appropriate stance for India to take in international negotiations on healthcare, given the significant role now being played by philanthro–capitalism?
5. Can PPPs be radically reassessed to ensure they meet social and not private goals?

[14] http://www.ppv.issuelab.org/resources/15662/15662.pdf, last accessed on 10 December 2019.

REFERENCES

Antia, Noshir H. 2009. *A Life of Change: The Autobiography of a Doctor*. New Delhi: Penguin.

Bajpai, Nirupam, and Jeffrey D. Sachs. 2004. 'National Common Minimum Programme of the Congress-led United Progressive Alliance: Policy Reform and Public Investment Requirements', Working Paper No. 22, Center on Globalization and Sustainable Development, New York. Available at https://academiccommons.columbia.edu/doi/10.7916/D8VX0PBV, last accessed on 10 December 2019.

Baru, Rama, V. 1998. *Private Health Care in India: Social Characteristics and Trends*. New Delhi: Sage.

Berman, Peter, A. 1998. 'Rethinking Health Care Systems: Private Health Care Provision in India', *World Development* 26(8): 1463–79.

Berman, Peter, and Rajeev Ahuja. 2008. 'Government Health Spending in India', *Economic and Political Weekly* 46(26/7): 209–16.

Bhagwati, Jagdish, and Arvind Panagariya. 2013. *Why Growth Matters: How Economic Growth in India Reduced Poverty and the Lessons for Other Developing Countries*. New York: PublicAffairs.

Bijoy, C.R. 2009. 'India: Transiting to a Global Donor', in *Special Report on South-South Cooperation: A Challenge to the Aid System?*, edited by A.J. Tujan. Manila, Philippines: IBON Books.

Corbridge, Stuart, John Harriss, and Craig Jeffrey. 2013. *India Today: Economy, Politics and Society*. Cambridge: Polity Press.

Das, Shankar, and Linda B. Cottler. 2017. 'The Health Care System in India', in *Health Care Systems in Developing Countries in Asia*, edited by Christian Aspalter, Kenny Teguh Pribadi and Robin Gauld. London: Routledge.

Dasgupta, Jasodhara. 2016. 'Whose Voice Really Counts? Experiences of Trying to Build "Voice" for Health Accountability in Uttar Pradesh, India', in *Feminist Subversion and Complicity: Governmentalities and Gender Knowledge in South Asia*, edited by Maitrayee Mukhopadhyay. New Delhi: Zubaan.

Deolalikar, Anil B., Dean T. Jamison, Prabhat Jha, and Ramanan Laxminarayan. 2008. 'Financing Health Improvements in India', *Health Affairs* 27(4): 978–90.

Dhingra, Bhavna, and Ashok Kumar Dutta. 2011. 'National Rural Health Mission', *Indian Journal of Pediatrics* 78(12): 1520–6.

Divan, Shyam. 2016. 'Public Interest Litigation', in *The Oxford Handbook of the Indian Constitution*, edited by Sujit Choudhry, Madhav Khosla and Pratap Bhanu Mehta. Oxford: Oxford University Press.

Drèze, Jean, and Reetika Khera. 2012. 'Regional Patterns of Human and Child Deprivation in India', *Economic and Political Weekly* 47: 42–9.

Fan, Victoria, Anit Mukherjee, Amanda Glassman, Yamini Aiyar, Avani Kapur, Smriti Iyer, H.K. Amarnath, Rifaiyat Mahbub, Yuna Sakuma, and Vikram Srinivas. 2014. 'Fiscal Federalism and Intergovernmental Transfers for Financing Health in India', Center for Global Development, Washington, DC.

Goswami, Debika, and Rajesh Tandon. 2013. 'Civil Society in Changing India: Emerging Roles, Relationships, and Strategies', *Development in Practice* 23(5–6): 653–64.

Hodges, Sarah. 2013. '"It All Changed After Apollo": Healthcare Myths and their Making in Contemporary India', *Indian Journal of Medical Ethics* 10(4): 242–9.

Hota, Prasanna. 2006. 'National Rural Health Mission', *Indian Journal of Pediatrics* 73(3): 193–5.

Husain, Zakir. 2011. 'Health of the National Rural Health Mission', *Economic and Political Weekly* 46(4): 53–60.

IAP (International Advisory Panel). 2006. 'Brief for the meeting held under the Chairmanship of Hon'ble Union Minister of Health & Family Welfare on 3 August 2006 to discuss the recommendations of the International Advisory Panel set up by Mr. Jaffery (sic) Sachs and colleagues from the Centre on Globalisation and Sustainable Development of the Earth Institute of Columbia University, New York'. Available at http://nhm.gov.in/monitoring/international-advisory-panel/minutes-of-the-international-advisory-panel.html, last accessed on 4 May 2020.

———. 2007. 'Record of discussions of the meeting of the International Advisory Panel (IAP) for NRHM held on 7.8.2007 under the Chairmanship of Union Minister for Health & FW'. Available at http://nhm.gov.in/monitoring/international-advisory-panel/minutes-of-the-international-advisory-panel.html, last accessed on 4 May 2020.

Illich, Ivan. 1976. *Medical Nemesis*. New York: Bantam Books.

Jeffery, Roger. 1982. 'New Patterns in Health Sector Aid', *Economic and Political Weekly* 17(37): 1495–503.

———. 1986. 'Health Planning in India: The Role of the Planning Commission', *Health Policy and Planning* 1(2): 127–37.

Jeffery, Roger, Craig Jeffrey, and Jens Lerche (eds) 2013. *UP: Identity Politics and Development Failure*. New Delhi: Sage.

Kay, Meera. 2015. 'The Unethical Revenue Targets that India's Corporate Hospitals Set their Doctors', *BMJ* 351: h4312.

Kingdon, John W. 1984. *Agendas, Alternatives and Public Policies*. Boston and Toronto: Little, Brown and Company.

Kohli, Atul. 1989. 'Politics of Economic Liberalization in India', *World Development* 17(3): 305–28.

Lefebvre, Bertrand. 2008. 'The Indian Corporate Hospitals: Touching Middle Class Lives', in *Patterns of Middle Class Consumption in India and China*, edited by Christophe Jaffrelot and Peter van der Veer. New Delhi: Sage.

———. 2010. 'Hospital Chains in India: The Coming of Age?' *Asie Visions*. Paris: IFRI.

———. 2013. 'Les Chaînes Hospitalières en Inde: Quels Modèles Pour Approcher la Diffusion Spatiale de ces Réseaux de Soins?' (Hospital Chains in India: Which Models to Approach the Spatial Diffusion of these Networks of Care?), in *Les réseaux dans le temps et dans l'espace* (Networks in Time and Space), edited by Laurent Beauguitte. (Paris: Actes de la deuxième journée d'études du groupe fmr (flux, matrices, réseaux) [Proceedings of the second day of study of the fmr group (flows, matrices, networks)]).

Narwal, Rajesh. 2015. 'Success and Constraints of the National Rural Health Mission: Is there a Need for Course Correction for India's Move towards Universal Health Coverage?', in *India: Social Development Report 2014: Challenges of Public Health*, edited by Council for Social Development. New Delhi: Oxford University Press.

Nayar, Kesavan Rajasekharan. 2012. 'Three Decades of ICSSR-ICMR Committee Report & the Re-assertion of Social Determinants of Health', *The Indian Journal of Medical Research* 136(4): 540–3.

Nishtar, Sania. 2010. 'The Mixed Health Systems Syndrome', *Bulletin of the World Health Organization* 88(1): 74–5.

Nundy, Samiran, Keshav Desiraju, and Sanjay Nagral. 2018. *Healers or Predators: Healthcare Corruption in India*. New Delhi: Oxford University Press.

Pai, Nirmala M. 1982. *Dr. T.M.A. Pai: A Brief Biography*. Manipal, Karnataka: Academy of General Education.

Qadeer, Imrana. 2013. 'Universal Health Care: The Trojan Horse of Neoliberal Policies', *Social Change* 43(2): 149–64.

Ramalingaswami, V., R.S. Arole, B.S. Cowasji, N.S. Deodhar, C.R. Jungalwalla, C.R. Krishnamurthi, J.P. Naik, V.N. Rao, S. Sankaran, Narottam Shah, V. Subhadra, K.N. Udupa, and N.H. Antia. 1981. *Health for All: An Alternative Strategy*. Pune: Indian Institute for Education.

Ramani, K.V., and Dileep Mavalankar. 2006. 'Health System in India: Opportunities and Challenges for Improvements', *Journal of Health Organization and Management* 20(6): 560–72.

Rao, M. Govinda, and Mita Choudhury. 2012. 'Health Care Financing Reforms in India.' Working Paper. New Delhi: National Institute of Public Finance and Policy.

Reddy, K. Srinath, Abhay Bang, Mirai Chatterjee, Jashodha Dasgupta, Anu Garg, Yogesh Jain, A.K. Shiva Kumar, et al. 2011. 'High Level Expert Group Report on Universal Health Coverage for India.' New Delhi: Planning Commission.

Reich, Michael. 2002. 'Reshaping the State from Above, from Within and from Below: Implications for Public Health', *Social Science and Medicine* 54(11): 1669–75.

Ridker, Ronald, and Philip Musgrove. 1999. 'Health Care in India: Learning from Experience', *OED Precis 187*. Washington, DC: World Bank.

Sengupta, Amit, and Vandana Prasad. 2011. 'Developing a Truly Universal Indian Health System: The Problem of Replacing "Health for All" with "Universal Access to Health Care"', *Social Medicine* 6(2): 69–72.

Shiffman, Jeremy, and R.R. Ved. 2007. 'The State of Political Priority for Safe Motherhood in India', *BJOG: An International Journal of Obstetrics & Gynaecology* 114: 785–90.

Shroff, Zubin Cyrus, Marc J. Roberts, and Michael R. Reich. 2015. 'Agenda Setting and Policy Adoption of India's National Health Insurance Scheme: Rashtriya Swasthya Bima Yojana', *Health Systems & Reform* 1(2): 107–18.

Singh, Prerna. 2014. *How Solidarity Works for Welfare: Subnationalism and Social Development in India*. New York & Cambridge: Cambridge University Press.

Sridhar, Devi, and Eduardo J. Gomez. 2010. 'Health Financing in Brazil, Russia, and India: What Role does the International Community Play?', *Health Policy and Planning* 26(1): 12–24.

Terwindt, Carolijn. 2014. 'Health Rights Litigation Pushes for Accountability in Clinical Trials in India', *Health and Human Rights* 16(2): e84–e95.

Tillin, Louise, Rajeshwari Deshpande, and K.K. Kailash. 2015. *Politics of Welfare: Comparisons across Indian States*. New Delhi: Oxford University Press.

Tillin, Louise, and Jane Duckett. 2017. 'The Politics of Social Policy: Welfare Expansion in Brazil, China, India and South Africa in Comparative perspective', *Commonwealth & Comparative Politics* 55(3): 253–77.

15

Healthcare Sector Financing in India

Abusaleh Shariff, Gulrez Shah Azhar, and Amit Sharma

The per capita household consumption expenditure has almost doubled since 2005 (World Bank 2018). Yet with the top 1% owning more than half of India's wealth, it is among the most unequal countries in the world (Credit Suisse 2019). There are many complex varieties of disparities and diversity in inequality based on occupations, rural–urban residence, gender, and socio-religious identities. Improvement in the quality of life for its citizens, therefore, is uneven and often haphazard.

The Indian population faces a wide variety of health conditions from undernutrition and anaemia, communicable and non-communicable diseases (NCDs), to trauma and environmental health conditions. According to the fourth National Family Health Survey (NFHS-4; reference year 2015–16), child undernutrition rates are at 38.4 per cent, and 53 per cent of all women aged 15–49 are anaemic. Nationally 8 per cent of men and 5.8 per cent of women have high blood sugar levels (>140 mg/dL) and 13.6 per cent men and 8.8 per cent of women have high blood pressure levels (systolic >140 mmHg and/or diastolic >90 mmHg). Just over 70 per cent of the population—mostly comprising women, children, and the old—is at high risk of facing extreme health conditions with none or low levels of healthcare access in India.

India's commitment to the recommendations of the Bhore Committee report of 1946 (Bhore, Amesur, and Banerjee 1946) has been to ensure access and use of healthcare services to the masses of whom about two-thirds were categorized as poor. The national government, with the support from the state governments through budgetary process, allocated public resources to cover health and health promotional costs all over India. The international budgetary benchmark is to allocate about 6 per cent of the GDP for health sector (Kumar et al. 2011; Savedoff 2007). In India, however, so far the allocations are in the range between 1.5 per cent and 2 per cent of GDP (Hooda 2013).

The public financing of healthcare in India, expressed as the domestic general government health expenditure as a percentage of GDP, is among the lowest in the world at only 1 per cent of GDP (WHO 2017) while out-of-pocket spending is as high.

Catastrophic expenditure on healthcare is the leading cause of poverty in India, and resent estimates show that it has pushed 60 million Indians below the poverty line in 2010 (Shepherd-Smith 2012). Of the out-of-pocket spending, expenditure on medicines alone accounts for 72 per cent of the total direct cost. Financial barriers led to roughly a quarter of the population unable to access health services during 2004, and over 35 per cent of patients admitted to hospital were pushed into poverty (Marten et al. 2014).

This persists despite India being a signatory to the Alma-Ata Declaration of 1978 calling for primary essential healthcare to be made universally accessible. The declaration affirmed that a fundamental human right—'health' is a state of complete physical, mental, and social well-being, and not merely the absence of disease or infirmity (WHO 1948). Calling the gross inequalities as politically, socially, and economically unacceptable it reminded the governments its responsibility in providing adequate health and social measures. It also emphasized on the attainment of the highest possible level of health as a most important world-wide social goal, and in recognition of its multidimensional nature, that its realization requires the actions of many other social and economic sectors in addition to the health sector.

With a constant refrain of lack of adequate resources for the health sector from the government, and huge gaps in the national health policy, the healthcare sector has been dominated by the private sector, hospital-based curative care with little regulation of quality and cost of care. With the recent announcement of a strong government health scheme it is important to revisit how the funds are and should be spent.

INDIA'S HEALTHCARE SECTOR AND FINANCING

Broadly, India's healthcare financing sector is divided into three parts: (i) government-provided public funds through budgetary mechanism; (ii) out-of-pocket expenditures that households make; and (iii) a small corporate and civil society (including bilateral and multilateral support) supported healthcare provisioning (see Table 15.1).

Note that the private sector healthcare provisioning is kept out of this list for the obvious reason that it does not necessarily contribute to the 'healthcare financing', since this sector survives on it through market-based and often exploitative pricing policies. There have been a few public–private partnership (PPP) initiatives in some states in the immediate past, yet their successes and contribution in healthcare financing is not clearly known.

The third-party insurance types of financing are not separately added into this list as its penetration in India is still in its incipient stage. A discussion of the recent Government of India initiative of mass-access public insurance—Rashtriya Swasthya Bima Yojana (RSBY)—can be found at the end of this chapter.

The healthcare sector is characterized by a multiplicity of providers, treatment systems, and payment mechanisms. Treatment providers are both licensed and unlicensed, with greater numbers of unlicensed providers seen in rural areas. Treatment systems include the government recognized modern allopathic medicine and the AYUSH[1] systems. Several unrecognized systems include traditional bone setters and faith healers. The allocation from the national budget for AYUSH has been increasing and stood at INR 1,429 crore[2] in 2017–18 underscoring its increasing importance. However, the allocation for Ministry of Health and Family Welfare (MoHFW) as a whole was INR 48,853 crore for the same period (Centre for Budget and Governance Accountability 2018).

Healthcare facilities exist in both the public and private sectors. The public healthcare system consists of the subcentres, primary health centres, community health centres, district hospitals, and the tertiary care centres. They are set up based on defined population and geographic criteria. The private healthcare system also consists of a wide range of facilities. They range from a single practitioner outpatient clinic, small nursing homes with few inpatient beds, to large multispecialty hospitals.

Table 15.1 Share of Healthcare Financing according to Sources

Source of Funds	Amount (in INR Crore)	Percentage of Total
Government Resources		
Union government	37,221	8.2
State governments	59,978	13.3
Local bodies	2,960	0.7
Households (Mostly out-of-Pocket)		
Households*	320,262	71.0
Other Sources		
Enterprises**	20,069	4.4
NGOs	7,422	1.6
External/donor funding	3,374	0.7
Total	451,286	100.0

* 67 per cent share of out-of-pocket; includes insurance contributions.

** includes insurance contributions.

Source: National Health Accounts Estimates for India 2017 (National Health Systems Resource Center 2017).

Note: NGO – non-governmental organization.

[1] AYUSH is an acronym for ayurveda, yoga and naturopathy, unani, siddha and homoeopathy.

[2] A crore equals 10 million. Money in India is often written in terms of crores in official government documents.

Table 15.2 Statement 1: Components of primary health care and respective dimensions

Components	State of Health to Which a Particular Component has Reference	Dimensions of a Particular Component of PHC
1. Promotive health care	Normal state of health	1. Nutritional balance and adequacy. 2. Clean and potable water. 3. Sanitation and public hygiene. 4. Private/personal hygiene.
2. Preventive health care	Normal state of health Symptomatic state of health	5. Mass prevention of immunizable diseases. 6. Post symptomatic prevention of locally endemic diseases.
3. Curative health care	Sick-ordinary Sick-persistent	7. Care and treatment of ordinary sickness. 8. Care and treatment of chronic sickness.

The Indian Public Health Standards (IPHS) govern the staffing and standards at various health facilities. There is a staffing imbalance between rural and urban areas and between states. In general, the southern states and urban areas have better staffing.

Human health consists of a complex set of components each of which requires a different strategy and treatment protocol (see Table 15.2). Based on such a requirement there are a hierarchy of institutions which are conceptualized and developed for over a century across the country, sustaining the predominantly rural nature of living and lifestyles of people and households (see Figure 15.1).

The costs of healthcare and their payment mechanisms are varied. Since health is a state subject, there are variations in state health policies and associated delivery mechanisms and price or cost of care. States which allocated higher health funding are observed to also attain better public health systems, while states with lower public-sector health funding tend to promote a larger private health sector. Recently there has been an increase in private sector participation in the public health system through PPP mechanisms for example, the RSBY and the Chiranjeevi Yojana in Gujarat. At the same time the central government also supports the state health departments through budgetary allocations and through 'vertical' health programmes and independently through the centrally sponsored schemes. These centrally sponsored programmes are typically for a single health condition for instance, control programmes for HIV, polio, and tuberculosis, and the National Health Mission (NHM).

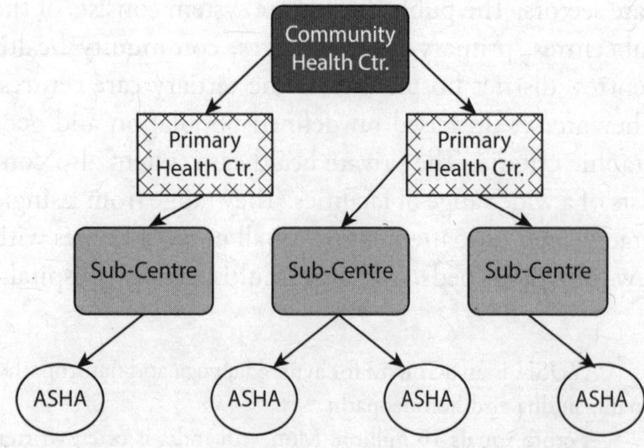

Figure 15.1 Community Level Health Policy Hierarchy

MORBIDITY AND TREATMENT PROFILE OF INDIA

To understand healthcare financing in India, it is imperative to understand the structure and incidence of ill health, sickness, and morbidity. Data on these parameters are routinely collected from the public and private hospitals but they are not amenable for use in research and analytical studies. Hospital-based data are episodic and selective of those who choose to seek treatment from a professional service provider. Such data suffers from selectivity bias and is unfit for use in health policy and planning analysis.

The government-sponsored NSSO surveys are a good source of dependable data collected from households and individuals across India. The NSSO's 71st Round (2014) canvassed a specialized questionnaire to assess the health and morbidity conditions of citizens all over India. Further cost of assessing various types of healthcare services was also incurred. Thus, NSSO is the best source to estimate and analyse the out-of-pocket spending of households.

Table 15.3 presents data suggesting that the morbidity prevalence is relatively higher in urban areas and amongst women. Often morbidity reporting is associated with relative higher-level education which is the

Table 15.3 Number (per 1,000) of Persons Reporting Any Ailments during Last 15 Days

Sector	Ailment	Male	Female	Combined Average
Rural	Short duration	44	54	49
	Chronic	36	45	40
	Any	80	99	89
Urban	Short duration	45	56	51
	Chronic	56	79	67
	Any	101	135	118

Source: Government of India (2015). National Sample survey Office, 'Key Indicators of Social Consumption in India'.
Note: Ailments for long duration (30 days or more) are referred as chronic ailments with a 15-day reference period, rest are short-duration ailments.

case in urban areas compared to rural parts of India. One therefore expects better reporting of morbidity in urban areas (based on higher levels of knowledge about the condition of sickness) and due to ease of accessing healthcare. Morbidity data is based on recall methods with multiple periods such as during last year, during last month, or last 15 days. Such recalls appear to be better in urban areas. However, it must also be noted that due to high population density in urban areas, there is a possibility of higher incidence of certain types of diseases and sickness, which can spread through contagion effects.

Rural areas report relatively less chronic conditions, whereas urban populace report substantially higher chronic conditions compared to short-duration morbidity. Over all 118 persons in urban areas and only 89 persons in rural areas reported suffering from an ailment during a reference period of 15 days per 1,000 people.

The higher incidence of morbidity amongst women is an important one. Since women get exposed to long durations of natal and postnatal episodes that require medical and healthcare assistance, overall relatively higher incidence is expected. A common economic categorization using the NSSO is to generate quintile classes of 'mean (monthly) per capita consumer expenditures' (MPCE). Proportion of ailing persons (per 1,000) during last 15 days by quintile class suggests that morbidity reporting increases as MPCE increases and is most pronounced in urban areas.

Overall public institutions (including hospitals) are utilized only by about 30 per cent of the sick population in rural and 21 per cent in urban areas. The dominant medical market is with the private doctors who manage small clinics often with no facilities for diagnostics, surgery, and inpatient care. Almost one half of all patients used these clinics (Table 15.4). A majority of patients choose allopathic medicine despite high policy promotion for AYUSH-linked indigenous systems of medicine. Note that a large proportion of these clinics are run by non-allopathic practitioners, often with no recognized education or degrees, who at best maybe described as quacks.

It is somewhat interesting to note that only two states namely Assam and Odisha have shown higher shares of treatment from the public institutions over the last two decades. However, in Assam, the average cost of hospitalization treatment in urban facilities is also high which needs to be explored further. It is worth preparing case studies for these two states which have shown a trend opposite to privatization of medical treatment.

Health Providers

Before delving into details on the costs of care aspects, it would be helpful to get a sense of the complex array of providers, their training and workforce maldistribution. The Medical Council of India (MCI) and the councils at

Table 15.4 Percentage Distribution of Spells of Ailment Treated During Last 15 Days by Level of Care

Level of Care	Rural			Urban		
	Male	Female	Persons	Male	Female	Persons
HSC, PHC, & Others*	10.6	12.3	11.5	3.5	4.2	3.9
Public hospital	15.9	17.5	16.8	17.4	17.3	17.3
Private doctor/clinic	52.7	48.9	50.7	48.9	50.8	50.0
Private hospital	20.8	21.3	21.0	30.2	27.7	28.8
Combined average	100.0	100.0	100.0	100.0	100.0	100.0

* includes auxiliary nurse midwifes (ANM), accredited social health activists (ASHA), anganwadi workers (AWW), dispensaries, community health centers (CHCs), mobile medical units (MMUs)
Source: Government of India (2015). National Sample survey Office, 'Key Indicators of Social Consumption in India'.

various states oversee the medical service providers. The MCI maintains the medical register, online faculty directory, and accreditation standards for medical colleges. Currently, the MCI and state medical councils have more than a million registered physicians. This number may not be a true reflection of the actual number of allopathic physicians since all registered physicians may not be practising clinically. Number of AYUSH practitioners is 0.74 million (AYUSH 2015), but many of them prescribe allopathic medicines.

Despite training almost 50,000 allopathic doctors a year, the doctor–patient ratio in India is 0.65:1,000, which is far below the WHO standards of 1 per 1,000. India also lags behind the WHO standard of 4.45 skilled health professionals per 1,000 population. The doctor–patient ratio has consistently remained low for long and the majority of allopathic providers are based in urban areas. In medical training there is an overemphasis on medical specialization. There is no 'gatekeeping' and the patients are free to visit specialist even for simple symptoms. There are extremely few family medicine or general practice residency training positions and there is stiff competition for specialty residency positions. Further, thousands of allopathic medical graduates spend several years after graduation to get into these training positions wasting opportunity cost. Even though the country trains a significant number of nurses, many move out of the country (due to factors such as low pay and poor working conditions), while the system is understaffed. Significant cost advantages can be achieved by deemphasizing specialization and through task shifting that is hiring and skill-building of non-medical workers.

COST OF CARE AND CONSTRAINTS OF HEALTH SECTOR FINANCING

India's growth story since its independence has innumerable surprises. One such surprise is the consistent and abysmally low levels of health sector financing despite sustained GDP growth and growth rates over the last two decades and more. While budgetary allocations go through constraints, it appears that this is due to a lack of consensus on health as a priority that health expenditure has remained suboptimal. The apathy of public policy has ensured that the out-of-pocket expenditures dominate the total expenditure. Health being a state subject also plays a role. While states are free to prioritize the service delivery protocols, they have generally failed to utilize the budget outlays and contribute their own share to the health budgets. Under conditions of financial austerity, health is among the first sectors to be axed with lowering of state support. Current recommendations (despite existing evidence) from academics close to the political dispensation calling for full cost recovery of healthcare provisioning are likely to gain traction (Kurian 2015).

Given the current increasing state support to RSBY, and the recent announcement of Ayushman Bharat Yojana or Pradhan Mantri Jan Arogya Yojana (PMJAY), a further expansion in private healthcare industry is underway. As evidence suggests, these private healthcare systems accentuate the already alarming income disparities. Though globally there are a few successful cost-recovery models available, such efforts in India have not yielded positive results due to issues relating to lack of unit cost estimations and adverse selection, which exert higher fiscal impact on poorer households, rural areas, and relatively backward regions of India. NSSO survey provides estimates of expenditures on non-hospitalized and hospitalized episodes separately (see Table 15.5).

On average, the total cost of non-hospital treatment per ailment has worked out to be INR 639 in urban and INR 509 in rural areas. But the cost of hospitalized episodes is rather high at INR 24,436 in urban and INR 14,935 in rural areas. The household expenditure is relatively higher for males for hospitalization and for non-hospitalization in urban areas (see Table 15.5). Further, Table 15.6 shows that the sick spend several times greater expenditure in private hospitals as compared to public hospitals for both rural and urban areas for both males and females. Although this may be a reflection of relatively poor quality health services in the public sectors facilities, the disproportionately higher costs in private sector institutions cannot be explained in terms of quality of care.

Table 15.5 Average Total Medical Expenditure (INR) for Treatment of Ailments

Gender	Rural	Urban	All
Non-Hospitalization Expenditure			
Male	502	683	
Female	515	604	
Combined average	509	639	
Hospitalization Expenditure			
Male	17,528	28,165	21,223
Female	12,295	20,754	15,292
Combined average	14,935	24,436	18,268

Source: Government of India (2015). National Sample Survey Office, 'Key Indicators of Social Consumption in India'.

Table 15.6 Average Medical Expenditure (INR) per Hospitalization at Public and Private Hospitals

Level of Care	Male	Female	All
Rural			
Public hospital	6,473	4,843	5,636
Private hospital	24,756	18,419	21,726
Combined average	17,528	12,295	14,935
Urban			
Public hospital	10,040	5,125	7,670
Private hospital	37,181	27,783	32,375
Combined average	28,165	20,754	24,436

Source: Government of India (2015). National Sample Survey Office, 'Key Indicators of Social Consumption in India'.

Table 15.7 Average Total Medical Expenditure (INR) for Non-Hospitalized Treatment per Ailing Person Suffering from Only One Ailment for Different Levels of Care

Level of Care	Rural		Urban	
	Male	Female	Male	Female
HSC, PHC & others*	309	314	347	386
Public hospital	407	505	372	411
Private doctor/clinic	560	600	672	646
Private hospital	773	810	1131	785
Combined average	549	589	741	629

Source: Government of India (2015). National Sample Survey Office, 'Key Indicators of Social Consumption in India'.

Likewise, for non-hospitalized treatment per ailing person, one can find larger expenditures in the case of private doctors/clinics and private hospitals as compared to public hospitals and HSC, primary health centres and others for both males and females and in both rural and urban areas (Table 15.7).

There is considerable interstate variation in health sector expenditures. Interestingly, the rural expenditures have consistently been lower than urban spending. And this limited expenditure is dominated by medical expenses with relatively little money going towards non-medical expenses (Table 15.8).

Table 15.8 Average Medical Expenditure (INR) and Non-Medical Expenditure (INR) because of Hospitalization per Hospitalization Case (excluding childbirth) for Select States

State	Rural			Urban		
	Medical	Non-Medical	All	Medical	Non-Medical	All
Andhra Pradesh	13,227	2,184	15,411	31,242	2,429	33,671
Assam	6,966	1,554	8,520	47,064	5,304	52,368
Bihar	11,432	2,194	13,626	25,004	3,054	28,058
Chhattisgarh	12,149	1,895	14,044	22,647	2,245	24,892
Gujarat	14,298	1,362	15,660	20,155	1,121	21,276
Haryana	18,341	2,604	20,945	32,370	2,847	35,217
Jharkhand	10,351	2,227	12,578	13,151	1,860	15,011
Karnataka	14,091	2,027	16,118	22,190	2,012	24,202
Kerala	17,642	1,743	19,385	15,465	1,652	17,117
Madhya Pradesh	13,090	2,236	15,326	23,993	2,381	26,374
Maharashtra	20,475	2,011	22,486	29,493	1,534	31,027
Odisha	10,240	2,376	12,616	19,750	2,963	22,713
Punjab	27,718	2,061	29,779	29,971	2,007	31,978
Rajasthan	12,855	2,755	15,610	16,731	1,616	18,347
Tamil Nadu	11,842	2,126	13,968	23,757	2,336	26,093
Telangana	19,664	2,019	21,683	20,617	1,966	22,583
Uttar Pradesh	18,693	1,901	20,594	31,653	1,749	33,402
West Bengal	11,327	1,514	12,841	24,875	2,374	27,249
All-India	14,935	2,021	16,956	24,436	2,019	26,455

Source: Government of India (2015). National Sample Survey Office, 'Key Indicators of Social Consumption in India'.

Table 15.9 Percentage Distribution of Total Household Expenditure by Different Categories of Expenditure

State	Rural			Urban		
	Doctor's Fee	Medicine	Others*	Doctor's Fee	Medicine	Others*
Andhra Pradesh	11.3	76.2	12.7	8.5	79.3	12.2
Assam	7.0	63.8	29.4	10.3	52.1	37.7
Bihar	12.0	71.9	16.1	15.0	62.9	22.2
Chhattisgarh	25.5	69.5	5.0	10.6	82.5	6.8
Gujarat	23.6	57.5	18.6	28.6	54.2	17.2
Haryana	10.3	72.7	17.2	15.5	67.3	17.1
Jharkhand	17.9	66.0	15.9	16.2	45.5	38.2
Karnataka	18.2	67.0	14.9	16.2	64.4	19.3
Kerala	11.2	73.8	15.1	10.2	74.6	14.9
Madhya Pradesh	14.4	68.6	17.0	15.2	71.4	13.4
Maharashtra	23.4	63.6	12.8	23.1	60.3	16.6
Odisha	4.8	74.9	20.3	6.2	79.2	14.8
Punjab	9.8	76.2	14.2	9.4	72.8	18.0
Rajasthan	10.2	82.4	7.4	20.9	67.4	11.8
Tamil Nadu	20.8	60.7	18.5	15.8	70.6	13.5
Telangana	11.8	69.4	18.8	13.5	71.6	14.8
Uttar Pradesh	12.8	76.1	11.2	14.9	70.9	14.3
West Bengal	15.5	69.8	14.7	15.5	68.7	15.8
All-India	13.6	71.5	14.7	15.6	68.0	16.4

* includes diagnostic tests.
Source: Government of India (2015). National Sample Survey Office, 'Key Indicators of Social Consumption in India'.

State-wide disaggregation of total expenditure by items of expense shows that medicines comprise the largest expenditure category, followed by doctors' fees and others (including diagnostic tests). Despite some interstate variations, the trends are similar across states and items of expenditure (Table 15.9). A substantial (just about two-thirds) share of all expenditures incurred in treating a sick person across India has been on purchase of drugs and medicines. There is a case for urgent analysis and control of drug pricing in India including issues relating to intellectual property rights, compulsory licensing, and manufacturing of generic medicines.

HOUSEHOLD HEALTH EXPENDITURES ACCORDING TO CONSUMPTION CLASS AND SOCIO-RELIGIOUS COMMUNITIES

Two dominant diversity dimensions plaguing India's development scene over the few decades since liberalization relate to the disparities in many social and economic indicators or broadly labelled as human development measures. Healthcare indicators form a dominant part of human development. The economic dimension is measured in through MPCE, while the social is measured through socio-religious categories (SRCs). Population distribution based on MPCE was analysed to calculate population quintiles where the 1st and 5th quintiles represented 20 per cent of the richest and the poorest households respectively. Across the MPCE quintiles, expenditures are higher for urban (as compared to rural) areas, and the amounts increase as the quintile class base increases. Table 15.8 shows that the major expenses are medical and other expenses constitute a small fraction of the total expenditure per hospitalization case. However, it is likely that the relatively poor—the households that fall under the first and second MPCE class spend disproportionately higher share of their monthly income on healthcare access.

Across MPCE quintiles for both rural and urban areas, majority of households use their income and/or savings for meeting hospitalization expenditure. This increases proportionately based on quintile class.

Table 15.10 Average Medical and Other Related Non-Medical Expenditure (INR) per Hospitalization Case for Each Quintile Class of Average Monthly per Capita Consumption Expenditure

Quintile Class of UMPCE	Medical		Other		Total	
	Rural	Urban	Rural	Urban	Rural	Urban
01	10,146	11,199	1,658	1,317	11,805	12,516
02	11,276	14,533	1,791	1,620	13,067	16,153
03	10,326	17,926	1,766	1,772	12,092	19,697
04	13,482	24,776	1,879	2,131	15,361	26,907
05	21,293	42,675	2,458	2,743	23,752	45,418
Combined average	14,935	24,436	2,021	2,019	16,956	26,455

Source: Authors' estimates based on data from unit level data of National Sample Survey Office's 71st round survey on social consumption relating to health (June 2014).

Alarmingly, almost a quarter of households across the board are forced to borrow money for meeting hospitalization expenditure (Table 15.9).

With low state support, most of the expenditure is out-of-pocket. The tables that follow show household medical expenditure, doctor's fees, and medicines as average totals and share of total household expenditure for SRCs, MPCE quintiles, gender and other sectors (rural versus urban).

Table 15.10 shows Average Medical and Other Related Non-Medical Expenditure (INR) per Hospitalization Case for Each Quintile Class of average monthly per capita consumption expenditure. As expected it shows higher expenditure for higher quintile classes and for urban areas as against rural areas.

Table 15.11 shows Percentage Distribution of Households Meeting Hospitalization Expenditure by Major Sources of Finance, as per Quintile Classes of UMPCE. Across MPCE quintiles for both rural and urban areas, majority of households use their income and/or savings for meeting hospitalization expenditure. This increases proportionately based on quintile class. Alarmingly, almost a quarter of households across the board are forced to borrow money for meeting hospitalization expenditure (India 2019).

Table 15.12 presents estimates of household expenditures for the SRCs and MPCE quintiles for in-patient and outpatient services separately for public and private institutions. The share of total medical expenditure in household expenditure is considerably higher on in-patient services and in private institutions as compared to public institutions. This observation stands true across SRCs, MPCE quintiles, gender, and sectors.

Table 15.11 Percentage Distribution of Households Meeting Hospitalization Expenditure by Major Sources of Finance, as per Quintile Classes of UMPCE

Quintile class of UMPCE	Income/ Savings	Borrowings	Sale of Physical assets	Contribution from Friends/Relatives	Others	All
			Rural			
01	65.6	26.8	1.1	5.3	0.5	100
02	67.1	25.8	1.4	4.8	0.5	100
03	68.1	25.3	0.6	5.1	0.5	100
04	68.8	26.0	0.4	3.8	0.8	100
05	68.1	23.1	0.9	6.9	0.7	100
Combined average	67.8	24.9	0.8	5.4	0.7	100
			Urban			
01	68.4	21.7	0.4	6.4	2.7	100
02	71.8	21.9	0.4	4.5	1.1	100
03	74.1	20.7	0.3	3.9	0.7	100
04	74.9	16.1	0.3	6.9	1.6	100
05	80.9	13.7	0.4	3.7	1.0	100
Combined average	74.9	18.2	0.4	5.0	1.3	100

Source: Authors' estimates based on data from unit level data of National Sample Survey Office's 71st round survey on social consumption relating to health (June 2014).

Table 15.12 Average Total Medical Household Expenditure by SRCs and MPCE Class*

Category		Public Institutions		Private Institutions	
		Outpatients	Inpatients	Outpatients	Inpatients
SRC	H-STs	3,012	238	25,820	739
	H-SCs	5,149	466	21,691	858
	H-OBCs	5,293	633	29,599	989
	H-Upper Castes	11,074	589	37,723	1,168
	Muslims	5,653	678	27,151	1,152
	All Others	11,120	1,005	35,755	1,493
MPCE quintile	Q1	4,058	551	20,462	861
	Q2	4,290	639	18,517	714
	Q3	5,454	445	22,847	879
	Q4	6,173	419	23,574	1,063
	Q5	15,088	843	45,942	1,406
Gender	Male	11,008	568	36,705	1,048
	Female	4,475	598	26,172	1,072
Sector	Rural	5,374	565	25,615	940
	Urban	9,223	633	37,995	1,245
Total		6,307	585	30,422	1,061

* Average calculated only for those households which reported any in-patient (or outpatient) case within past 365 (or 15) days.
Source: Authors' estimates based on data from unit level data of National Sample Survey Office's 71st round survey on social consumption relating to health (June 2014).

The outpatient expenditures too are marginally higher at private institutions across the board.

When expenditure by MPCE quintiles is analysed, it is quite clear that both the top and bottom quintile households spend a higher share of their expenditure on hospitalization at public health facilities than the middle quintiles. In comparison with other households, households in the bottom quintile spend significantly higher share of their usual household expenditure on hospitalization in private hospitals (36 per cent).

The total amount spent on in-patients in private institutions is approximately one quarter (24.6 per cent) of the total household expenditure, which is much higher than the in-patient expenditure at public institutions (7.2 per cent). There is a slight difference of 0.3 per cent in the expenditure of outpatients. This observation stands true across SRCs, MPCE quintiles, gender, and sectors (Table 15.13). While comparing medical expenditures incurred by various socio-religious groups, we observe that the share of medical expenditure on in-patients in public institutions is the highest for Hindu upper castes and the lowest for Hindu scheduled tribes (STs). But an issue to be taken seriously from this data is the fact that when there just about one fourth of all household expenditures is spent on one or more episodes of sickness in a household during a year. Such exorbitant expenditure burden on households may even push many families into the poverty trap.

The total household expenditures on male inpatients at both public and private institutions (12.7 per cent and 29.8 per cent respectively) are much higher than the share of household expenditures on female inpatients (5.1 per cent and 21 per cent respectively). This indicates gender bias in healthcare access. However, not much of a gender bias is found in expenditures on outpatient services in either of the types—public or private (Table 15.13).

DETERMINATION OF HOUSEHOLD EXPENDITURE ON HEALTH ACCORDING TO CONSUMPTION CLASS AND SOCIO-RELIGIOUS COMMUNITIES—A MULTIVARIATE ANALYSIS

In line with observations from Tables 15.10 and 15.11, the multivariate analysis re-confirms that considerable variation exits across SRCs, MPCE quintiles, gender and sectors. Total medical expenditure per hospitalization

Table 15.13 Share of Total Medical Expenditure in Household Expenditure (percentage)

Category		Public Institutions		Private Institutions	
		Outpatients	Inpatients	Outpatients	Inpatients
SRC	H-STs	4.5	0.4	26.2	0.9
	H-SCs	6.7	0.7	22.5	1.0
	H-OBCs	6.0	0.8	25.9	1.0
	H-Upper caste	10.5	0.5	24.9	0.9
	Muslims	6.4	0.7	22.4	1.1
	All others	10.6	1.0	23.2	1.1
MPCE quintile	Q1 (Bottom)	8.1	1.3	36.1	1.6
	Q2	6.1	1.0	24.6	1.0
	Q3	6.3	0.6	24.5	1.1
	Q4	5.9	0.4	21.3	1.1
	Q5 (Top)	9.7	0.6	24.8	0.8
Gender	Male	12.7	0.7	29.8	1.0
	Female	5.1	0.7	21.0	1.0
Sector	Rural	6.8	0.8	24.7	1.1
	Urban	8.3	0.6	24.4	0.9
Total		7.2	0.7	24.6	1.0

Source: Authors' estimates based on data from unit level data of National Sample Survey Office's 71st round survey on social consumption relating to health (June 2014).

case (in past 365 days) was taken as dependent variable in the linear ordinary least squares (OLS) regression.

Independent variables were coded as binary or categorical variables in the following manner:

- Sector where hospitalization happened: 0 if urban and 1 if rural;
- Gender of patient: 0 if male and 1 if female;
- Socio–religious categories of patient: 1 if Hindu SC (scheduled caste), 2 if Hindu ST, 3 if Hindu OBC (other backward classes), 4 if Muslims, 0 if all others including Hindu upper caste;
- Expenditure quintile of patient's household: 0 if from top quintile (80–100 per cent), 1 if second from top quintile (60–80 per cent), 2 if third from top quintile (40–60 per cent) and so on;
- Age groups of patients: 0 if age is between 20 and 39 years, 1 if age is between 0 and 5 years, 2 if age is between 5 and 19 years, 3 if age is between 40 and 59 years, 4 if age is 60 years and above.

Across the board expenditures are higher in private institutions compared to public institutions (Table 15.14). While higher expenditure for males and those living in urban areas is somewhat expected, expenditures across MPCE quintiles and SRCs show interesting trends. Regression results reveal that medical expenditure incurred on each hospitalization incidence in case of any type of hospital in rural India is INR 4,574 less than that in urban India, INR 655 less per case in rural government hospitals than in urban government hospitals, INR 5,623 less in case of rural private hospitals than in urban private hospital. This concludes that healthcare facilities are cheaper in rural India than in urban India. However, it does not indicate any possible difference that may exist in types and quality of treatments provided in rural and urban India. It is also evident that expenditure incurred per case of hospitalization of females is much less (in the range of INR 4,000 to INR 8,000) than per case expenditure incurred on males. This hints towards stark gender bias in healthcare. Similarly, per case expenditure increases significantly as age of the patient increases, as economic status (quintiles) of the patients rises irrespective of type of hospital (government or private) where the treatment has been taken.

Interestingly, expenditure incurred by Hindu STs in government hospitals is the least (INR 5,293 less per case than Hindu upper caste and others), followed by Hindu SCs (INR 4,237 less), Hindu OBCs (INR 4,222 less), and Muslims (INR 3,879). Muslims spend about INR 1,414 more than Hindu STs at

Table 15.14 Regression Models for Healthcare Expenditure

Category	All Cases	Government Hospitals	Private Hospitals	Public Health Facilities
Rural	−4573.973 (14.42) [−4602.24 – −4545.71]	−655.2256 (11.1) [−676.97 – −633.48]	−5623.396 (22.09) [−5666.69 – −5580.1]	−901.0623 (11.42) [−923.44 – −878.68]
Female	−7617.506 (13.98) [−7644.9 – −7590.11]	−4096.464 (10.89) [−4117.8 – −4075.13]	−8373.027 (21.43) [−8415.02 – −8331.03]	−4650.981 (11.1) [−4672.74 – −4629.23]
Age <5 years	−4848.576 (27.65) [−4902.77 – −4794.38]	−2590.047 (22.44) [−2634.03 – −2546.06]	−8281.517 (41.64) [−8363.13 – −8199.9]	−3005.764 (22.79) [−3050.43 – −2961.1]
Age 5–19 years	−1577.249 (21.82) [−1620.01 – −1534.49]	−424.3096 (15.95) [−455.57 – −393.05]	−3485.174 (34.91) [−3553.59 – −3416.76]	−848.1527 (16.1) [−879.71 – −816.59]
Age 40–59 years	5036.892 (17.16) [5003.26 – 5070.52]	2929.844 (12.99) [2904.38 – 2955.31]	5625.419 (27.01) [5572.48 – 5678.35]	2268.148 (13.11) [2242.45 – 2293.84]
Age 60+ years	7296.495 (18.86) [7259.53 – 7333.47]	2339.707 (14.76) [2310.78 – 2368.64]	8867.89 (28.97) [8811.12 – 8924.66]	1766.434 (15.01) [1737.01 – 1795.86]
Quintile 4	−13231.51 (19.3) [−13269.34 – −13193.69]	−5914.908 (16.48) [−5947.2 – −5882.61]	−13125.03 (28.49) [−13180.87 – −13069.19]	−5586.644 (16.91) [−5619.79 – −5553.5]
Quintile 3	−13787.33 (18.74) [−13824.06 – −13750.61]	−5157.295 (15.37) [−5187.42 – −5127.17]	−12776.24 (28.86) [−12832.81 – −12719.68]	−4957.347 (15.73) [−4988.18 – −4926.52]
Quintile 2	−15557.27 (20.99) [−15598.41 – −15516.12]	−5353.142 (16.28) [−5385.06 – −5321.23]	−14287.84 (34.74) [−14355.93 – −14219.75]	−5197.562 (16.48) [−5229.86 – −5165.27]
Quintile 1	−15126.68 (22.61) [−15171 – −15082.36]	−5553.759 (17.08) [−5587.23 – −5520.29]	−12205.71 (40.47) [−12285.02 – −12126.4]	−4767.098 (16.96) [−4800.35 – −4733.85]
H-STs	−4243.681 (28.99) [−4300.5 – −4186.86]	−5293.105 (19.35) [−5331.04 – −5255.17]	501.5587 (53.82) [396.08 – 607.04]	−5050.423 (18.79) [−5087.25 – −5013.6]
H-SCs	−5327.495 (19.89) [−5366.48 – −5288.51]	−4236.994 (13.97) [−4264.37 – −4209.62]	−4373.385 (33.53) [−4439.1 – −4307.67]	−3608.767 (14.04) [−3636.28 – −3581.25]
H-OBCs	−2315.316 (16.26) [−2347.19 – −2283.44]	−4222.29 (12.96) [−4247.7 – −4196.88]	−1931.769 (24.72) [−1980.21 – −1883.33]	−4131.865 (13.02) [−4157.38 – −4106.36]
Muslims	−4768.543 (20.65) [−4809.01 – −4728.08]	−3879.233 (14.73) [−3908.11 – −3850.36]	−3793.897 (33.65) [−3859.84 – −3727.95]	−3707.283 (15.01) [−3736.7 – −3677.86]
Constant	35703.93 (21.22) [35662.33 – 35745.52]	16029.52 (17.93) [15994.38 – 16064.66]	40984.91 (31.51) [40923.15 – 41046.67]	16264.6 (18.46) [16228.41 – 16300.78]

Source: Authors' estimates based on data from unit level data of National Sample Survey Office's 71st round survey on social consumption relating to health (June 2014).

Notes: (1) Dependent variable: Total out-of-pocket health expenditure in rupees. (2) Independent variables: Sector, Sex, Age group, MPCE quintiles, SRCs. (3) All the independent variables are (used as) categorical variables. (4) First category in each of the independent variables are omitted and coefficient of the omitted categories are to be interpreted as 1. (5) Omitted categories are: Urban, Male, Age 20–39 years, Quintile 5 (top), and All Other SRCs (everyone excluding H-SCs, H-STs, H-OBCs and Muslims). (6) Results are displayed in the format Coefficient (Standard Error) [Confidence Intervals] up to 2 significant digits. (7) All values are significant at P<0.01 (99% confidence interval).

government hospitals and INR 358 and INR 343 more than Hindu SCs and Hindu OBCs respectively. On the other hand, Hindu SCs spend least at private hospitals (INR 4,373 less than Hindu upper caste and others) followed by Muslims (INR 3,794 less than Hindu upper caste and others), Hindu OBCs (INR 1,932 less). Hindu STs spend more than everyone else on each private hospitalization case (INR 502 more than Hindu upper caste).

These patterns can also be understood using regression models for government hospitals, private hospitals, and public health facilities. Public health facilities include auxiliary nurse and midwife (ANM), accredited social health activist (ASHA), anganwadi worker (AWW), primary health centres, dispensary, community health centres, mobile medical unit, and public hospitals.

Medical Insurance

The NFHS-4 figure of 28.7 per cent households with any usual member covered by a health scheme or health insurance shows a healthy increase over the previous figure of 4.8 per cent during NFHS-3. A variety of medical insurance schemes both in the public and private sector are behind this increase. They include private insurance plans, and the RSBY. Other insurance schemes such as the Central Government Health Scheme (CGHS) and Employee State Insurance (ESI) have been in existence since many years and may not have contributed to this increase. ECHS could have registered an increase due to more and more defense force retirees. While the health coverage has increased, the depth of coverage (INR 30,000 per year under RSBY for the entire family) leaves much to be desired.

Tables 15.15a and 15.15b show insurance penetration by state for rural and urban areas. The coverage of health expenditure support was based on a combination of government-funded insurance scheme, employer-supported health protection, arranged by household with insurance companies and others.

Coverage varied across the states and rural/urban areas. For the majority of states, those not covered outnumber those with some sort of coverage. Among rural areas the states with lowest coverage included Arunanchal Pradesh, Assam, Delhi, Haryana, Madhya Pradesh, Maharashtra, Manipur, Punjab, Sikkim, Uttrakhand, Uttar Pradesh, Andaman & Nicobar, Chandigarh, and Lakshadweep. Government-funded insurance schemes had a good coverage in Telangana, Andhra Pradesh, and Mizoram. Urban areas had an overall better coverage of health expenditure support schemes. States such as Bihar, Manipur, Uttar Pradesh, Andaman & Nicobar Islands, Lakshadweep, and Puducherry had low coverage, while Andhra Pradesh, Chhattisgarh, Mizoram, Nagaland, and Telangana had a high coverage from government-funded insurance schemes.

Rashtriya Swasthya Bima Yojna

To protect poor (below poverty line or BPL) families from hospitalization-related catastrophic medical expenses, the Ministry of Labour and Employment launched the RSBY scheme. Its budget allocation was of INR 1,000 crore for financial year 2018 (Centre for Budget and Governance Accountability 2018). The scheme involves coverage of INR 30,000 per family per year. Smartcards have been provided at enrollment service centres to facilitate cashless transactions at the point of care in empanelled hospitals for almost 725 medical procedures. More than 41 million families (about 150 million people) out of a targeted 65 million families were enrolled in RSBY in September 2016. However, a recent evaluation of the scheme (Karan, Yip, and Mahal 2017) using the difference in econometric methodology shows that it had not provided any significant financial protection to poor households. They found that RSBY did not affect the likelihood, level, or catastrophic out-of-pocket spending for in-patient care. They also did not find any statistically significant effect of RSBY on the level of outpatient out-of-pocket expenditure and the probability of incurring outpatient expenditure. In contrast, the likelihood of incurring any out-of-pocket spending (inpatient and outpatient) rose by 30 per cent due to RSBY and was statistically significant. Although out-of-pocket spending levels did not change, RSBY raised household non-medical spending by 5 per cent. Overall, the results suggest that RSBY has been ineffective in reducing the burden of out-of-pocket spending on poor households.

Mobilizing Health Resources

Between preventive and curative healthcare, most of the infrastructure, workforce, and spending falls on the curative side. In 2013, the expenditure on preventive care was estimated at INR 40,627 crore (9.6 per cent of current health expenditure, that is INR 326 per capita) (National Health Systems Resource Centre 2016). This highlights the need for increased mobilization of resources towards preventive care (Kumar et al. 2011).

In the Union Budget 2018–19, the Government of India announced a 'revolutionary' programme, the National Health Protection Scheme (NHPS), which is also the world's largest health programme. The NHPS aims to cover 100 million poor and vulnerable families, and reach about 500 million people, providing a coverage of INR 5 lakh[3] per family per year for secondary

[3] A lakh is a hundred thousand, a tenth of a million. It is often used instead of hundred thousand in official Indian government documents.

Table 15.15a Insurance Penetration by State–Rural: Per Thousand Distribution of Persons by Insurance/Health Coverage Support for Different States and Union Territories

State/UT	Not Covered	Government-Funded Insurance Scheme	Employer-Supported Health Protection	Arranged by Households with Insurance Companies	Others	All	No. of Persons Surveyed	
							Estimated. ('00)	Sample
Andhra Pradesh	303	694	2	0	0	1000	336,261	5,482
Arunachal Pradesh	958	29	7	1	5	1000	9,907	1,942
Assam	980	6	12	1	0	1000	258,350	8,757
Bihar	935	57	8	0	0	1000	849,932	11,638
Chhattisgarh	598	397	5	0	0	1000	201,314	3,524
Delhi	971	19	1	10	0	1000	5,211	366
Goa	937	62	1	0	0	1000	5,849	470
Gujarat	880	96	1	24	0	1000	301,786	8,082
Haryana	977	20	2	1	0	1000	157,175	4,152
Himachal Pradesh	912	71	8	7	4.	1000	59,992	3,552
Jammu & Kashmir*	927	36	36	1	0	1000	78,273	4,003
Jharkhand	969	25	6	0	0	1000	236,827	4,884
Karnataka	927	45	16	3	9	1000	368,942	7,824
Kerala	572	388	26	12	2	1000	179,072	5,484
Madhya Pradesh	997	3	0	0	0	1000	491,909	10,416
Maharashtra	982	12	3	3	0	1000	572,664	14,072
Manipur	996	2	0	0	1	1000	16,946	4,002
Meghalaya	818	129	53	0	0	1000	24,643	2,931
Mizoram	263	705	31	0	0	1000	4,988	1,924
Nagaland	736	261	4	0	0	1000	12,631	1,650
Odisha	779	212	6	3	1	1000	340,257	8,186
Punjab	964	24	11	0	0	1000	164,502	4,044
Rajasthan	777	223	0	0	0	1000	466,751	9,645
Sikkim	999	1	0	0	0	1000	3,727	1,343
Tamil Nadu	807	184	4	5	0	1000	353,918	8,237
Telangana	265	729	5	1	0	1000	187,718	3,317
Tripura	860	127	7	5	1	1000	27,894	3,608
Uttarakhand	963	30	6	1	0	1000	146,6977	29,924
Uttar Pradesh	1,000	0	0	0	0	1000	62,858	1,756
West Bengal	846	146	4	4	0	1000	592,332	11,860
Andaman & Nicobar Islands	1,000	0	0	0	0	1000	2,828	827
Chandigarh	978	2	20	0	0	1000	318	311
Dadra & Nagar Haveli	787	206	4	3	0	1000	1,594	371
Daman & Diu	882	104	0	14	0	1000	350	288
Lakshadweep	1,000	0	0	0	0	1000	112	403
Puducherry	903	95	2	0	0	1000	4,735	298
All India	859	131	6	3	1	1000	7,849,544	189,573

* This refers to the erstwhile state of J&K before the creation of the two union territories of Jammu & Kashmir and Ladakh in 2019.
Source: Government of India (2015). National Sample Survey Office, 'Health in India'.

Table 15.13b Insurance Penetration by State–Urban: Per Thousand Distribution of Persons by Insurance/Health Coverage Support for Different States and Union Territories

State/UT	Not Covered	Government-Funded Insurance Scheme	Employer-Supported Health Protection	Arranged by hh with Insurance Companies	Others	All	No. of Persons Surveyed	
							Estimated '(00)	Sample
Andhra Pradesh	495	470	16	13	5	1000	147,020	5,154
Arunachal Pradesh	882	43	20	28	25	1000	1,874	1,052
Assam	929	53	8	10	0	1000	34,262	2,654
Bihar	966	24	3	1	6	1000	97,336	5,958
Chhattisgarh	650	346	3	1	0	1000	44,420	2,502
Delhi	827	89	19	64	0	1000	104,445	5,058
Goa	821	178	0	0	0	1000	8,874	446
Gujarat	828	36	15	121	0	1000	215,306	7,129
Haryana	844	73	10	73	0	1000	83,990	3,888
Himachal Pradesh	864	130	1	4	1	1000	6,504	840
Jammu & Kashmir*	888	47	14	45	6	1000	20,298	2,785
Jharkhand	941	21	38	0	0	1000	70,638	3,434
Karnataka	842	63	66	21	8	1000	226,697	6,903
Kerala	644	295	18	39	4	1000	146,483	5,745
Madhya Pradesh	947	38	8	6	1	1000	180,096	8,715
Maharashtra	855	48	27	69	1	1000	427,758	13,052
Manipur	992	8	0	0	0	1000	8,063	3,185
Meghalaya	682	230	77	6	5	1000	5,160	1,449
Mizoram	258	738	1	1	2	1000	4,170	1,940
Nagaland	693	306	1	0	0	1000	3,812	1,001
Odisha	869	87	29	16	0	1000	63,230	3,390
Punjab	910	47	36	6	0	1000	97,927	3,753
Rajasthan	764	226	7	2	0	1000	175,527	7,010
Sikkim	858	106	35	1	0	1000	920	757
Tamil Nadu	756	171	35	36	3	1000	347,074	7,853
Telangana	595	337	54	14	1	1000	112,331	3,265
Tripura	919	64	7	0	10	1000	7,351	2,369
Uttarakhand	942	43	11	3	1	1000	424,341	17,159
Uttar Pradesh	986	10	1	4	0	1000	17,886	1,421
West Bengal	800	110	32	57	1	1000	256,910	10,923
Andaman & Nicobar Islands	990	9	0	0	1	1000	1,362	407
Chandigarh	876	88	22	4	11	1000	8,191	563
Dadra & Nagar Haveli	880	1	113	6	0	1000	1,371	270
Daman & Diu	854	0	0	146	0	1000	2,063	249
Lakshadweep	991	9	0	0	0	1000	512	433
Puducherry	968	18	3	11	0	1000	7,271	819
All-India	820	120	24	35	2	1000	3,361,473	143,531

* This refers to the erstwhile state of J&K before the creation of the two union territories of Jammu & Kashmir and Ladakh in 2019.

Source: Government of India (2015). National Sample Survey Office, 'Health in India'.

and tertiary care hospitalization. While details are still awaited at the time of writing, there does not seem to be any substantial increase in allocation for the MOHFW in the Union health budget—perhaps the states will take on a greater share.

Global Trend

The WHO in its 2010 and 2013 annual health reports called for universal health coverage (UHC), stating that it leads to the best outcomes in relation to health spending. In India, similar to previous efforts (Lal 2005; Misra, Chatterjee, Rao 2003), the erstwhile Planning Commission had set up a High-Level Expert Group (HLEG) to provide recommendations towards UHC. The HLEG called for investments in health workers, the creation of public health and health management cadres, access to essential drugs, community participation, and action on social determinants of health. After two years of deliberations, the HLEG report was included in the Twelfth Five Year Plan as the health chapter. The government decided to implement this in a phased manner with one district from each state chosen to pilot the implementation. However, in a study of progress assessment of UHC among BRICS countries, it was found that India, despite the second highest rate of economic growth, has had the least improvement in public funding for health. Globally, countries with the best health outcomes have some sort of UHC provisioning (Marten et al. 2014).

In the US, the elderly, children, and the low-income families are covered through state Medicare plans, while the working population and their dependents are covered through employer-provided health insurance plans. There are separate schemes for active duty military persons and veterans. Despite insurance coverage there are some degrees of co-payments and deductibles which the patient is expected to pay. Out-of-pocket (without any health insurance plan coverage) patients end up paying extraordinarily higher rates for care. However, the system comes under considerable criticism since the health expenditures are the highest in the world, while the health outcomes are among the lowest in OECD countries. Currently there is considerable debate over the Affordable Care Act (commonly known as Obamacare) which provides state subsidies to insurance companies for those who are unable to buy the plans, ability to young people to stay on their parents plans, and a compulsory enrollment mandate to increase the risk pool. The current administration has made several attempts to 'repeal and replace' Obamacare with 'something better'. However, till now none of the replacement bills have successfully passed the Congress.

Local Trends

The mohalla (community) clinics in Delhi provide a useful case study of healthcare experiment deserving a mention. The Delhi state government plans to open 500 mohalla clinics, and it already has 100 functional clinics for patient care (Government of NCT of Delhi 2015). The providers are paid by the government on a per patient basis and patients are provided free medicines from an essential medicines list. Initial reports suggest that these clinics have been quite popular. The state government has also started paying for diagnostic and surgical procedures. Andhra Pradesh, Karnataka, Rajasthan, and Tamil Nadu too have schemes of their own for varying levels of cost coverage; however, they are mostly for accessing tertiary care services.

WAY AHEAD

When viewed from a broad perspective, it appears that the health market in India whether under public control or under public supervision (private) is not sensitive to the affordability and capacity to pay issues. This has kept a large amount of our population at risk. This is explained by Table 15.13 which presented the expenditure as a share of household MPCE according to quintiles and SRCs. Similar interpretation emerged from Table 15.14 where we assess independent impact using regressions. With the systematic neglect of the public sector and an increasing role of private sector, this is likely to have adverse health impacts on the population.

Using data from several sources, this chapter reviewed health financing in India. We reviewed India's healthcare sector and financing, describing the morbidity and treatment profile, analysing the cost of care and constraints of health sector financing, disaggregating the household health expenditures according to consumption class and SRCs, and also performed multivariate analyses. We have identified gaps and shown the limitations of existing bas insurance-based schemes in reducing out-of-pocket health spending by poor households and described extant health insurance schemes, global, and local trends. In line with the global call to action on universal healthcare, we urge upon readers the need for a fair and equitable healthcare system for a country that a fifth of humanity resides in.

POLICY RECOMMENDATIONS

1. First and foremost, policy must bring focus on improving and creating new-world standard public health and curative care institutions across rural and urban India. This is not the same as opening new hospitals.
2. One-fourth of all household expenditures is spent on healthcare should there be one or more episodes of sickness in a household during a year. Such exorbitant expenditure burden on the households may even push many families into the poverty trap.
3. When expenditure by MPCE quintiles are analysed, it is quite clear that the bottom quintile (8.1 per cent) and the top quintile (9.7 per cent) households spend a relatively higher share of their household expenditure on hospitalization in public health facilities than the middle quintiles (see Table 15.13). In comparison with other households, bottom quintile households spend significantly higher share of their usual household expenditure on hospitalization in private hospitals (36 per cent).
4. There is large gender bias in healthcare access which must be addressed both at the institutional and household levels.
5. A substantial (just about two-thirds) share of all expenditures incurred in treating a sick person has been on purchase of drugs and medicines. There is a case for urgent analysis and control of drug pricing in India including issues relating to intellectual property rights, compulsory licensing, and manufacturing of generic medicines.
6. Health sectors must be opened to the international investors under the PPP model and strong regulatory mechanisms must be placed with support from multilateral institutions such as the WHO.
7. Tripartite insurance systems must become a reality in India within the next decade.

REFERENCES

AYUSH. 2015. 'Summary of AYUSH Registered Practitioners (Doctors) and Population Served as on 1.1.2015'. Available at http://ayush.gov.in/sites/default/files/Medical%20Manpower%20Table%202015.pdf, last accessed on 23 February 2020.

Bhore, J., R. Amesur, and A. Banerjee. 1946. 'Report of the Health Survey and Development Committee'. New Delhi: Government of India.

Centre for Budget and Governance Accountability. 2018. 'Union Budget Analysis Tool 2017–18'. Available at http://unionbudget2017.cbgaindia.org/, last accessed on 23 February 2020.

Credit Suisse. 2019. *Global Wealth Report 2019*. Zurich: Crédit Suisse.

Government of NCT of Delhi. 2015. *Annual Plan 2015–16*, volume II. New Delhi: Planning Department, Government of India.

Hooda, S.K. 2013. 'Changing Pattern of Public Expenditure on Health in India: Issues and Challenges'. ISID-PHFI Collaborative Research Centre, Institute for Studies in Industrial Development, New Delhi.

IIPS (International Institute for Population Sciences) and ICF. 2017. National Family Health Survey (NFHS-4), 2015–16: India. Mumbai: IIPS and ICF.

Karan, A., W. Yip, and A. Mahal. 2017. 'Extending Health Insurance to the Poor in India: An Impact Evaluation of Rashtriya Swasthya Bima Yojana on Out-of-Pocket Spending for Healthcare'. *Social Science & Medicine*, 181: 83–92.

Kumar, A.S., L.C. Chen, M. Choudhury, S. Ganju, V. Mahajan, A. Sinha, and A. Sen. 2011. 'Financing Health Care for All: Challenges and Opportunities', *The Lancet* 377(9766): 668–79.

Kurian, O. 2015. *Financing Healthcare for All in India: Towards a Common Goal*. New Delhi: Oxfam India.

Lal, P.G. 2005. 'Report of the National Commission on Macroeconomics and Health'. National Commission on Macroeconomics and Health, Ministry of Health & Family Welfare. New Delhi: Government of India.

Marten, R., D. McIntyre, C. Travassos, S. Shishkin, W. Longde, S. Reddy, and J. Vega. 2014. 'An Assessment of Progress towards Universal Health Coverage in Brazil, Russia, India, China, and South Africa (BRICS)'. *The Lancet* 384(9960): 2164–71.

Misra, R., R. Chatterjee, and S. Rao. 2003. *India Health Report*. New Delhi: Oxford University Press.

National Health Systems Resource Centre. 2016. National Health Accounts Estimates for India 2013–14. Ministry of Health and Family Welfare. New Delhi: Government of India.

———. 2017. National Health Accounts Estimates for India. Ministry of Health and Family Welfare. New Delhi: Government of India.

———. 2019. National Health Profile 2019. Ministry of Health and Family Welfare. New Delhi: Government of India.

National Sample Survey Office (NSSO). 2015. 'Key Indicators of Social Consumption in India', NSS

71st Round, June 2014, Government of India, New Delhi.

Savedoff, W.D. 2007. 'What should a country spend on health care?', *Health Affairs* 26(4): 962–70.

Shepherd-Smith, A. 2012. 'Free Drugs for India's Poor', *The Lancet* 380(9845): 874.

World Bank. 2018. 'Household Final Consumption Expenditure Per Capita (Constant 2010 US$)', World Bank National Accounts Data and OECD National Accounts Data Files, Washington, DC.

World Health Organization (WHO). 1948. 'Preamble to the Constitution of WHO as Adopted by the International Health Conference, New York, 19 June–22 July 1946'. Geneva: World Health Organization.

———. 2017. 'Global Health Expenditure Database'. Geneva: World Health Organization.

16

Private Sector in Health

William Joe, Pallavi Joshi, and Sunil Rajpal

The health system can be understood as comprising six building blocks: (i) service delivery; (ii) health workforce; (iii) information and surveillance mechanisms; (iv) medical products, vaccines, and technologies; (v) financing; and (vi) leadership and governance (WHO 2007). In India, the private sector in health is inextricably linked to each domain and assumes high strategic relevance for development of health systems. The successive National Health Policies (NHP) of 1983, 2002, and 2017 have also increasingly recognized the private sector as a key partner in health development (Government of India 2017). Over the last few decades, a dynamic private sector has facilitated rapid expansion of healthcare services including infrastructure and human resources. These are expected to complement the pro-poor public sector efforts for achieving universal coverage of healthcare services. But such patterns are more explicit in countries such as Sri Lanka (Rannan-Eliya and de Mel 1997), whereas in case of India, even the poor resort to private health services due to the defunct state of public health facilities (Banerjee, Deaton, and Duflo 2004). Nevertheless, the private sector has gradually evolved and now exhibits leadership in pharmaceutical and medical technological advancements and its distribution.

With huge presence, the private sector now assumes an instrumental role in health and economic development (Government of India 2017). Yet, the private sector is often seen as iniquitous for shortcomings linked to urban-centric presence, pro-rich bias, malpractices, and supernormal-profit motives in healthcare provision. The concerns intensify manifold because of a weak regulatory framework and a fragmented market structure with considerable heterogeneity in inputs, services, and quality of care. This chapter reviews the salient features of private sector in health in India and outlines critical policy issues while reconciling the views on private sector growth and its welfare implications. The rest of the chapter is organized as follows: the next section presents an international perspective on the role of private sector in health. The second section describes the presence of private sector in healthcare provisioning in India. Section three adopts an equity perspective and highlights the relative contribution of public and private sectors in healthcare utilization and financing. The fourth section revisits the prominent policy concerns associated with private sector in India and also briefly discusses the approach of NHP 2017 towards the private sector. The last section concludes with actionable policy recommendations.

PRIVATE SECTOR IN HEALTH: INTERNATIONAL PERSPECTIVE

The private sector includes the entire set of private sector individuals, institutions, and entities that are directly and indirectly engaged in provisioning of healthcare services (Mackintosh et al. 2016). With growing population and diversified health needs, it is instrumental for governments to devise prudent mechanisms to collaborate with the private sector for strengthening health systems and accelerating progress towards the Sustainable Development Goals (SDGs) Agenda 2030. In most countries, the private sector is involved in all spheres of healthcare delivery including treatment provision, insurance management, and outsourcing of medical and non-medical supplies. Importantly, the structure and composition of public and private sector can vary across health systems and has varying implications on progressivity in health financing and equity in health outcomes.

As such, the institutional arrangements for health system financing allow categorization of countries under four broad types of health systems (Reid 2009): (i) Beveridge model (tax-based financing); (ii) Bismarck model (universal multi-payer system); (iii) National Health Insurance model (government-run insurance programme); and (iv) Out-of-pocket (OOP) model. The UK, Germany, Canada, and India are examples of such health systems, respectively.[1] It may be noted that both public and private sectors have important roles to play under each system. For instance, the National Health Service (NHS) of the UK is largely funded by general taxation but healthcare delivery structure outlines an important role for general practitioners from the private sector. Similarly, Canada follows a single payer system but allows competitive purchasing of health services through private sector. However, in most of the developing countries healthcare is financed through a regressive OOP model with a predominant share of the private sector.

Given the variations, it is critical to understand the evolving character of the private sector globally and exploring the policy alternatives to achieve objectives of universal health coverage (UHC). In this regard, Mackintosh et al. (2016) present an alternative approach to classify the role of private sector based on: first, size and pattern of private health expenditure; second, the scale and level of the private sector enterprises in healthcare provisioning; and third, the accessibility of the public sector determined by a reliance on user fees. Based on these metrics India is identified to have a dominant private sector because of excessive reliance on private sector, from both supply- and demand-side perspectives, as well as limited role of public sector financing in healthcare provisioning.

In general, private sector is criticized for unduly affecting availability of skilled human resources in the public sector and also leading to catastrophically high health expenditures (Horton and Clark 2016; Sengupta and Nundy 2005). Contractual arrangements or PPPs are also perceived as biased arrangements that can undermine strengthening of public health systems. But restricting the scope of private sector can be linked to suboptimal outcomes and it is important to identify and promote effective partnerships between the public and private players (McPake and Hanson 2016; Montagu and Goodman 2016). In plural health systems, such as India, health system development and the attempts toward UHC can sustain well with effective public sector stewardship that recognizes and harnesses the potential of partnership with private sector players.

While public health spending is necessary to improve population health outcomes, private sector spending can also play an instrumental role. A higher share of private sector in total health expenditure can be discussed under two possible scenarios: One, where high private health expenditure is accompanied by higher levels of life expectancy. Two, where private health spending is not necessarily linked to consistent life expectancy improvements. Cross-country analysis (Figure 16.1a) shows that high levels of per capita private health expenditure is associated with higher life expectancy at birth but it is also important to note that smaller increments in health spending at lower levels are associated with substantial life expectancy gains. But private health spending beyond a particular level is not necessarily associated with higher incremental gains in life expectancy. The increments in private health expenditure is mainly determined by three factors namely, price of medical care technology, health financing principles, and the higher willingness to pay from improvements in economic well-being. In fact, Figure 16.1b indicates that private health expenditure increases with improvements in per capita GDP.

High levels of private health spending can be beneficial but it is important to ensure progressive health financing mechanisms to achieve efficiency gains in health outcomes. But amidst heterogeneities, policy-makers face an uphill task to coordinate and collaborate

[1] In case of India, despite various government health schemes and disease programmes, 70 per cent OOP makes it more of an OOP model.

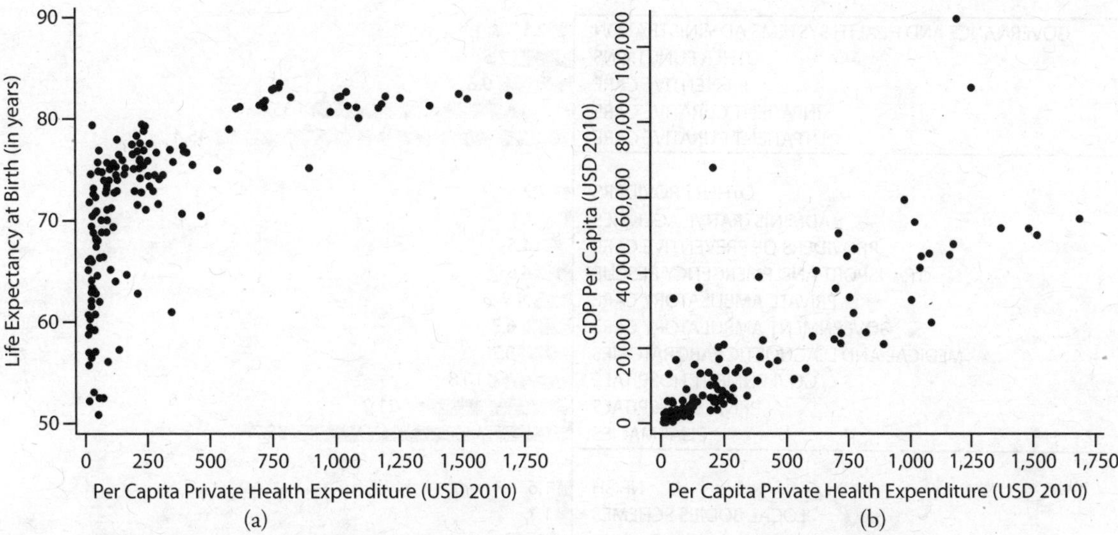

Figure 16.1 Association of Private Health Expenditure with Key Developmental Indicators, 2014

Source: World Development Indicators. https://datacatalog.worldbank.org/dataset/world-development-indicators, last accessed on 4 March 2020.

with the private sector. The WHO (2000) recommends strategic purchasing as a policy tool that can allow rational service mix, provider mix, and volume of medical and non-medical health services to maximize societal objectives. This consideration has merit as private sector can provide a range of medical and non-medical health services at competitive prices and quality (Figueras, Robinson, Jakubowski 2005; McPake and Banda 1994; Preker and Harding 2007; Vining and Globerman 1999). While strategic purchasing of non-medical services is more acceptable than medical services (Vining and Globerman 1999), poor evidence-base on nature of competition and its impact on quality, equity, and efficiency of healthcare services can make this field of policymaking highly indecisive and uncertain (Gilson and Raphaely 2008). The political economy of the health sector further undermines the assumption of fair competition and provides limited scope to rule out opportunism in contracting-out of services.

PRIVATE SECTOR IN INDIA: FACTS AND FIGURES

As per the National Health Accounts (NHA), the share of total health expenditure in GDP has increased marginally from 0.95 per cent in 2004–5 to 1.13 per cent in 2014–15. The increase is associated with the launch of National Rural Health Mission (NRHM) that enhanced government spending in total health expenditure from 22.5 per cent 2004–5 to 29.0 per cent in 2014–15. During this period the share of household out-of-pocket expenditures in total health spending has decreased from 69.4 per cent to 62.6 per cent. Correspondingly, there are small increments in social security expenditure on health (from 4.2 per cent to 5.7 per cent) and private health insurance expenditure (from 1.6 per cent to 3.7 per cent). These facts reveal that healthcare financing in India, based on direct household spending, continues to be a predominant feature even as there are modest efforts to institutionalize and organize health spending through risk-pooling mechanisms. The health financing situation, however, can improve in coming years because of the recent Union Budget 2018 announcement to cover 100 million poor households under the Ayushman Bharat Yojana—National Health Protection Scheme (NHPS).

Figure 16.2 presents the distribution of current health expenditure by healthcare functions, healthcare providers, healthcare financing schemes, and sources of financing. In healthcare provisioning, private hospitals account for one-fifth share whereas pharmacies as retail sellers have the highest share amounting to over one-third of total current health expenditure. Similarly, most of the health expenditure is incurred for outpatient and inpatient curative care and the bulk of these services are provided through the private sector. However, in the last two decades, health insurance has emerged as an important service provided by the private sector with significant collaborations in delivery of several public health insurance schemes. The Insurance Regulatory

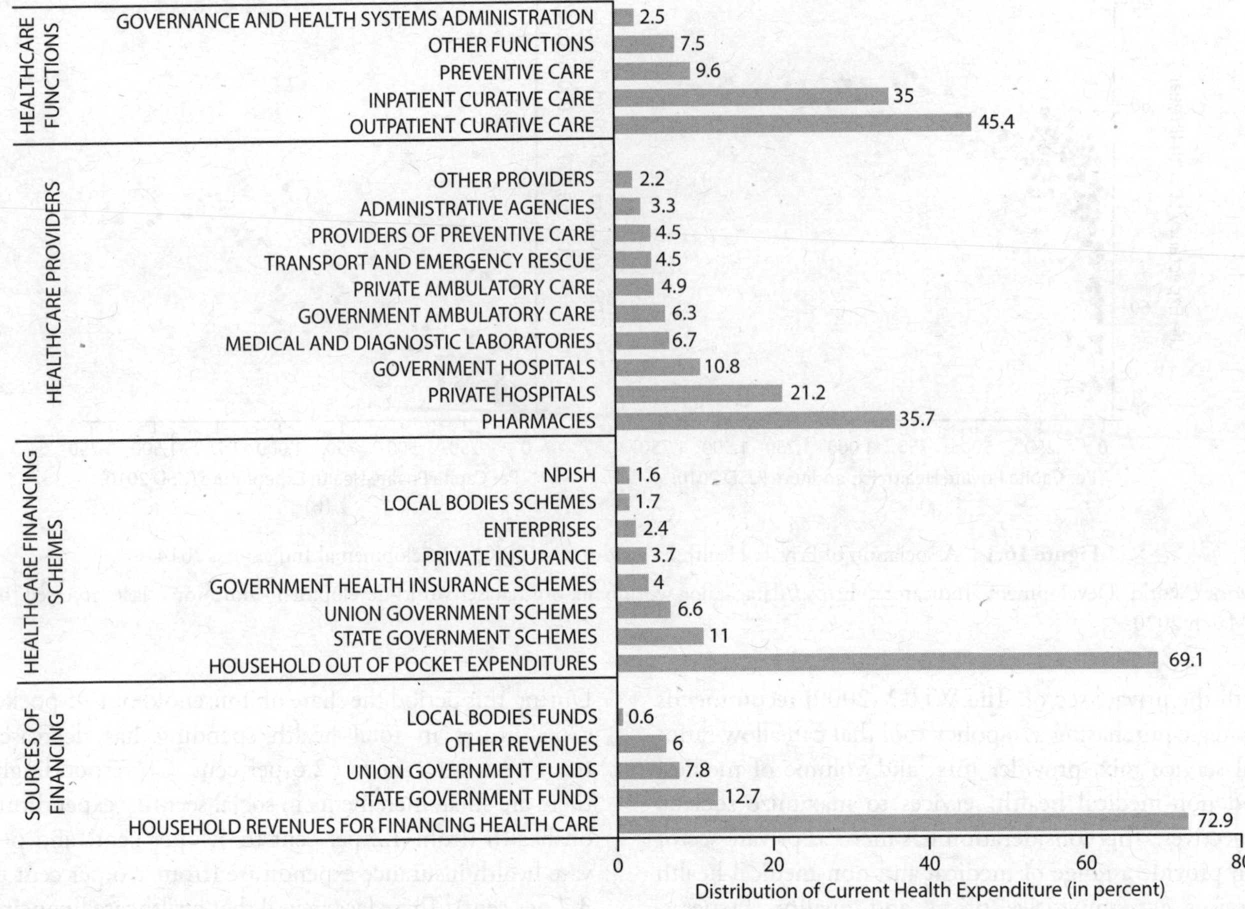

Figure 16.2 Distribution of Current Health Expenditure, 2013–14

Source: National Health Accounts 2013–14. (NHSRC, Ministry of Health and Family Welfare, 2016).
Note: NPISH - Non-Profit Institutions Serving Households.

and Development Authority (IRDA) reports that health insurance market in India is witnessing significant annual growth with overall premium of over INR 345 billion in 2016–17. A total of 437.5 million individuals were covered by health insurance policies, of which 77 per cent were covered under government-sponsored health insurance and the rest were covered under various group and individual policies issued by general and health insurers (IRDA 2016–17). In 2015–16, 358 million persons in India were enrolled under various (government or private) insurance schemes and policies (Table 16.1). The bulk of these insured persons (273 million), however, are enrolled under various government-sponsored insurance schemes.

Public and private sector have almost similar share in terms of number of individual family floater policies. Yet, the risk pool captured under the current insurance net is skewed and suboptimal. Expansion in coverage is critical from both pricing as well as equity perspective. In particular, an efficient pooling mechanism can also allow effective regulation and also offer the scope for both public and private sectors for provisioning of healthcare with greater quality and accountability. The insurance sector, however, can expect huge impetus post the budgetary announcements on NHPS with unprecedented coverage limits. The success of NHPS will require considerable focus on the implementation mechanisms including premium structure as well as the role and responsibilities of regulators and the third-party administrators.

Figure 16.3 presents a decadal profile of increase in number of medical education institutions and the overall enrolment or intake capacity. In 2014, India had a total of 385 medical institutions with a major share (54 per cent) of the private sector. Jointly, these institutions account for an enrolment/intake capacity of over

Table 16.1 Health Insurance Policies, Persons Covered and Gross Premium, 2015–16

Type of insurance	Indicator	Public Sector	Private Sector	Total
Government-sponsored scheme including RSBY	No. of Policies	277	156	433
	Persons (in '000)	219,671	53,601	273,272
	Premium (INR Lakh)	202,578	44,826	247,404
Group insurance schemes excluding government-sponsored schemes	No. of Policies	347,310	41,258	388,568
	Persons (in '000)	40,886	16,153	57,039
	Premium (INR Lakh)	858,784	303,268	1,162,052
Individual family floater	No. of Policies	2,126,298	2,959,096	5,085,394
	Persons (in '000)	6,719	9,136	15,855
	Premium (INR Lakh)	171,763	291,963	463,726
Individual floater other than family floater	No. of Policies	3,604,730	2,736,806	6,341,536
	Persons (in '000)	9,288	3,510	12,798
	Premium (INR Lakh)	325,940	245,633	571,573
Total	No. of Policies	6,078,615	5,737,316	11,815,931
	Persons (in '000)	276,563	82,399	358,962
	Premium (INR Lakh)	1,559,065	885,689	2,444,754

Source: National Health Profile of India, 2017. Central Bureau of Health Intelligence, Ministry of Health and Family Welfare.
Note: A lakh is equivalent to 0.1 million.

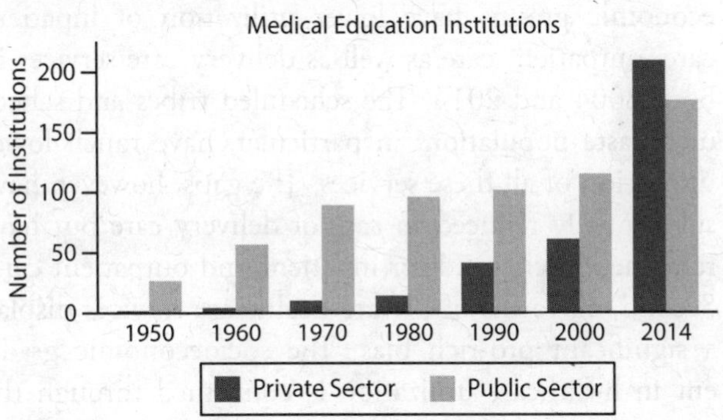

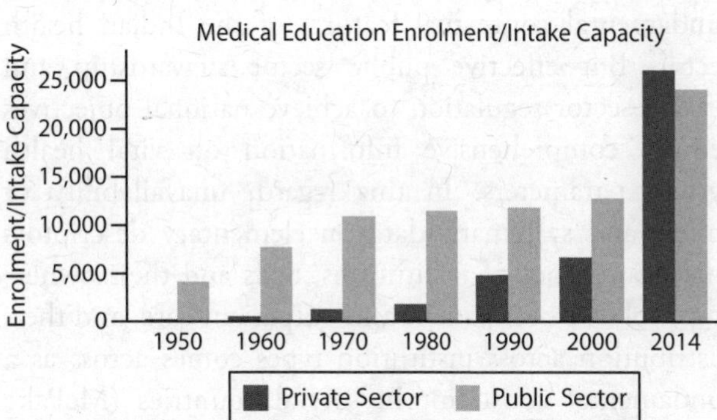

Figure 16.3 Medical Education Institutions and Enrolment/Intake Capacity across Public and Private Sectors, India 1950–2014
Source: Choudhury (2014).

50,000 medical students (52 per cent share of private sector). The role of private sector in medical education has witnessed exponential growth since the 1990s. It is also worth noting that between 1970 and 2000 there were limited investments for establishment of new public sector medical institutions but since 2000 there is a 50 per cent growth in their numbers. Yet there are substantial shortfalls resulting in huge pool of unqualified rural medical practitioners and quacks attending to illnesses or curative care procedures. The proliferation of such practices across various states reveals the scarcity and skewed distribution of human resources for health in India and highlights the huge demand for cost-effective healthcare.

Similarly, private healthcare facilities in India display substantial heterogeneity. It is estimated that India has over one million private healthcare enterprises but only about 25 per cent of these establishments are with employees whereas over 750,000 are own account enterprises (Table 16.2). Sole practitioners (doctors, nurses, and midwives) constitute bulk of the private sector, although lack of comprehensive data about the formal and informal providers at the system level restricts insights on their distribution. Since 2000–1 the share of allopathic enterprises and hospitals has increased, though only two-thirds of all medical facilities have a formal registration (Mackintosh et al. 2016). But with increasing corporatization and inflow of capital

Table 16.2 Percentage Share of Different Enterprise Types in India, National Sample Surveys 2000–1, 2006–7, and 2010–11

Establishment type	Own account enterprises			Establishment with employees		
	2000–1	2006–7	2010–11	2000–1	2006–7	2010–11
Hospital service	0.7	1.2	3.6	15.4	14.9	25.7
Medical and dental practices	52.1	55.5	63.3	58.4	47.1	48.9
Indian system of medicine	28.7	24.2	23.0	13.2	18.1	12.9
Nursing and physiotherapy	15.3	14.4	5.2	1.5	7.3	1.9
Diagnostics or pathology	1.4	2.3	2.4	9.2	11.3	9.0
Others	1.8	2.4	2.5	2.3	1.4	1.7
All	100	100	100	100	100	100
Total number of enterprises	1,075,000	785,000	736,000	229,000	268,000	285,000

Source: Mackintosh et al. (2016).

investments, the private sector has gradually developed establishments that can provide healthcare across a range of medical specialties.

The growth tendency displayed by the private sector is also acknowledged in the NHP 2017 as one of the fundamental contextual features of the Indian health sector. But effective public sector stewardship and private sector regulation to achieve national objectives require comprehensive information on vital health system parameters. In this regard, unavailability of timely and systematic data on elementary descriptors such as number of institutions, beds and their ownership, volume of inpatient and outpatient care, and their distribution across institution types comes across as a fundamental constraint in several countries (McPake and Hanson 2016). India is no exception and there is very limited information to comprehensively describe the private sector, particularly the supply-side features.

PRIVATE HEALTHCARE UTILIZATION AND EXPENDITURE

Table 16.3 (a and b) shows that utilization of inpatient care across both public and private sector facilities in India has increased from 28 cases per 1,000 persons in 2004 to 37 cases per 1,000 persons in 2014. Similarly, outpatient care use has increased from 75 cases per 1,000 persons in 2004 to 85 cases per 1,000 persons in 2014. In 2014, the private sector accounted for about 60 per cent share in total inpatient care, 75 per cent share in total outpatient care, and 35 per cent share in delivery care services. Clearly, the private sector has an overwhelming share in provision of outpatient and inpatient care including delivery care.

It is observed that inadequate public health investments and the gross neglect of public health sector has intensified inequalities in healthcare utilization and financing. Two clear patterns of healthcare inequities are evident from Table 16.3. First, marginalized socioeconomic groups have lower utilization of inpatient care, outpatient care as well as delivery care services in both 2004 and 2014. The scheduled tribes and scheduled caste population, in particular, have much lower utilization of all these services. The gaps, however, have substantially reduced in case of delivery care but have remained unchanged for inpatient and outpatient care. Second, all forms of private healthcare services display a significant pro-rich bias. The socioeconomic gradient in healthcare utilization is confirmed through the concentration index[2] for utilization of inpatient, outpatient, and delivery care services across public and private sector (Table 16.3). The concentration index has a distinct positive value for utilization of all three types of healthcare services from private sector whereas the index is significantly negative for the public sector.

Table 16.4 reports the OOP expenditure incurred by households in 2004 and 2014. For comparability, the estimates are presented in 2014 prices. On average, the overall inpatient care expenditure has increased from over INR 15,000 to INR 20,000 but bulk of the increment is associated with the private sector. In fact, in 2014 the average inpatient care expenditure in private sector is almost four times that of the public sector. The

[2] The concentration index is widely used to examine socioeconomic inequalities in healthcare whereby a negative (positive) value of the index reflects pro-poor (pro-rich) concentration of the concerned health variable.

Table 16.3a Utilization of Inpatient and Outpatient Care Services by Socioeconomic Background (per 1,000 persons)

Criteria	NSS 2004			NSS 2014		
	Public	Private	Combined	Public	Private	Combined
Inpatient Care Services						
Wealth Quintile						
Lowest Quintile	9.0	7.4	16.3	11.6	9.6	21.2
Second Quintile	10.9	11.2	22.1	14.7	15.9	30.6
Third Quintile	12.6	16.4	29.0	17.0	21.8	38.8
Fourth Quintile	13.8	24.5	38.2	15.7	31.2	46.9
Highest Quintile	12.2	32.9	45.1	13.9	48.8	62.7
Social Group						
Scheduled Tribes	9.8	6.9	16.7	15.2	10.4	25.6
Scheduled Castes	14.1	11.7	25.8	18.5	18.7	37.3
Other Backward Classes	10.6	18.5	29.1	12.7	25.1	37.7
Others	11.3	20.3	31.6	14.1	26.5	40.6
All	11.5	16.7	28.2	14.4	22.9	37.3
Concentration index	–0.127	0.108		–0.150	0.128	
Standard error	(0.004)	(0.003)		(0.003)	(0.003)	
Outpatient Care Services						
Wealth Quintile						
Lowest Quintile	13.6	32.7	46.3	15.8	34.3	50.1
Second Quintile	15.6	47.4	62.9	20.8	47.2	68.0
Third Quintile	17.2	54.2	71.4	19.1	59.7	78.8
Fourth Quintile	21.6	73.8	95.3	25.7	83.3	109.0
Highest Quintile	21.6	101.9	123.5	26.2	123.1	149.3
Social Group						
Scheduled Tribes	14.8	25.5	40.3	23.0	24.9	48.0
Scheduled Castes	19.0	48.7	67.6	22.5	54.0	76.5
Other Backward Classes	15.9	56.8	72.7	21.6	64.1	85.7
Others	18.6	72.3	90.9	18.1	83.0	101.0
All	17.3	57.5	74.8	20.9	63.8	84.7
Concentration index	–0.080	0.0418		–0.096	0.068	
Standard error	(0.006)	(0.002)		(0.006)	(0.002)	

Source: Authors' compilation using NSS data for the respective given years.

gap between public and private outpatient care is much less and partly reflects the limited needs as well as vast heterogeneity of the private sector. For instance, about 50 per cent of the spells of ailments are treated by fragmented private doctors and clinics whereas one-fourth of such care is accounted by the private hospitals. Nevertheless, a distinct socioeconomic gradient in healthcare expenditure is apparent across both public and private sector and across type of care.

The NHP 2017 thus rightly accords high priority to curb the incidence of catastrophic healthcare expenditure. Since these catastrophic payments are overwhelmingly concentrated among the poor, health insurance can have an important role for enhancing financial protection and fairness while seeking private healthcare services, particularly inpatient care.

STRATEGIC AND POLICY CONCERNS

Welfare is a common terminology in the economics literature as well as routine sociopolitical discourse and is concerned with the policy benefits accruing to specific

Table 16.3b Utilization of Institutional Delivery Care Services by Socioeconomic Background (in per cent)

Criteria	NFHS 2005–6			NFHS 2015–16		
	Public	Private	Institutional	Public	Private	Institutional
Wealth Quintile						
Lowest Quintile	8.4	4.4	12.7	51.9	7.9	59.8
Second Quintile	14.1	9.5	23.6	60.6	14.8	75.5
Third Quintile	22.5	16.8	39.4	58.9	26.3	85.2
Fourth Quintile	27.2	30.8	58.0	49.8	40.9	90.8
Highest Quintile	23.9	60.0	83.8	34.2	61.3	95.5
Social Group						
Scheduled Tribes	19.4	13.6	33.0	60.1	18.5	78.6
Scheduled Castes	11.9	6.0	17.9	56.1	12.1	68.3
Other Backward Classes	16.2	21.5	37.8	50.5	29.5	80.0
Others	21.8	31.2	53.0	44.7	39.4	84.1
All	18.0	20.9	38.8	52.1	27.1	79.2
Concentration index	0.21	0.46		0.05	0.37	
Standard error	(0.005)	(0.004)		(0.001)	(0.001)	

Source: Authors' compilation using NFHS data for the respective given years.

individuals and groups. However, health and healthcare investments have high merit than certain other forms of expenditure and introduces an element of extra-welfarism of this otherwise intrinsically private good. Such distinct meritorious good should be subsidized for an equitable distribution and for enhancing the benefits to society. This implies that health systems should emphasize on increasing health investments to achieve this socially desirable objective. In this context, the High-Level Expert Group (HLEG) Report on UHC for India (HLEG 2011) made several recommendations regarding healthcare financing. In particular, the HLEG called for increasing public health expenditure (central and state governments combined) from the existing level of 1.2 per cent of GDP to at least 2.5 per cent by the end of the twelfth Five-Year Plan, and to at least 3 per cent of the GDP by the end of the year 2022. While government expenditure can play a critical role in increasing the overall health spending, major efficiency gains are feasible if existing levels of spending are institutionalized through risk pooling and insurance mechanisms in India. Importantly, private sector can accelerate progress towards UHC whereby active public health management policies can shape the approach towards healthcare delivery (Horton 2016). Such an increase is warranted not only to meet the pervasive challenge of primary healthcare but also to strengthen secondary and tertiary care in the country. But expansion of private sector is not necessarily devoid of irrational profiteering. India is at a critical juncture in health development and the tilt towards the private sector mandates effective regulation to achieve the national objectives of equitable and affordable healthcare. This section briefly reviews a few strategic concerns that have significant bearing on India's health system including the private sector.

Strategic Purchasing under NHP 2017

Inadequate public sector investments and inefficiencies in service delivery and quality have reshaped individual preferences for the private sector. The NHP 2017 acknowledges these facts and envisages an unprecedented role for the private sector for health development in India. The NHP recommends an internationally recognized framework of strategic purchasing to harness the synergy between public and private sector (WHO 2000). This has relevance because with effective regulations such arrangements have the potential to swiftly expand healthcare delivery with efficient pricing and acceptable quality standards. This move under NHP has received widespread attention but robust evaluations are necessary to develop consensus on its merits and demerits.

In this context, it is worth noting NITI Aayog's intent to develop a PPP model for treatment of chronic

Table 16.4 Household Out-of-Pocket Expenditure on Inpatient, Outpatient, and Delivery Care Services by Socioeconomic Background (INR at 2014 prices)

Criteria	NSS 2004			NSS 2014		
	Public	Private	Combined	Public	Private	Combined
Inpatient care						
Wealth Quintiles						
Lowest Quintile	6,556	14,012	9,891	6,556	20,896	13,150
Second Quintile	6,686	14,670	10,715	6,097	17,480	12,128
Third Quintile	7,634	16,005	12,369	6,539	22,558	15,682
Fourth Quintile	9,085	19,918	16,013	7,199	23,835	18,411
Highest Quintile	14,526	30,584	26,226	14,242	42,376	36,367
Social Group						
Scheduled Tribes	6,801	14,620	10,013	4,185	26,818	13,520
Scheduled Castes	6,156	17,471	11,272	6,713	20,668	13,864
Other Backward Classes	8,271	18,645	14,856	6,066	26,154	19,551
Others	11,347	24,922	20,048	11,993	34,347	26,825
All	8,597	20,734	15,791	7,638	27,959	20,288
Outpatient care						
Wealth Quintiles						
Lowest Quintile	551	544	544	521	699	642
Second Quintile	526	652	620	515	607	574
Third Quintile	547	774	723	356	678	601
Fourth Quintile	705	747	736	355	796	689
Highest Quintile	697	1,053	988	412	905	816
Social Group						
Scheduled Tribes	417	494	467	442	656	554
Scheduled Castes	524	648	613	374	640	565
Other Backward Classes	623	741	716	449	760	681
Others	670	917	864	467	813	748
All	604	783	741	437	755	676
Delivery Care						
Wealth Quintiles						
Lowest Quintile	1,713	5,637	3,084	2,187	14,750	4,495
Second Quintile	2,328	7,824	4,302	2,553	15,427	6,204
Third Quintile	2,722	7,742	5,326	3,165	15,498	7,913
Fourth Quintile	3,043	12,584	8,363	3,344	18,932	10,991
Highest Quintile	4,431	15,600	13,270	4,714	27,459	21,043
Social Group						
Scheduled Tribes	1,659	8,245	3,666	2,187	11,785	3,993
Scheduled Castes	2,018	8,706	4,476	2,535	18,656	6,551
Other Backward Classes	2,617	9,826	6,567	2,581	18,346	8,803
Others	3,254	12,715	8,874	3,641	20,387	11,269
All	2,567	10,734	6,767	2,758	18,730	8,508

Source: Authors' compilation using data from NSSO (2014).

non-communicable diseases (NCDs) at select district hospitals. Quintessentially, it involves sharing of public resources (funds and infrastructure) to improve functioning of district hospitals and reduce out-of-pocket expenditure. Prima facie, this strategy has merit but overall resource support and incentive design is critical for enhancing equity in access and financing. The policy has to undergo a litmus test in providing comprehensive outpatient and inpatient care based on social insurance or government insurance financing. Besides, the political economy of strategic purchasing can be rather complex. For instance, scope for opportunism in contracting-out of services or fair competition will be conditioned by the regulatory environment and stewardship in designing socially beneficial strategic purchasing.

Expansion of quality services and infrastructure in underserved areas comes across as a formidable challenge. Innovative financial and managerial design will be required to correct these geographical imbalances—a task where the public sector finds repeated failures. These concerns are also linked to cost escalations such that ensuring UHC through strategic purchasing may have huge fiscal implications. The private sector can propose various services for collaborations but needs can also be based on electoral agenda and nature of redistributive politics. For instance, health clientelism is resonating across several Indian states and healthcare is a prime component of several election manifestos. However, it maybe cautioned that such strategies should display fiscal sustainability as excessive commitments (and malpractices) are known to have adverse implications (Reddy and Mary 2013).

Regulation of the Private Sector

Private sector in health is often used colloquially as a singular entity. The private sector has wide heterogeneity, ranging from small clinics to large specialized corporate hospitals, from informal health practitioners to registered private practitioners, local pharmaceutical companies to multinationals, pathology labs to large diagnostics facilities, and from pharmacy institutes to universities. While the national health policies have stressed upon framing and implementing effective regulatory interventions to increase efficiencies and uniformity in service delivery of the burgeoning private sector, they have only peripherally captured the contours of its plurality. The initial discussions on the regulation of private sector essentially focused on doctors and institutions/facilities, and it is only recently that issues related to pharmaceuticals, diagnostics, medical education, and research are emphasized (Baru 2013). But in the absence of comprehensive data for private health sector—on finance, clinical establishments, human resources, pharmacies, and pharmaceutical manufacturing units in the country—it is difficult to monitor and regulate the sector.

The regulations should initiate by re-examining medical education and practice and its regulation based on the Indian Medical Council (IMC) Act, 1956. Although, the National Medical Commission Bill 2017 seeks to replace the existing Indian Medical Council (IMC) Act, 1956, further efforts are necessary for improving ethical standards for medical services and ensuring quality of medical education, fee, training, and registration under the aegis of the National Medical Commission. Similarly, an institutional focus on public health cadre (such as in Tamil Nadu; see Gupta et al. 2010) for technical and managerial functions can augment the regulatory capacity of the health system including planning and collaborations with the private sector.

Even though a large proportion of population avails private healthcare services, the quality and cost of the services provided at large have been a cause for concern. High variance in fee by doctors, hospitals, and diagnostic facilities; irrational prescription of medicines; negligence of treatment protocol among some private facilities are some of the serious issues confronting private healthcare delivery. This entails serious repercussions on the trust of people in the health system. It is to mitigate these concerns and ensure quality and safe healthcare delivery, proactive regulation of health sector, and particularly[3] private sector is advocated. With the aim of bringing uniformity to health services in the country, the Clinical Establishments (Registration and Regulation) Act, 2010 (CEA) was introduced by the central government to regulate not only clinical establishments in the private sector, but in the public sector, in all recognized systems of medicines. The CEA is an important regulatory tool to improve quality standards of facilities and services across the country. However, the CEA is yet to be adopted by several states including those which have state-specific provisions for the regulation of the private sector. Besides, there have been huge regional variations

[3] Unlike the majority of the private sector in health, the public health sector is required to follow minimum standards and is under public audit owing to bureaucratic procedures (see Duggal and Nandraj 1991). Nonetheless, public health sector is equally in the regulatory ambit of the broader healthcare regulations.

in enforcing of the act due to poor updating of existing regulations, lack of formulations of rules/bylaws to enforce the act, and constant opposition by medical professional bodies.

As regulation is a dynamic process, it requires constant reiteration and updating with the changing characteristics of the health sector. Timely and systematic revisions of the regulatory framework are necessary to allow effective regulation of emerging issues and medical innovations. For instance, in a writ petition (W.P. No. 31385 of 2016) involving negligence of rules and regulations by a hair transplant clinic in Chennai leading to the death of a medical student, the Madras High Court noted that the present regulations are 'incapable' of regulating such private facilities. Even after 20 years of the Tamil Nadu Private Clinical Establishments (Regulation) Act, 1997, there are no rules framed by the state legislature to enforce the said act. While the CEA takes cognizance of the wider scope and nature of the private healthcare sector, states with pre-existing legislations on health facilities have not been successful in making concomitant revisions (Nandaraj 2012). Since law enforcement is directly linked to accountability, older legislations tend to lose their relevance in the present context—this is particularly true in the cases of registration requirements for the establishments and penal provisions on the contravention of legislations. There are also governance-related issues in some states where the state councils and district registration authorities have not been notified to enforce the act because of various bureaucratic and infrastructural (human resources, finances, and technical capacity) bottlenecks (Nandraj 2015). In places where the act is enforced, there are no inspections, and there are only monetary penalties and no imprisonment (Nandraj 2015). Additionally, processing of complaints against doctors have been very slow, and there is low evidence on whether any action is taken against the doctors (Phadke 2016).

Manufacture and sale of pharmaceuticals is another critical area for regulations to ensure availability and access to safe medicines. The regulatory framework for pharmaceuticals in India is complex as multiple nodal agencies are involved in the regulatory process—including the Central Drugs Standard Control Organization (CDSCO), Union Ministry of Health and Family Welfare (MoHFW) and State Drug Regulatory Authorities (SDRAs); the Department of Pharmaceuticals, Union Ministry of Chemical and Fertilizers; and the Department of Biotechnology, Union Ministry of Science and Technology.[4] Ensuring safety, efficacy, and quality of pharmaceuticals is the prerogative of the CDSCO and SDRAs. Both the agencies are responsible to enforce the Drugs and Cosmetics Act, 1940 (DCA) and the rules thereof. However, regulators face the perennial challenge of uniform enforcement of DCA due to varying regulatory capacities (financial, human resources, and infrastructural) of the SDRAs—which are primarily responsible for monitoring the introduction of new drugs, and manufacture and sale of the drugs in the country (Chowdhury et al. 2015). Uniform interpretation of DCA is a problem with dearth of procedural guidance at various levels, lack of proper channels for interface between industry and regulator (Wattal et al. 2017). Further, prices of medicines are regulated at the national level by the National Pharmaceutical Pricing Authority (NPPA). At present, Drug Price Control Order (DPCO), 2013 forms the legal basis to regulate prices of medicines, listed in the National List of Essential Medicines (NLEM) prepared by the MoHFW. Nevertheless, efforts are warranted to standardize pricing across a range of pharmaceutical drugs. For instance, Srinivasan and Phadke (2013) suggest that pricing of combination drugs and drug innovations under similar therapeutic class is necessary to ensure better access to medicines in India. Besides, the government has to strike a balance between the methodological approach towards pricing on one hand and the ease of implementation and monitoring on the other. The shift from cost-based pricing towards a market-based pricing under National Pharmaceutical Pricing Policy, 2012 has been a major concern over the years as it may have no impact on pricing of non-NLEM drugs.

Nonetheless, the Draft Pharmaceutical Policy (2017) has highlighted the need to streamline and regulate distribution and marketing of drugs to increase accessibility and affordability of drugs. The policy also states that there is a need to regulate prevailing practices that undermines the effectiveness of pricing practice. These include improving the overall structure and functioning of NPPA; desirable interventions to address varying industry practices (namely, a company manufactures a

[4] Department of Industrial Policy and Promotion (DIPP) regulates patents and the exports of drugs are governed by Directorate General of Foreign Trade under and the Union Ministry of Commerce and Industry. The Department of Biotechnology, Union Ministry of Science and Technology (DST) works along with the CDSCO to frame guidelines for the regulation of biosimilars.

salt on a given production line and sells it under different brand names at different prices); controlling trade margins addressing differential prices for the same drug and the mark-ups for retailers, distributors, and stockists and so on. Thus, the government has a crucial role in establishing pricing norms for drugs, diagnostics, consultations, and treatment procedures.

Integration with National Programmes

The private health sector can be leveraged to actively participate in delivery of priority national health programmes. In the past, the government has collaborated with the private sector to implement major health financing schemes such as Rashtriya Swasthya Bima Yojana (RSBY). With ongoing epidemiological transition, there is a further need to address the financing concerns concomitant to the treatment of chronic diseases. For instance, the Revised National Tuberculosis Control Programme has outlined strategy to work with the private sector providers to ensure higher case detection and treatment adherence. Incentive mechanisms are usually the preferred approach to link the private sector with national programmes but there is huge potential for collaboration in a range of public health services including primary care. This may help address the resource requirements, particularly human resources and basic infrastructure, for implementation of the interventions. Collaboration with private sector is also desirable to develop transparent drug pricing norms for major public health programmes that target chronic diseases such as diabetes, hypertension, cancer, and tuberculosis. Similarly, fostering relationship from a convergence point of view particularly under initiatives such as Swachh Bharat Abhiyan, Poshan Abhiyaan, and Ayushman Bharat Yojana are also necessary.

RECOMMENDATIONS

With economic growth and advancing medical technology, household healthcare expenditures display a peculiar non-diminishing marginal utility of healthy life at almost all ages. From this perspective, high healthcare OOP expenditure in India is not just a necessity but also reflects the rising aspirations to get the highest level of care available. But given minuscule insurance coverage, a pro-rich pattern of private healthcare services is expected to manifest in the form of higher OOP healthcare expenditure that partly reflects higher cost of services in the private sector, and in part indicates higher willingness to pay. While the public sector continues to be a significant source of healthcare utilization for the poor and systematic government investments are necessary to ensure access to all types of services of high quality. The choice of health investment directly through the public sector or via supporting private sector engagements remains an instrumental concern and should be approached from both equity and efficiency perspective. While growing medical tourism and increasing ability to pay of the richer sections has led to expansions in network of corporate hospitals across metropolitan cities. But some recent instances have contributed to huge public outcry against unfair pricing and practices across corporate hospitals. With a dominant role of the private sector in both formal and informal healthcare, there is a need to reorient the policies with a carrot-and-stick approach.

As India embarks on the road to UHC, the following areas should be prioritized for action to strengthen health systems by harnessing the synergistic public–private mix in India.

1. Given the widespread presence and resource advantages of the private sector, various national health schemes and programmes should actively consider partnering with the private sector delivery of cost-effective services, particularly for marginalized socioeconomic groups across underserved areas. Partnering with the private sector for rapid scale up of the NHPS in terms of financing and service provision is an important area and has been successfully demonstrated by certain states. This can reduce the levels of OOP expenditure and lower the incidence of catastrophic expenditure. Similar potentials exist under the programmes for treatment of NCDs. Collaborations for infrastructure development under Swachh Bharat Abhiyan, Poshan Abhiyaan, and Ayushman Bharat Yojana are important opportunities.
2. Involvement of private sector in healthcare provisioning (doctors and hospitals) across preventive and curative care is instrumental to achieve policy goals of UHC. Strategic purchasing of both preventive and curative care services should be extensively piloted across states to arrive at a reasonable mix of insurance schemes, gatekeeping provisions, and coverage of services. These efforts can expand the network of health and wellness centres by providing greater pool of

human resources for healthcare delivery. The private sector should also be invited to contribute towards the insurance premium risk pools.

3. Increasing intake capacity for medical education is critical to meet the shortage of doctors and nursing staff as well as to cater to the increased demand for diverse types of healthcare specialties. PPPs in medical education should be actively pursued to develop medical education based on private capital investments and effective public sector regulation. Increased supply of human resources of health can reduce the supply-side cost push of medical services and induce greater competition in terms of quality and prices for medical consultations. Partnering with district hospitals in upgrade and expansion of medical education are pivotal areas.
4. At present, there is a wide lacuna in the data of private health sector, either it is restricted to some studies or it is quite dated, failing to reflect the present-day magnitude and scope of the sector. While broad data on private health financing is available, data for other variables including clinical establishments such as clinics, hospitals, practitioners, and so on is rather sparse. A comprehensive database is also lacking because 'health' is the state subject and is the prerogative of states to compile such information, and such data is not captured centrally. The CEA was introduced to ensure uniformity in data, however, it has not been implemented and/or has not been enforced by various states. Hence, ensuring availability of comprehensive data and inclusion of private clinical establishments in surveillance mechanisms needs to be strengthened in order to gauge the presence of private sector in the health systems, introduce more targeted policies and regulatory reforms. In this regard, a legislation could be introduced by MoHFW in the form of a portal, mandating data collection, sharing, and linking, with adequate guidelines for various stakeholders. Provision of such a portal can also be introduced through the envisioned National Electronic Health Authority and State Electronic Health Authorities (under the draft Digital Information Security in Healthcare Act, 2017).
5. It is important to develop permanent institutional mechanisms for consensus building across government, professional associations, and patient representatives on pricing norms and conditions. The need for such regulations is strongly felt in the wake of recent controversies around inconsistent treatment and billing protocols in some major private sector establishments as well as the presentations by private healthcare representatives seeking rationalization of pricing interventions. Pricing of pharmaceutical products to cover a large basket of drugs and monitoring of quality of medicines deserve further attention.
6. All states should develop a public health management cadre that can play both regulatory and supervisory roles to provide technical support and to assist implementation of health policies and regulation of the private sector.
7. The private sector heterogeneity in quality of human resources and services should be reduced by expanding the reach of the formal sector and by monitoring of efforts for adopting fair normative standards and practices for pricing, quality, and accountability of healthcare services. Integrating formal and sole private sector practitioners to facilitate gatekeeping mechanisms can be an important way forward towards ensuring successful implementation of Ayushman Bharat Yojana.

REFERENCES

Banerjee, A., A. Deaton, and E. Duflo. 2004. 'Health, Health Care, and Economic Development: Wealth, Health, and Health Services in Rural Rajasthan', *The American Economic Review* 94(2): 326.

Baru, Rama V. 2013. 'Challenges for Regulating the Private Health Services in India for Achieving Universal Health Care', *Indian Journal of Public Health* 57(4): 208–11.

Choudhury, P.K. 2014. 'Role of Private Sector in Medical Education and Human Resource Development for Health in India', ISID Working Paper 169, Institute for Studies in Industrial Development, New Delhi.

Chowdhury, N., P. Joshi, A. Patnaik, and B. Saraswathy. 2016. 'Administrative Structure & Functions of Drug Regulatory Authorities in India', ICRIER Working Paper 309, Indian Council for Research on International Economic Relations, New Delhi.

Figueras, J., R. Robinson, and E. Jakubowski. 2005. *Purchasing to Improve Health Systems Performance*. United Kingdom: McGraw-Hill Education.

Gilson, L. and N. Raphaely. 2008. 'The Terrain of Health Policy Analysis in Low- and Middle-income Countries: A Review of Published Literature 1994–2007', *Health Policy and Planning* 23(5): 294–307.

Government of India. 2017. National Health Policy 2017. New Delhi: Ministry of Health and Family Welfare. Available at https://www.nhp.gov.in/NHPfiles/national_health_policy_2017.pdf, last accessed on 2 November 2017.

Gupta, M.D., B.R. Desikachari, R. Shukla, T.V. Somanathan, P. Padmanaban, and K.K. Datta. 2010. 'How might India's Public Health Systems be Strengthened? Lessons from Tamil Nadu', *Economic and Political Weekly*, 46–60.

Horton, R. and S. Clark. 2016. 'The Perils and Possibilities of the Private Health Sector', *The Lancet* 388(10044): 540–1.

Mackintosh, M., A. Channon, A. Karan, S. Selvaraj, E. Cavagnero, and H. Zhao. 2016. 'What is the Private Sector? Understanding Private Provision in the Health Systems of Low-income and Middle-income Countries', *The Lancet* 388(10044): 596–605.

McPake, B. and E.E.N. Banda. 1994. 'Contracting Out of Health Services in Developing Countries', *Health Policy and Planning* 9(1): 25–30.

McPake, B. and K. Hanson. 2016. 'Managing the Public–Private Mix to Achieve Universal Health Coverage', *The Lancet* 388(10044): 622–30.

Montagu, D. and C. Goodman. 2016. 'Prohibit, Constrain, Encourage, or Purchase: How should We Engage with the Private Healthcare Sector?', *The Lancet* 388(10044): 613–21.

Nandraj, Sunil. 2012. 'Unregulated and Unaccountable: Private Health Providers', *Economic & Political Weekly* 47(4): 12–17.

Preker, A.S. and A. Harding. 2007. 'Political Economy of Strategic Purchasing', in *Public Ends, Private Means: Strategic Purchasing of Health Services*, edited by A.S. Preker et al. World Bank Publications, pp. 13–52.

Rannan-Eliya, R.P. and N. de Mel. 1997. 'Resource Mobilization in Sri Lanka's Health Sector', Data for Decision Making Project. Boston: Harvard School of Public Medicine.

Reddy, S. and I. Mary. 2013. 'Rajiv Aarogyasri Community Health Insurance Scheme in Andhra Pradesh, India: A Comprehensive Analytic View of Private Public Partnership Model', *Indian Journal of Public Health* 57: 254–9.

Reid, T.R. 2009. *The Healing of America: A Global Quest for Better, Cheaper, and Fairer Health Care*. The Penguin Press.

Sengupta, A. and S. Nundy. 2005. 'The Private Health Sector in India: Is Burgeoning, but at the Cost of Public Health Care', *BMJ* 331(7526): 1157.

Srinivasan, S. and A. Phadke. 2013. 'Pharma Policy 2012 and its Discontents', *Economic and Political Weekly* 48(1): 38–42.

Vining, A.R. and S. Globerman. 1999. 'Contracting-out Health Care Services: A Conceptual Framework', *Health Policy* 46(2): 77–96.

Wattal, V., P. Joshi, A. Arora, and A. Mehdi. 2017. *International Cooperation for Registration of Medicines: Opportunities for India*. New Delhi: Academic Foundation.

World Health Organization (WHO). 2007. 'Everybody's Business—Strengthening Health Systems to Improve Health Outcomes: WHO's Framework for Action'. Geneva: WHO. Available at http://www.who.int/healthsystems/strategy/everybodys_business.pdf, last accessed on 2 November 2017.

17

Strategic Analysis of India's Private Hospital Sector

Akshat Kumar, Rohit Gupta, and Lawton R. Burns

An analysis of any country's healthcare industry typically centres on its hospital sector. Hospitals constitute two of the three arms of healthcare delivery: primary, secondary, and tertiary.[1] While primary care addresses the needs of individuals on an ambulatory basis by the clinician of first contact (often a primary care physician, nurse practitioner, or physician assistant), secondary and tertiary services are typically offered through referrals to specialists and sub-specialists located in hospital inpatient and outpatient departments. According to the data in India's National Health Accounts (NHA), primary care constituted 45.5 per cent of current health expenditures in 2013–14, while secondary and tertiary care accounted for 34.8 per cent and 17.1 per cent, respectively (MoHFW 2016).

In India, hospitals offer both allopathic and traditional Indian (or AYUSH: Ayurvedic, Yoga and Naturopathy, Unani, Siddha, Homeopathy) medicine. Combined, these accounted for 30 per cent of all healthcare spending at the start of the new millennium (based on 2001–2 NHA data) and ranked second in all spending behind drugs (38 per cent) (Burns 2014). The most recent NHA data for 2013–14 shows the picture has not changed much since 2002—32 per cent of 'current health expenditures' are on hospitals versus 39.6 per cent on pharmaceuticals.[2] Overall, healthcare delivery (excluding pharmaceuticals) accounts for the major share of spending, accounting for 47.7 per cent of current expenditures (MoHFW 2016).

GROWTH OF INDIA'S HEALTHCARE INDUSTRY

Tailwinds to Growth

The present size and growth rate of India's healthcare industry have far exceeded expectations (Burns, Srinivasan, and Vaidya 2014). By 2017, analysts estimated that the total spending in India's healthcare industry had reached USD 160 billion. The market size accelerated

[1] A fourth category, quaternary care, is an extension of tertiary care in reference to advanced levels of medicine which are highly specialized and not widely accessed. Experimental medicine and some types of uncommon diagnostic or surgical procedures are considered quaternary care.

[2] 'Current health expenditures' are defined as non-capital spending, estimated to be 93 per cent of total spending.

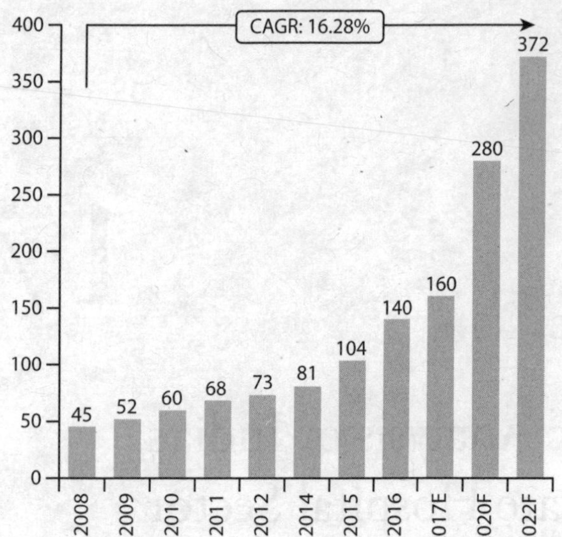

Figure 17.1 Healthcare Sector Growth Trend (in billion USD)

Source: Frost and Sullivan, Deloitte, LSI Financial Services, TechSci Research, and IBEF.org.
Notes: E – estimate; F – forecast.

from a compound annual growth rate (CAGR) of 16.5 per cent (2008–20 overall) to 22.9 per cent during the last five years of this period (2015 to 2020). This will result in an industry spend of USD 372 billion by 2022 (IBEF 2019). Based on the current growth trend depicted in Figure 17.1, India will rank among the top three healthcare markets globally in terms of incremental growth by 2022 (IBEF 2019).

A major driver of spending growth has been a change in the structure of healthcare delivery over the past several decades. Following Independence, the government-funded hospital system dominated care delivery in India. Today, by contrast, the majority of hospital expenditures occur in the private sector of healthcare delivery. Figure 17.2 shows that the government's contribution to total healthcare spend decreased from 34 per cent to 20 per cent between 2005 and 2018. At the same time, total healthcare spending as a percentage of India's gross domestic product (GDP) gradually increased from 4.3 per cent to 4.7 per cent. While this is far below the global average of 9.9 per cent, the private sector contributed more than 80 per cent of the spending and has emerged as the dominant player in the healthcare industry. Government spending on healthcare has remained more or less stagnant, remaining between 1.3 per cent and 1.5 per cent of GDP (Ministry of Finance 2016).

Several other structural factors have driven this more than expected growth of private sector spending (see Figure 17.3). These include *economic factors* such as high GDP growth and increasing national income, which have helped fuel healthcare utilization as a luxury good by the ever-expanding upper middle class. India overtook China in GDP growth in 2015 and reached 7.1 per cent in 2016; however, the country has suffered several consecutive quarters of falling growth since early 2016. Structural factors also include *demographic factors* such as a growing population (and a growing population that is working and productive). India is expected to overtake China in population size by 2028 (if not sooner), and to continue growing until 2061. Other

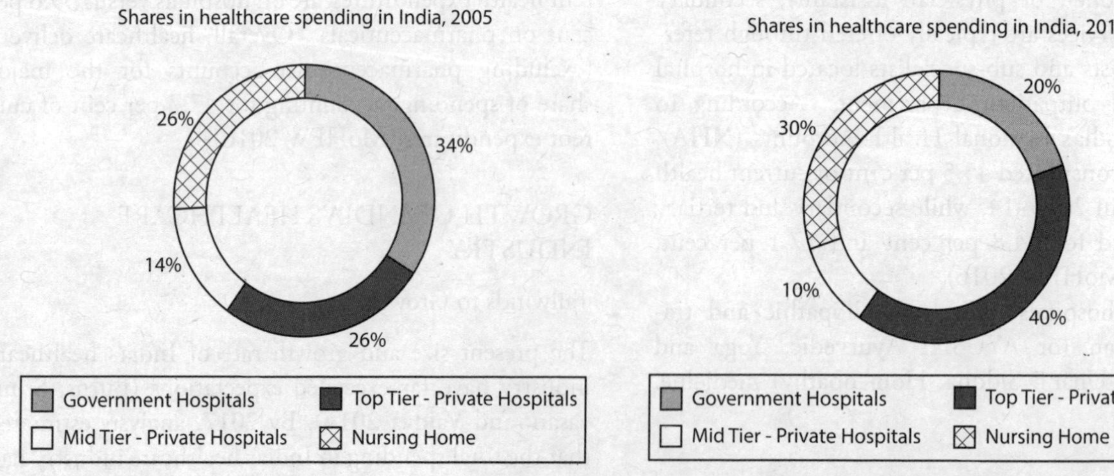

Figure 17.2 Public versus Private Shares of Spending on Healthcare 2005 and 2015

Source: 2005 data: A report on 'Indian Hospital Services Market Outlook' by consultancy RNCOS, Grant Thornton, LSI Financial Services, OECD, TechSci research. 2018 data: https://www.whatsnextcw.com/wp-content/uploads/2019/11/CW_India-Healthcare_Report_2019.pdf.

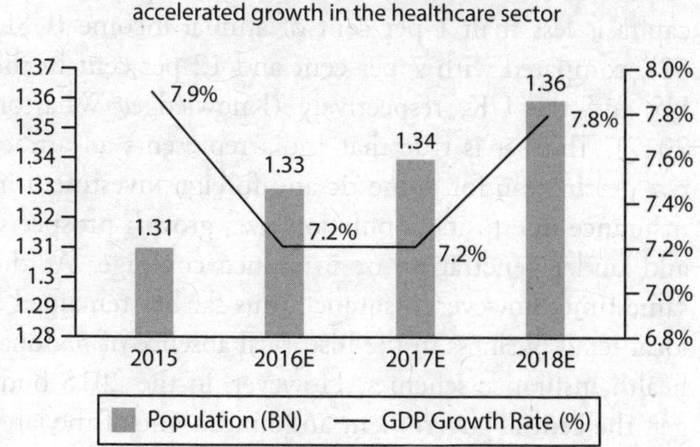

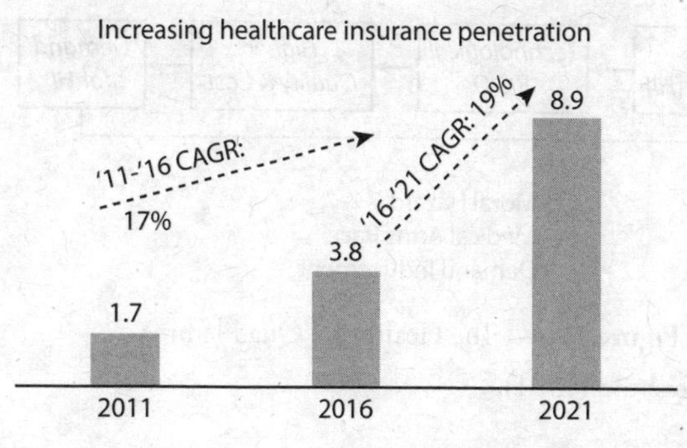

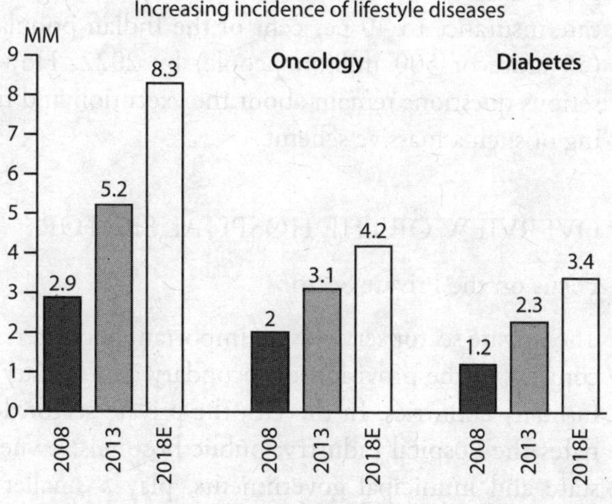

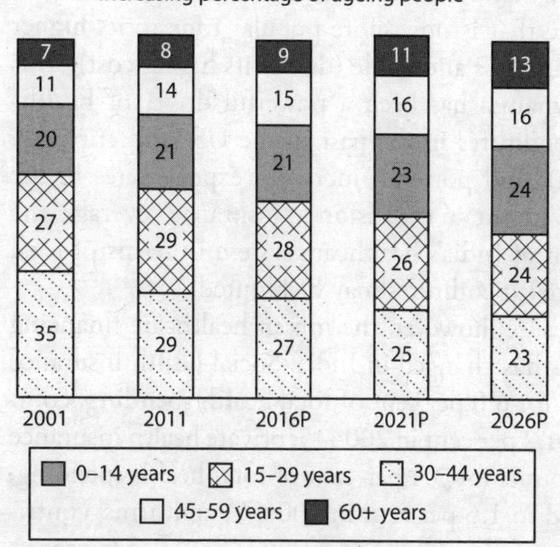

Figure 17.3 Demographic Changes in India

demographic drivers include an ageing population (due to increasing life expectancy and falling rates of fertility) and higher prevalence of chronic lifestyle-based diseases, which increase demand for healthcare. Finally, they include *increased penetration by private insurance* that makes healthcare utilization of the private sector more affordable.

Headwinds to Growth

Despite these positive forces, India's healthcare sector and overall economy face some strong headwinds to expansion. One such headwind is inertia in India's overall healthcare financing. Household spending as a percentage of total health expenditures has remained quite high: 67.7 per cent in 2013–14 compared to 71.1 per cent in 2004–5. By contrast, third-party payments financed through social insurance, private insurance, and firms have barely increased from 11.5 per cent in 2004–5 to 11.8 per cent in 2013–14, despite an increase in healthcare insurance penetration (MoHFW 2016).

Why is this important? A heavy reliance on out-of-pocket spending will limit the expansion of the healthcare sector for several reasons. First, the growth in the cost of healthcare typically exceeds the growth in GDP and disposable income, making healthcare less affordable over time. Second, families that rely on out-of-pocket spending typically consume less healthcare. Third, families typically prefer to save their limited incomes for future healthcare expenditures rather than purchase private health insurance.

Evidence from the US clearly shows that insurance drives 'the healthcare quadrilemma' (see Figure 17.4). According to this model, expansions in insurance

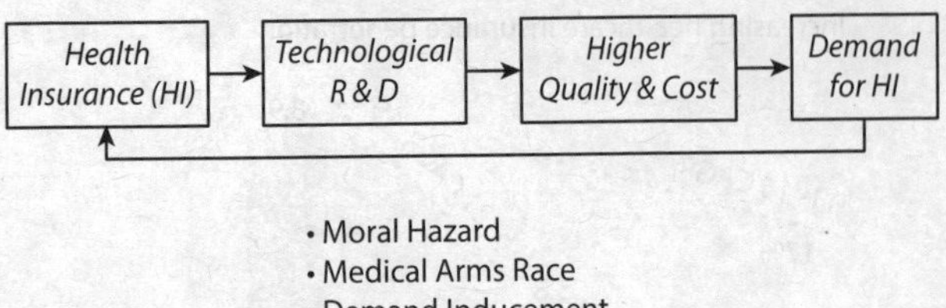

Figure 17.4 The Healthcare Quadilemma

Source: Weisbrod (1991).

coverage foster greater investment in technological research and development (R&D) which, in turn, lead to higher quality and cost of care. These, in turn, lead to more expensive healthcare which, in turn, cycles back to increase demand for more insurance coverage to finance healthcare that is now more popular (due to its higher quality) and less affordable (due to its higher cost). This causal dynamic has been a powerful driver of healthcare expenditures in the past in the US (and currently in China), and portends increased expenditures in the future. Without an expansion in insurance coverage, the expansion of India's healthcare system in terms of total healthcare expenditures may be blunted.

To be sure, however, the mix of healthcare financing payments has changed in India. Social health insurance accounts for 6.0 per cent of total health spending, compared to 4.2 per cent in 2004–5; private health insurance now accounts for 3.4 per cent of total health spending, compared to 1.6 per cent in 2004–5; and firms' contribution has fallen from 5.7 per cent to 2.4 per cent as insurance coverage has increased (MoHFW 2016).

At the same time, the absence of a significant healthcare quadrilemma may be a blessing in disguise for the Indian healthcare sector. The US experience suggests an insurance-driven market can lead to uncontrollable (and ultimately unsustainable) increases in costs that exceed GDP growth. Therefore, the inertia in healthcare financing in India may help to curb costs at the point of care. At the same time, however, this inertia places reimbursement pressure on private providers, which can threaten the quality of care and potentially lead to higher corruption.

It is also important to mention that while India's economy enjoys strong tailwinds in terms of population and economic growth, such growth potential has not yet been manifested in several related economic sectors. According to a recent report, India remains underinsured at just 3.9 per cent compared to the global average of 6.3 per cent; much of this coverage is in life insurance. Moreover, the annual insurance premium per capita is less than 1 per cent of annual income (USD 52), compared with 7 per cent and 12 per cent in the US and the UK, respectively (Knowledge@Wharton 2017). Thus, it is true that India represents an attractive destination for domestic and foreign investment in insurance due to its population size, growth prospects, and under-penetration of insurance coverage. At the same time, however, insurance thus far has remained a local retail business in the historical absence of national health insurance schemes. However, in the 2018 budget, the central government announced one of the largest government-funded healthcare programmes called the National Health Protection Scheme (NHPS). The programme sets an ambitious target of providing healthcare insurance to 40 per cent of the Indian population (50 crore or 500 million people) by 2022. However, serious questions remain about the execution and funding of such a massive scheme.

OVERVIEW OF THE HOSPITAL SECTOR

Focus on the Private Sector

The private sector serves as an important and interesting contrast in the provision of secondary and tertiary care in many countries. In the US, the private sector dominates the hospital industry; public hospitals, owned by state and municipal governments, play a smaller role in treating the population with commercial insurance and focus more on treating the poor and the indigent. The private sector in the US is heavily weighted towards nonprofit private hospitals as opposed to for-profit ('investor-owned') hospitals due to the historical roots of the industry in community-based and philanthropic sponsors (for instance, churches).

In China, by contrast, the public sector dominates in the provision of hospital care. This reflects the nationalization of hospitals (and government employment of physicians) under the Maoist regime in the 1950s. Only in the past few decades private, for-profit owners have been allowed and are now, publicly encouraged. This change in policy seeks to expand hospital bed capacity in the face of rising demand and ability to pay for healthcare (Burns and Liu 2017).

In India, state and local governments have traditionally operated medium and large-sized hospitals, while small hospitals (often referred to as 'nursing homes') were privately operated by entrepreneurial physicians. From the 1980s, for-profit chains consisting of medium-sized secondary hospitals began to form and spread through the country's large cities. The private sector grew in tandem with encouragement from the World Bank, the International Monetary Fund (IMF), and others, who questioned the efficiency of health provision through the public sector. The number of private health enterprises rose sharply after 1990 during the liberalization of the Indian economy, and particularly after 2000 following the rollout of liberalization policies in the country's healthcare sector.

One interesting contrast between China and India is that public hospitals are regarded as higher in quality in the former, while for-profit hospitals are regarded as higher in quality in the latter. This perception has only recently emerged in India during the post-liberalization phase. More than 20 years ago, patients used to prefer public hospitals for all complicated and critical care. However due to higher investments in technology and manpowe, patient preferences have shifted towards the private sector. Another factor favouring private hospitals is the desire for quality and respectful treatment on the part of the poor, who are willing to borrow to finance this care. There are, nevertheless, some national premier public institutes—the All India Institute of Medical Sciences (AIIMS) in Delhi and the Postgraduate Institute of Medical Education and Research (PGIMER) in Chandigarh, for instance—that continue to deliver world class medical education and research to the benefit of large volumes of patients at subsidized costs. Thus, there are examples of a few public institutions offering world-class care, just as private hospitals offer care that is highly variable in both quality and cost. The only constant in this equation is the variability in standards of care across both public and private hospitals.

Rise of India's Private Hospital Sector

India's healthcare sector, especially in the provision of hospital services, has come to be dominated by the private sector. This reflects two forces: private sector investment and stagnation in public sector spending. Survey data from waves of the National Sample Survey Office (NSSO), conducted under the auspices of the Government of India, chart the growth of 'unorganized service sector enterprises'. These enterprises include physicians, hospitals, nursing homes, dentists, laboratories, and a host of other formal and informal practitioners. The data shows an explosion in the formation of private enterprises from roughly 80,000 during 1981–90 to more than 630,000 during 2001–10. Comparing these same epochs, the number of private hospitals grew from 8,123 to 52,240, accounting for 7.8 per cent of total private healthcare enterprises (Hooda 2015).

Over time, privately owned hospitals have displaced their counterparts in the public sector. Between 1988 and 2000, the share of hospitals in the private sector rose from 55.9 per cent to 74.9 per cent; between 1988 and 2013, the share of hospital beds in the private sector grew from 30.4 per cent to 50.7 per cent. Between 1987 and 2014, the share of inpatient care treatments rendered in the private sector grew from 40.0 per cent to 68.0 per cent, while the share of outpatient treatments remained roughly constant at 77 per cent (Hooda 2015). These statistics are consistent with other, more recent data indicating that private healthcare accounts for anywhere from 60 per cent to 74 per cent of India's total healthcare expenditures (IBEF 2017; Malik, Solanki, and Menon 2016).[3] India's hospital industry generated anywhere from USD 63 billion to USD 80 billion in revenues in 2015, with a 24.2 per cent trailing five-year CAGR.

This displacement has been partly financed by rising out-of-pocket costs borne by patients, which have recently become a source of public outrage and media coverage. Going forward, India will do well to chart its own unique path of an innovative balance between (a) higher quality, higher cost private care; and (b) lower quality, lower cost public care. Public–private partnerships (PPPs), supply chain, and delivery system innovations to cut costs and improve quality for larger patient volumes, may help progress towards this goal.

Horizontal Integration and Concentration

Perhaps the biggest trend in the hospital sector in most countries since the middle of the past century has been horizontal integration into multi-unit chains (also known as multi-hospital systems). This trend began in the US in the late 1960s following the passage of Medicare and Medicaid, which extended health insurance coverage to two new segments of the population (the elderly and the poor, respectively). Four investor-owned (for-profit) hospital systems quickly entered the market, particularly in southern US states that had less organized labour and thus lower labour costs. This expansion in insurance coverage precipitated the healthcare quadrilemma portrayed in Figure 17.4 and the massive

[3] IBEF's estimate is 74 per cent. Edelweiss' estimate is USD 48 billion out of USD 85 billion.

escalation in national health expenditures in the US from 1965 to 1985. Some analysts argue that this series of events explains why healthcare spending in the US nominally and as a percentage of GDP far exceeds the rest of the world.

One way to operationalize the horizontal integration of a healthcare sector is its degree of 'concentration'. This can be measured in several alternate ways including the percentage of the market controlled by the 'top four' players (the Herfindahl–Hirschman Index [HHI]),[4] the number of multi-unit chains, the percentage of facilities belonging to multi-institutional chains, and the percentage of hospital beds in such chains. While such statistics are readily calculable in the US at both local and national levels, the available data from India do not permit most of these calculations.

What little data we have suggests that approximately 80 per cent of India's hospital industry is 'unconcentrated', defined as small, independent facilities, many of them single-specialty in nature. Indeed, the NSSO data referenced above segments private health enterprises in India by those with a single worker, those with two to five workers, those with six to 10 workers (called 'medium'), and those with 11+ workers (called 'large') (Hooda 2015). According to this data, only 2.9 per cent are medium and only 1.8 per cent of private enterprises are large. If we focus only on hospitals, 53 per cent have six or more workers. World Bank data suggests that only 30 per cent of India's hospitals have more than 150 beds; many hospitals have fewer than 30 beds. The supply of beds is also low relative to the country's large population: India has only 0.7 beds per thousand people compared to 2–4 beds per thousand in other emerging markets. In summary, the Indian hospital market remains highly fragmented despite the spate of mergers and acquisitons as discussed later in the chapter.

Diversification of Services

Another way to analyse hospitals is in terms of their service mix (or diversification). Most hospitals in the US are general medical–surgical facilities that treat patients across a range of clinical areas (such as medicine, surgery, obstetrics, pediatrics, ophthalmology, and so on). Historically, a handful of US hospitals catered to specific population segments (for example, children's hospitals) or diseases (for example, tuberculosis, psychiatric disorders), but they have remained a minority. From the 1980s, a new crop of US hospitals developed around single specialities (for example, cardiac care, orthopedics, women's health) with substantial physician ownership, often financed by Wall Street capital. Such facilities became more widely known as 'focused factories'. Public concerns over possible 'cherry-picking' and diversion of healthier patients to such facilities and away from general medical–surgical hospitals led to a moratorium on focused factories in 2003 and their legal prohibition in 2010.

The story is quite different in India. Indian hospitals run under various degrees of service diversification. Hospital corporations or trusts can run both single-speciality hospitals (for example, eye hospitals) and multi-speciality (general medical–surgical) hospitals. There are few statistics on the service mix of India's hospitals, but there are several well-known case studies of single-speciality facilities (for example, Narayana Health, Vaatsalya, Aravind, L.V. Prasad, and so on) (Burns 2014). Indeed, some of these facilities are repeatedly offered to their US counterparts as 'lessons to be learned' (Richman and Schulman 2017).

Governance Models

There is also great diversity among Indian hospitals in terms of their governance. Indian hospitals operate under the three models of governance described in the following paragraphs.

Trust and Management Services Company Model

In this model, a trust procures land from the government and constructs a hospital upon it. The trust may then manage the hospital itself or may engage professional service providers to run and manage the hospital. This model includes certain restrictions on expansion and requirements to render services to poor patients.

Corporate Hospital Model

In this model, a company buys the land and then constructs the hospital upon it. This model requires more funding to finance the cost of the land, which is quite expensive. As a result, highly-reputed and well-established corporate houses tend to use this model. The corporate house hires a management services company

[4] The HHI is a commonly accepted measure of market concentration. It is calculated by squaring the market share of each firm competing in a market, and then summing the resulting numbers, and can range from close to 0 to 10,000.

to run and manage the hospital. This model is preferred among investors.

Physician Group Model

In this model, groups of successful doctors from different disciplines collaborate to start large hospitals. The doctors utilize a partnership, limited liability partnership (LLP), or private limited company. Though these doctors are comfortable with bank debt, they seem to be increasingly amenable to private equity investment as well. This model is fast emerging in Tier 2 and Tier 3 cities.

MAJOR PRIVATE HOSPITAL CHAINS

India's hospital sector is best known internationally for its private hospital systems, not its public-sector institutions. This is partly due to several case studies by Harvard Business School (and other universities) on such institutions as Apollo, Fortis, and Narayana Health (Herzlinger and Virk 2008; Khanna, Rangan, and Manocaran 2005; Oberholzer-Gee, Khanna, and Knoop 2007). We provide a brief overview of several of the biggest players in Figure 17.5 and in the following paragraphs.

Apollo Hospitals Group

The Apollo Hospitals Group is India's largest nationwide, multi-speciality chain of hospitals. Apollo has vertically integrated beyond hospitals to include standalone pharmacies, diagnostic clinics, and primary clinics. Apollo began in 1983 as a 150-bed hospital in Chennai, Tamil Nadu, and was founded by Prathap Reddy, a cardiologist with considerable clinical experience in the US. The hospital, the first for-profit facility in India, subsequently grew from 150 to 600 beds.

Apollo initially concentrated much of its capacity in southern India but has since diversified geographically. Starting from its base in Chennai, Apollo has focused on (i) organic growth rather than acquisitions; and (ii) building tertiary and quaternary hospitals in several tier 1 cities. In 1988, Apollo built a second hospital in Hyderabad. By 2000, Apollo had added six more facilities in Delhi, Madurai (Tamil Nadu), Visakhapatnam (Andhra Pradesh), Aragonda (Andhra Pradesh), and

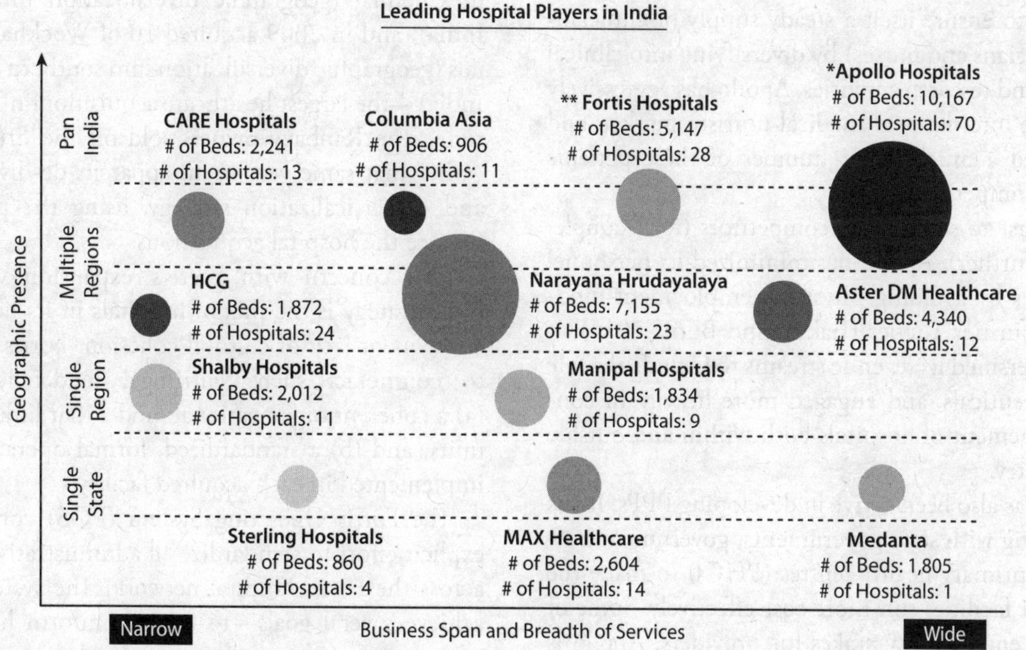

Figure 17.5 Private Hospital Business Span and Breadth of Service

* Beds as on 30 June 2019, ** Fortis presentation (Demerger of hospitals business of Fortis into Manipal) as of March 2018, publicly available on Fortis Healthcare Ltd.'s website and https://www.apollohospitals.com/apollo_pdf/AHEL-Investor-Presentation-June19-INR.pdf.
Source: Company Reports, CRISIL Research.

a specialty facility in Chennai. By 2004, it had added facilities in Mysuru (Karnataka), Ahmedabad (Gujarat), Bilaspur (Chhattisgarh), Kolkata (West Bengal), and also in Sri Lanka, in the capital Colombo. Between 2004 and 2010, Apollo doubled its overall capacity from 4,000 to 8,000 beds; with a jump in operating revenues from USD 147 million to USD 457 million.

As of 2019, Apollo has 10,167 beds—25 per cent added in the past three to four years—spread across 70 hospitals, along with more than 2,500 pharmacies. Apollo has the highest market share (28 per cent) in terms of operational beds among its listed Indian peers. Apollo's average revenue per occupied bed (ARPOB) grew roughly 9 per cent per annum over the past five years, owing to average annual price hikes of 3–4 per cent and a roughly 4 per cent increase driven by a more complex case mix and shorter hospital stays (higher patient turnover). It has sought to develop high local market share to drive utilization, scale economies, and charge premium prices. Being the market leader, Apollo enjoys the advantage of being the price setter across all regions.

Apollo strives for efficiency in delivering healthcare services, particularly through tightly controlled operating costs and high utilization of equipment. It seeks to grow its revenues by expanding outside of the tier 1 cities into the tier 2 and tier 3 markets. Moreover, it has sought to ensure itself a steady supply of clinicians (both physicians and nurses) by diversifying into clinical education and research activities. Apollo has aggressively targeted the international medical tourism market, and has garnered a much larger number of these patients relative to competitors.

In contrast to some of its competitors (for example, Fortis; see further), Apollo has minimized its personnel expenditures by avoiding physician employment models, at least in tier 1 cities (Bakshi and Burns 2014). It has also diversified its revenue streams to include the sale of pharmaceuticals, and engaged more heavily in contract management of hospitals both within and outside of the country.

Apollo has also been active in developing PPPs. It has been working with state governments, government hospitals, and primary health centres (PHCs) to make the government facilities run more cost-effectively. Some of these PPPs entail equity stakes for providers. Apollo is also helping run some government teaching hospitals and develop government trauma centres; the latter are sorely needed to handle the high number of traffic accident victims in India.

Fortis Healthcare

Fortis Healthcare was established in 1996 by the owners of Ranbaxy, one of India's largest pharmaceutical companies and one of the world's top generic pharmaceuticals manufacturers. Ranbaxy's owners envisioned Fortis as a vertically integrated, 'end-to-end' healthcare organization with capabilities in drug research, clinical trials, laboratory services, and healthcare services delivery. During the earlier years of its operation, Fortis focused on the hospital business, building up a large chain of tertiary care facilities. Several years ago, they began to sell off some of their non-hospital assets and disaggregated.

The first Fortis hospital was opened in 2001 in Mohali, a city in the northern Indian state of Punjab. The state's per-capita income is among the highest nationwide and is home to one of the largest populations of affluent non-resident Indians. Like its American investor-owned counterparts, Fortis Healthcare system targeted more lucrative geographic markets from the start.

Fortis built its first few hospitals on a greenfield basis, diversifying into New Delhi in 2003–4. As with investor-owned systems in the US, however, Fortis expanded largely through acquisitions of other systems. In 2005, Fortis acquired Escorts' hospitals (three owned and one managed in Delhi), thereby tripling its bed capacity. In 2008, Fortis acquired a stake in Malar Hospitals in Chennai (geographic diversification into southern India), and in 2009 acquired 10 of Wockhardt's hospitals (geographic diversification into southern and eastern India)—the largest healthcare acquisition in India at the time. The Ranbaxy owners sold off the drug business earlier that same year in an apparent de-diversification and de-verticalization strategy, using the proceeds to finance the hospital acquisitions.

One concern with Fortis's 'expansion via acquisition' strategy is the mix of hospitals in its network and consequent lack of cultural cohesion. Fortis has sought to counteract such centrifugal tendencies through (a) a coherent organizational model that links operating units; and (b) a standardized, formal operating system implemented in each acquired facility.

The Fortis Operating System (FOS) constitutes an explicit effort to standardize all administrative processes across the Fortis hospital network. The system aims to achieve several goals—to ensure uniform high quality of patient-facing processes to make them more patient-centric, embed best practices in operational efficiency, facilitate performance management across all hospital sites, and positively impact the system's bottom line.

The ultimate goal is to help Fortis scale up its hospital network faster and with the right quality of care. Fortis executives believe this effort will enable the system to pursue its 'ability mantra': provide service that is predictable, service that is on time, and service that is available for all—in effect, conquer its own version of the 'iron triangle of healthcare' (Burns 2014).

The FOS developed initially at Fortis Hospital in Mohali out of a major investment in information technology (IT). It is used to manage hospital capacity, patient flow, facility services, and performance monitoring. It concentrates on the major ARPOB drivers—specialty mix, pricing, length of stay, bed turnover, patient volume, and procedure volume. This is Fortis' key operating metric, reflecting their heavy preoccupation (shared by other hospital systems in India) with efficient, low-cost, and high-volume operations. In keeping with this strategy, full occupancy and efficiency trump brand image. Indeed, the fastest and easiest way to achieve scale economies is by increasing utilization of existing capacity, for example, by decreasing length of stay, decreasing procedure times, increasing bed and procedure room turnover rates, and increasing patient volume. Nevertheless, full occupancy synergistically promotes brand image—high volumes give Fortis' facilities the public perception of being 'busy places' and thus highly demanded sites of care.

As a result of its focus on maximizing ARPOB, Fortis is able to quickly implement new processes and monitor those processes in the acquired hospitals. Such processes include an array of access measures (such as percentage of patients waiting beyond the appointment time, and percentage of same-day consultations), throughput measures (such as turnaround time for laboratory results, percentage of X-ray reports ready within 30 minutes, and percentage of critical call-outs not communicated to clinicians), and output measures (such as percentage of planned discharges, percentage of discharges before 11 a.m., and overall discharge time).

Healthcare information technology (IT) acquired from a Boston-based hospital system (Partners Healthcare) forms the backbone of Fortis' system for electronic medical records (EMRs), patient safety, and quality compliance. As a result, patients' medical records are easily transferred between the hub and the spoke hospitals. The continuous monitoring of outcomes also allows systems to be modified to increase efficiency and make them more convenient for the patient. For example, Fortis reduced the lab turnaround time for results from over seven hours to one hour.

In 2018, IHH Healthcare Berhad, a Malaysian-Singaporean private healthcare group, acquired a controlling stake in Fortis Healthcare (31 per cent) for INR 40 billion. This is the first major investment by a foreign company for a primary controlling interest in a private hospital chain in India. The Fortis Board also approved appointment of 4 IHH nominees on its 7 member reconstituted board. The deal got the approval of the anti-trust regulator Competition Commision of India. With this, IHH was successfully able to outbid other private equity firms, especially the offer from a consortium of Manipal Health Enterprises and TPG Capital. According to Bhavdeep Singh, former CEO of Fortis, the strategy going forward is to grow the hospital and diagnostics businesses, and to focus on the system's two customers—patients and their providers.

Max Healthcare

Max India was established in 1985 as a public limited company with a mission to establish niche, 'life-centred' businesses in insurance, healthcare, and clinical research. Max Healthcare, the healthcare delivery business of Max India, opened its first outpatient facility in 2000 and its first hospital in 2002, and then quickly expanded its presence in northern India.

Like Apollo and Fortis, Max offers specialty care institutes in several clinical areas: heart and vascular, neurosciences, orthopaedics, cancer, plastic and reconstructive surgery, minimal access and bariatric surgery, obstetrics and gynaecology, and paediatrics. The Max network began as a hub-and-spoke model (HSM) with primary and secondary care facilities spread across Delhi feeding into its state-of-the-art tertiary care facility at Saket, New Delhi. Over the years, it has evolved into a truly networked architecture where each hospital occupies a nodal position in the network with its unique strengths and characteristics.

Unlike Apollo and Fortis, Max Healthcare has not followed a national and international expansion strategy. Instead, it has remained more regionally focused on the north Indian landscape. Max follows the 'Shatabdi' strategy—their new hospitals come up along the route of the Shatabdi Express train. This enables the organization to leverage the entire network and to allocate its resources most efficiently (clinical and non-clinical) among all its hospitals.

Revenues are driven through innovative marketing techniques, largely geared towards walk-ins and international patients, and supported by robust operating processes. These processes allow the organization to drive efficiencies in various areas such as discharge turnaround times and supply chain (such as procurement) efficiencies.

Two key differentiators for Max have always been its emphasis on clinical excellence and the keen focus on service quality. These enable the company to deliver a holistic patient experience and drive higher brand recall. Clinical excellence efforts at Max are geared towards achieving 100 per cent patient safety and, increasingly, measuring clinical outcomes and attaining global benchmarks. Continuous training ensures that the clinical staff is up to date with best practices. In recent times, Max has also focused on leveraging IT management systems such as an EMR system in order to further its clinical excellence agenda. The implementation of the EMR system has begun to show early benefits encompassing cost efficiencies, improved resource utilization, process standardization, and, more importantly, improved quality of patient care.

Service excellence efforts are focused on ensuring a consistent patient experience across all Max facilities. To this end, Max has designed and implemented standard operating procedures for all customer touchpoints. The staff undergoes extensive training in all nonclinical areas such as front office, finance and billing, housekeeping, and so on, and is periodically audited and re-trained wherever required.

Max believes that its people are its greatest strength and works towards creating a unique value proposition at various levels across the managerial, administrative, and clinical workforce. Its culture of service, patient care, hospitality, and doing the right thing is integral to the vision and values of the organization. The company therefore endeavours to hold all its employees to these high standards.

In 2018, Radiant Life Care Private Limited, a hospital management company promoted by Abhay Soi and backed by global investment firm KKR, acquired a majority stake in Max Healthcare from Max India. This led to demerger of Max's non healthcare assets (Max Bupa and Antara Senior Living) into a separate entity owned by Max India. Radiant Life Care already ran two successful hospitals—BLK multi-speciality hospital in Delhi and Nanavati in Mumbai. The combination of Radiant and Max Healthcare would create the largest hospital network in North India, which will become one of the top three hospital networks in India by revenue and the fourth largest in India in terms of operating beds. The combined business is expected to provide significant growth potential and compelling business synergies. The Radiant group is known for taking over 'sick units' and making them profitable through sound management.

Narayana Health

Narayana Health (originally Narayana Hrudayalaya) was started in Bengaluru by Mother Teresa's cardiac surgeon, Devi Shetty, in 2001. His mission was to lower the cost of heart surgery and other tertiary care in order to make it affordable for a greater percentage of the Indian population. Cardiac surgeries in the US can cost up to USD 50,000; in India, by contrast, they typically cost USS 5,000 to USD 7,000. Shetty not only managed to reduce the cost even further to USD 1,800, but also implemented schemes to help patients pay these (lower) medical bills.

Narayana's business model is based on several components. First, outpatients who seek care at the facilities finance the care of inpatients; margins on the outpatient side approach 80 per cent, while inpatient margins are negligible.

Second, Shetty focuses on high volumes and patient throughput, based on reductions in lengths of stay and the productivity of his surgeons. By 2012, his Bengaluru hospital performed 35 heart surgeries a day; with a goal to reach 50–60 surgeries per day. Shetty employs cardiac surgeons and pays them a fixed salary at rates comparable to those at other hospitals. However, he requires them to treat more patients, thereby reducing the professional cost per procedure. To promote efficiency, computerized tomography (CT) scanners and magnetic resonance imaging (MRI) machines are used for 14 hours a day (compared to eight hours per day usage at most hospitals); higher utilization reduces the cost per test. To smooth out patient demand, patients are charged lower rates for tests conducted in late evening. All these strategies serve as a source of natural scale economies (that is, spreading higher volume over fixed capital and labour costs).

Third, Narayana surgeons specialize in only three or four types of operations; younger surgeons, by contrast, do anywhere from 10–15 different types of procedures. The focus and specialization provides not only a source of additional scale economies but also continual learning, thereby improving the quality of patient outcomes.

In addition, Shetty places great emphasis on the ability of large volumes to drive down costs for hospital vendors, which then pass savings along to his facilities in the form of lower input prices. The large volume of surgeries at Narayana thus allows Shetty to achieve savings in consumables and equipment. Narayana Hrudayalaya saves 40 per cent on gloves by importing them by the container-load from Malaysia. Shetty's team also convinced an equipment vendor who wanted to use Narayana as a referral to park its catheterization laboratory at the hospital free of charge.

The system also foregoes extraneous amenities (for example, air-conditioning in cooler climates), reducing hospital capex and operational costs compared to rival systems. According to Shetty's son Viren, an engineer and director at the hospital, 'The way we design the hospitals and our close monitoring of our projects help us to keep a very tight control of our construction costs.'

The Narayana organization has gone beyond cost-saving innovations. In the early 2000s, a famine in the region caused problems with affordable healthcare for farmers. To increase access to healthcare, Shetty proposed a micro-health insurance scheme to increase patients' ability to pay. The Karnataka State Government launched the Yeshasvini micro-health insurance plan (run by an independent contractor) in 2003. Farmers paid INR 60 annually to obtain coverage for 1,650 different types of surgeries. The plan initially covered 1.7 million farmers, and has since expanded to cover 3 million farmers (2017–18) at a premium of INR 300 per year. Enrollees account for about 10 per cent of Narayana's patients; another 15 per cent of patients receive discounts depending on their ability to pay. Shetty also offers luxury private and semi-private rooms for procedure recovery as part of a high-end package priced at USD 4,000 to USD 5,000, which helps to subsidize the procedures for patients who cannot pay. To understand their ability to offer discounts and subsidies while maintaining financial viability, the management team studies profit-and-loss performance on a daily basis, allowing them to assess the discounts they can offer the next day without adversely impacting profitability.

Narayana operates under an asset-light business model, and is predominantly an affordable healthcare provider. Its multi-unit chain of 23 multispeciality hospitals and seven heart centres ranks Narayana as a top-three player (by 2019's bed count) in India's hospital industry, with 7,155 beds. It has a pan-India presence, and most of its hospitals have multispeciality offerings, with a focus on cardiac and renal care. Given its focus on the affordable income category, around 65 per cent of its capacity is geared toward general wards. It adds new hospitals and beds to its network with low capital investment through revenue share agreements, lease agreements, and managed care contracts.

Medanta Hospital

Medanta—The Medicity, located in Gurugram, Harayana, was founded in 2009 by Naresh Trehan, an eminent cardiac surgeon. It is one of India's largest multispeciality institutes with six centres of excellence, 1,520 operational beds (including over 350 critical care beds), and 37 operation theatres catering to over 20 specialties. Medanta has also partnered with other hospitals in Ranchi and Indore.

Its flagship facility in Gurugram has 1,250 operational beds. It has one facility each in Indore (95 beds) and Ranchi (175 beds). It also features operational clinics and other services that include Medanta Mediclinic (DLF Cybercity, Gurugram; and Defence Colony, New Delhi), Neuroscience Clinic in Patna, an airport clinic at Delhi Airport, and air ambulance services. Medanta has plans to expland further: it opened a 1,000-bed facility in Lucknow in 2019 and laid foundation stones of a 700-bed hospital in Noida (both in states of UP). In fiscal year (FY) 2016, Medanta earned revenues of USD 227 million. It enjoys high occupancy and ARPOBs, resulting in some of the highest EBITDA margins and ROCEs across industry.[5] In 2016, it achieved an EBITDA of USD 54 million (23.7 per cent EBITDA margin).

Manipal Hospital

Founded in 1991, Manipal was India's third largest healthcare group, with more than 4,900 operational beds across 15 hospitals and eight locations (as of March 2016). Manipal's specialties include oncology, cardiology, cosmetic surgery, orthopaedics, and rheumatology. Manipal is selectively exploring both organic and inorganic growth strategies in international markets including the Middle East, where the group has an education business footprint, and in Malaysia. Manipal earned revenues of USD 288 million revenue in FY17 and EBITDA of USD 38 million (13.3 per cent EBITDA margin). As noted above, Manipal is merging with Fortis Hospitals to become the largest hospital chain in the country.

[5] 'EBITDA' refers to a company's earnings before interest, depreciation, and taxes. 'ROCE' refers to return on the capital employed, and is measured by earnings before interest and taxes (EBIT) divided by capital employed.

CARE Hospital

The CARE Hospitals Group operates 13 hospitals with 2,241 beds, serving six cities across five states in India. CARE is the regional leader in tertiary care in south/central India and among the top five pan-India hospital chains. CARE Hospitals delivers comprehensive care in more than 30 specialities in tertiary care settings. CARE is a complete healthcare ecosystem, with related components of education, training, and research. A network of telemedicine hubs in rural Andhra Pradesh and Maharashtra deliver care at the doorstep to hundreds of thousands of people. These activities are managed by its partner, CARE Foundation. Adopting a service-oriented delivery model, its core purpose is 'to provide care that people trust'.

CARE Hospitals was founded in 1997 by B. Soma Raju and a team of India's leading cardiologists. The founders developed Asia's first indigenous coronary stent, the 'Kalam–Raju stent,' named after A.P.J. Abdul Kalam, former president of India, and Raju, CARE's chairman and managing director. CARE Hospitals has developed several innovations in an effort to make healthcare affordable for all, while ensuring clinical outcomes at par with international standards.

KIMS Hospital

Founded in 2004, KIMS operates a network of multispeciality hospitals in Andhra Pradesh and Telangana, with approximately 1,600 beds spread across five hospitals including one tier 1 location (Hyderabad, Telangana) and several tier 2 and 3 locations (Nellore, Rajahmundry, and Srikakulam in Andhra Pradesh). The company is led by Bhaskar Rao, a renowned cardio-thoracic surgeon. It earned revenues of USD 90 million and EBITDA of USD 18 million (EBITDA margin of 20.6 per cent).

Aster Medicity

As one of the newer players on the block, Aster Medcity is a quaternary healthcare centre in the southern Indian city of Kochi, Kerala. It is owned and managed by Aster DM Healthcare, a Dubai-based healthcare conglomerate founded by Azad Moopen. It is a USD 85 million waterfront facility and one of the largest in the state of Kerala with a capacity of 670 beds. It has been operational since 2014 and has expanded gradually to a 12-hospital chain with 4,340 beds under the Aster DM Healthcare company name.

IMPORTANT MACRO TRENDS

There are at least four macro-level trends unique to India that deserve specific mention. These include the pivotal role of nonprofit/trust hospitals, the growth of medical tourism, the shift towards HSM, and the increased penetration of private hospitals into tier 2 and tier 3 cities. These are discussed in the following paragraphs.

Pivotal Role of Nonprofit/Trust Hospitals

India's hospital sector has traditionally included a set of so-called 'Trust hospitals', which are equivalent to the nonprofit hospitals in the US. Since the country's Independence, these hospitals have played a pivotal role in the hospital sector. The underlying principle is simple. The government provides land at subsidized rates to a private entity; the entity earns profits from some segments of the population; those profits are used to provide subsidized care to people who otherwise could not afford it. Some of the earliest Trust hospitals in the capital city of Delhi were Sir Ganga Ram Hospital (SGRH), M.C.K.R. Hospital and Research Institute, and the Tirath Ram Shah Hospital. SGRH and Dayanand Medical College and Hospital (DMC, Punjab) are two of the largest Trust hospitals which have continued to proliferate in the post-liberalization era and play a pivotal role in shaping the hospital ecosystem in northern India.

Sir Ganga Ram Hospital, New Delhi

SGRH was first established at Lahore, Punjab (Pakistan) in 1921 by the philanthropist Sir Ganga Ram. After the Partition, the Sir Ganga Ram Trust Society constructed a hospital at its present location in Rajendra Nagar, New Delhi, in April 1954. Today, SGRH is a multi-speciality 675-bed hospital with two affiliated hospitals and 180 additional beds.

SGRH prides itself in being a 'People's Own Hospital', where economically stronger patients subsidize the treatment of the economically weaker section of the society. The Sir Ganga Ram Trust Society had been providing free treatment to patients admitted on 20 per cent of the total bed strength right from the inception of this hospital in 1954, even without any statutory directive from the Government of India at the time of allotment of land.

Dayanand Medical College and Hospital, Ludhiana, Punjab

DMC Ludhiana was conceived as a medical school in 1934 by an Indian army captain. Since 1964, it has been one of northern India's premier tertiary care centres and medical colleges. It has gradually expanded over the years to its current bed capacity of 1,048 beds. In 2001, DMC opened a single specialty facility (DMC Heart Centre) to provide sophisticated cardiac care.

Other Single-Speciality Centres

Additional single-speciality centres of excellence have proliferated over the recent years. Two targeted specialties are ophthalmology (such as Centre for Sight, Amar Eye Centre, Shroff Eye Centre in Delhi) and diabetes (Mohan Diabetic Centre in Chennai, Apollo's sugar clinics in Hyderabad). Other successful models—including the Fortis Escorts Heart Institute (New Delhi), the Asian Institute of Gastroenterology (Hyderabad), the Institute of Liver and Biliary Sciences (New Delhi)—have also grown remarkably in recent years. The biggest challenge for these emerging single-speciality hospitals is the requirement of support services from other specialities that patients may need. Consequently, in recent years, many of these single-speciality hospitals have diversified to become multi-speciality providers.

Growth of Medical Tourism

Medical tourism has long been posed as a growth driver of India's private hospitals. During the early 2000s, US consultants projected large, escalating expenditures by Western patients travelling to Asian destinations for cheaper care of comparable quality. Most of these projections were vastly inflated. Consultants failed to consider that US insurers (both commercial and public) may not pay for non-US healthcare, and that US providers might be unwilling or reticent to refer patients to global care sites due to issues of care continuity (Burns, Jayaram, and Bansal 2014). Despite the relative underperformance, the growth story of India's medical tourism industry is impressive.

Nevertheless, hope springs eternal. In 2015, India's medical tourism sector was estimated to be worth USD 3 billion, much lower than earlier forecasts. It is projected to grow to USD 12.5 billion by 2022 at a CAGR of ~20 per cent (see Figure 17.6). According to the Confederation of Indian Industries (CII), the primary driver of this growth is cost-effectiveness, that is, treatment from accredited facilities at par with developed countries at much lower cost. According to a report published in 2015, India has one of the lowest cost and highest quality of all medical tourism destinations (Nasdaq Market News 2016).

Shift to Hub-and-Spoke Model

With 70 per cent of Indians living in rural areas and making less than USD 3 per day, innovative models are required to serve the healthcare needs of the majority. The HSM has an innovative architecture that emphasizes optimal utilization of scarce healthcare resources in rural areas (Devarakonda 2016).

Harvard Business Review cited this model as a key innovative approach to provide high quality care at a lower cost (Govindarajan and Ramamurti 2013). According to the authors, 'in order to reach the masses of people in need of care, Indian hospitals create hubs in major metro areas and open smaller clinics (the spokes) in more rural areas which feed patients to the main hospitals (the hub), similar to the way that regional air

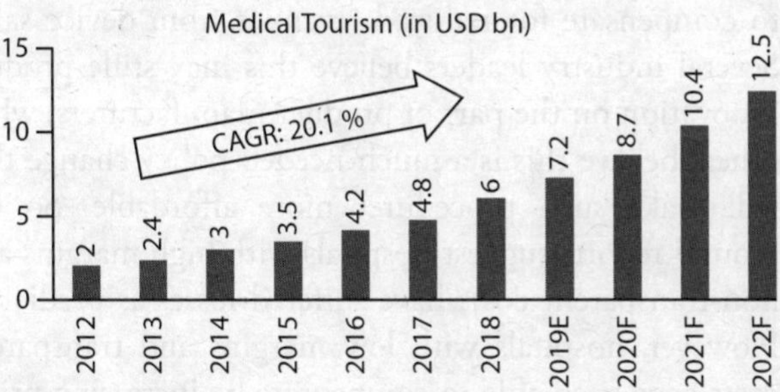

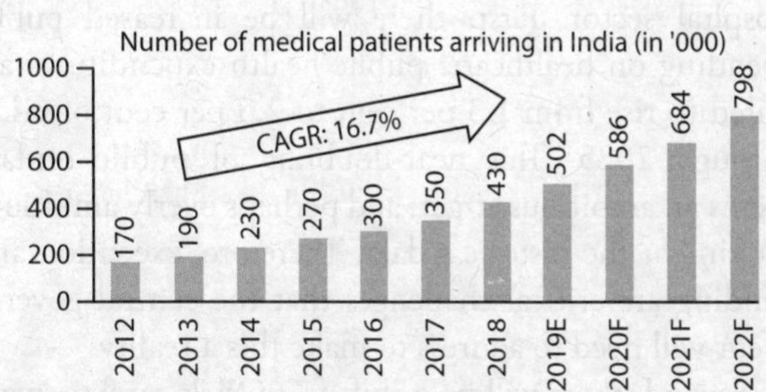

Figure 17.6 Medical Tourist Arrivals in India

Source: https://www.whatsnextcw.com/wp-content/uploads/2019/11/CW_India-Healthcare_Report_2019.pdf .

Notes: E – estimate; F – forecast.

routes feed passengers into major airline hubs'. There is little research in both the US and India regarding the competitive performance or advantage of the HSM approach. What little evidence that does exist suggests that locally-organized systems (which develop an HSM around a tertiary hospital) may achieve lower costs of care compared to more regionally-dispersed systems where patient referrals across facilities are impeded by sheer distances (Burns et al. 2015).

All the big hospital chains have experimented with this model in one form or the other. For example, multi-unit chains such as Apollo, Max Healthcare, and Fortis operate primary clinics as some of their spokes. Patient referrals from primary care clinics play a major role in total admissions at a tertiary care centre. They have also developed smaller secondary hospitals in Tier II and Tier III cities as spokes (feeders) to their tertiary hospitals in tier 1 cities. However, operational inefficiencies, regulatory hurdles, low margins and lack of leadership have slowed widespread adoption of these models by existing big healthcare systems.

Increased Penetration into Tier 2 and Tier 3 Cities

There is substantial demand for high-quality and specialty-based healthcare services in tier 2 and 3 cities. To encourage the private sector to establish hospitals in these cities, the government relaxed the taxes on these hospitals for the first five years (IBEF 2017). Vaatsalya Healthcare was one of the first hospital chains to target these cities for expansion. Apollo Hospitals is one of the largest players to enter these cities with its Apollo Reach initiative.

IMPACT OF RECENT POLICY CHANGES

The National Health Policy (NHP) 2017 has and will have several important implications for India's private hospital sector. First, there will be increased public spending on healthcare: public health expenditures are slated to rise from 1.3 per cent to 2.5 per cent of GDP through 2025. This near-doubling of public outlays seems an ambitious target, and perhaps overly ambitious looking at the historical data. Therefore, execution and funding are critical challenges that the central government will need to address to make this a reality.

Second, there will be a shift from 'sick care' to 'wellness' with a new focus on 'comprehensive primary healthcare services'. Third, as in the case of China, there is now a public focus on privatization. The government wishes to align the growth of the private healthcare sector with public health goals through a 'positive and proactive' engagement.

On the face of it, this is a positive development that signals the government's intention to increase its overall expenditures on healthcare as a percentage of GDP. It also recognizes the potential of PPPs in solving the complex challenges of India's healthcare system. A focus on preventive healthcare and wellness is also a welcome sign. Historically, however, there has been a huge gap between policy aims and achievements in India (and in other Asian countries like China as well) (Burns, Srinivasan, and Vaidya 2014). Hence, we will need to wait and see how many of these well-intentioned promises are actually realized.

The introduction of the NHP may carry some headwinds for private hospitals. The profit margins of private hospitals used to be driven by high margins on medical devices (such as cardiac stents, orthopaedic implants) and other higher-end consumable products. However, in February 2017, the Government of India placed coronary stents on its Essential Drugs List. Then, in August 2017, the country's National Pharmaceutical Pricing Authority (NPPA) issued orders setting price ceilings on orthopaedic knee implants (INR 54,720 to INR 113,950, exclusive of the Goods and Services Tax) in order to 'check unethical profiteering and exploitative pricing at the cost of the patients in an unregulated market' (Worstall 2017).

The move was designed to make healthcare more affordable and accessible to its low-income population. However, some fear that one impact might be the removal of high-priced implants from the Indian market by vendors, which will actually decrease access to higher-end technology. This can significantly affect the bottom line of private hospitals, who may now need to change their revenue model and corporate strategy. Some hospitals may hike the costs charged for related services (such as hospital stays and/or physician fees) in order to compensate for reduced revenues from device sales. Several industry leaders believe this may stifle product innovation on the part of product manufacturers, while others believe this is a much-needed policy change that will make such procedures more affordable. So far, ground reports suggest hospitals with high margins and non-transparent costs have suffered losses as predicted. However, hospitals with low margins and transparent costs have been able to compensate by increasing prices of other ancillary services. It remains to be seen how the policy implications will play out in areas like affordability, high tech innovation and hospital growth.

Some Indian states have taken comparable actions to contain the costs of private hospitals. The 2017 amendments proposed to the Karnataka Private Medical Establishments Bill would regulate hospital reimbursement for specific procedures to public insurance levels, prohibit them from balance-billing patients for any additional costs, and penalize physicians for negligence (in surgical cases) with fines or imprisonment. Providers countered by arguing that price-setting would hurt the medical tourism business and their business models, which rely on cross-subsidization of public patients by private-paying patients. Doctors in the state responded with a one-day strike (IANS 2017).

Overall, while the Indian population obtains at least 70 per cent of their healthcare services from the private sector, that sector has been increasingly identified as a major culprit in high-cost healthcare. The recent NSSO report indicates that private hospitals charge three times more than public hospitals for an admission; in some cases, such as eye care and obstetrics/neonatal care, the difference can be at least sixfold or eightfold, respectively (Hooda 2015). Moreover, a performance review of the country's private hospitals by the Comptroller and Auditor General suggests that most facilities may be avoiding state income taxes and not living up to their obligations to devote dedicated bed capacity to low-income patients who cannot pay (*The Hindu* 2017).

FUTURE OUTLOOK: THREATS AND OPPORTUNITIES

Three Major Risks

Going forward, India's hospital sector faces three major risks. First, due to the costs of land, equipment, and construction, the private hospital sector faces high capital needs and a long gestation period. It thus cannot quickly fill the needed bed capacity to handle the country's growing and underserved population. Second, due to the lack of a well-developed medical technology sector, the hospital sector is dependent on imports for medical equipment—estimated to be as high as 70 per cent (Burns et al. 2014). However, a 2014 regulation allowing 100 per cent foreign direct investment (FDI) in the medical equipment sector may reduce the overall import bill. Third, the country faces a shortage of qualified doctors and healthcare workers. There are currently fewer than ten 10 doctors per 10,000 people. Part of the reason for the shortage is loss of doctors to Western countries; another cause is the shortage and maldistribution of medical colleges across Indian states. High geographical variability in density of doctors is a related but separate problem.

Three Opportunities

The country also faces three opportunities. First, India's high growth rate, driven by stable structural economic and demographic factors, makes it one of the most lucrative emerging markets industries in the world. Second, the NHP 2017 recognizes the private sector as a key player, even in primary care. In addition, if the NHPS materializes, it will provide the funding for innovative PPPs to provide sustainable primary care in rural India and in tier 2 and 3 cities. Third, there are important opportunities to develop a medical tourism sector that can augment hospital revenues with private paying patients and allow facilities to treat patients with public insurance coverage.

The hospital sector in India is poised to rapidly expand through private investments. These will come not only from the nation's large for-profit systems profiled above, but also from external firms that enter through relaxed laws governing FDI, as well as from private equity firms that partner with local firms (Kumar 2014). The hospital sector is also expecting to grow through an anticipated influx of foreign medical tourists. Both trends, if witnessed, signal expansion and heightened competition in the sector.

The sector will also undergo significant organizational transformation as major players develop 'health cities', diversify into adjacent healthcare services businesses (for example, primary clinics, diagnostics, pharmacies), and diversify vertically into the health insurance business. As we have learned in the US, hospital providers have not historically developed the capabilities to run such businesses; indeed, they have lost a lot of money in these types of diversification moves. Even in the absence of diversification, the hospital systems in India will likely face the same challenges of horizontal integration confronting the multi-hospital chains in the US. These include the difficulties in extracting scale economies from multi-plant operations, the difficulties in standardizing clinical operations and achieving clinical integration with medical staff across sites, and the challenge of getting multiple units to act in concert in a previously decentralized healthcare system. India's systems are relying heavily on performance metrics, performance dashboards, and IT to provide some of this cohesion. Evidence from the US suggests that while IT is an important tool for gathering and analysing data, its impact on improving the cost-effectiveness of care is still unclear and undemonstrated.

TOP FOUR POLICY RECOMMENDATIONS FROM US/CHINA EXPERIENCE

Following are the recommendations that India must implement in order to benefit from the US/China examples.

1. *Spend adequately on primary healthcare*: In the US, primary care has traditionally represented only a fraction of healthcare spending, but directly or indirectly drives the downstream costs (90 per cent or even more). Proactively and aggressively spending on primary healthcare can have more sustainable long-term benefits. The US is beginning to learn from its mistakes by increasing attention to different primary care initiatives (for example, patient-centred medical homes, Direct Primary Care).
2. *Focus on patient-centric care*: Healthcare has multiple stakeholders. While creating new organization forms and systems of care, it can be easy to lose sight of the end customer (the patient). Policies should foster innovation and incentivize private players to engage patients in more consumer-centric care using technology. Some examples: tele health clinics and kiosks, virtual physician visits, price transparency, customer satisfaction measures, and cutting edge wellness programmes.
3. *Achieve the quadruple aim*: Ten years ago, a US physician called for pursuit of the 'triple aim'—reduce the per capita cost of care, improve the patient's experience of care, and promote the health of the population (Berwick, Nolan, and Whittington 2008). More recently, other physicians have advocated a fourth aim—reduce physician burnout and improve the physician's work satisfaction (Bodenheimer and Sinsky 2014). Healthcare is ultimately delivered by people. Doctors, nurses, and other frontline staff form the backbone of any healthcare delivery system. Countries must create systems that attract and retain top talent.
4. *Increase spending on medical research*: India has its own unique demographics and disease challenges. The central government must support long-term research to improve the health of its population. This effort will buttress the first three policy goals.

REFERENCES

Bakshi, Ajay and Lawton Burns. 2014. 'The Medical Profession in India', in *India's Healthcare Industry: Innovation in Delivery, Financing, and Manufacturing*, edited by Lawton Burns, pp. 141–68. Cambridge, UK: Cambridge University Press.

Berwick, Donald, Thomas Nolan, and John Whittington. 2008. 'The Triple Aim: Care, Health, And Cost', *Health Affairs* 27(3): 759–69.

Bodenheimer, Thomas and Christine Sinsky. 2014. 'From Triple to Quadruple Aim: Care of the Patient Requires Care of the Provider', *Annals of Family Medicine* 12(6): 573–576.

Burns, Lawton R. (ed.) 2014. *India's Healthcare Industry: Innovation in Delivery, Financing, and Manufacturing*. Cambridge, UK: Cambridge University Press.

Burns, Lawton R., Prashanth Jayaram, and Richa Bansal. 2014. 'Medical Tourism: Opportunities and Challenges', in *India's Healthcare Industry: Innovation in Delivery, Financing, and Manufacturing*, edited by Lawton Burns, pp. 219–89. Cambridge, UK: Cambridge University Press.

Burns, Lawton R. and Gordon Liu. 2017. *China's Healthcare System and Reform*. Cambridge, UK: Cambridge University Press.

Burns, Lawton R., Jeffrey McCullough, Douglas Wholey, Gregory Kruse, Peter Kralovec, and Ralph Muller. 2015. 'Is the System Really the Solution? Operating Costs in Hospital Systems', *Medical Care Research and Review* 72(3): 247–72.

Burns, Lawton R., Tanmay Mishra, Kalyan Pamarthy, and Arunavo Roy. 2014. 'The Medical Device Sector in India', in *India's Healthcare Industry: Innovation in Delivery, Financing, and Manufacturing*, edited by Lawton Burns, pp. 500–37. Cambridge, UK: Cambridge University Press.

Burns, Lawton R., Bhuvan Srinivasan, and Mandar Vaidya. 2014. 'India's Hospital Sector: The Journey from Public to Private Healthcare Delivery', in *India's Healthcare Industry: Innovation in Delivery, Financing, and Manufacturing*, edited by Lawton Burns, pp. 169–218. Cambridge, UK: Cambridge University Press.

Devarakonda, S. 2016. 'Hub and Spoke Model: Making Rural Healthcare in India Affordable, Available and Accessible', *Rural and Remote Health* 16: 3476. Available at https://www.rrh.org.au/public/assets/article_documents/article_print_3476.pdf, last accessed on 14 November 2017.

Govindarajan, Vijay and Ravi Ramamurti. 2013. 'India's Secret to Low-Cost Health Care', *Harvard Business*

Review, 15 October. Available at https://hbr.org/2013/10/indias-secret-to-low-cost-health-care, last accessed on 15 November 2017.

Herzlinger, Regina and Pushwaz Virk. 2008. 'Fortis Healthcare (A)', HBS Case #9-308-030. Boston, MA: Harvard Business School Publishing.

The Hindu. 2017. 'Most Private Hospitals Evade Tax: CAG', 28 July. Available at http://www.thehindu.com/news/national/most-private-hospitals-evade-tax-cag/article19380559.ece, last accessed on 15 November 2017.

Hooda, Shailender K. 2015. *Private Sector Healthcare Delivery Market in India: Structure, Growth, and Implications*. New Delhi: Institute for Studies in Industrial Development.

India Brand Equity Foundation (IBEF). 2017. *Healthcare*. 3 May. Available at https://www.ibef.org/download/Healthcare-May-2017.pdf, last accessed on 15 November 2017.

———. 2019. *Healthcare*. October. Available at https://www.ibef.org/download/Healthcare-October-2019.pdf, last accessed on 15 November 2019.

Indo-Asian News Service (IANS). 2017. '40,000 Private Hospitals Closed in Karnataka as Doctors Protest Medical Bill,' *Hindustan Times*, 3 November. Available at http://www.hindustantimes.com/india-news/40-000-private-hospitals-closed-in-karnataka-as-doctors-protest-medical-bill/story-c1PrVNZy2xckDC6RON7EMI.html, last accessed on 15 November 2017.

Khanna, Tarun, V. Kasturi Rangan, and Merlina Manocaran. 2005. 'Narayana Hrudayalaya Heart Hospital: Cardiac Care for the Poor', HBS Case #9-505-078. Boston, MA: Harvard Business School Publishing.

Knowledge@Wharton. 2017. 'Is India's Insurance Market Coming of Age?', 9 November. Available at http://knowledge.wharton.upenn.edu/article/indias-insurance-market-coming-age/, last accessed on 15 November 2017.

Kumar, Aman. 2014. 'Opportunities in Healthcare Private Equity in India', in *India's Healthcare Industry: Innovation in Delivery, Financing, and Manufacturing*, edited by Lawton Burns, pp. 424–40. Cambridge, UK: Cambridge University Press.

Malik, Deepak, Rahul Solanki, and Archana Menon. 2016. *Healthcare*. Edelweiss Securities. 7 October. Available at https://www.edelresearch.com/showreportpdf-34289/HEALTHCARE_-_SECTOR_REPORT-OCT-16-EDEL, last accessed on 12 January 2020.

Ministry of Finance. *Indian Public Finance Statistics 2015–2016*, August. New Delhi: Government of India. Available at http://dea.gov.in/sites/default/files/IPFS%20English%202015-16.pdf, last accessed on 15 November 2017.

Ministry of Health and Family Welfare (MoHFW). 2016. *National Health Accounts: Estimates for India 2013–14*. New Delhi: Government of India.

Nasdaq Market News. 2016. *Medical Tourism Market Report: 2015 Edition. Latest Industry Shares, Trends, Growth, Survey, Insights, Outlook: ReserachMoz*, January. Available at https://www.pm360online.com/medical-tourism-market-report-2015-edition-latest-industry-shares-size-trends-growth-survey-insights-outlook-researchmoz/, accessed on 14 November 2017.

Oberholzer-Gee, Felix, Tarun Khanna, and Carin-Isabel Knoop. 2007. *Apollo Hospitals – First World Health Care at Emerging-Market Prices*, HBS Case #9-706-440. Boston, MA: Harvard Business School Publishing.

Richman, Barak and Kevin Schulman. 2017. 'What U.S. Hospitals Can Still Learn from India's Private Heart Hospitals', *NEJM Catalyst*, 3(3), 25 May. Available at https://catalyst.nejm.org/us-hospitals-learn-india-heart-hospitals/, last accessed on 15 November 2017.

Weisbrod, Burton A. 1991. 'The Health Care Quadrilemma: An Essay on Technological Change, Insurance, Quality of Care, and Cost Containment', *Journal of Economic Literature* 29: 523–52.

Worstall, Tim. 2017. 'India's Mistake in Cutting Knee Implant Costs—Price Fixing Simply Doesn't Work,' *Forbes*, 17 August.

18

The Public Health System in Uttar Pradesh

Systemic Malaise, Diagnostics, and a Set of Prescriptions

Santosh Mehrotra with Anurag Priyadarshi

Uttar Pradesh (UP) has among the worst health indicators of any state in India. If UP does not achieve the global health-related Sustainable Development Goals (SDGs), India will not; if India will not, nor will the world. This is because if UP was a country, its population would make it the sixth most populous country in the world.

UP's public health system will need to address different kinds of challenges in the near future. First, UP is undergoing multiple health-related transitions. There is a dual challenge that UP faces. These relate to premature mortality, morbidity, and disability underlying sharply rising non-communicable disease (NCDs) but at the same time ongoing communicable disease conditions. Second, as per the latest 2014 report of National Sample Survey Office (NSSO), nearly 80 per cent of all outpatient visits and about 60 per cent of all hospital episodes occur in the private sector. However, critical public health services such as immunization, provision of maternal and child health services, prevention of communicable diseases programmes, management of outbreaks, epidemics, and disasters and surveillance continue to be delivered largely through the public health system. This is yet another reason why the state is at a critical juncture, as it tries to rebuild the public health system, and, with this objective, had in 2018 prepared a draft State Health Policy (SHP).[1]

This chapter addresses three issues in respect of UP's health system—infrastructure, human resources, and governance—with a greater focus on governance. But it begins with the first two issues because if the severe shortages of public health infrastructure and health-related human resources are not resolved first or at least simultaneously, systemic change in the governance of the health system cannot convert a poorly functioning public/private health system into an optimal one. While the focus of this chapter is on the governance system in the health sector, we need to put the governance issues in UP in context.

This chapter is organized as follows. The first section begins with a conceptual framework that is the basis of the rest of the analysis (see Mehrotra and Delamonica 2007; Mehrotra 2016). Section two examines very briefly the health and nutrition outcome indicators for UP, and compares them to those prevailing

[1] As of January 2020, this is still a draft document.

in the rest of India. The focus is on the comparison with other poorer states (mostly northern and eastern states of India). The next section briefly discusses the infrastructure shortages relative to norms that exist in UP, and how those compare with other states. The fourth section discusses the human resource shortages in UP, again comparing with other states, as well as the national average. Section five examines the fragmentation of the public health delivery system, created by the multiplicity of institutions that deliver public health services. The next section discusses the dysfunctionality that arises from the lack of cross-sectoral coordination among ministries/institutions whose effectiveness will largely be responsible for how the social determinants of health outcomes play out (favourably or adversely). Section seven examines how data collection and use, and e-governance generally, could improve the governance of UP's health system. The chapter concludes with five policy recommendations.

THE SYNERGY AMONG SOCIAL SERVICES

Interventions in health, nutrition, water and sanitation, fertility control, education, and income complement each other—and positively affect the life of an individual. This increases the impact of any one from investments in any other (see Figure 18.1).

Figure 18.1 represents this notion of synergy. On the horizontal rows, the various social services are

Social services inputs/processes	Human development outcomes/outputs: Knowledge	Family size	Health Status	Nutritional Status	Healthy living conditions
Education		↲	↲	↲	↲
Family Planning	↲				
Health	↲	↲		↲	
Nutrition	↲	↲	↲		
Water and sanitation					

Figure 18.1 The First Synergy between Social Service Inputs and Human Development Outputs

Source: Mehrotra and Delamonica (2007); Mehrotra (2016).

represented as inputs or interventions—education, family planning, health, nutrition, and water and sanitation. The vertical columns represent the human development outcomes or outputs—knowledge, family size, health status, nutrition status, and healthy living conditions. The dark-shaded cells show the direct and obvious relationship between inputs and outputs. The light shaded cells are the ones where there is a relationship, but an indirect one, between a certain intervention and an outcome—for example, the use of contraception (that is family planning), by helping the spacing of children, indirectly benefits the health status of the mother as well as the child.

The arrows represent feedback effects from human development outcomes to the inputs/processes. For example, the improved health status of a child improves her ability to learn, just as improved nutritional status does. Similarly, reduced family size improves the chances that a poor family will be able to afford education for all the children rather than merely the boy(s) in the family, and so on.

Since the connections presented here are central to our arguments about synergies, a more in-depth review of these connections is needed. First of all, it has to be recognized that all these relationships are based on evidence discovered several years ago. However, probably in part due to overspecialization within the disciplines represented on the matrix, they are all too often presented separately. By integrating them, it becomes clear that their separate effects, the ones often reported, are only partial. In fact, the impact of any one form of investment is increased in the presence of the others, proving the advantages of integrated approaches.

Notice that *educational inputs* have an impact on all types of human development outcomes. The positive effects of education are intuitive and well known. First, parents, especially mothers, make better use of information and reproductive healthcare facilities if they are more educated. Thus, more widespread education is associated with a lower fertility rate. Better nutrition and healthcare is provided by educated parents for themselves and their children. Various routes ensure this result. The general knowledge acquired at school increases understanding of modern health practices and scientific beliefs, which make mothers (and fathers) more open to using healthcare centres. Households with educated mothers spend a higher proportion of their income on food and health services. In addition, the capacity to acquire new knowledge and change behaviour accordingly is higher among those who attended school, as evidenced by the differential diffusion of HIV/AIDS among educated and uneducated women (Vandemoortele and Delamonica 2000). As a result, health investments are more efficient in the presence of a more literate population (Caldwell 1986).

In countries where parents have been exposed during their school years to nutrition information combine different foods to obtain better nutritional outcomes. Also, mothers take better care of their nutritional needs during pregnancy, avoiding low birth weight (ACC/SCN 2000). Basic education also facilitates the rapid adoption of improved hygienic behaviour. This not only improves health outcomes but also enhances the impact of investments in water and sanitation systems.

In summary, education, and in particular girls' education, contributes to enhance the impact of other sectoral interventions. All of these, in turn, result in good nutrition and health, increasing the likelihood children will attend school and become better students. For instance, with lower fertility, parents can devote more attention to their children's studies and afford more food and school supplies which improve learning. In addition, access to clean water and safe sanitation (that is healthy living condition) helps girls—when girls need less time in household chores like fetching water, they have more opportunities to attend school. Also, they have more time and energy to study and do well in school, avoiding repetition or dropping out.

Family planning, by providing easy access to contraceptive means, enables the mother to space births, thus lowering the health risk to herself and the child, reducing infant and maternal mortality, and improving the healthy development of the child. Thus, lower fertility has a positive implication for improving health and increasing life expectancy. Another important complementary outcome of intervention in health, education, water/sanitation, and family planning is a rapid demographic transition. As children survive, families voluntarily curtail the number of future births. This is not the place to enter the debate on the relative impact of supply of contraceptives versus desired family size in family planning (Bongaarts 1994; Cassen 1994; Pritchett 1994). However, it is clear that lower infant and child mortality plays a major role in reducing fertility rates (Caldwell 1986), as does education, the availability of information on reproductive healthcare, and its accessibility (Cochrane 1979).

As population growth slows down, school systems find it easier to absorb all children. Teacher–pupil ratios can be reduced without unduly burdening budgets and construction costs can also be reduced releasing resources for other measures to enhance school quality.

As in the case of the health and nutrition sectors, the availability of information on and access to family planning services will not, on their own, reduce fertility as much as it might be needed or desired. They are more effective when couples are more educated and child survival rates are higher.

It is also very well established that lack of good *nutrition* critically interacts with *health*. For instance, control of diarrhoea and measles is very important not only for health outcomes but also in reducing malnutrition (by improving the capacity to absorb and retain caloric intake). By the same token, an insufficient intake of total calories, vitamins, and proteins weakens children's immune systems. This would make them vastly more vulnerable to the onset and consequences of infectious diseases. Interventions in health promote good nutrition and interventions in nutrition promote good health.

Moreover, micronutrient deficiencies and illness can have devastating consequences for the cognitive development of a child. For instance, iron deficiency or anaemia reduces cognitive functions, iodine deficiency causes irreversible mental retardation, and vitamin A deficiency is the primary cause of blindness among children. Girls are unfairly disadvantaged in many of these cases because they have to undergo monthly menstruation cycles, when they lose blood, sometimes excessively, without having counselling support or medical advice. They are more likely to suffer from iodine or iron deficiency.

While it is clear that good health and nutrition have benefits which reinforce each other, the above examples also show that they impact positively on fertility control and education. But it is also clear that good health, the protection against disease, and proper nourishment cannot be produced by health services or food alone.

Safe water and adequate sanitation also play a fundamental role in determining health conditions. Access to safe water and sanitation dramatically reduces the incidence of diarrhoea and many other diseases that kill millions of children and adults each year. Another effect of better access to water takes place through the reduced effort in carrying water, a burden that is usually unduly borne by females. Given the traditional roles they play in most societies, when women have more time, they can apply it to better infant and child care.

This leads to positive health results. Finally, especially for women, more time is available for pecuniary productive activities. This direct impact of water and sanitation improvements positively affects productivity not only through improved health outcomes, but by releasing time, thereby enabling women to undertake economic activities, even if these activities are home based. This is less publicized than the effect of higher levels of education and better health on productivity.

The presence of toilets, safe water, and hygienic conditions at school can reduce some constraints on sending children, especially girls, to school. Separate toilets for girls are known to be a consideration for parents because of privacy and security concerns for post-pubescent girls. Backed by proper hygienic behaviour such as hand-washing and the use of soap, access to safe water and adequate sanitation reduces morbidity from infectious diseases and increases the nutritional status of children, which furthers their learning abilities.

In summary, each intervention has ramifications which lie outside its 'sector' and adds up to a virtuous circle of social and economic development. This is different from the existence of an externality, although they are, of course, present. Unlike the traditional treatment of externalities, which are usually exceptions, these interactions are pervasive.

This is a multi-dimensional synergetic system. No wonder it results in a complex process, at which most developing countries have not yet succeeded. From an instrumental point of view, the benefits do not automatically accrue to all and markets alone would not ensure universal access, hence there is a need for the public sector to step in and finance these services, and also to probably provide them, especially at the most basic/primary levels in rural areas, where quality private services are missing.

In sum, interventions in health, nutrition, water and sanitation, fertility control, education, and income complement each other and positively affect the life of an individual. This increases the impact of any one form of investments in any other. It is because there have been serious shortcomings in respect of each one of these dimensions of basic social service delivery in UP that its health outcomes are much worse than in the rest of even the poorer states in India. Although these problems are prevalent nationwide (Rao 2017), they are more exaggerated in UP. This is discussed in the next section.

HEALTH OUTCOMES IN UP: MUCH WORSE THAN INDIA

Table 18.1 presents data for outcome/process indicators for UP, India, and other poorer states. UP's literacy rate is 69 per cent compared to India's 74 per cent, but health indicators (infant mortality rate [IMR], under-five mortality rate [U5MR]) for UP were worse than not only India, but also other major poorer states in 2005–6 (National Family Health Survey or NFHS-3), but remain worse in 2015–16 (NFHS-4). For process indicators such as share of children fully immunized too there is little cause for cheer, as only half of all UP's children are immunized. The female fertility rate for India has shown a sharp decline between 2005–6 and 2015–16, from 2.7 births per woman of age between 15 and 49 years (the reproductive years) to 2.2 births, and this is the only outcome indicator in which UP (2.7) is now doing better than Bihar (3.5).

In respect of nutrition indicators (see Table 18.2), UP is doing better than Bihar, but only slightly. UP's situation remains grim in 2015–16: 40 per cent of children are still underweight, 46 per cent are stunted, and 18 per cent are wasted, and only stunting has seen a 10 percentage point fall over the 10 years between NFHS-3 and NFHS-4. These rates are only worse in Bihar, though not much different than in UP.

These health and nutritional outcome indicators are the result of a combination of factors: (a) shortages in infrastructure of public health; (b) shortages in human resources in public health; and (c) serious governance failures. We discuss each of these in turn in the next few sections.

SHORTAGES IN HEALTH INFRASTRUCTURE, EQUIPMENT, AND SUPPLIES

UP suffers from a shortfall in functional sub-centres, primary health centres (PHCs), and community health centres (CHCs) as per its population, as Tables 18.3, 18.4, and 18.5 show. These tables present the grim reality of the state of health infrastructure in UP. Table 18.3 shows that only a quarter of sub-centres, PHCs, and CHCs are in place, compared to the norms. Table 18.4 shows that the situation is even worse on the ground because according to the Ministry of Health and Family Welfare (MoFHW), none of the sub-centres are as effective and functional as they could be, and under 5 per cent of the PHCs (based on the Indian Public Health Standards [IPHS] norms) are functional. Table 18.5 demonstrates that the number

Table 18.1 UP vs Poorer States: Key RMNCH+A* indicators

S. no	Indicators	India			Uttar Pradesh			Bihar			Madhya Pradesh			Rajasthan		
		NFHS-4	NFHS-3	Diff	NFHS-4	NFHS-3	Diff	NFHS-4	NFHS-3	Diff	NFHS-4	NFHS-3	Diff	NFHS-4	NFHS-3	Diff
1	IMR	41.0	57.0	–16.0	64.0	73.0	–9.0	48.0	61.0	–13.0	51.0	69.0	–18.0	41.0	65.0	–24.0
2	U5MR	50.0	74.0	–24.0	78.0	96.0	–18.0	58.0	84.0	–26.0	65.0	93.0	–28.0	51.0	85.0	–34.0
3	%age of mothers who had full antenatal care	21.0	11.6	9.4	5.9	2.7	3.2	3.3	4.2	–0.9	11.4	4.7	6.7	9.7	6.3	3.4
4	%age of institutional deliveries	78.9	38.7	40.2	67.8	20.6	47.2	63.8	19.9	43.9	80.8	26.2	54.6	84.0	29.6	54.4
5	%age of children aged 12–23 months fully immunized (BCG, measles, and 3 doses each of polio and DPT)	62.0	43.5	18.5	51.1	23.0	28.1	61.7	32.8	28.9	53.6	40.3	13.3	54.8	26.5	28.3
6	%age of female sterilization married women 15–49 yrs	36.0	37.3	–1.3	17.3	17.3	0.0	20.7	23.8	–3.1	42.2	44.3	–2.1	40.7	34.2	6.5
7	%age of total unmet need for FP for married women 15–49 yrs	12.9	13.9	–1.0	18.1	23.1	–5.0	21.2	23.9	–2.7	12.1	12.1	0.0	12.3	15.7	–3.4
8	%age of unmet need for spacing married women 15–49 yrs	5.7	6.1	–0.4	6.8	9.0	–2.2	9.4	10.4	–1.0	5.7	5.4	0.3	5.7	7.3	–1.6

* RMNCH+A refers to Reproductive, Maternal, Newborn, Child and Adolescent Health.
Source: Respective NFHS surveys.

Table 18.2 UP vs Poorer States: Key Nutrition Indicators

S. no	Indicators	India			Uttar Pradesh			Bihar			Madhya Pradesh			Rajasthan		
		NFHS-4	NFHS -3	Diff.	NFHS-4	NFHS-3	Diff.	NFHS-4	NFHS-3	Diff.	NFHS-4	NFHS-3	Diff.	NFHS-4	NFHS-3	Diff.
1	%age of mothers who consumed iron and folic acid for 100 days or more	30.3	15.2	15.1	12.9	6.0	6.9	9.7	6.3	3.4	23.6	7.1	16.5	17.3	8.7	8.6
2	%age of all women aged 15–49 years who are anaemic	53.0	55.3	–2.3	52.4	49.9	2.5	60.3	67.4	–7.1	52.5	55.9	–3.4	46.8	53.1	–6.3
3	%age of children exclusively breastfed for 6 months of age	54.9	46.4	8.5	41.6	51.3	–9.7	53.5	28.0	25.5	58.2	21.6	36.6	58.2	33.2	25.0
4	%age of children aged 6–8 months receiving solid or semi-solid food and breastmilk	42.7	52.6	–9.9	32.6	41.2	–8.6	30.7	54.5	–23.8	38.1	46.0	–7.9	30.1	38.7	–8.6
5	%age of children under 5 years who are underweight	35.7	42.5	–6.8	39.5	42.4	–2.9	43.9	55.9	–12.0	42.8	60.0	–17.2	36.7	39.9	–3.2
6	%age of children under 5 years who are stunted (low height for age)	38.4	48.0	–9.6	46.3	56.8	–10.5	48.3	55.6	–7.3	42.0	50.0	–8.0	39.1	43.7	–4.6
7	%age of children under 5 years who are wasted (low weight for height)	21.0	19.8	1.2	17.9	14.8	3.1	20.8	27.1	–6.3	25.8	35.0	–9.2	23.0	20.4	2.6

Source: Respective NFHS surveys.

Table 18.3 Shortfall of Health Infrastructure in UP (values in absolute numbers)

	Sub-centres	PHCs	CHCs
Required	31,200	5,194	1,298
Available	20,521	3,497	773
Shortfall	34%	33%	40%

Source: MoHFW (2017b).

Table 18.4 Non-Functionality of PHCs and CHCs in UP (in numbers)

Sub-centres	Sub-centres functioning per IPHS norms	PHCs	PHCs functioning per IPHS norms
20,521	0	3,497	170

Source: MoHFW (2015b).

Table 18.5 Health Infrastructure in India, especially UP, Bihar, TN, and Kerala

	India	UP	Bihar	TN	Kerala
Districts	640	75	38	32	14
Sub-centres	155,069	20,521	9,729	8,712	4,575
PHCs	25,354	3,497	1,802	1,368	824
CHCs	5,510	773	148	385	225

Source: MoHFW (2017b).

of sub-centres, PHCs, and CHCs is much smaller in UP compared to that in Tamil Nadu (TN) and Kerala. At the same time, the outcome indicators are much worse in UP than in these other states. In other words, the need in UP is greater, but the infrastructure, in sheer quantitative terms, is much less.

When compounded with the human resource shortages (the next section), it is hardly surprising that the outcome indicators shown in the previous section are among the worst in UP. The governance problems (the subsequent sections) in the public health system only serve to compound the problems for the patients.

HUMAN RESOURCE SHORTAGES AND THE RELATED QUALITATIVE ISSUES

In UP, as on 2017, the density of allopathic doctors is estimated to be 3.2 while that of nurses is 3 per 10,000 population. This translates to one allopathy doctor catering to a population of 3,185 in the state as against the norm of 1 doctor per 1,000 population. Similarly, one nurse caters to a population of 3,067 as against the World Health Organization (WHO) norm of one nurse per 500 population.

The Quantitative Evidence in Respect of HR Shortages

This section examines the human resource shortages from a variety of perspectives in the form of tables. We discuss each of these tables and what they reveal separately.

Table 18.6 compares UP's doctor strength to that of India, and particularly of Kerala and TN. What is remarkable is that while UP has a population over twice as large as Kerala or TN, that it had less doctors in total than TN in 2007, and over the next seven years till 2014 TN had increased its doctors by a larger number than UP had.

A more worrying situation is revealed by Table 18.7, which normalizes the same data for doctors per 1000 population in each state. In 2007, the number of doctors was barely a third of the average in India, and a quarter of that of Kerala and TN. The ratio per 1,000 had barely improved in UP by 2017, while the ratio had improved significantly from already much higher levels in Kerala and TN.

Similarly, when we examine Table 18.8, it is clear that UP has a serious shortage of all kinds of personnel for the health system, whether it is doctors, specialists, or paramedics (particularly in the lower level facilities).

Table 18.6 State-wise Number of Doctors Possessing Recognized Medical Qualifications

As of	UP	Kerala	TN	India
2007	51,978	35,109	78,574	731,439
2014	65,343	44,515	102,328	938,861
2016	65,343	51,063	118,275	1,005,281

Source: MoHFW (2017b).

Table 18.7 Ratio of State-wise Number of Doctors Possessing Recognized Medical Qualifications to Population (per 1,000 people)

As of	UP	Kerala	TN	India
2007	0.278	1.047	1.197	0.648
2014	0.309	1.263	1.490	0.758
2016	0.299	1.431	1.704	0.792

Sources: The population values for the year 2007, 2014, and 2016 are taken from the population projections for India and states. See MoHFW (2006, 2017b).

Table 18.8 Huge Gaps in HR at CHCs and PHCs in UP compared to India

Type of medical and paramedical staff	UP vs India	Required [R]	Sanctioned [S]	In Position [P]	Vacant [S – P]	%age of shortfall
Doctors at PHCs	UP	4,509	3,497	2,209	1,288	51.0
	India	34,750	25,308	27,421	–2,113	21.1
Surgeons at PHCs	UP	773	529	112	417	85.5
	India	5,396	3,320	896	2,424	83.4
Obstetricians & Gynaecologists (OB&GY) at CHCs	UP	773	524	115	409	85.1
	India	5,396	3,249	1,296	1,953	76.0
Physicians at CHCs	UP	773	523	103	420	86.7
	India	5,396	2,772	918	1,854	83.0
Paediatricians at CHCs	UP	773	523	154	369	80.1
	India	5,396	2,484	968	1,516	82.1
Total Specialists (Surgeons, OB&GY, Physicians and Paediatricians)	UP	3,092	2,099	484	1,615	84.3
	India	21,584	11,661	4078	7,583	81.1
Radiographers at CHCs	UP	773	230	82	148	89.4
	India	5,396	4,167	2,150	2,017	60.2
Pharmacists at PHCs & CHCs	UP	4,270	2,952	2,883	69	32.5
	India	30,704	28,268	23,131	5,137	24.7
Laboratory Technicians at PHCs & CHCs	UP	4,270	1,331	963	368	77.4
	India	30,704	22,626	17,154	5,472	44.1
Nursing staff at PHCs and CHCs	UP	8,908	4,497	4,412	85	50.5
	India	63,080	74,098	65,039	9,059	–3.1
Health assistants (Female)/ LHV at PHCs	UP	3,497	3,781	1,916	1,865	45.2
	India	25,308	22,993	13,372	9,621	47.2
Health Assistants (Male) at PHCs	UP	3,497	5,757	954	4,803	72.7
	India	25,308	23,505	12,616	10,889	50.2
Health workers (Female)/ ANM at sub-centres	UP	20,521	23,580	20,265	3,315	1.2
	India	153,655	178,480	193,191	–14,711	–25.7
Health workers (Female)/ ANM at PHCs	UP	24,081	27,334	23,731	3,603	1.5
	India	178,963	195,672	212,185	–16,513	–18.6
Health assistants (Male) at sub-centres	UP	20,521	9,080	3,152	5,928	84.6
	India	153,655	93,002	55,657	37,345	63.8

Source: MoHFW (2015b).

While there are shortages in India generally, there is a systematic pattern showing shortages being worse in UP. Moreover, UP shows a pattern of not filling sanctioned posts. It is equally important that the numbers of human resources required as per norms is well above those that have been sanctioned by the state government. So when the filled posts are much lower than even the sanctioned posts, one can see how serious are the shortages of medical staff in UP.

Table 18.9 shows that the number of AYUSH[2] doctors in UP is much more respectable compared to both

[2] AYUSH refers to Ayurveda, Yoga and naturopathy, Unani, Siddha, and Homoeopathy.

Table 18.9 State-wise Numbers of AYUSH Registered Practitioners, 2014

Stats	UP	Kerala	TN	India
Total	81,320	36,836	33,783	771,468
Per 1,000 population	0.373	1.033	0.487	0.608

Note: The population for the year 2016 has been arranged from the population projections for India and states.
Sources: MoHFW (2006, 2017b).

India as well as the high-performing states of Kerala and TN (even though per 1,000 population even AYUSH practitioners are too few in UP relative to India and high-achieving states). This has implications for how they are currently deployed, and we discuss this issue in the next section on governance within the public health system.

Tables 18.10–18.11 reveal that the situation is rather grim in respect of para-medical staff in UP compared to not only Kerala and TN but also on average in India. Although UP has a much larger population there are only a fifth of the registered nurses or midwives as there are in Kerala or TN. The same applies to lady health visitors or pharmacists.

Table 18.10 State-wise Number of Auxiliary Nurse Midwife, Registered Nurses/Midwives, Lady Health Visitors, and Pharmacists

State/India	ANM	RN and RM	LHV	Pharmacists
UP	48,542	52,080	2,763	30,276
Kerala	30,047	231,457	8,507	29,487
TN	56,434	251,704	11,178	58,466
India	821,147	1,900,837	56,264	741,548

Source: MoFHW (2017b).
Notes: ANM = Auxiliary Nurse Midwife; RN/RM = Registered Nurse/Registered Midwife; LHV = Lady Health Visitors.

Table 18.11 Ratio of State-wise Number of Registered Nurses and Pharmacists in India to the Population (per 1,000 people)

State/India	ANM	RN and RM	LHV	Pharmacists
UP	0.222	0.239	0.127	0.139
Kerala	0.842	6.488	0.238	0.826
TN	0.813	3.627	0.161	0.843
India	0.647	1.498	0.443	0.584

Sources: MoHFW (2006, 2017b).
Notes: (a) The population for the year 2016 has been arranged from the population projections for India and states.
(b) ANM = Auxiliary Nurse Midwife; RN/RM = Registered Nurse/Registered Midwife; LHV = Lady Health Visitors.

Measures Required to Address the Human Resource Issues in UP

One can see that fixing the governance issues in the public health system in UP will not resolve the serious structural problems that beset the government-funded health sector. In fact, it is obvious that without solving the infrastructural and human resource problems of the system, addressing the governance issues will be like tinkering at the margins of the problem. The following actions could be considered.

Utilizing AYUSH Doctors

In order to meet the shortage of doctors it could be considered that the government can recruit the existing AYUSH doctors and offer them a foundation course. AYUSH doctors should be used to man the national health programmes. Even the PHCs should be staffed by AYUSH doctors. The system needs specialists only at the CHC level. The AYUSH system, especially Ayurveda and homoeopathy, play an important role in the healthcare delivery system of Kerala. As of now most of these AYUSH institutions function as stand alone facilities and have not been co-located within PHCs, CHCs, and district-level facilities (MoHFW 2014). In a similar way the co-located AYUSH systems within PHCs, CHCs, and district level facilities can help in a better delivery of health services in the state. In Madhya Pradesh and Odisha, AYUSH human resources are being effectively used to plug human resource gaps at PHCs and efforts have been made towards building their competencies and multi-skilling. Both states report positive feedback from such multi-skilling. In other states an average of 10–14 per cent outpatient load is taken care of by AYUSH systems and most of the states report adequate availability of AYUSH medicines.

In UP, the public health system currently employs 3,000 AYUSH providers, working at the PHC and CHC levels to provide specialized services in their domain. In the recent past, nearly nine million patients received care through AYUSH providers, illustrating the widespread demand and acceptability for these services. Recently, an additional 2,800 have been recruited for placement at PHC and CHC levels to fill in the critical gap at frontline facilities, to address the shortage of allopathic doctors.

Provision of Walk-in Interviews

Doctors' appointments are caught up in the bureaucracy and procedures of the Public Services Commission. There should be a provision for walk-in interviews in order to speed up the process. There was provision for walk-in interviews even for such highly skilled professionals as Air India pilots. For sanctioned posts the budget normally exists and therefore appointments can easily be made. There is a very large number of sanctioned posts that remain unfilled in UP. With unfilled posts, it is not possible for health facilities such as the PHCs, CHCs, and district hospitals to function 24×7. If public health facilities do not function 24×7, there being little prospect of their getting utilized more than they are currently utilized. A very important reason for private or out-of-pocket (OOP) expenditure on health being high is because the private facilities normally have 24×7 services, which (at least in 2012) was true for only 50 per cent of all government facilities. Walk-in interviews for appointment to doctor positions should become a regular practice.

Deployment and Transfers of Doctors

A new system of transfers of doctors will emerge now. Four new categories of districts for purposes of transfers of doctors—A, B, C, and D—have been created. If a doctor is currently located in C or D category district (less preferred), in the next posting, he/she will get preference to be located in district A or B (which are more preferred by doctors in terms of posting). There is now also an online application process for transfer. This should improve the deployment of doctors to less preferred districts, while serving as a dampener upon the 'transfer and promotion industry' that operates marked by widespread corruption. Another method that has been used—if a doctor has a rural posting for three years he will get up to a 30 per cent weightage in promotion consideration. Moreover, to fill the sanctioned posts faster, the state government undertook two steps in 2017: first it has increased the retirement age from 60 years to 62 years. Second, there is now cabinet approval for walk-in interviews for doctors. As a result, 1,000 vacant posts of doctors were to be filled by conducting such interviews.

Special Incentive-Based Salary for Specialists

The Provincial Medical Service (PMS) has found it difficult to retain specialist doctors in the cadre. General doctors with an MBBS and specialist doctors are paid the same in the PMS, with the result that the PMS tends to lose specialists. They are not permitted to do private practice in government. Therefore, there is a case for offering special incentive-based salary for specialists so that the PMS does not lose specialists.

Timely Hiring of Personnel

Our consultations with a number of policymakers as well as stakeholders in the public health revealed a number of additional concerns. There are 13 medical colleges in UP but only three have regular principals. The rest are all appointed on a temporary and ad hoc basis. In the absence of full-time regular appointment of principals, it is hard to see how medical colleges can be governed effectively. All principals in medical colleges must be appointed on a regular basis within three months of the post falling vacant.

Much infrastructure has been built but human resources needed to run the hospital or facilities are not hired. Several actions are necessary. First, the number of seats in medical colleges need to increase but the Medical Council of India (MCI) has to approve this increase. It is not clear why there is need for an MCI approval; this is a job of the state government and professional bodies within the state rather than the MCI. Second, there is scope for introducing a public health course to man lower level staff positions. Third, there are not enough specialists with Doctor of Medicine and Master of Surgery qualifications and more posts need to be created for them. Finally, just like in the education sector we have lower level contractual teachers called Shiksha Mitra who are locally hired, it is essential that the auxiliary nursing midwives (ANMs) must be also locally hired so that absenteeism rate is lower and attendance higher.

Longer Tenures for Director Generals

Most director generals of health have a tenure which does not normally exceed beyond six months as they tend to retire soon thereafter, as they tend to be appointed at the end of their careers, or they are shunted through political pressure. This is not good for the administration of the directorate and for morale generally within the directorate. The director general of health must have a minimum tenure of two years. Some mechanism should be found to accommodate those who have the seniority but do not have a length of service left over to allow them two years in the position of director general of health.

Change in Hospital Administration

Chief Medical Officers (CMOs) who are doctors usually turn out to be administratively not very proficient in administrative matters. They normally come to a meeting with administrative staff and it is the latter who, on account of their institutional memory and networks, are able to control their CMOs. Some administrative staff in fact have a reputation of being a 'law unto themselves'. Hospital administration, if it is to improve, cannot be run by such people. There is a case now for appointing professionals in hospital management to run hospitals. In fact, the administration of medical colleges, community health centres and district hospitals could then become more professional.

Hiring of Contractual Staff

Paramedics belongs to the category of class III and class IV employees, and like all regular hospital staff have job security for life. They cannot be held to account by doctors, and it is next to impossible to discipline them. It was the view of several stakeholders that it is essential that paramedic appointments must be made contractual. If the fear is that there are no good agencies that will perform this task of finding paramedic contractual staff on a regular basis and transparently, then one can expect such agencies will develop over a period of time. They can help to hire paramedics for the public health system.

Similarly, there is no reason for UP to have regular nursing staff since it has been very difficult to discipline them. A class III nurse gets a salary of INR 25,000 per month. By contrast, in a corporate private sector hospital a nurse may get a salary of INR 10,000 per month. Despite the difference in salary, unfortunately the nurses in government hospitals do 'little work'. Hence the suggestion that nurses could be hired in larger numbers on a contractual basis. It is very difficult to discipline regular staff. Contractual staff could be hired with the promise that if they perform well, they could become tenured into regular jobs over a period of time. That would require human resource policies to be altered—performance would have to be objectively measured, and good performance would be rewarded with increasingly longer contracts and higher pay, eventually culminating in regular positions.

ADDRESSING COORDINATION FAILURE WITHIN THE HEALTH DEPARTMENTS

Until the early 2000s in UP (and in other states of India) there was only one department in the health sector. The division into two departments came in 2002 at the instance of a Government of India directive. All states now have a Department of Medical Education and a Department of Health. This has created fragmentation in the governance of the public health system.

In UP, however, the fragmentation is even greater. As though the fragmentation resulting from the 2002 action of the Indian government was not bad enough, we now have for the last several years a third department dealing with health which is the Department of Family Welfare that does not exist as a separate entity in other states. Postings in the National Health Mission (NHM) located in the Department of Family Welfare are much sought after because NHM mission funds are much greater than the state government's own resources. Moreover, within the three departments related to health there is no there is no institutional mechanism for ensuring that the five or six institutions (Health Directorate, the NHM, the Technical Support Unit, the State Innovations in Family Planning Services Project Agency, and the State Institute of Health and Family Welfare) which are part of the department can coordinate with each other.[3]

We would therefore recommend that there should ideally be one commissioner for health who would supervise all three secretaries of the three different health departments. This arrangement would be comparable to what is prevailing in the agriculture department in UP. There is an agricultural production commissioner who has 13 departments reporting to him. Similarly, there is an industrial development commissioner which has the following departments reporting to him—small industries, heavy industries, labour, and udyog bandhu. Similarly, there is a social welfare commissioner, who looks after the interests of backward classes, scheduled castes (SCs) and scheduled tribes (STs).

The above action may not still solve the problem if there is an absence of coordination mechanisms between

[3] The Common Review Mission to UP in 2017 noted the following: 'The state needs to make an effort for convergence between National Health Mission and Directorate' (MoHFW 2017: 22). Unfortunately, the 8th Common Review Mission had also recognized the same problem in 2014: 'In UP integration within Directorate appears as a problem, manifesting itself at state and district management' (MoHFW 2014: 152).

various institutions within the departments. Hence, it will be essential to introduce a mandatory meeting of the heads of institutions to be presided over by Commissioner for Health Services (the post for which has to be created by a Cabinet decision). In Kerala, convergence between Directorate of Health Services and the State Health Mission is commendable. District Programme Managers (for NHM) are selected from Kerala Medical Services (MoHFW 2014: 171). The state's approach discourages parallel systems of service provision and programme management. This is reflected across all levels with increased integration and ownership of NHM initiatives within the health department/directorate of the state (MoHFW 2014). Clearly, UP will need to adopt the Kerala model with regard to intra-department convergence/coordination.

Separate Public Health Management Cadre

There is fragmentation within the Department of Health, with all its varied institutions[4] having very different reporting structures. In addition, there is the Rashtriya Swasthya Bima Yojana (RSBY) (now Ayushman Bharat), which has its own reporting structure. With such multiplicity of organizations dealing with public health, half the time of officers at the senior level is taken up with administrative issues. For the doctors particularly this is a problem because administration detracts them from their medical practice. A separate public health management cadre is necessary for administering the public health system.

In certain public facilities a position of hospital manager was created, and once appointed, they are performing well. They mostly come with a background of Master of Public Health and not Bachelor of Medicine and Bachelor of Surgery (MBBS), or sometimes they are AYUSH doctors. Appointing such administrators will take the pressure away from current doctors who are finding it difficult to combine medicine practice along with hospital administration. There are too few doctors in any case, as we have noted earlier. The appointment of these new hospital managers was resisted by some PMS doctors but most are quite happy.

[4] Technical Support Unit, State Institute for Family Planning, the National Health Mission (NHM), UP Health Systems Strengthening Project (funded by the World Bank), State Institute of Health and Family Welfare, and the Directorates for Health and for Family Welfare.

Adoption of the Discom Model

UP is the most populous state in the country, and its health profile changes in different parts of the state. It is very difficult for a single directorate of health to manage a large system, which is dealing with some of the worst health and nutrition outcome indicators in the country. India needs four directorates of health in a state as large as UP. There are four electricity distribution companies (also called discoms) in UP responsible for different regions of UP. In other words, the discom model has to be similarly adopted for the health sector. The health system administration has to be seen to be more accountable, and closer to the people. A decentralization of the apex organization in the state, like the directorate, needs to benefit from decentralization.

Issues in the Financing of the UP Public Health System

The overall health budget in UP is one of the lowest in the country at INR 790 per capita, which stands in sharp contrast to the national average of INR 1,538 per capita. With over 15 per cent of the country's population, UP accounts for only 9 per cent of India's public health spending which gets reflected in the adverse health outcomes. Some other states such as Bihar have recently significantly increased their health sector funding by using the flexibility allowed by the 14th Finance Commission recommendations (which devolved greater central tax revenues to the states 2015 onwards). However, the UP government seems to be unwilling to use a larger part of the additional revenue now available to increase its abysmally low health spending. UP's public health expenditure should at least be brought to levels of the national average per capita spending. The UP SHP commits to increasing its own allocation to health, in the light of the increase of 14th Finance Commission funds to each state, including UP. This is essential because of the very poor outcome indicators in UP, especially compared to poorer states.

Additionally, the financial allocation system within the state is very inflexible, and does not allow local level leeway in use of resources. There should be flexibility in granting funds to different institutions with differing needs. For instance, every CHC is given a similar grant across the board of INR 200 million (20 crore) per annum. Similarly, most CMOs are ignorant of the flexibility they can exercise in the use of funds and in what areas there remain constraints. Regular training of CMOs is needed with regard to financing issues.

Similarly, medical colleges are given a grant but there is no flexibility in the use of funds; so electricity bills have been mounting and not enough money has been given for paying off the electricity bills. Money, however, is available under other heads but it cannot be utilized to meet the pending electricity bills. As a result, services are adversely impacted and public health is affected.

A big problem with regard to finance is that infrastructure has been built but there is no provision for meeting the recurrent cost or even hiring staff to make the infrastructure operational. Similarly, when infrastructure or a hospital building is created, the health department is never involved in the building plans of the hospital facilities. Never involving professionals during the planning phase and before these facilities are created results in underutilization of facilities. This is quite unlike the private sector where professional doctors are involved in the planning of hospital facilities, or when such infrastructure is created. The UP SHP should ensure that doctors must be involved in all future facility building plans. In addition, no facility should begin construction unless staff positions, departments to be opened, and operation and maintenance costs have been provided for in the Health Department budget for the year in which the facility is to become operational.

Also, Japanese encephalitis (JE) and acute encephalitis syndrome (AES) have been major causes of deaths in UP over the last few years. The number of children dying from these diseases in the last few years remains persistently high—661 deaths in 2014, 521 in 2015, and 694 in 2016. This was a 33 per cent increase in the deaths from 2015. One would normally expect a substantial hike in resources for 2017 to take care of expected patients as well as preventive efforts. The reality in UP is the exact opposite. The proposed funds as well as actual allocation provided by the Union health ministry to the state government under the NHM had been significantly reduced. The demands by UP for AES/JE for 2016–17 was INR 304 million (30.4 crore), of which only INR 101.9 million (10.19 crore) was approved by the Centre. However, in the year 2017–18 the budget demand was reduced to INR 200 million crore but the amount approved by the Centre was further cut to just INR 57.8 million (5.78 crore), which is 29 per cent of the proposed amount. For specific disease-related financial allocations, there is need for holistic planning, so that (a) financial allocations for addressing the sanitary conditions in the Terai belt of UP (where the AES/JE is most concentrated) are enhanced; (b) at the time of outbreak of the disease (which tends to be concentrated in the monsoon months when the vector is able to breed easily) financial allocations are made to panchayats and to urban local bodies (ULBs), with strict monitoring of the use of funds through social audits.

Drug Procurement

The NSSO 2014 round of survey reported that patients visiting public health facilities in UP were receiving medicines free or partly free only to the extent of 42 per cent in the outpatient care facilities, while it was 54 per cent in inpatient care facilities. On the other hand, patients visiting public health facilities in TN and Rajasthan reported receiving medicines free in outpatient care settings to the extent of 92 per cent and 79 per cent respectively. In inpatient care settings, the respective shares for these states were 97 per cent and 92 per cent respectively, while the all-India average was reportedly nearly 60 per cent for outpatient and 68 per cent for inpatient facilities.

While UP health department has many institutions, the one institution that was needed on an urgent basis (and has been needed for decades) was a central drug procurement corporation (CDPC)—in 2017 it finally got one. Tamil Nadu has had one for decades, and it has made possible that all health facilities receive drugs from the central supply depot. In UP, by contrast, the system of drug procurement was decentralized to the district level. This has many disadvantages. First, it raises costs since bulk drug purchases can help the government to reduce unit cost of drugs. Second, it encourages decentralized corruption, which is impossible to control precisely because it is so decentralized across the administration at each location. In UP, procurement of drugs has faced problems, according to the NHM Common Review Mission (CRM) reports. Approximately 35 per cent to 40 per cent of the items remained unsupplied without any written communication by the suppliers (MoHFW 2014: 187).

Coordination can make procurement processes more efficient. There are lessons to be learnt from the experience of states like TN and Kerala. Kerala has a transparent and robust system of procurement through a central procurement agency. The Kerala Medical Services Corporation Limited has adopted e-tendering, pre-offer meeting, and payments through online bank transfers. District drug warehouses were available in all 14 districts. A CDPC in UP can promote the sale of only generic drugs, which are often deliberately in short supply in the current system. Moreover, there can be provision for free drugs to those living below the poverty line (BPL), marginally deprived people, and emergency patients only. UP's plan is to follow the Rajasthan model for this purpose. The proposal is that services (for example, diagnostics) should also be part of procurement and not just medicines.

CROSS-SECTORAL COORDINATION FOR BETTER PUBLIC HEALTH OUTCOMES

We noted in the first section that health outcomes are the result of interventions in other 'sectors': nutrition, water and sanitation, family planning, and even education. As against the national literacy rate of 74 per cent, the literacy rate in UP was 67.7 per cent. Of that, male literacy was 77.3 per cent (national 84 per cent), while female literacy stood at 57.2 per cent (national 65 per cent).

India has worse nutritional indicators than the average sub-Saharan African malnutrition rate. UP has among the worst indicators for any state in India. The nutritional outcomes in UP have shown little improvement between 2005–6 (NFHS-3) and 2015–16 (NFHS-4).

Underlying poor nutritional outcomes is the social determinant of health—sanitation. Rural sanitation remains a serious problem in India, although very significant gains have been made since 2014, thanks to a new approach and much greater focus on it, especially but not only by the prime minister. India accounted for 60 per cent of the global population that defecates in the open; half of India's population defecated in the open in 2011. According to Census 2011, only 31 per cent of rural households had an individual toilet. According to the Management Information System of the Government of India, the share of rural households (which is where the problem is concentrated though not confined to rural areas) with individual household latrines (IHHL) has risen to 100 per cent in every state by 2019–20, on account of the Swachh Bharat Abhiyan (SBA), from 39 per cent in October 2014, enabling the UP government, rightly or wrongly, to declare the state as an Open Defecation Free (ODF) state.[5] A Quality Council of India survey in late 2017 claims over 90 per cent use of toilets (Quality Council of India 2017). The NSS 76th Round (2018), however, shows a different picture. In other words, the difficulty is that survey data offers a different picture from the administrative data regarding ownership of household latrines. In India, barely 30 per cent of households draw their drinking water from a hand pump, and most receive piped supply; UP households have much greater reliance on a poorer source like hand pump (71 per cent). Also, NSS 2018 reports only 46 per cent of households had a latrine in rural UP in December 2018, while that share is 63 per cent in India. In fact, despite the SBA, 48 per cent of UP households have no access at all to latrines—so inevitably they defecate in the open. In other words, there is clearly a long way to go in respect of achieving a UP free of open defecation.

Earlier the focus on sanitation programme used to be on building toilets but never was there a similar focus on community mobilization. Much greater attention is needed for creating and sustaining public level awareness about toilet use. That requires the triggering of behaviour change. Only 100 people have been trained in the community-led total sanitation methodology when in fact we need 100,000 people, one for every village. This is a very low-cost way of ensuring behavioural change; the state needs to pay only INR 100 per person. Just as the government created a category for accredited social health activists (ASHAs) and anganwadi workers (AWWs) to work as as service providers, we now need new people who will trigger behavioural change for improving the situation regarding to open defecation.

However, the matter of sanitation goes beyond mere building/use of toilets. If health outcomes are to improve, general cleanliness and hygiene are also important. For instance, one reason why the Gorakhpur district is overwhelmed by AES/JE just around the monsoon period is because of the appalling conditions of environmental health and sanitation, which is caused by water collecting in the Terai belt around the town. The SBA has to focus its activities in the Terai districts of UP, especially in the vicinity of Gorakhpur.

Given these sets of concerns it is natural we should be worried about effective coordination between the various departments . This is necessary if the requisite health outcomes are to be achieved in UP. Effective governance in the public health sector requires first, that there is effective coordination between major departments of the state government that impact health outcomes—the Department of Health and Family Welfare; the Department of Women and Child Development (important on account of Integrated Child Development Services [ICDS], which is supposed to impact nutritional

[5] As per the website of SBA. See https://sbm.gov.in/sbmReport/home.aspx, last accessed on 15 January 2020. Similarly, the website states that UP became 99.27 per cent free of open defecation (self-declared by village pradhans).

outcomes of women and children); and Department of Drinking Water and Sanitation.

There is a second level of governance of the public health system that is critical for good outcomes—coordination between the State Department of Health on the one hand, and the local bodies on the other (Panchayati Raj Institutions [PRIs] for rural areas, and ULBs for urban areas). In fact, one of the reasons for Kerala's health sector success story is precisely this convergence of services at the local level of government.

There is a third level of governance of the public health system that is an issue across India—the existence of vertical national programmes (HIV/AIDS, malaria, tuberculosis, and so on) financed from central funds, and the more regular public health systems (financed largely by the state). These are all issues present in UP.

The larger political economy of UP is not the subject of this chapter; however, a brief digression on that subject here would not be out of place. I have argued elsewhere (Mehrotra 2006), that despite the rise of identity politics in UP in the last quarter century, it did not necessarily contribute to the improvement in social services—quite unlike other states such as TN and Kerala. The emergence of identity politics in these southern states in the twentieth century had resulted in social outcomes improving dramatically. Perhaps one important reason for that outcome in the south was that there emerged in those two states a two-party system in its electoral politics, each major party competing with the other to provide improved social services. However, unfortunately in UP the identity politics simply led to the fragmentation of the votes among four major parties. These parties, when in power, focused their energies upon using their power to merely distribute patronage to the caste groups supporting them electorally, with precious little positive outcomes for the rest of the population.

The NHM's CRM reports have also raised these issues repeatedly. It is imperative for the states to have a convergence across various departments in order to build a robust health system. It is seen that all the national programmes clubbed together present a very complicated picture at the field level, particularly in subcentres (MoHFW 2014: 159). Strong institutional convergence was not seen between village health nutrition and sanitation committees (VHNSCs) and gram panchayats (MoHFW 2017: 10). A number of actions would help in ensuring greater coordination between sectors, as the next few paragraphs show.

Better Linkage between Health Functionaries and PRIs and ULBs in UP

Not only has very little decentralization occurred in any sector in UP (unlike in Kerala), but the district staff are lacking in public health skills. UP District Programme Manager Unit (DPMU) staff is overburdened by the number of programmatic interventions for a variety of programmes. Lack of public health skills among district staff limits potential for health system strengthening in districts (MoHFW 2017: 225). Given the absence of accountability and lack of skills of district staff to local community, the DPMU gets overburdened.

The VHNSC in UP has not been functioning on a regular basis, nor is it effective. While effective convergence is reported from several states between ASHAs, ANMs, and AWWs for organizing VHNSC meetings, convergence between the health, ICDS and Jal Nigam (which incorporates the public health engineering function) departments appears to be a challenge at the block and district level. In UP an 'AAA' platform[6] (for ASHAs, ANMs, and AWWs) is being implemented in 25 high priority districts for effective convergence between frontline workers (MoHFW 2014: 11), but not in other districts. The VHNSC is an important instrument to ensure coordination and synergy between state interventions in health, nutrition, and sanitation measures at the local level. This we know can work, and has been shown to work in other states.

Thus, PRIs play an active role in VHSNCs in many states, with Kerala reflecting the most well-defined and institutionalized systems. Involvement of the PRIs in the Rogi Kalyan Samiti (RKS) was seen in Odisha, Kerala, Chhattisgarh, Mizoram, and TN (MoHFW 2014: 10); but not in UP. So RKS needs to be revitalized in UP.

In Kerala, effective convergence was observed between health institutions and local governance structures (PRI/ULBs), as seen in the palliative care programmes (MoHFW 2014: 171). Convergence extends beyond programmatic efforts to additional financing—state funds to PRI are equivalent to the untied funds provided through the NHM (MoHFW 2014: 171).

In UP, the ULBs and PRIs are very weak. So while in other states such as Kerala they have been used effectively

[6] The AAA platform, seen in UP as a form of convergence at the level of the sub-centre, has potential to serve as a site for coordinated service delivery, population enumeration, and screening.

to strengthen the public health system, it has not been successfully replicated in UP in the short run.

Decentralized governance in the health system is possible. In Kerala, community health care and support is effectively integrated into the PRI system. In the palliative care initiative, a panchayat-appointed community health nurse, supported by the ASHA in the community and the junior public health nurse at the sub-centre, provides home-based care. In order to decentralize care for patients with mental illness, funds for drugs are routed through PRIs with follow-up care provided at the PHC. PRIs also provide mobility support for outreach services and facility maintenance (MoHFW 2014).

From the perspective of UP, the PRIs should conduct social audits of health services. The role that they can be given in the public health system is to carry out social audit at the village level of health services.

Other Cross-Sectoral Interventions Proposed

The communication of messages relating to health, nutrition, and sanitation for the community could be improved through the school system in UP. This will require collaboration between the Department of Health and the Department of School Education. States of TN and Kerala have their own school health programmes. The 8th and 9th CRMs note that there is little evidence of the involvement of education in imparting health messages in UP (MoHFW 2014, 2017).

Sanitation in and around hospitals is extremely poor. This issue is also important from the perspective of hospital-acquired infections, and more specifically the spread of antimicrobial resistance—UP's health systems are already overburdened. The sanitary conditions are terrible primarily on account of the much larger crowd in public health facilities than what the facility is capable to serve. A system study is needed. For instance, one result could be that registration of all patients should take place just outside the hospital, rather than inside the hospital which results in unnecessary overcrowding and creates unsanitary conditions.

Social practices among the population adversely impact health outcomes among illiterate and poor patients. There is a need for mapping out such practices. For instance, in a personal communication with a member of public health staff, it was discovered that the female baby is often bathed in cold water at birth, while the male baby is bathed in warm water. This kind of practice would result in premature neonatal mortality for female children but not for male children.

DIGITIZING THE HEALTH SYSTEM

Generating Intelligence

It was noted by senior staff that there is excessive data being generated—more than can be usefully analysed and used by decision makers. The lower-level staff have to fill hundreds of forms, often in different formats. But one of the major challenges to the health system is that the Health Management Information System and Mother and Child Tracking System data are not being used for planning and monitoring purposes (MoHFW 2017: 263). In UP it is seen that the there is no institutionalized mechanism to track non-functional equipment (MoHFW 2017: 4). Governance is abstract in character, an architecture dealing with multiple organizations. It can be simplified by application of information and communication technology (ICT), which can enable health-related information being made available on the web, create PPP model, help customer contact, allocate patient to different levels of healthcare, provide electronic forum for patient interaction, and build an e-prescription system. Intersectoral coordination too is a problem that could be better addressed if each part of the governance system was 'talking to each other' through a platform where such information was regularly shared and available to each player in the system. That, however, would require that using such information available on the platform to solve health-system-related issues becomes incentivized in the HR performance evaluation system for the staff that will use the system. Other means for improving governance and efficiency through the use of information technology include:

1. Computerization of hospitals (registration, outpatient, inpatient, laboratory, imaging section, and record section) are initial steps that UP government could adopt. Quality assurance by total quality management, and medical and nursing audits supported by computerization of all processes such as store, pharmacy, finance and purchase section, inventory, and administrative machinery would save money, time, and transcend human error.
2. Automated information management tools such as internet, web-based libraries, electronic medical records (EMRs), electronic health records (EHRs), and computerized prescriptions are important components. EMRs or EHRs integrates patients' data with decision-making

system; these contain complete history by patient–computer interaction and records sensitive issues such as addiction, abnormal sexual behaviour, STD and HIV, mental illness, and suicidal tendency. Ultimately EMR leads to data mining for newer scientific developments. EMR also enables easy communication of patient data between different professionals like gram panchayat specialists, care teams, and pharmacies. Interoperability will be an issue if EMR formats and other aspects of health surveillance are not synchronized nationally and internationally—the UP government should work with the central government to deal with this issue.

The recruitment process in several states such as Kerala, Punjab, and Odisha have been streamlined by adopting innovative measures such a web-enabled procedures, decentralized recruitments, direct walk-in interviews, and the constitution of specially empowered committees for expediting recruitment processes. UP should adopt the same methods to improve transparency in recruitment processes.

Digitalized office procedures through digital document filing system at district health societies have enhanced financial and administrative efficiency in Kerala, for example (MoHFW 2014). Kerala uses IT in several initiatives—Jatak and Janani Software for community-based management of severely/acutely malnourished children, and HR Apps to manage employee leave status at district level (MoHFW 2014: 171). The same digital document filing system can be adopted in UP.

A few states such as TN, Maharashtra, and Delhi have taken initiatives using ICT in the health system and achieved progress. UP needs to follow suit by adopting the good practices, for which examples are discussed in the next few paragraphs.

Wipro for Delhi Municipal Corporation (DMC)

Wipro provided Hospital Information System (HIS) to six hospitals of DMC. This HIS has 28 modules meeting the hospital needs. Automating these functions has helped DMC handle large numbers of patients and helps them in providing better patient care. An electronic patient folder will enable the doctors to have ready access to past episodes and information of the patient, thus ensuring efficient patient care.

Tata Consultancy Services (TCS) for the TN Government

The TN government has allotted funds to TCS to develop a suitable solution to maintain EMR. ICT is employed in medical college hospitals in TN to manage inpatient and outpatient details, medical records, office automation, and lab and pharmacy services. Such electronic dataflow lends accuracy.

In TN, a chart of all pregnant women is maintained to monitor and follow up on each mother to invite her for delivery in a primary health facility through 'Phone to Heart Touch Approach' wherein the 108 staff calls the expecting woman a week before and a week after the expected date of delivery to motivate her for institutional delivery (MoHFW 2014: 66). Though there has been an increase in the rate of institutional deliveries in UP to 68 per cent of all births (NFHS-4, 2015–16), the Kerala share is 100 and TN share 99 percent; in India the share is 79 per cent. Following these practices can encourage better engagement of women with the public health system.

Hewlett Packard in Maharashtra

In January 2007 with INR 10 billion (1,000 crore) funding, automation project of 19 government hospitals and 14 medical colleges started. Private tech companies were engaged by the government for system integration and doctors' training. There has been remarkable change in patient experience towards e-healthcare and computerization (Mahapatra et al. 2007).

Equipment Management and IT

Rajasthan's equipment management software e-Upkaran sets a good example (MoHFW 2017: 4). E-Upkaran is a comprehensive software to improve the inventory management and maintenance services of equipment in hospital. This covers all the 2,500 facilities in Rajasthan, including medical colleges and hospitals across all districts. Mapping has been completed in the state (MoHFW 2014). These measures can improve efficiency and effectiveness in UP as well.

Tracking of the Health System

The health system began tracking health inputs, processes, and outputs in UP about 10 years ago. Before the NRHM, there was no tracking at all, but now it has become excessive. The pro forma of monitoring formats is complex. For instance, district ranking is carried out and shared in a booklet with the district magistrate of each district of UP. There is no explanation for the criteria used for the ranking and why the district magistrate needs it. Rather what would be much more useful is a one-pager which consists of a few key indicators, which could be used by senior administrators at district headquarters and in Lucknow for monitoring purposes. What is needed in fact is simple data in one format and digitized so that the district magistrate can make use of that data. The ANM could be trained to fill out and submit this data so that it could be regularly collated for passing on to higher level.

***

UP's poor health outcomes are due to a combination of limited infrastructure, serious human resource shortages, and governance failures, which this chapter has examined. Given this combination of problems with the health system per se, and the underlying social determinants of health (nutrition, sanitation), as well as the much lower educational levels of the population, the synergies that we explained in at the start of the chapter do not operate in the case of UP. Following the diagnosis of the malaise of the public health system, this chapter also made a number of suggestions or 'presctiptions' with respect to these weaknesses in the public health system. The latter have led to the predominance of private providers and the rising out-of-pocket expenditure for households.

After the National Health Policy was announced by the Union government in 2017, the UP government decided to articulate its own health policy. Given that the State Health Policy, two years later (at the time of writing in January 2020) was still not a public document, there is a case for all these suggestions to be implemented.

The medical college in Gorakhpur—BRD Hospital—saw an increase in the number of deaths of children in the 2010s; this is tragic because any government medical college/hospital stands at the pinnacle of the public health system of any Indian state, the peak of a 5-tier system (sub-centre, PHC, CHC, district hospital, medical college). Patients should reach a medical college after they have exhausted all possibilities at lower levels of care; it is a tertiary level referral facility. Most deaths in Gorakhpur were and are occurring in the case of neonatals, which suggest that the neonatal units are not functioning effectively. By contrast, the CRM have noted that the special newborn care units (SNCU) in Kerala, Odisha, Telangana, and Madhya Pradesh have good infrastructure and functionality. In Madhya Pradesh, 30 SNCUs out of 53 have been accredited by the National Neonatology Forum. UP needs to follow suit.

Another observation from the Gorakhpur case is that lower level facilities in UP's public health system are dysfunctional or non-existent in large parts of the state. Naturally, the higher-level facilities get overburdened with case load. However, Common Review Missions (of the National Health Mission) have noted that in almost all states the utilization of district-level facilities (district hospitals, general hospitals) is high due to availability of a complete range of primary and secondary care services at the district level. Availability of comprehensive secondary care is at the level of the district hospitals in most states, but in TN and Kerala secondary care services is available at sub-distict/taluka level (MoHFW 2014: 3). In Kerala, sub-centres conduct NCD clinics, demonstrating a model for the non-high focus states to move towards the provision of a more comprehensive primary health care package. If a similar situation does not begin to prevail very soon in UP, the tertiary-level hospitals are going to get overwhelmed, a problem compounded by a shortage of staff.

Unfortunately, the risk is that the way decisions are playing out, the shortage of funds may prevent any but the most limited reforms from being implemented. The Union government in early 2018 announced the extension of the hospitalization insurance (RSBY) from just over 100 million members to 500 million over the next few years. However, given the dysfunctional state of the public health system, it is unlikely that public providers will be able to meet the needs even of hospitalization, thus benefiting the private sector clinics and hospitals, and entrenching even further the predominant role that private providers play.

Improving the sub-centres and calling them health and wellness centres may not solve the problem of preventive and basic curative care, given that multiple health transitions (growing NCDs, continuing high incidence of communicable diseases, high unmet need for family planning) are taking place in India and particularly UP. The public health system needs an effective referral system from these health-and-wellness centres to PHCs, CHCs, and district hospitals. If not, sick people will still clock up large and growing OOP costs on account of outpatient consultations, diagnostics, and medicines, and on private curative care, further raising out-of-pocket expenses, thus increasing poverty.

REFERENCES

Administrative Committee on Coordination / Sub-Committee on Nutrition (ACC/SCN). 2000. 'Nutrition throughout the Life Cycle', *Fourth Report on the World Nutrition Situation*. Geneva: UN Administrative Committee on Coordination/Sub Committee on Nutrition.

Caldwell, J.C. 1986. 'Routes to Low Mortality in Poor Countries', *Population and Development Review* 12(2): 171–220.

Cochrane, S.H, 1979. *Fertility and Education: What Do We Really Know?* Baltimore MD: Johns Hopkins Univerity Press.

Ministry of Health and Family Welfare. 2014. 8th *Common Review Mission Report*. New Delhi: Government of India.

———. 2015a. *National Health Profile, 2015*. New Delhi: Government of India.

———. 2015b. *Rural Health Statistics, 2014-15*. New Delhi: Government of India.

———. 2017. *9th Common Review Mission Report*. New Delhi: Government of India.

Mahapatra, S., R. Das, M. Patra. 2007. 'Current e-Governance Scenario in Healthcare Sector of India', paper presented at a conference in Cairo, Egypt.

Mehrotra, S. 2006. *Well-Being and Caste in Uttar Pradesh. Economic and Political Weekly* 41(40): 4261–71.

Mehrotra, S. and E. Delamonica. 2007. *Eliminating Human Poverty: Macro-economic and Social Policies for Equitable Growth*. London: Zed Press.

Mehrotra, S. 2016. *Seizing the Demographic Dividend: Policies to Achieve Inclusive Growth in India*. New Delhi: Cambridge University Press.

Quality Council of India. 2017. *A Survey of SBM Toilet Usage*. New Delhi: Quality Council of India.

Rao, Sujatha K. 2017. *Do We Care? India's Health System*. New Delhi: Oxford University Press

Vandemoortele, J. and E. Delamonica. 2000. 'The "Education Vaccine" against HIV/AIDS', *Current Issues in Comparative Education* 3(1): 6–13.

Part V
Health Sector Regulation

19

Regulation of Drug Products in India

Lessons from the United States and the European Union

Richard Kingham and Vasudha Wattal

India has a long history of regulation of drugs and related healthcare products, dating at least to the enactment of the Drugs and Cosmetics Act of 1940 (DCA) and the Drugs and Cosmetics Rules of 1945 (DCR). This history compares favourably with that in the US (which first imposed general requirements for premarket approval of drugs in 1938) and the EU (which first imposed such requirements in the 1960s). In recent decades, India has become the largest supplier of generic drugs to the world.[1] Given the high quality of its educational institutions in science and technology and the increasingly significant role played by Indian scientists and business persons in multinational pharmaceutical companies, there is good reason to believe that, in the coming decades, India could also become a leader in the development and manufacture of innovative drugs.

Recent reports (such as Chokshi, Mongia, and Wattal 2015; Chowdhury et al. 2015; Mongia et al. 2017; Wattal et al. 2017) have, however, identified significant challenges that India must confront if it seeks to enter the ranks of the leading countries in drug development and manufacturing, or even to assure its own citizens of a reliable supply of drugs that meet the highest standards of quality, safety, and efficacy. This chapter describes the key issues that have been identified, briefly summarizes the manner in which the US and the EU have met similar challenges, and outlines the elements of a possible reform programme taking a cue from these experiences.

This chapter concentrates on drug products, rather than medical devices and related products, because some of the most recent research has had a similar focus. It does not discuss potential reforms of the regulatory system for clinical trials, nor does it address special classes of drug products, such as ayurvedic medicines. Drug regulatory systems in the EU, US, and elsewhere have traditionally recognized the special issues presented by products such as herbal ingredients and homoeopathic medicines and established distinct systems of regulation to deal with them.

CURRENT CHALLENGES TO THE DRUG REGULATORY SYSTEM IN INDIA

Under the current regulatory system, responsibility for regulation of drugs is divided between the national

[1] For recent years trade statistics, see https://pharmexcil.com/trade-statistics, last accessed on 1 February 2020.

authority (the Central Drugs Standards Control Organization, or CDSCO) and the state drug regulatory authorities (SDRAs) in each of the states and union territories in India. The CDSCO has responsibility for registering imported drugs, 'new drugs',[2] and selected categories of drugs such as biologics. The SDRAs supervise other products, including generic drugs, accredit manufacturers and distributors, carry out the great majority of inspections of manufacturing facilities,[3] maintain state laboratories to test samples of distributed drugs, and investigate and prosecute law violations.

The reports issued by the Health Policy Initiative at Indian Council for Research on International Economic Relations (ICRIER) have identified significant challenges to these systems (Chokshi, Mongia, and Wattal 2015; Chowdhury et al. 2015; Wattal et al. 2017). We both were part of ICRIER's research in different capacities—Richard as an advisor and Vasudha as a researcher. Among the challenges highlighted were the following:

- The division of responsibilities between CDSCO and the SDRAs creates the potential for inconsistency in the interpretation and application of regulatory requirements. In addition, there is significant room for improvement in communications between the national and state authorities and among the state authorities themselves.
- There is great disparity in the capabilities and staffing of inspectorates among the SDRAs. Many SDRAs lack the minimum number of trained inspectors to carry out their responsibilities,[4] and there is over-reliance on contractual arrangements.
- Infrastructure at the national and state levels requires significant improvements, especially vis-à-vis deployment of information technology (IT) capable systems, and training and qualifications of staff in the state drug laboratories.
- There is a lack of transparency in the review and decision-making processes and inadequate provision for guidance and advice to applicants to ensure that they submit the information required for product approvals and other regulatory actions.
- There appears to be a high dependence on external reviewers, suggesting understaffing of relevant experts within the regulatory authorities in relation to the size of the market.
- Although there is debate as to the extent of the problem, it appears that a substantial number of substandard and/or counterfeit drugs are offered for sale on the market.[5]
- Track-and-trace requirements (which are one of the methods of reducing the risk that counterfeit products will enter the market and of ensuring traceability when defects are discovered in legitimate drugs) are currently under discussion for the domestic market (track-and-trace mechanisms have already been put in place by the Ministry of Commerce and Industry for the export of medicines from India), but there is at present no agreement on their feasibility or on alternative methods (for example, imprinted dosage forms or product pedigrees).[6]

[2] New drugs are defined to include (a) those which have not been used to a significant extent under proposed conditions of use in India or that have not been recognized as safe and effective by the licensing authority; (b) those already approved by the licensing authority but which are proposed to be approved for new claims; and (c) fixed-dose combinations of two or more previously approved drugs. Drugs lose their 'new' status four years after approval.

[3] While most inspections are carried out by state authorities within their jurisdictions, some inspections are carried out jointly by inspectors from SDRAs and CDSCO (for example, inspections of facilities that hold certificates of pharmaceutical products or that manufacture vaccines, biosimilars, or large-volume parenteral drugs.

[4] In 2003, the Mashelkar Committee recommended that there be one inspector for every 50 manufacturing facilities and every 200 retail pharmacies in a state. In 2015, a report by Chokshi and others (2015) found that even this minimal standard was not met in a number of states.

[5] In this chapter, 'counterfeit' drugs are products manufactured and distributed without complying with applicable government approvals, while 'substandard' drugs are products that are subject to relevant approvals, but that do not meet applicable quality requirements (for example, as to their purity, quantity of active ingredients, or bioavailability). The DCA makes no explicit mention of the term 'counterfeit', and instead uses terms such as 'spurious', 'misbranded', and 'adulterated' to indicate willful trademark infringement. For a detailed discussion on the definitions, see Chokshi et al. (2015). The most recent National Drug Survey 2014–16, carried out by the National Institute of Biologicals under the aegis of the Ministry of Health and Family Welfare (Government of India), reports an estimate of not of standard quality (NSQ) drugs to be 3.16 per cent and spurious drugs to be 0.0245 per cent. The report can be accessed at: https://mohfw.gov.in/documents/reports/drugs-survey-report, last accessed on 6 March 2018.

[6] On India's serialization and traceability initiative for pharmaceuticals, ICRIER along with Alliance for Global Pharmaceutical

- There is an absence of clear and uniform interpretation of requirements for good manufacturing practice (GMP) for drug products.

EXPERIENCE FROM THE US AND THE EU

The US and the EU drug regulatory systems did not spring full-blown in their existing form, but instead evolved over many decades, with periodic adjustments based on experience and changing demands of patients, governments, and other stakeholders. In the history of those systems, one can find the counterpart of virtually every challenge that currently confronts India and, accordingly, lessons can be drawn for the Indian context. We take up individual discussions on both regions.

United States

Many of the drug regulation laws enacted in the US have been the result of major public health scandals.[7] The first such law[8] was passed in 1902 following fatal incidents involving contaminated serums and vaccines (Coleman 2016). That statute required licensing of facilities in which biologics were manufactured for distribution in interstate commerce, but imposed no such requirements for non-biologic drugs. The first general federal law governing foods and drugs, enacted in 1906, prohibited the sale of adulterated drugs but established no requirement for premarket approval or licensing of manufacturing facilities.[9] The federal courts were empowered to impose legal sanctions when drugs were found to violate the minimal standards of the statute (for example, if they did not meet professed standards of purity or quality). To support this function, the predecessor of today's Food and Drug Administration (FDA) relied heavily on laboratories staffed by government chemists who tested samples obtained from inspections or in the market place.[10]

In 1938, following another public health scandal (Hutt, Merrill, and Grossman 2014), in which nearly 100 persons died after receiving an elixir of sulfanilamide containing the deadly poison diethylene glycol, the US Congress enacted the Federal Food, Drug, and Cosmetic Act.[11] Among other things, that statute required manufacturers to submit new drug applications (NDAs) for review by FDA before introducing products to the market. Such applications became effective within 90 days unless FDA made an affirmative decision that a drug was unsafe. The NDA requirement was limited to products that contained active ingredients not previously used in marketed drug products or that represented significant changes to such products, and pre-enactment drugs were excluded from the NDA requirement under a 'grandfather clause'. When drugs had been marketed under NDAs for a reasonable period of time (such as four or five years), FDA often determined that they were no longer 'new' and permitted identical, similar, or related products to enter the market without NDAs. Thus, generic versions of innovative products were commonly introduced with no prior government review (Merrill and Hutt 1980: 371–2).

Following the thalidomide incident of 1962 (when thousands of children in Europe and hundreds in the US

Serialization (RxGPS) had held a consultative meeting of industry and government stakeholders in April 2017. The deliberations at this meeting were produced in the form of a white paper, which included key recommendations for the Government of India with respect to serialization of pharmaceuticals for export and domestic market. The recommendations of this document are summarized in the article here: http://www.expressbpd.com/pharma/pharma-technology-review/making-sense-of-serialisation/389701/, last accessed on 6 March 2018.

[7] Although the US is a federal system comprising 50 ostensibly sovereign states, over the past hundred years or so, the federal government has assumed primary responsibility for most regulation of drugs. Many states maintain 'mini' food and drug laws, but none have substantial resources to enforce them. Most states issue largely ministerial licences for drug facilities within their territories, and all states regulate the practice of pharmacy, including certain aspects of so-called compounding pharmacies. Otherwise, FDA takes the lead in assuring that drugs which enter the market are subject to necessary approvals and comply with requirements for GMP.

[8] 32 Stat. 728 (1902). The current version of the law is now codified as 42 U.S.C. §262. Enforcement of the law was originally entrusted to a laboratory of the Marine and Public Health Service, which was later incorporated in the agency that became the National Institutes of Health. In 1972, responsibility for enforcement of the Biologics Act was transferred to the Food and Drug Administration. See Coleman (2016).

[9] Food and Drugs Act of 1906, 34 Stat. 768. Enforcement of the act was entrusted to an agency within Department of Agriculture that eventually came to be known as the Food and Drug Administration. After a series of government reorganizations, FDA became an agency of the Department of Health and Human Services.

[10] The agency originally entrusted with enforcement of the law was known as the Bureau of Chemistry. For many years thereafter, FDA's scientific resources were largely confined to chemical analysis of foods and drugs in the market place.

[11] 52 Stat. 1040 (1938). The statute is currently codified at 21 U.S.C. §§201 *et seq.*

were born with severe birth defects after their mothers received the tranquilizer during pregnancy), the US Congress once again revisited the statutory requirements for drug regulation. New drugs could now be marketed only after FDA approval, and the law was amended to require proof of efficacy in addition to safety. The US Congress directed FDA to review all drugs that entered the market under the old NDA system between 1938 and 1962 to determine whether they met the new efficacy requirement. The US Congress also made a major change relating to drug quality: drugs would be deemed to be adulterated if they were not manufactured and stored in accordance with current GMP, even if there was no evidence that such products were substandard in purity or other aspects of quality.[12]

Following enactment of the 1962 amendments, FDA initiated a series of programmes that largely transformed drug regulation in the US. As part of the review of efficacy of pre-1962 drug products, FDA required manufacturers of 'me too' drugs (that is, drugs which copied existing innovative products), including generics, that had not previously been subject to NDAs to submit applications and market their products in accordance with them. The agency also promulgated regulations setting out detailed requirements for GMP,[13] and compliance with those regulations and guidance issued under them now became the main focus of quality assurance. Although FDA maintained laboratories to test samples in the marketplace, the primary emphasis was on assurance of quality through premarket review of manufacturing methods (set out in NDAs), inspections of manufacturing facilities prior to and following approval, and vigorous enforcement when recurrent GMP issues were detected.[14] In addition, FDA recognized the importance of limited clinical studies to ensure that generic drugs would be bioequivalent to reference products, issuing regulations in 1977 that contained detailed requirements for such testing.[15] Today, with very limited exceptions, all prescription drugs sold in the US are subject to full or abbreviated NDAs that have been reviewed by FDA, and all drugs in the market place are required to comply with provisions of GMP.[16]

To enforce compliance with requirements for GMP, FDA maintains a staff of several thousand inspectors,[17] located in offices around the US and in selected foreign countries. Inspectors are highly trained and work according to detailed policies governing inspections, under the supervision of FDA's headquarters offices.

Finally, it is worth noting that the US, like India, has experienced problems with counterfeit drugs, which are typically distributed by criminal organizations that make no effort to comply with requirements for NDAs, GMP, or other provisions of US drug law.[18] Legislation enacted in the 1960s empowers FDA to investigate drug counterfeiters, and federal prosecutors can initiate criminal proceedings and other enforcement actions against them. Provisions enacted in 2013 require recordkeeping

[12] Drug Amendments of 1962, 76 Stat. 780.

[13] 21 C.F.R. Parts 210–11.

[14] FDA relies mainly on informal enforcement mechanisms, including notices of inspectional observations and warning letters to industry, but it can also invoke statutory powers to interdict import of drugs from non-compliant manufacturers located outside the US and refer cases to the Department of Justice for formal judicial proceedings, including injunction actions. In recent settlements of court cases relating to GMP violations, financial penalties of as much at USD 750 million have been imposed, and manufacturers have been subjected to onerous requirements, including third-party supervision of product-release decisions and regular FDA inspections (paid for by manufacturers). See US Department of Justice press release, 9 January 2020, at https://www.justice.gov/opa/pr/justice-department-recovers-over-3-billion-false-claims-act-cases-fiscal-year-2019, last accessed on 1 February 2020.

[15] The requirement for pre-market approval of generic drugs was ratified by the US Congress when it enacted the Drug Price Competition and Patent Term Restoration Act of 1984 (commonly known as the Hatch–Waxman Act), Public L. 98–417. Such drugs are subject to abbreviated new drug applications (ANDAs) that contain full details as to manufacturing processes and data necessary to demonstrate bioequivalence to reference drugs. FDA has issued detailed guidance documents concerning the test methods required to demonstrate bioequivalence.

[16] Many nonprescription drugs containing old and well-established active ingredients are marketed pursuant to over-the-counter (OTC) drug monographs issued by FDA which contain requirements for active ingredients, dosages, and instructions for use. 21 C.F.R. Parts 330–69. Nonprescription drugs must also comply with the same requirements for GMP as apply to prescription drugs.

[17] As of May 2017, FDA's Office of Global Operations, which conducts inspections in the US and abroad, had a total of 5,065 employees. See FDA website at https://www.fda.gov/aboutfda/centersoffices/officeofglobalregulatoryoperationsandpolicy/default.htm.

[18] The statute defines a counterfeit drug, in part, to mean 'a drug which, … without authorization, bears the trademark, trade name, or other identifying mark … of a drug manufacturer … and which thereby falsely purports or is represented to be the product of … such other drug manufacturer'. 21 U.S.C. §321(g)(2).

systems, including drug 'pedigrees', that should greatly reduce the scope for counterfeit drugs.[19]

Europe

Most European countries did not adopt premarket approval requirements for drugs until the thalidomide incident in the 1960s, and they were, to some extent, able to benefit from the experience (and mistakes) of the US. The framework directive for drug regulation issued by the predecessor of the EU in 1965 did not distinguish between 'new' and 'old' drugs but instead required marketing authorizations (the equivalent of US NDAs) for all 'proprietary medicinal products' (that is, finished pharmaceutical products) based on proof of safety, efficacy, and quality.[20] Provisions adopted in 1986 established standards for approval of generic medicinal products, for which full quality dossiers and data demonstrating equivalence to reference products are required.[21]

The regulatory system adopted in Europe contemplates an almost completely closed system, with government authorizations for manufacturers, importers, and distributors. In nearly all member states, retail sale of medicinal products is permitted only by pharmacies, which are also subject to government licensing requirements.[22]

Current European legislation establishes requirements for GMP and sets out the concept of the 'qualified person' (QP), an employee or contractor of the manufacturing authorization holder who certifies that each batch of medicinal products released for sale conforms to the requirements of the marketing authorization and GMP. EU and member state laws set standards for the education and experience of QPs, require that they be registered by the member state in which they perform their services, and impose legal responsibility on them for ensuring that products released under their supervision meet applicable quality requirements.[23] The EU has also established requirements for a good distribution practice (GDP), which apply to wholesalers and similar intermediaries in the distribution chain.[24]

EU member state inspectorates have substantial powers to ensure compliance with GMP requirements. They can, for example, revoke GMP certificates for manufacturing facilities (including facilities outside the EU), so that QPs will not certify any batches of drugs originating from those facilities. They can also suspend or revoke manufacturing authorizations for facilities within the EU, thereby making further manufacturing operations unlawful until compliance issues are resolved to the satisfaction of the inspectorate.

The EU also had to deal with a problem that did not face the US FDA: the regulatory system is based on the expectation that inspections of manufacturing establishments will be carried out by officials of the individual member states, among which there were historical disparities in regulatory systems and capabilities.[25] It was thus critically important that the EU establish benchmarks for qualification and experience of inspectors, common procedures for inspections, systems for recognition of inspections among the member states, and methods of communicating inspectional findings across the member states. The methods by which this was accomplished in the EU can serve as a model for a large nation such as India that is organized as a federal system in which the states play a major role in pharmaceutical inspections and enforcement.[26]

[19] These requirements are contained in the Drug Quality and Security Act, Pub. L. 113–54.

[20] Council Directive 65/65 of 26 January 1965 on the approximation of provisions laid down by law, regulation, or administrative action relating to proprietary medicinal products, 1965 J.O. (No. 22) 369, reprinted in 1972 O.J. (1965–66) at 20 (special English edition). The directive has since been superseded by European Parliament and Council Directive 2001/83 (EC) as amended. See European Commission Eudralex website at https://ec.europa.eu/health/sites/health/files/files/eudralex/vol-1/dir_2001_83_consol_2012/dir_2001_83_cons_2012_en.pdf.

[21] Council Directive 87/21/EEC of 22 December 1986, amending Directive 65/65/EEC. 1987 O.J. (No. L 15) 36.

[22] A handful of member states permit the sale of a limited number of nonprescription medicinal products by outlets other than pharmacies. The UK regime, which is among the most liberal ones, permits certain nonprescription drugs to be sold in supermarkets, but the list of such products is short and, in many cases, there are restrictions on the number of doses that can be contained in a single package.

[23] See European Parliament and Council Directive 2001/83/EC as amended, title IV. The principles of GMP, originally adopted in 1991, are currently set out in Commission Directive 2003/94/EC of 8 October 2003.

[24] Guidelines of 5 November 2013 on GDP of medicinal products for human use, 2013 O.J. C 343/1 (23 November 2013).

[25] In some member states with federal systems, inspectors do not even work for the national government but are employed by the federal states or autonomous regions, which may differ by the number and quality of their inspectors.

[26] Details concerning these arrangements can be found in volume 4 of the European Commission's Eudralex website at https://ec.europa.eu/health/documents/eudralex/vol-4_en.

RECOMMENDATIONS BASED ON THE DISCUSSION

Many reports (Department-Related Parliamentary Standing Committee on Health and Family Welfare 2012; Mashlekar et al. 2003; Mongia et al. 2017; NIB 2016; Wattal et al. 2017) have set out recommendations for improvements in the regulatory system for drugs in India, and it is not the purpose of this chapter to repeat them. Instead, what follows is a series of recommendations that draws specifically on the experience of the US and the EU in dealing with challenges currently faced in India. The aim is to identify the features that are best suited to the needs of the Indian industry and its regulators. There is a particular focus on measures that can help assure the quality of products and protect patients against receiving substandard or counterfeit drugs.

Establishing a Closed System of Drug Distribution

India may wish to consider the EU model for controlling the importation, manufacture, and distribution of drugs. That model contemplates licensing requirements for all entities involved in the process, including importers, manufacturers, distributors and wholesalers, and the points of retail sale or administration. A key element of such a system is a legal requirement, imposed on each licencee at each stage of the process, to demand evidence from its suppliers that they hold required licences and are otherwise in compliance with applicable regulatory provisions, and to provide similar evidence of compliance to their customers down the supply chain. Any drug within the supply chain in the possession of an entity (other than the ultimate consumer) which is not in compliance with these requirements is automatically deemed to be unlawful, and the person in possession of the drug is deemed to be an offender. Such a system substantially reduces the need for testing of samples of drugs in the marketplace and lessens the burden of proof in enforcement proceedings relating to counterfeit drugs.[27]

[27] Further consideration of this approach should take account of the pharmaceutical distribution systems in India and the role of 'carrying and forwarding agents' (CFAs), who are nodal points of contact between the pharmaceutical manufacturers and the retailers in each state. Although drug distribution systems in India have not been extensively examined in the literature, some issues have been raised in Jeffery (2007).

Improve the Capability of Industry and Government to Assure Drug Quality

The EU and US systems both recognize that the primary responsibility for assuring the quality of drugs rests with manufacturers, who must build quality into each stage of the manufacturing process. Other measures, including testing of finished products, periodic internal audits, government inspections, and testing by government laboratories, play an important but secondary role. The key functions of government are, therefore, to ensure that manufacturers fully understand their responsibility, encourage and facilitate voluntary compliance, and punish repeated or serious instances of non-compliance with dissuasive penalties.

Several specific measures may assist in the accomplishment of these goals:

- Establish clear government standards for GMP, including detailed guidance for specific aspects of quality systems.[28]
- Initiate government-sponsored educational programmes to ensure that all manufacturers understand the requirements of GMP. Some such programmes have in fact already been initiated by the Department of Pharmaceuticals (under the Ministry of Chemicals and Fertilizers) and the Indian Drug Manufacturers Association (an association of small and medium drug manufacturers in India). Beginning in 2015 they have collaboratively been conducting country-wide workshops to train officials within small and medium enterprises. More work is, however, required.
- Each batch of finished drug products manufactured or imported by Indian companies should be certified by a qualified person or QP registered with relevant state or national government regulatory authority and having educational qualifications and experience set out in law. As in the EU, the QP should bear personal legal responsibility if non-compliant products are released for sale.
- Marketing authorization applications for all drug products should be submitted, preferably to the

[28] Guidance issued by the EU may provide a starting point, since it is clearly organized and readily accessible. See part I of volume 4 of the Eudralex website, https://ec.europa.eu/health/documents/eudralex/vol-4_en.

national regulatory authority,[29] to ensure that all applications are reviewed by relevant experts and to maintain consistency in approval decisions for all drugs, including generics. Dossiers for generic versions of reference products previously authorized as 'new' drugs should contain full quality sections, in the same detail as those submitted for new drugs,[30] coupled with data to demonstrate therapeutic equivalence to reference products.[31] To facilitate these requirements, the national regulator should issue detailed guidance for the content and format of applications and establish systems for providing pre-submission advice, where appropriate, to ensure that applications meet expectations and can be reviewed efficiently.

- Pre-approval inspections for all drugs, carried out by national or state authorities as appropriate, to confirm that facilities and equipment are as claimed in applications and compliant with GMP. Although such inspections are already carried out, it is important to ensure that they address not only general issues of GMP but also focus on details of facilities, manufacturing methods, in-process controls, and other commitments made in marketing authorization applications. Deviations from such commitments may affect the quality of finished products, including, in the case of generic drugs, equivalence to reference products.
- Conduct periodic, risk-based inspections of drug manufacturing facilities to assure continuing compliance with GMP and provisions of marketing authorizations. Such an approach was announced by the CDSCO in 2016, and training programmes were conducted over the course of the year.[32] It is critically important that this initiative be fully implemented at both the state and national levels.
- Establish measures to improve the capability of state regulatory authorities to carry out inspections, including training programmes sponsored by the national authorities, establishment of agreed procedures for inspections and inspection reports, and similar measures.[33]
- Establish GDP to ensure that drugs are transported and held by distributors and retailers under conditions adequate to protect their quality and potency, coupled with inspections and enforcement measures to encourage compliance with good distribution practices.[34]
- Enhance enforcement powers, including effective penalties for dealing with manufacturers, distributors, and retailers that fail to comply with applicable licence requirements. At present, licence suspensions are often imposed for short periods, whereas suspensions in the EU normally continue until a facility has been re-inspected and determined to be in full compliance with applicable legal requirements, including GMP and specifications in marketing authorizations.
- Invest towards a real-time, preferably online, mechanism for communication and coordination among national and state regulatory authorities

[29] If the state regulatory authorities continue to review certain applications, including those for generic drugs, it will be important to ensure that they have sufficient qualified reviewers. Ideally, state authorities should not rely on external reviewers, as this will significantly increase the risk of inconsistency in the quality of reviews. In addition, the national authorities should establish detailed guidelines for review processes and operate training programmes to ensure consistency among the state regulatory review processes.

[30] Appendix IA to Schedule Y of the DCR appears to require less detail as to the manufacturing processes for drugs already approved in India than for those not previously approved. If so, this is not consistent with the practice in the EU and US, which requires the same level of detail as for innovative products.

[31] The need for bioequivalence studies was considered by the CDSCO in 2017. As a first step, such data have been made mandatory for drugs that fall under class II and class IV of the Biopharmaceutics Classification System. As of now it is not clear whether the national or state regulators will review the data; if the states have this responsibility, it will be important to ensure that they have the necessary expertise. The relevant amendment to the DCR is set out at https://cdsco.gov.in/opencms/opencms/system/modules/CDSCO.WEB/elements/download_file_division.jsp?num_id=OTgy, last accessed on 28 January 2020.

[32] The relevant public notice can be accessed here http://cdsco.nic.in/writereaddata/Public%20Notice26_5_2016.pdf.

[33] Documents in the Eudralex website give a good idea about how these efforts have been carried out in the EU. See European Commission, *Compilation of Community Procedures on Inspections and Exchange of Information* (EMA/572454/2014/Rec 17) at http://www.ema.europa.eu/docs/en_GB/document_library/Regulatory_and_procedural_guideline/2009/10/WC500004706.pdf.

[34] EU guidelines for good distribution practices may provide a useful starting point. See note 26 and Eudralex website at http://eur-lex.europa.eu/legal-content/EN/TXT/?uri=uriserv:OJ.C_.2013.343.01.0001.01.ENG&toc=OJ:C:2013:343:TOC.b

to share inspection findings and coordinate,[35] coupled with establishment of an inspections working party, composed of representatives of national and state inspectorates, which would hold frequent meetings to coordinate policy initiatives, approve new guidance and procedural documents, and carry out similar tasks.

***

It is recognized that some of the proposals set out in this chapter would entail significant investments of time, financial resources, and personnel at both the national and state levels. It is advised, however, that implementation of procedures along the lines suggested is essential if India wishes to assure that drugs supplied to its citizens are safe, effective, and of suitable quality and to take its rightful place among the world leaders in the development and manufacturing of both new and generic drug products.

REFERENCES

Bogaert, P., & D. Geradin. 2014. *EU Law and Life Sciences*. New York: Institute of Competition Law.

Coleman, T.S. 2016. 'Early Developments in the Regulation of Biologics', 71 Food & Drug Law J. 544.

Chokshi, M., R. Mongia and V. Wattal. 2015. 'Drug Quality and Safety Issues in India', ICRIER Working Paper (September), ICRIER, New Delhi

Chowdhury, N., P. Joshi, A. Patnaik, and B. Saraswathy. 2015. 'Administrative Structure and Functions of Drug Regulatory Authorities in India', ICRIER Working Paper (September), ICRIER, New Delhi.

Department-Related Parliamentary Standing Committee on Health and Family Welfare. 2012. *59th Report on the functioning of the Central Drugs Standard Control Organization (CDCSO)*. New Delhi: Rajya Sabha Secretariat. Available at http://164.100.47.5/newcommittee/reports/EnglishCommittees/Committee%20on%20Health%20and%20Family%20Welfare/59.pdf, last accessed 28 January 2020).

Hutt, P., D. Merrill, and L. Grossman. 2014. *Food and Drug Law: Cases and Materials* 4th edition.

Jeffrey, R. 2007. *Pharmaceutical Distribution Systems in India*. Edinburgh: The Centre for International Health Policy.

Kingham, R. 2017. *The Life Sciences Law Review*, 5th edition. London: Law Business Research.

Mashelkar, R.A. et al. 2003. *Report of the Expert Committee on a Comprehensive Examination of Drug Regulatory Issues, Including the Problem of Spurious Drugs*. New Delhi: Ministry of Health and Family Welfare.

Merrill R., and P. Hutt, *Food and Drug Law: Cases and Materials* (1st ed. 1980).

NIB (National Institute of Biologicals). Survey of the extent of problems of spurious and not of standard quality drugs in the country 2014–16. Noida (Uttar Pradesh). National Institute of Biologicals, Ministry of Health and Family Welfare, Government of India.

Mongia, R., D. Pokhriyal, S. Rao, and A. Mehdi. 2017. *Challenges and Prospects for Clinical Trials in India: A Regulatory Perspective*. New Delhi: Academic Foundation.

Wattal, V., P. Joshi, A. Arora, and A. Mehdi. 2017. *International Cooperation for Registration of Medicines in India: Opportunities for India*. New Delhi: Academic Foundation.

[35] A major mechanism for such communications in the EU is the EudraGMP website, which contains both public information on licensed manufacturing facilities and nonpublic information, available only to regulators, concerning inspections, enforcement actions, and similar matters. See http://eudragmdp.ema.europa.eu/inspections/displayWelcome.do.

20

Regulation of Medicines

Promoting Global Supply Chain Security

Susan Winckler and Alissa McCaffrey

Inputs to health status are broad and diverse, and there is a case to be made for promoting health prior to injury or illness, but sometimes there is no substitute for medical care, including pharmaceutical treatment. A key manufacturer and exporter of pharmaceuticals, India has emerged as a leader in the global pharmaceutical market. Pharmaceuticals manufactured in India are exported to more than 200 countries, and make up 40 per cent of the generic demand in the US.[1] Foreign pharmaceutical investment of nearly INR 916 billion (USD 14 billion) since 2010 has helped stimulate massive growth in the Indian pharmaceutical industry.[2] The third largest in the world by volume and fourteenth largest by value (approximately INR 1.95 trillion, or USD 30 billion),[3] the value of the Indian pharmaceutical market is expected to reach INR 3.6 trillion (USD 55 billion) by 2020.[4]

To help maintain its status as a leader in the global pharmaceutical market and promote an image of safety and security for its exported products, India has taken important initial steps to ensure the security of the pharmaceutical supply chain and the quality and authenticity of Indian pharmaceutical products worldwide. Passed into law in 2011, the Indian pharmaceutical serialization and traceability requirements were among the first in the world. Over the past several years, serialization and traceability requirements have been increasingly adopted by other markets around the world as a means of securing the pharmaceutical supply chain and protecting patient access to safe and effective medications. Serialization and traceability of pharmaceutical products create more transparency and visibility of each product in the pharmaceutical supply chain and therefore enable stakeholders to catch duplicative and unauthorized serial numbers. Though these functionalities depend on system accuracy and sustainability, a well-implemented,

[1] Indian Brand Equity Foundation (IBEF), *India Pharmaceutical Industry.* Available at http://www.ibef.org/industry/pharmaceutical-india.aspx (last accessed on 4 March 2020).

[2] India Department of Pharmaceuticals (IDP), *Indian Pharmaceutical Industry—A Global Industry*. Available at: http://pharmaceuticals.gov.in/pharma-industry-promotion (last accessed on 4 March 2020).

[3] IDP, *Indian Pharmaceutical Industry—A Global Industry.*

[4] IBEF, *India Pharmaceutical Industry*, updated March 2017.

well-tested, and accurate model can provide great public health benefits. In developing and implementing such systems, India is at the forefront of pharmaceutical supply chain security worldwide. However, it will only remain at the forefront if the continued implementation is done in an effective, efficient manner that facilitates cross-border trade.

SUPPLY CHAIN SECURITY AND TRACEABILITY

Threats, Risks, and the Need for Enhanced Security

A breach of the pharmaceutical supply chain can have serious health consequences including product shortages that delay appropriate patient treatment, and medical complications for those who receive ineffective or damaged product that could, in severe cases, result in death. The market for counterfeit drugs has expanded in recent years, posing a risk to patients since counterfeit drugs are substandard products and also physically indistinguishable from safe, valid products. In addition, when drugs are diverted or stolen from the supply chain, they may be intentionally altered or damaged due to improper storage or exposure to contaminants. Therefore, the quality and safety of the product cannot be assured or maintained. According to the World Health Organization (WHO), the existence of substandard and falsified (SF) medical products affect every region of the world, and medicines from all major therapeutic categories.[5]

While serialization and the use of serialized data (that is, traceability), described below, is an important, and potentially necessary, tool for improving supply chain security and preventing falsified medications from being distributed to patients, serialization and traceability alone are insufficient to protect the supply chain. Systems and processes for serialization and traceability are intended to be implemented on top of a series of fundamental supply chain protections such as good distribution practices (GDPs), which provide for a baseline level of quality and safety in the purchase, receipt, storage, and export of pharmaceuticals for human use, authorized trading partner requirements, which institute a process for registering/licensing legitimate supply chain entities, and enforcement authorities, which provide in-country entities with the legal authority and responsibility to enforce supply chain security requirements upon entities manufacturing, transferring, supplying, and dispensing pharmaceuticals.

WHAT IS SERIALIZATION?

Serialization is the process by which products are marked with a unique identifier—typically a unique number or alphanumeric code. That unique serial number, along with other related information, is typically encoded in a barcode affixed to the package that can be read electronically (see, for example, Figure 20.1). As a general matter of practice, the barcode includes the serial number, a product number (referred to as a Global Trade Item Number or GTIN), the date of expiry, and the batch number of the product. This barcode and data elements (collectively referred to here as the 'unit identifier') are affixed to the lowest saleable unit—the smallest amount of product intended for sale to a dispensing entity (that is, pharmacy). In our example, '(21)' represents the serial number, '(01)' is product number, '(17)' the date of expiry (given in YYMMDD format), and '(10)' is the batch number of the product.

PACKAGING LEVELS AND SERIALIZATION

There are three main levels of packaging for pharmaceutical products moving through the supply chain, each with its own serialization requirements.

- Primary level—the level of packaging in direct contact with the product (for example, blister card, vial, single therapy kit, and ampule).
- Secondary level—a package containing one or more primary packages, or a group of primary packages containing a single item. The secondary package is often the smallest level intended to be sold to the dispenser/pharmacy (that is, the saleable unit). In some instances (for example,

Figure 20.1 A serial number representation
Source: Image courtesy of GS1 Global.

[5] The WHO, *Substandard and Falsified (SF) Medical Products*, updated 2018. Available at http://www.who.int/medicines/regulation/ssffc/en/.

a bottle of tablets without an outer carton), the primary package and the secondary package can be the same.

- Tertiary level—the logistic unit (for example, shipper, carton, case, pallet, and tote) containing one or more primary/secondary levels of packaging.

General industry consensus is that the unit identifier should be affixed to each saleable unit, often the secondary package. Product serialization at the primary level is costly and has not been pursued or successfully achieved by any other global market. Many manufacturers estimate that the addition of primary package serialization (when the secondary package is the serialized saleable unit) would cost up to USD 1 million per packaging line, and most manufacturers use many lines to package products. Serialization of the primary package may not even be technically feasible in some instances because of product size or packaging material. Furthermore, serialization of the secondary package is the smallest level of serialization needed for the most basic traceability functionality (that is, point-of-dispense verification).

THE VALUE OF SERIALIZATION AND TRACEABILITY

Serialization itself provides virtually no benefit to the supply chain, rather, it is the use of that serialized data in a traceability system that enhances supply chain security.[6] The infrastructure and processes that leverage serialized data to improve supply chain security are collectively referred to as a 'traceability system'.

Traceability systems can provide an audit trail of the path of a pharmaceutical package from the current entity/owner back to the manufacturer. The serialization of pharmaceuticals, and application of the unit identifier (as described before), enables traceability systems and processes. For example, once a unique serial number is affixed to an individual product package (that is, serialization), systems can then be developed to generate a report from the supply chain of when each trading partner purchased and sold the package carrying that unique serial number (that is, traceability). Although serialization requires large investments of time and resources, with the appropriate infrastructure and technology the data acquired from serialized product can be leveraged to address challenges, such as counterfeiting and product diversion, by increasing transparency and control throughout the pharmaceutical supply chain. Further, knowledge of where a product has been and which entities had ownership of a product as it made its way through the supply chain has great utility for product investigations (for example, this can help identify where an illegitimate product entered the legitimate supply chain) and recalls (that is, can allow for more precise and rapid recall) of pharmaceutical products if necessary (Brown, Nichols, and Chang 2015).

Importantly, the relative benefits of traceability systems vary depending on the specifics of implementation including the specific data discovery and data reporting models, the adherence of supply chain entities to global norms and in-country requirements, and the level of enforcement across industry of a standardized serialization and traceability approach.

TRACEABILITY MODELS FOR SERIALIZED PRODUCT

There are two main models of traceability used globally: a verification model (typically at the point-of-dispense) and a tracing model.

In a verification model, product serial numbers are authenticated at the end of the supply chain. At the most basic level, this model has only two components. First, manufacturers must affix a serial number to a product package and maintain a repository or database of the serial numbers they commission (or generate). This is done by manufacturers as part of the serialization process. Second, dispensers must have a mechanism in place by which the unit identifier on the product can be 'verified' against the data commissioned or generated by the manufacturer. By only involving manufacturers and dispensers, this model limits the number of stakeholders that must integrate their data systems to a traceability system. Other supply chain partners (that is, wholesale distributors, third party logistics or 3PLs) are not required to scan, upload, transmit, or otherwise connect to a data communication pathway.

While the complexity of serialization and verification should not be understated, verification is the least complex of the various approaches that can be taken, and results in significant benefits to patient safety and supply chain security. In fact, serialization without point-of-dispense verification, at minimum, does little to advance patient safety. A point-of-dispense verification

[6] RxGPS, *Serialization Primer*, 29 March 2016. Available at http://www.rxgpsalliance.org/wp-content/uploads/2016/03/Serialization-Primer-032916.pdf.

model increases the likelihood that adulterated or counterfeit product will be identified and removed from the supply chain *before* it is delivered to a patient. After the product is delivered, it becomes impossible to ensure that the damaged or ineffective product is not used by a patient.

A traceability system is significantly more complex to implement than verification. First, traceability requires the capture (that is, scanning and recording of product data in a standardized format) and maintenance of significantly more data. A traceability system, however, requires *every* company that owns a product to capture and maintain data about each serialized unit. It is a significant operational burden to scan and capture the data, and a significant information technology burden to maintain the related data repository. As noted earlier, a verification model requires only the manufacturer to capture and maintain information about each individual serialized unit—an activity that is part of existing serialization processes. Second, a traceability model significantly increases the number and complexity of data connections needed. A traceability system requires that every member of the supply chain connect to some type of data exchange, not just manufacturers and dispensers.

A traceability system provides modest additional security value to the supply chain beyond verification, but comes at a significant cost. For example, in the event that a counterfeit product enters the supply chain, a verification model is likely required to identify that product as counterfeit and prevent it from being dispensed to a patient, while the addition of traceability will also facilitate an investigation of where that product penetrated the legitimate supply chain. This is a modest benefit to patient safety and supply chain security, but is significantly more complex, as depicted by Figure 20.2.

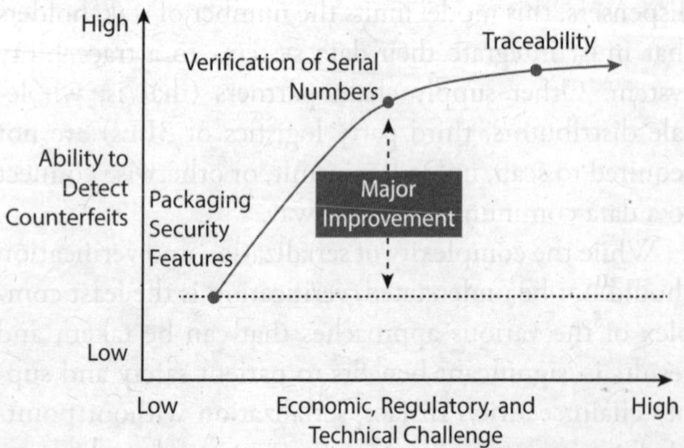

Figure 20.2 The Indian Approach to Supply Chain Security

GOALS

As a significant global exporter of pharmaceutical products, India's image as a safe and secure manufacturer of drugs is incredibly important. It was in response to questions threatening this image that the India serialization requirements for exported product were first developed with the stated purpose to 'address counterfeit and ineffective product recall challenges, which effects the entire healthcare supply chain, from manufacturers all the way to patients, wholesalers, distributors, exporters and healthcare providers.'[7]

There is also a desire on the part of Indian regulators to facilitate development of a system to 'authenticate the genuineness of drugs' being produced and dispensed domestically (that is, within India). This desire was the impetus for draft domestic serialization requirements.

EXPORT REQUIREMENTS

On 10 January 2011, the Directorate General of Foreign Trade (DGFT), announced the adoption and implementation of a traceability system incorporating serialization for all pharmaceutical products exported from India. Specifically, exported drug products must carry a one or two-dimensional barcode encoding the unit identifier. For all products manufactured on or after 1 April 2016, non-small scale industry (non-SSI) manufacturers must serialize the secondary and tertiary package. Small scale industry (SSI) manufacturers were required to serialize all product packages at the secondary and tertiary level as of 1 April 2017. Serialization of the primary package is optional for exported products. Manufacturers must aggregate[8] lower-level packaging to higher-level packaging and upload this 'parent-child' information to a central database.

According to the export requirements, manufacturers may apply for an exemption that would remove

[7] Implementation Guidelines for Coding & Labelling Pharmaceuticals and Drugs Using Global Supply Chain Standards to Meet Directorate General of Foreign Trade's (DGFT's) Authentication, Track and Trace Requirements, Version 1.3, at 5 (August 2015). Available at http://dava.gov.in/davahq/files/DGFT_Drug_Track_N_Trace_Implementation_Manual.pdf, last accessed on 24 January 2020.

[8] Aggregation associates a set of 'contained' or 'child' objects (for example, cases) within a 'containing' or 'parent' entity (for example, pallet). The parent identifier identifies the aggregation and the 'children' contained within the parent entity.

their obligation to serialize the primary and secondary packaging levels. Exemptions are reserved for drugs exported to a country where the government of the importing country has mandated or formally notified its intention to mandate its own serialization requirements.[9] Manufacturers must obtain written approval from the Indian government to avail themselves of this exemption.

While the export requirements have not been officially revoked or amended, as of February 2020, the Centre for Development of Advanced Computing (CDAC) has proposed that exported product data no longer be reported to the Drugs Authentication and Verification Application (DAVA) portal, but to the Integrated Validation of Exports of Drugs from India and its Authentication (iVEDA) portal.

DRAFT DOMESTIC REQUIREMENTS

On 3 June 2015, The Department of Health and Family Welfare issued a proposed amendment to the Drugs and Cosmetics Rules (DCR), 1945. The proposed amendment would require manufacturers to serialize the primary, secondary, and tertiary packaging levels. Manufacturers would also be required to maintain parent–child (that is, aggregation) data and information about the movement of their products through the supply chain and upload that data to a central database. Responsibility for the correctness, completeness, and timeliness of data reported to the central portal would be assigned to the manufacturer. This draft amendment has not been revised or finalized.

DAVA DATABASE/iVEDA DATABASE

The Indian system utilizes a centralized database model. In a centralized model, all data are accessed from a central storage repository. All supply chain participants move a copy of their data to the database for storage and for the purposes of verification queries. Then, when a barcode is scanned (for example, for a verification request at the point-of-dispense), the information encoded can be cross-checked with the database containing known serial numbers.

[9] As of May 2018, these countries include: Saudi Arabia, Russia, the European Union, the United States, Turkey, and Nigeria.

AREAS OF ATTENTION

Generally speaking, there are four key steps on the pathway to a well-regulated, secure pharmaceutical supply chain using serialization and traceability. The first is the development of market-specific, yet globally aligned, requirements by the government of a given market. The second is the development of systems and processes to meet the requirements (much of which is carried out in the private sector). Third is the implementation of the requirements by utilizing the necessary systems and processes, and fourth is ongoing revision, modification, and enforcement of the requirements. Each of these steps comes with important considerations gleaned from the various markets that have undergone similar processes, or from the unique circumstances or considerations specific to particular market, such as India.

THOUGHTFULLY DEVELOPED SERIALIZATION REQUIREMENTS

Serialization of pharmaceuticals can have various applications in the marketplace, but there are also many supply chain problems for which serialization may not be the appropriate solution. Serialization is just one important tool that can advance the security of the legitimate supply chain and reduce fraud. Also, the multiple approaches to traceability (for example, verification and full traceability) vary in ease, cost, and duration of implementation. Therefore, it is imperative that a country identifies its goals and objectives prior to the development of a serialization or traceability mandate in order to identify the best way to achieve the stated goals.

An understanding of the full economic and regulatory impact of requirements for serialization and traceability is also important when finalizing serialization and traceability requirements. The proposed requirements for domestic product in India contemplate a traceability system, which provides some added benefit beyond authentication but imposes regulatory requirements on all members of the supply chain and requires the collection and maintenance of significantly more data. An alternate approach, used in the European Union, is the 'end-point authentication' model which combines a point-of-dispense verification with additional security checks to verify the authenticity of a drug within the pharmacy before it is dispensed to the patient. This approach requires significantly less data to be collected and maintained and places less of a burden on the supply chain. An economic impact assessment for domestic requirements under consideration could help regulators understand the full impact—both costs and benefits—of alternative approaches to serialization and supply chain security so a model that appropriately limits costs while also protecting patients can be implemented. A regulatory impact assessment for the serialization and traceability requirements currently in effect for exports will also help to understand the impact of those requirements.

Serialization and traceability requirements should be developed with the appropriate global context and consideration for the challenges and successes experienced by other markets implementing similar controls. The importance of globally consistent and/or interoperable requirements cannot be overstated. Stakeholder input early in the regulatory process can also help to ensure that any requirements can be implemented by industry in an efficient, effective manner that is consistent with their existing systems and processes. The technical details of implementation require a deep understanding of the existing systems and processes, which can only be provided by those industry members. Successful and efficient implementation requires this input from impacted stakeholders early in the process when requirements are first being formulated, and also through public feedback on draft requirements.

SYSTEMS SHOULD BE DESIGNED TO MEET THE REQUIREMENTS

The technological infrastructure required to facilitate any level of serialization is complex and requires a significant investment of time and resources, particularly on the part of pharmaceutical manufacturers who must reconfigure all of their packaging lines to serialize product. Further, the infrastructure for storing and sharing data requires clear specifications, complex software development, impressive storage capacity, and important security checks and protocols. For India, the functioning and security of the central database is the responsibility of the government. In other markets, the private sector maintains its own data and is responsible for developing the appropriate systems and processes for data security, storage, and sharing.

Technological solutions should not dictate regulatory requirements or the resulting implementation of those requirements. In India, a number of operational challenges have arisen as a result of the way the DAVA portal and database were developed and structured. In many instances, the structure of the portal and database are forcing industry members to act in a manner that is not consistent with the regulatory requirements and runs counter to well-established data and information integrity principles for regulated industry.

For example, industry was advised to generate 'fictitious', 'dummy', 'virtual', or 'fake' data for certain data fields within DAVA database because these fields are not able to be marked optional and no data are technically required for these fields, which entirely contradicts basic principles of good regulatory practices, and specifically Current good manufacturing practices (GMPs). Fake data also presents an opportunity for fraud, deception, and illegal practices which undermines the entire system: if a counterfeiter acquires any fake serial numbers uploaded to a central database and uses them to label counterfeit products, those counterfeit products would be verified by the database as being *legitimate*—allowing exploitation of the very system developed to curtail these types of activities. This issue was a result only of the structure of the DAVA database. It is not a specific regulatory requirement, but became a 'requirement of regulators' because of the DAVA database construct. The iVEDA Portal was designed to fix many of the challenges of the DAVA database. However, once again the new technology will be dictating requirements as the Indian law for serialization and reporting has not been revised. Instead of dictating the means of compliance, technology solutions should be designed to meet relevant regulatory and business requirements.

IMPORTANCE OF EXPERIENCES OF OTHER MARKETS

Several countries have made substantial progress toward implementation of serialization and traceability, and the experiences of the public and private sectors in those countries should inform the development of serialization and traceability capabilities in other countries. By leveraging these experiences, markets can create efficiencies that will lower implementation costs and increase the speed and ease of implementation. A key lesson learned among countries implementing serialization and traceability is that requirements should facilitate, not impede, cross-border trade.

The first step in facilitating cross-border trade is implementation of serialization requirements that are consistent and aligned with global data standards because a single product often moves between and among multiple markets. Global standards facilitate international commerce through interoperability and promote competition and expansion. Standards create a common language among different systems which enables those systems to communicate in a common and understandable format. However, global standards are beneficial and achieve the intended effect only if they are implemented fully and without variation. The use of country-specific standards—*including country-specific variations to global standards*—is a barrier to global trade.

Further, the requirements of the country where the product will be dispensed should supersede any other product labelling requirements. The value of serialization is the ability to leverage traceability systems and processes to verify the authenticity of packages introduced into commerce. Therefore, any serialization requirement should be set by the country where the packages will be authenticated (and introduced into commerce). Requirements applicable to exports have significant potential to create confusion or conflict with the requirements of other markets, and could also create security risks. For example, the use of serialization data in a country other than the country dispensing the product (for example, an exporting country where product is manufactured) makes the serialization data susceptible to fraudulent use in the country of distribution. The requirements of one country should not jeopardize patient safety in another country.

One way to implement requirements that are tailored to a specific market while still receiving the benefit of global interoperability is by offering exemptions for product intended for export to countries where pharmaceutical serialization or traceability is already in place. While permitted in the Indian export requirements, exemptions are not easily achieved by industry and require application by each individual manufacturer for each of its products. If an importing country has mandated serialization, then any manufacturer exporting to that country also needs to abide by the mandate and apply serialization to their products. The current process only slows and complicates issuance of the exemptions as established by law. A simpler alternative would be to publish and maintain a list of countries that have mandated or formally notified an intention to mandate barcoding requirements and then automatically exempt all exports, by any manufacturer, to those countries from all requirements except barcoding for the tertiary package. This type of country-by-country exemption would also significantly reduce the workload of processing many applications from many manufacturers for the same exemption.

REQUIREMENTS SHOULD BE CONTINUALLY REFINED

The last step in facilitating the transition to a more secure supply chain through serialization and traceability requirements is the enforcement of those requirements. Similar to the use of global standards, serialization and traceability requirements are only effective so long as they are fully implemented by all relevant trading partners and stakeholders.

As systems and processes are implemented, there should be a clear process for industry to raise implementation or technical concerns to the relevant government entities. Every new regulatory system encounters the need for adjustments, reforms, and modifications throughout the implementation process. As public- and private-sector stakeholders implement new regulations, technical challenges and unforeseen issues arise. Ongoing communication with stakeholders throughout the implementation process is critical for successful and timely adoption of any requirements.

Thorough and appropriate training of the individuals carrying out that enforcement is also necessary to ensure that enforcement is standard across various regions. Clear, consistent, and frequent communication between the regulator and the individuals or entities responsible for enforcement will also help ensure that enforcement does not conflict with the stated requirements in any way. For example, customs officials have recently told industry members that previously acquired product exemptions are no longer valid for product being exported today. India's export requirements, and the subsequent regulations, make no mention of exemption expiration or limitation. Therefore, DGFT should alert customs officials/port authorities that exemption documents, regardless of when acquired, are active and valid.

FIVE KEY POLICY RECOMMENDATIONS

Pharmaceutical serialization and traceability are highly technical regulatory systems that have a deep impact on international trade. Over the past five years, there has been a dramatic increase in related regulatory requirements adopted by other countries. Much can be learned from these experiences, but much can also be learned from the experience of implementing the Indian export requirements. Implementation of the export requirements has surfaced several challenges for industry. Regulators must recognize these challenges and have the flexibility to adjust requirements to achieve full, successful implementation. As the Government of India seeks to further the implementation of India's serialization and traceability requirements, either for exported or eventually for domestic pharmaceutical products, there are five key recommendations to keep in mind, as discussed in the following paragraphs.

Develop a Comprehensive Approach to Supply Chain Security

Currently, India's system for serialization and traceability is incomplete. Serialization and traceability requirements for exported product do not paint the full picture of a secure supply chain. Yet, there are important challenges with the export requirements that should be better understood and alleviated prior to implementation of any serialization or traceability requirements for domestic product. If and when the Government of India chooses to pursue domestic requirements, regulators should solicit stakeholder input early in the regulatory process (that is, before the laws and regulations are developed) and throughout its implementation.

Serialization and traceability are useful additions to a comprehensive strategy to promote pharmaceutical supply chain security and promote patient safety. The Government of India should continue to invest in additional solutions to enhance safety and security such as licensure requirements for legitimate trading partners and proper, consistent enforcement of serialization and traceability requirements across the entire country. Early and continuous engagement with industry can help the regulators ensure that systems and processes for serialization and traceability are consistent with existing industry business practices, do not impede global trade, and promote the safety and security of both the Indian pharmaceutical supply chain and Indian products around the world.

Leverage Global Standards and Allow Appropriate Flexibility for a Globalized Economy

Global standards are critical to the development of regulatory systems that support and advance global trade. This is especially true with regard to serialization and traceability—systems and processes that are built for the generation and exchange of data among various entities with regard to product handled by multiple trading partners, often across several countries. GS1 is a globally-recognized standards-setting body that has developed a standardized approach to identifying and serializing pharmaceutical products. As India has recognized, the GS1 global standards are broadly considered the preferred standard for pharmaceutical serialization and the exchange of serialization data.

To date, implementation of the Indian export requirements has not been fully consistent with GS1 global standards for GTIN construction or the labelling of various packaging levels. As such, confusion with the application of GS1 standards to Indian exports has led to significant logistical challenges: the placement of multiple barcodes on a single product, the use of two different GTINs on one product, and so on. The addition of multiple datamatrices has caused scanning confusion in importing countries, threatens the accuracy of serialization data within and outside of India, and therefore has the potential to delay product transport and sale. Full implementation of GS1 global standards can help maintain the flow of product out of India and to patients around the world, thereby preventing shortages and other adverse events.

Develop Technological Infrastructure Tailored to the Supply Chain Security Strategy

Traceability of serialized product is predicated on the ability of a downstream trading partner to verify that the serial number on a product was commissioned by the manufacturer of that product. In combination with other controls and checks, this verification can authenticate a product and deem it safe for dispense and use by patients. Technology for traceability can best support product identification through timely and secure transmission of serialization data to the relevant and appropriate entities, and by ensuring manufacturers have the most up-to-date information about their products as they flow through the supply chain.

For example, the manufacturer and other parties responsible for the product need access to data regarding authentication attempts to best detect supply chain security concerns. If multiple verifications are attempted with regard to a single unit, the manufacturer should have access to that information in order to investigate the legitimacy of those attempts. Of course, access to authentication data must be balanced against privacy interests of stakeholders and patient safety. This means that access must be secure, password-protected in some fashion, and limited to those entities that have the capacity to resolve data errors and address any suspect product concerns resulting from notable data discrepancies. It may also mean that certain parts of the data are redacted.

Ensure Appropriate Data Reliability, Integrity, and Security

Verification, or other forms of traceability, are only as reliable and secure as the underlying serialization data. In addition to enforcement of GMPs and GDPs, in using a centralized database as the source data for verification requests and product traceability, the Government of India has the obligation to secure the central database.

Implementation of the serialization and traceability requirements for exported product have exposed some challenges and security concerns with using the DAVA portal and database, which should be rectified within the iVEDA system.

A way to limit access to serialized data is by limiting verification capabilities to licensed, or otherwise authorized, pharmaceutical supply chain trading partners. In contrast, patient-level authentication of serial numbers would complicate the process of data access management. Product authentication by patients would necessitate a database that is accessible by any person in a country to attempt a product verification. This would open the database to significant risk of unauthorized access, which would completely undermine supply chain security.

Have a Clear and Phased Implementation Process

Adoption and implementation of any traceability system should be phased in over time, starting simple and achieving benefits before considering additional functionalities. The initial phase of traceability or track and trace should be limited to serialization. The second phase of implementation should be point-of-dispense verification of the serial numbers encoded in the barcodes, as this functionality is essential to securing the supply chain and protecting patients, yet much less complex than full scale traceability. Only after the safety and security benefits of verification are realized should traceability requirements be considered in light of the improvements in supply chain security already realized through verification.

Successful implementation of any new regulatory system requires continuous feedback, evaluation, and adjustment. As the details are implemented, new and unforeseen issues are certain to arise. Throughout the implementation process, it should be verified that the systems are proceeding as anticipated and are actually capable of achieving intended objectives. The gradual or phased implementation of new regulatory requirements allows such feedback, evaluation, and adjustment. If phased correctly, this approach also allows industry and regulators to spread out costs and to control the costs of implementation by preventing investment in systems that ultimately have to be replaced.

Further, all compliance deadlines should be based on the date of publication of final, clear guidance. Industry cannot begin implementation until a complete and final set of requirements is available. This includes instances when new requirements indicate a change in scope from a previously published law, regulation, or guidance, given that these types of changes will significantly impact the implementation process. Changes in scope should be written and published through a formal rule-making process, and compliance deadlines should be revised accordingly.

***

India has made great progress in securing the pharmaceutical supply chain, particularly for product manufactured in India intended for export. While there is still much progress left to be made, especially for domestic product, existing systems and processes for compliance with the India export requirements should first be improved. A lack of data security in the central database could, itself, serve to detrimentally impact India's image as a secure, global exporter.

Only when the current systems and processes for serialization and traceability are modified and implemented fully (in phases), and the corresponding impact on supply chain security is assessed, should additional requirements be put in place. If and when India seeks to implement domestic serialization and traceability requirements, regulators should seek to engage industry early in the process, learn from global experiences, and implement requirements that are founded on global standards.

A secure supply chain stimulates in-country manufacturing activity and increases the confidence of importers in product coming from India. As a leader in pharmaceutical supply chain security, India will serve as an example for those markets looking to implement their own systems for serialization and traceability.

REFERENCE

K.D. Brown, E.L. Nichols, and C.F. Chang, *Improving Pharmaceutical Supply Chain Security: The Costs and Benefits of Global Standards*. A report prepared for the Asia Pacific Economic Corporation (APEC) Business Advisory Council, April 2015.

21

Under Trial

Clinical Research Regulations in India

Rahul Mongia

From a net importer of pharmaceuticals to an industry manufacturing over USD 25 billion worth of pharmaceuticals, the stellar rise of the Indian pharmaceutical industry is unparalleled amongst emerging economies. The establishment of the Abbreviated New Drug Application (ANDA) pathway in 1984 that allowed entry of 'generics' into the US also opened the floodgates for generics into other ICH (International Council on Harmonization of Technical Requirements for the Registration of Pharmaceuticals for Human Use) and ROW (rest of the world) markets. This meant that by proving 'bioequivalence'[1], the time-consuming and capital-intensive[2] step of generating 'safety' and 'efficacy' data via clinical trials became redundant for granting marketing authorization for generics. Bolstered by the flexibilities imparted by the ANDA pathway, the Indian pharmaceutical firms then operating under a 'process patent' regime in vogue since India's Patent Act of 1970, used their reverse engineering capabilities to enter developing and developed markets alike. By the turn of the twenty-first century, India exported generics to over 150 destinations and hailed as the pharmacy of the world (Pradhan and Sahu 2008). However, with the arrival of a global product patent regime, the foreign transnational pharmaceutical firms already in the 'patent drug' business began to look towards 'pharmerging economies'[3] as future growth avenues, while the large Indian pharmaceutical firms began to move from plain vanilla generics

[1] Generic drugs cannot be marketed without regulatory and clinical demonstration of 'bioequivalence', that is, the demonstration that the generic drug not only is chemically identical to a new drug, but also has identical effects within the human patient (therapeutic equivalence).

[2] Currently the cost of novel drug development is worked out by incorporating 'sunk costs' and 'time costs' incurred in undertaking failed global clinical trial programmes. These costs represent almost two-thirds of the total drug development costs. The 3rd Pharmaceutical Congress Asia, 2016, held in Singapore, opened with a corporate presentation where the current cost of novel drug discovery was quoted to be in excess of USD 3 billion. This figure is higher than the currently contested estimate by almost USD 0.6 billion. For a more detailed explication, see DiMasi, Grabowski, and Hansen (2016).

[3] 'Pharmerging economies' is a commonly used term to refer countries that are characterized by ascribing relatively lower positions amongst global pharmaceutical markets but having the potential for rapid growth in sales, that is, emerging.

towards 'specialty generics', 'patented drugs', and 'biopharmaceuticals/biosimilars'. This meant that the large pharmaceutical firms in emerging economies started to or strived to undertake global clinical trials in order to introduce novel drugs, while the foreign transnational pharmaceutical firms started offshoring clinical trials to the emerging economies as part of global clinical trial programmes. These developments together have brought clinical research and hence clinical trials at the centre of debate on drug regulation in emerging economies. The Indian case is particularly interesting.

While the procedure for conducting clinical trials was introduced in the Indian regulations as early as 1988,[4] it was not until 2005, however, that India began to be perceived as the country of choice for undertaking global clinical trial programmes.[5] To add to this perception India was naturally bestowed with the much-desired prerequisites for conducting clinical research and drug development—a large and diverse patient pool (trial participants), a highly skilled and polyglot workforce of qualified scientists (investigators), medical colleges (sites), and so on (Mongia et al. 2017). However, marred by an unpredictable regulatory regime amidst reports of few unethically conducted clinical trials, the clinical research activity in India dropped as quickly as it rose—only 19 trials were approved in 2013, a drop of roughly 93 per cent from 2012 (262 trials), and a fraction of its peak of 500 trials in 2010 (Mongia et al. 2017).

This chapter attempts to lay down the locus of clinical research regulation in India. In order to understand the nature and dynamics of the current clinical research regulatory milieu, this chapter is divided as follows. The next section charts an overview of the developments in the Indian clinical research ecosystem over the years. Section three elaborates on the current regulatory review procedure for clinical trials in India. The fourth section delves into the nature of trials being undertaken in the country and describes the recent upheaval in drug regulatory milieu in India. The last section concludes the chapter.

THE INDIAN CLINICAL RESEARCH ECOSYSTEM

Since Independence, several Indian pharmaceutical companies have grown to proportions that rival the growth encountered by the 'chaebols' and 'keiretsus' in the Asian tiger economies in the latter half of the twentieth century.[6] This is perhaps due to the sustained growth witnessed by the pharmaceutical sector that transcended the earlier 'import substitution' based protective economic regime, as well as the later export-led liberalized economic regime. However, this growth was neither assimilated stochastically nor inclusively as only the top 10 pharmaceutical firms currently make up for more than a third of the market, which is largely dominated by branded generics and constitutes nearly 70 per cent of the overall market (Pharmatrac Data 2016). While in 2016, the global generics market opportunity tapped by Indian firms stood at a whopping USD 26.1 billion, the future growth avenues are poised to move from the plain vanilla solid oral generics to niche specialty pharma products[7] involving

[4] In September 1988, the Eight Amendment of 1988 [G.S.R. 944(E) [No. X-11011/1/87-DMS&PFA] repealed Rules 30A, 69B, and 75B, and inserted a new Part XA (Rules 122A–122E) into the Drugs and Cosmetics Rules (DCR), 1945, titled 'Import or manufacture of new drug for clinical trials or marketing'. A new Schedule Y was also inserted, titled 'Requirements and guidelines on clinical trials for import and manufacture of new drug'.

[5] The removal of the phase lag and adoption of a product patent regime under the Agreement on Trade Related Intellectual Property Rights (TRIPS Agreement) are instrumental in the build-up of this perception. Phase lag removal meant that concurrent recruitment for global clinical trial programmes was legally allowed in India, while the adoption of a product patent regime meant that the obligation to file for marketing authorization in lieu for recruiting trial participants could be fulfilled with adequate safeguards to intellectual property held by the sponsor of these trials.

[6] This nature of this rise is comparable because in almost all instances, significant capital formation occurred in the so-called peripheral economies, which prospered at the expense of the core economies. In pharmaceuticals, the core economies are represented by the ICH markets, while India represents one of such peripheral economies.

[7] Specialty products includes generics based on new therapeutic entities (NTEs)/super generics and complex generics. Super generics is referred to enhanced version of approved drugs, which could be developed through a new route of administration, strength, dosage form, and combinations or device innovations to address specific patient needs. While complex generics are defined according to USFDA as off patent versions of drugs that involves complex APIs (active pharmaceutical ingredients) such as peptides or natural source products, complex formulation process (injectables), a unique route of administration, or a drug-device combination (drug eluting stents), and therefore offer a high barrier to entry. These drugs have a high degree of

complex/super generics and biosimilars, which have heightened regulatory requirements for proving clinical safety and efficacy. In order to navigate these headwinds several pharmaceutical companies are now collaborating with transnational pharmaceutical firms, while the latter are looking towards the pharmerging economies as future growth avenues. This evolution in the global pharmaceutical industry with the arrival of a more harmonized global drug regulatory landscape has warranted an escalation for conducting clinical research, especially in countries like India.

However, it is interesting to note that back in the 1980s when there was no regulatory framework for conducting clinical trials in the India, the Indian Council for Medical Research (ICMR) did release the first ever policy statement on 'ethical considerations involved in research on human subjects'. It was highlighted in the policy statement that the country is soon to foresee a rapid growth in clinical research and hence a regulatory framework for ethical conduct of such research is indispensable. Thereafter, the 1986 pharmaceutical policy of India was one of the first official documents to emphasize the concern of several clinically untested pharmaceutical products being present in the domestic market. It was only in 1988 with the eighth amendment that 'Schedule Y' was appended with Part XA to the DCR that laid down the procedure and guidelines on clinical trials for import and manufacture of new drugs in India (Roderick et al. 2014). However, it was not until 2005 that the definition for clinical trials in India was first spelled out via the insertion of rule 122DAA.[8] According to the rule, a clinical trial is 'a systematic study of a *new drug*' (emphasis added), while the term 'new drug' was defined in the eighth amendment (1988) itself in Rule 122E as an entity that has 'not been used in the country to any significant extent'. The cutoff limit for the term 'significant extent' was explained as 'four years from the date of its first approval or its inclusion in the Indian pharmacopoeia whichever is earlier'. As a consequence of this exceptionally distinct definition, most pharmaceutical manufacturers in India wait for four years (from a drug's first introduction in India) in order for the drug to lose its new drug status,[9] making sponsored clinical trials the province of select top Indian pharmaceutical firms.

By the turn of the twenty-first century and almost two decades after the first policy statement ICMR finalized the first set of guidelines for 'ethical biomedical research on human subjects' in the year 2000. A year later the official Good Clinical Practices (GCP) guidelines were released by the National Drug Regulatory Authority (NDRA),[10] which then became the gold standard for conducting clinical research on humans in India. However, the biggest reform to the clinical trial regulations was only brought in 2005 with amendments in the Schedule Y of the DCR 1945, which removed phase lag[11] for conducting clinical trials in India. This along with adoption of a product patent regime via TRIPS in the same year sent a strong signal to the global community that India would soon transform into a one-stop shop for all drug development needs.[12] This opened the floodgates for clinical research in India, which until then was mostly done either as clinical studies by academics or for proving bioequivalence for drugs for export markets. It is not surprising that from the year 2005 onwards, India witnessed a phenomenal growth in both local and global clinical trials only to stymie a few years later (see Figure 21.1).

This sudden spurt in clinical research-related activities in the presence of a fairly untested matrix of clinical research actors, agencies, guidelines, and regulations led to an unfavourable public opinion in India as several clinical research organizations were blamed for conducting trials without due concern for procedural and ethical issues. All these reports of unethical clinical research

tacit knowledge associated with their manufacturing and few bulk suppliers in the market.

[8] This was inserted via G.S.R. 32(E), dated 20 January 2005.

[9] After a drug loses its new drug status no additional animal or human data is generally required for marketing approval.

[10] CDSCO or Central Drugs Standards Control Organization is the NDRA in India. It is the central authority to approve new drugs and clinical trials in India.

[11] Any typical new molecular entity graduates through three phases before it can be marketed. The first phase typically generates the safety profile of a drug, while phase two and three generate and confirm the efficacy profile of a drug, respectively. A phase lag here means that phase II trial could be conducted in India only after Phase III trials were completed elsewhere. Schedule Y of the DCR was amended in 2005 to remove this lag and allow concurrent global clinical trials. This was perhaps introduced initially to ensure that only those drugs are introduced in India where a preliminary safety and efficacy data exists.

[12] Globally, clinical trials are conducted as part of multinational clinical development for novel drug discovery. These are concurrent trials unlike the phase-lagged local trials or the bridging studies that were done in India.

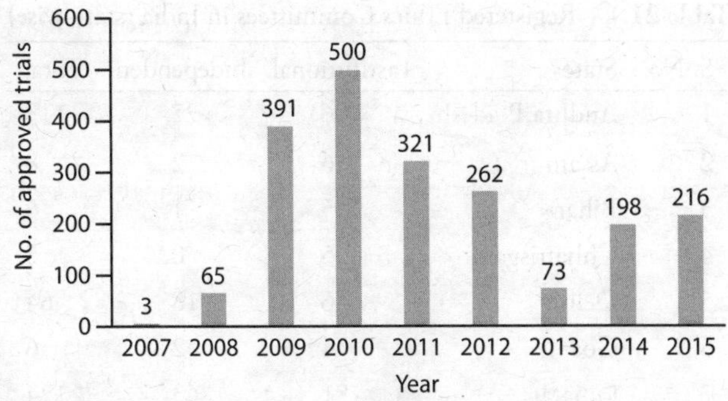

Figure 21.1 DCGI approved clinical trials in India

Source: CDSCO (Compiled from Clinical Trials Registry of India Data).

activities culminated into a petition[13] being filed with the Supreme Court of India against the inadequate regulations for conducting clinical trials in India (Mongia et al. 2017). As a result, a flurry of interim orders and directions were given to the NDRA resulting in frequent changes in clinical trial regulations creating an uncertain regulatory milieu. As a consequence, the sudden rise witnessed in the conduct of clinical trials in India came to a near halt, as discussed earlier.

While the petition is still pending before the Supreme Court of India, clinical trial regulatory milieu has witnessed quite frequent and abrupt changes. Starting in 2013, six major regulatory requirements that were imposed :

1. Examination of serious adverse events (SAEs) and procedures for payment of compensation in case of clinical-trial-related injury or death
2. Audio-visual recording of the informed consent process
3. A cap on the number of trials an investigator could simultaneously undertake[14]
4. The requirement of a minimum threshold of public medical institutions (with pre-defined standards) to be chosen as clinical trial sites[15]
5. Inspection and monitoring of clinical trials
6. Registration and accreditation requirements for ethics committees

Most of these reforms although deeply desired, were rendered counterproductive in the absence of adequate regulatory guidance on specific issues, clarity on legal terminologies, and a sound communication strategy. In order to better comprehend the nature and impact of these requirements a cogent description of the clinical trial review process is provided in the following section.

THE CLINICAL TRIAL REVIEW PROCEDURE AND OTHER REGULATORY REQUIREMENTS

India's regulatory review and approval process for introduction of new drugs has undergone a significant transformation over the past few years. In line with most drug regulatory jurisdictions all clinical trial applications must be granted approval from the NDRA and ethics committee(s) respectively. In India both the Drug Controller General of India (DCGI) and ethics committee approvals are mandatory for a sponsor to initiate a clinical trial, except in the case of clinical trials for academic/research purposes that are non-regulatory in nature, where only the latter's review suffices.[16] The DCGI review and approval process may be conducted in parallel with the Ethics Committee (EC) review. Both the review processes are briefly discussed below.

The DCGI Review

The DCGI's review and approval process within the CDSCO operates as a three-tiered system. Clinical

[13] *Swasthya Adhikar Manch* v *Union of India*, Writ Petition (Civil) 33 of 2012. The growing pressure amidst the order by the Supreme Court in the Swasthya Adhikar Manch petition paved way for the Government of India proposing amendments to the current Drugs and Cosmetics Act (DCA), 1940 by tabling a new bill. The draft of the Drugs and Cosmetics (Amendment) Bill, 2015 came into the public domain on 31 December 2014 and public comments were invited till 12 January 2015. This draft has now been withdrawn and instead a complete overhaul in the DCA was envisioned.

[14] This requirement was taken off with the August 2016 CDSCO order, which is available at http://www.cdsco.nic.in/writereaddata/restricion%20of%20conducting%20three.pdf.

[15] This requirement was also taken off with the August 2016 CDSCO order, which changed the requirement that trials be conducted at sites with more than 50 hospital beds to simply requiring the ethics committee to decide whether the site is suitable. See http://www.cdsco.nic.in/writereaddata/requirement%20of%2050%20bedded%20.pdf.

[16] It should be emphasized, however, that clarity on this aspect has emergence only in 2016, as a specific notification was issued by the CDSCO. In 2013, even the academic community was unsure on whether a regulatory approval should be sought for self-sponsored clinical studies of non-commercial interest or not.

trial applications (CTAs) and new drugs are initially evaluated by the subject expert committees (SECs),[17] and their recommendations are then reviewed by the technical review committee (TRC) that has been constituted under the Directorate General of Health Services (DGHS). The TRC consists of experts from various therapeutic areas. The DCGI grants clinical trial approval and new drug approvals based on the TRC's recommendations. The honourable Supreme Court of India mandated that a system be established to supervise clinical trials by constituting an apex committee under the chairmanship of the Secretary of Health and Family Welfare, which constitutes the third and the final layer for a CTA (see figure 21.2). The stated goal of the three-tiered process is to evaluate all new clinical trial applications in India on the following parameters:

- Assessment of risk versus benefit to the patients
- Innovation vis-à-vis existing therapeutic options
- Unmet medical need in the country

Ethics Committee Approval

India has a decentralized process for the ethical review of clinical trial applications, and requires an ethics committee's (EC's) approval for each trial site. Most ECs are based at clinical or academic institutions and hospitals. There are also independent ECs that function outside institutions for those researchers who have no institutional attachments or who work in institutions with no EC, however currently, they are allowed to review only bioavailibility/bioequivalence studies. There are a total of over 1,000 registered ethics committees with CDSCO (as on 1 January 2016)—836 of them are institutional ECs; the rest 243 are independent ECs (see Table 21.1).

If a multicentre trial is being conducted and the same clinical protocol is being used for all the sites, an EC that approves one trial site may also grant approval to another site within the study. However, the approving EC must also be willing to accept responsibility for overseeing the studies at each of the approved sites. Furthermore, the site must be willing to accept the EC's oversight role in this arrangement.[18]

Table 21.1 Registered Ethics Committees in India (state-wise)

S. No.	State	Institutional	Independent	Total
1	Andhra Pradesh	86	27	113
2	Assam	6	2	8
3	Bihar	5	1	6
4	Chhattisgarh	5	0	5
5	Delhi	46	18	64
6	Goa	4	2	6
7	Gujarat	81	43	124
8	Haryana	12	1	13
9	Himachal Pradesh	2	0	2
10	Jammu & Kashmir	2	0	2
11	Karnataka	84	28	112
12	Kerala	52	5	57
13	Madhya Pradesh	13	0	13
14	Maharashtra	184	75	259
15	Mizoram	1	0	1
16	Odisha	12	0	12
17	Puducherry	7	1	8
18	Punjab	20	1	21
19	Rajasthan	31	4	35
20	Sikkim	1	0	1
21	Tamil Nadu	86	25	111
22	Uttarakhand	5	1	6
23	Uttar Pradesh	48	7	55
24	West Bengal	43	2	45
25	Jharkhand	1	0	1
	Total	837	243	1080

Source: Compiled from CDSCO data as of January 2016.

A clinical trial, intended for academic purposes, that studies a new indication or route of administration

[17] In line with the current practice at several NDRAs, advisory committees for review of clinical trial applications were established in 2011 as the New Drug Advisory Committees (NDACs) at CDSCO. In 2014, these were renamed SECs as they were reorganized on the lines of expertise in different therapeutic areas. Members of any SEC are drawn randomly from a pool of experts (mostly academicians/key opinion leaders) working as consultants for the NDRA.

[18] In the draft of new drugs and clinical trial rules, 2018, it has been proposed that independent (registered) ECs will be able to review protocols for clinical trial sites where a local EC is absent, given that the EC registration address is within the same city or within 50 km radius of the clinical trial site. Independent ECs will be able to review protocols of bioavailibility/bioequivalence (BA/BE) studies as well. Such protocols may also be reviewed by ECs of other sites.

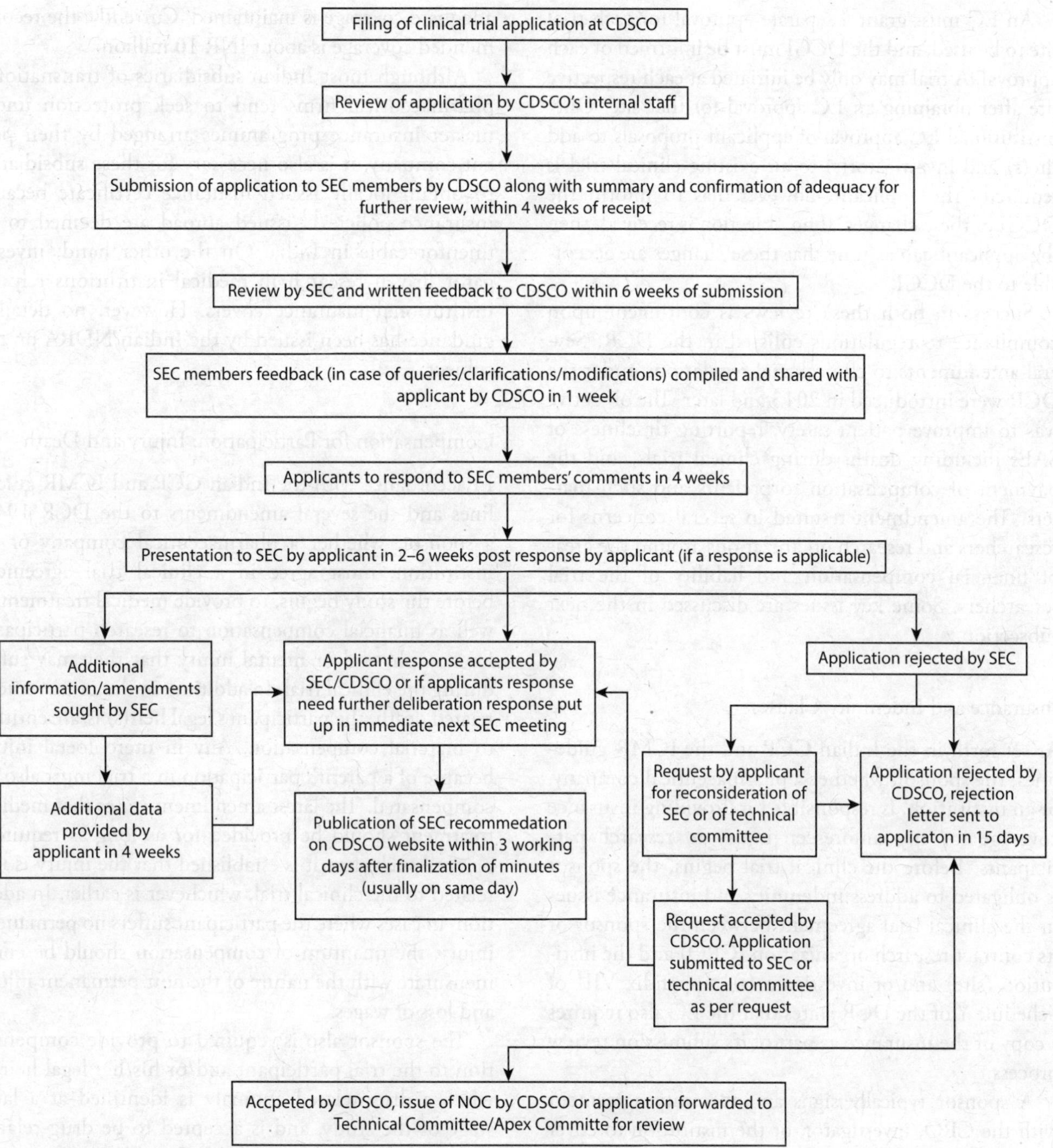

Figure 21.2 Process of review process of Clinical Trial Application in India
Adapted from 'Handbook for applicants and reviewers of clinical trials of new drugs in India', ICMR-CDSCO, January, 2017.

or new dose or dosage of an already approved drug formulation does not require DCGI approval as long as:

- the trial is approved by the EC; and
- the data generated is not intended for submission to the licensing authority (DCGI).

The EC has to inform the DCGI about the academic trials it has approved and about cases where there could be an overlap between the clinical trial intended for academic purposes and those for regulatory purposes. If the DCGI does not comment to the EC within 30 days from receiving EC notification, it is presumed that DCGI permission is not required.

An EC must grant a separate approval for each trial site to be used, and the DCGI must be informed of each approval. A trial may only be initiated at each respective site after obtaining an EC approval for that site. Only institutional EC approval of applicant proposals to add site(s) and investigator(s) to an existing clinical trial is required. The applicant, however, has to inform the DCGI of these changes. If no objection is received, then the applicant can assume that these changes are acceptable to the DCGI.

Success in both these reviews is contingent upon compliance to regulations enlisted in the DCR. Several amendments to clinical trial regulations under the DCR were introduced in 2013 and later. The objective was to improve patient safety, reporting timeliness of SAEs including deaths during clinical trials, and the payment of compensation to patients and such matters. The amendment resulted in several concerns for researchers and research organizations around the areas of financial compensation and liability of the trial researchers. Some key issues are discussed in the next subsection.

Insurance and Indemnity Clauses

As set forth in the Indian GCP and the ICMR guidelines, the sponsor, whether a pharmaceutical company, or an institution, is responsible for providing insurance coverage for any unforeseen injury to research participants. Before the clinical trial begins, the sponsor is obligated to address indemnity and insurance issues in the clinical trial agreement between the sponsor or its contract research organization (CRO) and the institution (site) and/or investigator(s). Appendix VIII of Schedule Y of the DCR states that the EC also requires a copy of the insurance as part of its submission review process.

A sponsor typically signs an indemnity agreement with the CRO, investigator, or the institution to cover any risks related to study-related participant injuries arising out of any act, omission, negligence or misconduct by the CRO, investigator, or the institution. The sponsor, in turn, also needs to obtain insurance coverage to cover any costs that may be incurred as a result of providing this indemnification.

In India, insurance is generally issued as a certificate from a locally based insurance company that is best able to ensure that coverage limits and terms comply with country-specific laws and regulations. The insurance certificate should be reviewed periodically to ensure adequate coverage is maintained. Currently, the recommended coverage is about INR 10 million.

Although most Indian subsidiaries of transnational pharmaceutical firms tend to seek protection under master insurance programmes arranged by their parent company, it is also necessary for these subsidiaries to obtain locally issued insurance certificate because insurance policies[19] issued abroad are deemed to be unenforceable in India. On the other hand, investigator driven research in medical institutions rely on institutional insurance covers. However, no detailed guidance has been issued by the Indian NDRA on the subject.

Compensation for Participation: Injury and Death

In accordance with the Indian GCP and ICMR guidelines and the several amendments to the DCR 1945, a sponsor, whether a pharmaceutical company or an institution, must agree in a clinical trial agreement before the study begins, to provide medical treatment as well as financial compensation to research participants for any physical or mental injury that they may suffer during the clinical trial. In addition, in the case of study-related death, the participant's legal heir(s) is/are entitled to material compensation. Any in utero foetal injury because of a parent's participation in a trial must also be compensated. The latest amendment states that medical treatment should be provided for as long as required, or until such time it is established that the injury is not related to the clinical trial, whichever is earlier. In addition, in cases where the participant suffers no permanent injury, the quantum of compensation should be commensurate with the nature of the non-permanent injury and loss of wages.

The sponsor also is required to provide compensation to the trial participant and/or his/her legal heir(s) when a drug-related anomaly is identified at a later stage of the study, and is accepted to be drug-related and resulting in injury or death. In addition, it is mandated that the sponsor should provide ancillary care to participants suffering from any other brief illness during the trial at the same hospital or trial site, whenever required.

As per the several amendments to Rule 122DAB of the DCR, the sponsor is responsible for compensating

[19] However, in practice, for most instances, compensations are paid directly by the sponsor and formal claims from the insurance companies are rarely pressed for.

the research participant and/or his/her legal heir(s) if the injury or death has occurred due to any of the following reasons:

- Adverse effects of investigational product(s) (IPs)
- Any clinical trial procedures involved in the study
- Violation of approved protocol, scientific misconduct, or negligence by the investigator/sponsor/CRO, or other responsible parties
- Failure of an IP to provide intended therapeutic effect where, the standard care, although available, was not provided to the participant as per trial protocol
- Use of a placebo in a placebo-controlled trial where, the standard care, although available, was not provided to the participant as per trial protocol
- Adverse effects due to concomitant medication administered as per the approved protocol
- Injury to the child in-utero due to a parent's participation in a clinical trial

The participant may be paid for the inconvenience and time spent, reimbursed for expenses incurred, and receive free medical services in connection with his/her participation for as long as required. The sponsor should also include a statement regarding the participant's right to compensation for ancillary care for unrelated illness or appropriate referrals in the clinical trial agreement.

In the case of a foreign sponsor, he/she must appoint a local representative or a CRO to fulfill the appropriate responsibilities as governed by the Indian regulations. The foreign sponsor must also enter into an agreement with his/her local representative stating that, as the sponsor, he/she will be responsible for medical treatment expenses as well as financial compensation in the case of trial-related injury or death of trial participants.

The first amendment of 2013 indicated that the sponsor should provide financial compensation and medical treatment as per the recommendations of the EC, the Expert Committee (constituted by the DCGI), where applicable, and ultimately the DCGI.

However, the latest amendment, which amended the first amendment, indicates that the sponsor must report, after due analysis, any SAEs/serious adverse drug reactions (SADRs) during a clinical trial within 14 days of the occurrence of the SAE/SADR to the DCGI and the EC(s) that accorded approval to the study protocol. The EC then submits its report with financial compensation recommendations within 30 days to the DCGI. Within 150 days of the occurrence of the adverse event, the DCGI must determine the cause of injury or death and make the final decision on the quantum of compensation to be paid by the sponsor or his/her representative.

The sponsor or his/her representative is required to pay the compensation to the participant or his/her legal heirs (in the case of death) within 30 days of receipt of the DCGI order. The orders provide a compensation formula in the case of death and a different one in the case of an SAE other than death. With these formulae in place, India becomes the only country to do so for the purpose of providing compensations for injuries or death related to a clinical trial.

In the event that a sponsor fails to provide compensation to a research participant for trial-related injuries or to his/her legal heir(s) in case of death, the DCGI may, after giving an opportunity to show cause why such an order should not be passed, by a written order, suspend or cancel the clinical trial and restrict the sponsor/CRO/local representative of a foreign sponsor from conducting any further clinical trials in India, or take any other action deemed fit under the rules.

Informed Consent Process

In all Indian clinical trials, a freely given, informed written consent is required to be obtained from each participant to comply with the requirements laid down in the Indian GCP and ICMR guidelines, and Schedule Y.

As per the GCP and ICMR guidelines, and Schedule Y, the informed consent form (ICF) and patient information sheet are viewed as essential documents that must be reviewed and approved by the EC and supplied to the licensing authority, the DCGI, prior to beginning a clinical trial. The ICF and patient information sheet are ultimately integrated into one document referred to as the ICF.

The investigator(s) should provide study information to the participant and/or his/her legal representative(s) or guardian(s) as well as to an impartial witness. The ICF content should be brief and clearly presented, without coercion or unduly influencing a potential participant to enroll in the clinical trial.

Participant information should be presented in both written and oral form, whenever possible, and in non-technical and understandable terms. When written consent as a signature or thumb impression is not possible, verbal consent may be taken after ensuring its documentation by an impartial witness, or through audio/video means.

Effective 31 July 2015, the DCR amendment states that investigator(s) must obtain an audio–video recording of the informed consent process for vulnerable participants in clinical trials of a new chemical entity or new molecular entity, including the procedure of providing information to the participant and his/her understanding of the consent. This audio–video recording should be retained in the investigator's files.[20]

According to the ICMR guidelines, any change in the ICF due to a protocol modification or an alteration in treatment modality, procedures, or site visits, should be approved by the EC and submitted to the DCGI before such changes are implemented. The participant and/or his/her legal representative(s) or guardian(s) will also be required to re-sign the revised ICF.

As stated in the respective guidelines, the ICF should be written in English and in a local language that the participant is able to understand. The document should be scientifically accurate as well as sensitive to the participant's social and cultural context.

The ICF should be signed and personally dated by the participant and the investigator(s). If the participant is incapable of giving an informed consent, his/her legal representative(s) or guardian(s) should sign and date the ICF. In cases where the participant and/or his/her legal representative(s) and/or guardian(s) are illiterate, an impartial witness, who should be present during the entire informed consent discussion, should sign and date the ICF. By signing the consent form, the witness attests that the ICF and any other written information provided, was accurately explained to, and understood by, the participant and/or his/her legal representative(s) and/or guardian(s), and that informed consent was freely given by the participant and/or his/her legal representative(s) and/or guardian(s). A copy of the signed ICF is retained by the investigator(s), and one copy should be given to the participant for his/her record.

[20] In cases where clinical trials are conducted on anti-Human Immunodeficiency Virus (HIV) and anti-Leprosy drugs, the investigator(s) must only obtain an audio recording of the IC process. The investigator(s) is also required to retain the audio recording for his/her records.

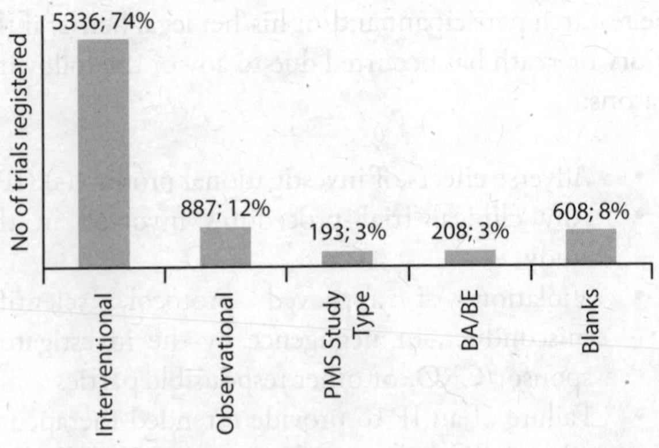

Figure 21.3 Registered Clinical Trials in India–Trial Type Profile

Source: Mongia et al. (2017).

Notes: Interventional – Active intervention on trial participation; Observational – No active intervention, such as: Epidemiological survey; PMS-Post-Marketing Surveillance to generate long-term safety profile (not to be confused with Phase 4 Trials); BA/BE – Bioavailability/Bioequivalence studies, for introducing generics or filing ANDA applications abroad; Blanks – Study type not assigned.

CONTEMPORARY INDIAN CLINICAL RESEARCH SCENE AND ALLIED REGULATIONS

In India, out of 7,232 registered clinical studies,[21] 74 per cent or 5,336 studies are classified as interventional trials (see Figure 21.3). Out of these interventional studies, only 2,522 or 48 per cent studies involve administration of allopathic entities—drugs/small molecules (2,065, or 39 per cent); biologics (256, or 5 per cent) and vaccines (201, or 4 per cent). The other half of the studies[22] involves interventions either based on alternate systems of medicine (AYUSH), probiotics or surgical procedures/use of medical devices (constituting non-drug) and so on (see Figure 21.4).

Out of the 2,522 interventional studies on allopathic entities, 902 studies or 37 per cent are sponsored by

[21] Trials registered in the Clinical Trials Registry of India (CTRI) from 2007 till 2 September 2016. The year of conduct of trials and the year of registration need not be the same because the mandatory registration of clinical trials was not done before 15 June 2009. Hence, several studies have been registered retrospectively and likewise prospectively.

[22] The chapter restricts the analysis of only the former category of interventions involving small molecules, biologics, and vaccines. The latter category of interventions, although relevant to clinical research, are out of the scope of the discussion presented here.

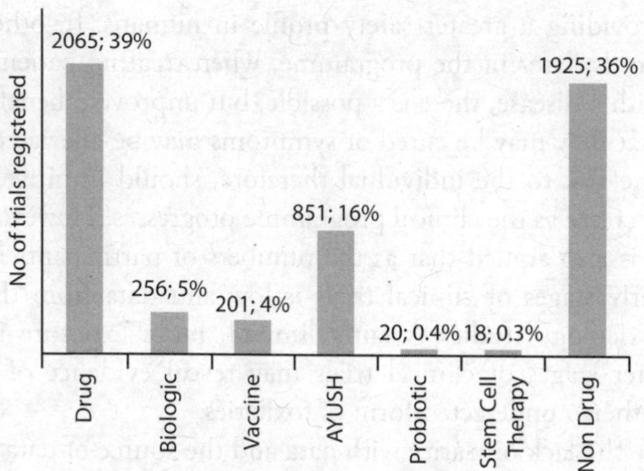

Figure 21.4 Registered Clinical Trials in India—Intervention Type Profile

Source: Mongia et al. (2017).

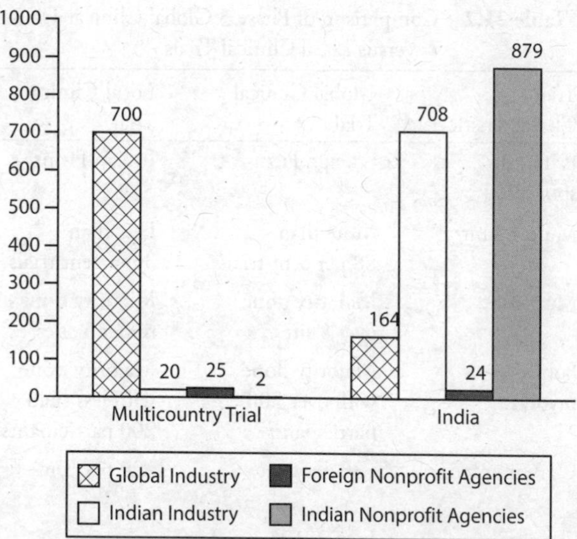

Figure 21.6 Registered Clinical Trials (in numbers)—Sponsor Site Profile

Source: Mongia et al. (2017).

national and international nonprofit agencies combined. Trials sponsored by foreign transnational firms are not very far behind as they constitute 864 studies or 34 per cent of the total, while the Indian pharmaceutical firms have sponsored 728 studies constituting 29 per cent of the total interventional trials under study (see Figure 21.5).

Over 81 per cent of the trials sponsored by foreign firms are multi-country, multicentric trials, while 97 per cent of the trials sponsored by both Indian firms as well as nonprofit agencies (Indian and foreign combined) respectively are locally instituted multicentric trials (see Figure 21.6).

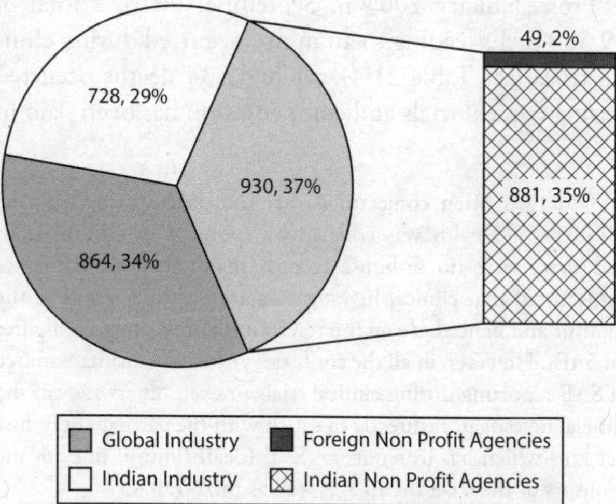

Figure 21.5 Registered Clinical Trials in India—Sponsor Profile

Source: Mongia et al. (2017).

Over 66 per cent of these trials are comprised of either Phase 3 or Phase 4. Out of the studies labelled as only Phase 3 studies (1,092 total), over 53 per cent are sponsored by foreign firms, mostly representative of global clinical trials, while 35 per cent of these are sponsored by Indian firms, mostly representative of bridging studies, the remaining 12 per cent Phase 3 trials are sponsored by nonprofit agencies (see Figure 21.7 and Table 21.2).

The data clearly shows a shift as the biggest contributor to the recent rise in the number of clinical trials in India are multi-country, multicentric, concurrent global clinical trials as they constitute a sizeable number of the

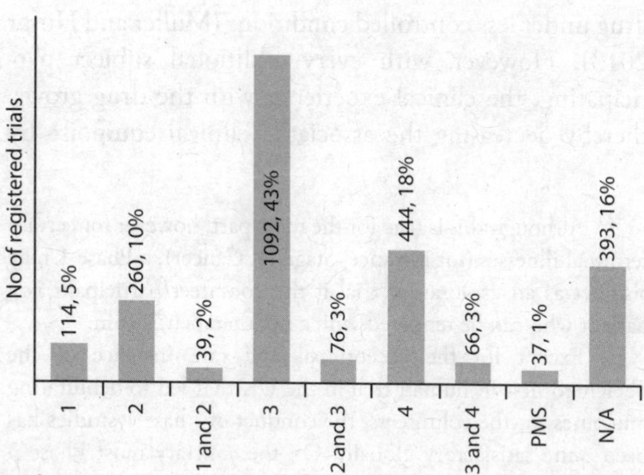

Figure 21.7 Registered Clinical Trials in India—Phase Profile

Source: Mongia et al. (2017).

Table 21.2 Comparison of Phase 3 Global Clinical Trials versus Local Clinical Trials

Trial Characteristic	Global Clinical Trial	Local Clinical Trial
Primarily sponsored by	Foreign Firms	Indian Firms
Multi-country	More than 88 per cent trials	Less than 3 per cent trials
Multi-site	Majority done over 8 sites	Majority done under 5 sites
Subjects involved	Majority done with over 500 participants	Majority done with less than 200 participants
CTA approved	~86 per cent (1 January – 30 June 2012)	~99 per cent

Source: Mongia et al. (2017).

total clinical studies being undertaken in India. The petitioners in the honourable Supreme Court of India pose active opposition to the very concurrent global clinical trial programmes while posing little or no concern for local clinical studies.

The leading contributor to this perception is the degree of risk involved along a clinical development programme and trials in general. To illustrate, for first-in-human studies such as Phase 1 studies, in most cases there is no clinical benefit to the individual,[23] while there is always some degree of risk involved. However, this is minimized by the small amounts of drug that is administered and the careful monitoring of the volunteer for any adverse signs caused by the drug.[24] The risk to the population increases as a trial advances, with more participants given greater cumulative amounts of the drug under less controlled conditions (Muller and Husar 2013). However, with every additional subject participating, the clinical experience with the drug grows, thereby decreasing the associated clinical equipoise by providing a greater safety profile in humans. In other words, later in the programme, when treating patients with a disease, there is a possible, but unproven, benefit that they may be cured or symptoms may be alleviated. The risk to the individual therefore, should intuitively decrease as the clinical programme progresses. However, it is also argued that as the numbers of participants in early stages of clinical trials is low and data from the toxicology studies is fairly limited, more exposure in later stages of clinical trials may reveal evidence of a hitherto undetected form of toxicities.

The lack of clarity with data and the source of data[25] on the occurrence of total number of SAEs during clinical trials in India further complicates the issue. In a Ministry of Health note[26], it was initially said that a total 1,514 participants had died between 2008 and August 2010 during clinical trials in India. In the second iteration[27] and it was said that between 1 January 2005 to 30 June 2012, 57,303 participants took part in clinical trials and 39,022 of these trials were completed. A total of 11,972 SAEs (see Table 21.3) occurred during this period and 2,644 deaths occurred during these clinical trials,[28] out of which 80 (about 3 per cent) were related to these trials. In 44 cases of deaths, compensation was paid while there was no data for compensation records previous to 2008. It was further said that between 1 January 2005 and 2012 end, 2,868 deaths occurred during clinical trials, even though only 89 (about 3 per cent) out of these were related to clinical trials. It was further stated that from January 2005 to December 2013, a total of 14,320 SAEs had occurred during clinical trials and 3,458 deaths occurred during this period.

From January 2005 to September 2016, a total of 19,583 SAEs leading to an injury occurred during clinical trials (see Table 21.4), while 4,534 deaths occurred during clinical trials and compensation has been paid in

[23] Although this is true for the most part, however for certain terminal illnesses (for instance, Stage IV Cancer), a Phase 1 may also act as an exploratory trial if the volunteer/participant is a patient who can be rendered with a net therapeutic gain.

[24] Except for the exceptional and rare instance of the TeGenero first-in-human trial in the UK that led to debilitating outcomes for the volunteers, the conduct of Phase 1 studies has been quite satisfactory globally. On the contrary most Phase 3 trials are conducted in outpatient settings, while all Phase 1 trials are conducted in inpatient settings under highly controlled conditions, rendering more protection for the participant.

[25] It was often conjectured that the data provided by the Ministry of Health was collated by sponsors of clinical trials and there were no in-house records maintained. It is further conjectured that clinical investigators are on the payrolls of the sponsor and hence have an interest in under reporting the figures on SAEs. However, in all the countries visited the ultimate source of SAE reporting during clinical trials or even otherwise was the clinical investigator (directly in touch with the participant or his/her kin) which has to report an SAE (death/injury) to both the sponsors of the trial; the ECs as well as the NDRA.

[26] See *Swasthya Adhikar Manch* v *Union of India*.

[27] *Swasthya Adhikar Manch* v *Union of India*.

[28] The latter figure on SAEs leading to death is mutually exclusive to the former figure of total SAEs leading to injuries.

Table 21.3 SAEs (death) reported during the period of 2005 to 2016

S No.	Year	No. of SAEs leading to death during a CT	No. of deaths related to clinical trial	No. of compensation paid cases
1	2005	128	5	5
2	2006	137	2	2
3	2007	136	4	4
4	2008	288	8	8
5	2009	637	16	16
6	2010	668	22	22
7	2011	438	16	16
8	2012	436	16	17
9	2013	590	NA	45
10	2014	443	NA	21
11	2015	381	NA	4
12	2016*	252	NA	Under examination
Total		4, 534		160+

* Till 30 September 2016
Source: Mongia et al. (2017).

Table 21.4 SAEs (injury) reported during the period of 2005 to 2016

S. No.	Year	No. of SAEs leading to injury during a CT (not caused due to or related to)		No. of related SAEs	No. of compensation paid cases
1	2005			1	NA
2	2006			22	NA
3	2007			14	NA
4	2008	11,972		46	NA
5	2009			86	NA
6	2010			85	NA
7	2011			140	NA
8	2012	Jan–June	1,226	112	NA
		July–Dec		NA	NA
9	2013	1,122		NA	145
10	2014	1,326		NA	94
11	2015	2,359		NA	55
12	2016*	1,578		NA	Under Examination
Total		19,583			

* Till 30 September 2016
Source: Mongia et al. (2017).

over 160 cases, while the same was under examination for the year 2016 (see Table 21.3).

It is important that a distinction is made between deaths/injuries occurring during a clinical trial and deaths/injuries related to such a trial. Globally, a sponsor is liable to pay compensation only in the cases where an analysis for 'relatedness'[29] attributes an SAE with the investigational product. In most regulatory jurisdictions, wherever possible the sponsor of a clinical trial usually covers for the injury/death associated with the trial for a medicinal product. Several regulatory jurisdictions, by virtue of being former British colonies, follow the Association of British Pharmaceutical Industries (ABPI) guidelines, which not only define when to provide for compensation, these also define and limit the liability by expressly mentioning when not to provide for such compensation. The latter has been missing from the Indian rules, which has been the cause of much confusion and loss of positive perception.

Besides, the connotation associated with the term compensation in most other jurisdictions is that of a payment for immediate harm. However, in the Indian rules, compensation is to be paid also in case of an injury or death discerned at a later stage.[30] In the absence of specific guidance on specific therapeutic areas, this translates into a limitless liability for the sponsors of clinical trials. When the Rule 122DAB was first inserted, the use of language such as, 'providing free medical management to clinical trial as long as required in case of any injury irrespective of whether the injury is related to clinical trial or not', 'providing financial compensation in case of injury or death due to failure of investigational product to provide intended therapeutic effect', and 'use of placebo in placebo controlled trial', only added to the uncertainty.

Compensation in the Indian setting is tied to an analysis for 'relatedness', where the relatedness needs to be proven with the investigational product, which not only includes the drug under study but also the comparator

[29] In an analysis for relatedness, a chosen 'causality' scale is reduced to the binary scale of 'relatedness' where an SAE (death or injury) is either related or not related to the investigational product.

[30] See for instance, heading 4 under agenda no. 1, minutes of the 68th meeting of Drugs Technical Advisory Board (DTAB), New Delhi 16 February 2015. Available at https://cdsco.gov.in/opencms/opencms/en/dcc-dtab-committee, last accessed on 4 March 2020. Also refer to the new draft on 'New Drugs and Clinical Trial Rules, 2018'.

arm, that is, either an 'active control/standard of care' or an 'inactive control/placebo'. This definition is akin to that in parlance in the European Union, where an investigational medicinal product also includes both the test and the comparator arms.

However for the purpose of paying compensation, the term used in the ABPI guidelines is that of a 'medicinal product'. This subtle difference translates into dropping compensation for the comparator arm. Further, the ABPI guidelines categorically mention that in case of harm/injury/death associated with the standard of care, which would have been administered/prescribed to the patient/participant in the normal course of clinical practice, would not attract a compensation from the sponsor of the trial. The Indian rules, however, function on the ethical principle of reciprocity, where by participating in a trial, a participant may be compensated for a trial-related injury even when it arises by the use of a reference product in the comparator arm, although this has not been expressly mentioned in the rules.[31] The need for detailed guidance is felt in this regard.

***

The unpredictability with risk 'in' and 'across' a clinical trial programme can play havoc with public policy stances in developing countries, which becomes all the more acute because clinical trials increasingly occur on a global scale as industry and sponsors in developed countries move trials to developing countries. The petition filed by the NGO Swasthya Adhikar Manch in the Supreme Court of India rests on this very concept that concurrent global drug development poses higher risks, while drug-lagged clinical development via bridging trials is a safer option and poses less harm. From a health policy perspective, the question remains to be decided whether a regulatory jurisdiction in such a condition should allow the early participation of its citizens in a global clinical development programme or wait until the sponsor applies for a marketing authorization and ask for a bridging trial. India is an example where the latter approach has been adopted for the most part of the history of clinical research for novel drug discovery. The end result being most trials in India are Phase 3 trials to confirm efficacy of the drug on Indian population. However, as the situation began to change, the regulatory overhaul in 2013 stymied the shift towards the global approach.

While India still continues to debate the relevance of a local clinical research infrastructure regulated, other drug regulatory jurisdictions are busy legislating laws that allow terminally ill patients try experimental therapies (including drugs, biologics, and devices) that have just completed Phase 1 testing but have not been approved by the NDRAs. These have been dubbed as 'right to try' and 'right to hope' for such patients. This gap in perception speaks volumes about the therapeutic cultures prevailing amongst different drug regulatory jurisdictions and consequently the need to factor these intricacies for ongoing and future policy reforms.

31 However, this is expressly mentioned in the Ranjit Roy Committee report. Also, in the draft of new Drugs and Clinical Trial Rules, 2018, a difference has been explicated between an investigational new drug (constituting only the intervention arm) and an investigational product (constituting both the intervention arm as well as the control/placebo arm), which although is in line with ABPI guidelines, for compensation for injury/death related to a trial, the term investigational product has been used. Hence, Compensation is proposed to be paid for investigational product, which includes the 'standard of care arm' as well.

REFERENCES

Chaudhury R.R. et al. 2013. 'Report of the Prof. Ranjit Roy Chaudhury Expert Committee to formulate policy and guidelines for approval of new drugs, clinical trials and banning of drugs', July. New Delhi: Ministry of Health and Family Welfare.

DiMasi, Joseph A., Henry G. Grabowski, and Ronald W. Hansen. 2016. 'Innovation in the Pharmaceutical Industry: New Estimates of R&D Costs', *Journal of Health Economics* 47(May): 20–33.

ICMR (Indian Council of Medical Research). 2017. *Handbook for Applicants and Reviewers of Clinical Trials of New Drugs in India*. New Delhi: ICMR.

Mongia, Rahul, Deepmala Pokhriyal, Seema Rao, and Ali Mehdi. 2017. *Challenges and Prospects for Clinical Trials in India: A Regulatory Perspective*. New Delhi: Academic Foundation.

Pradhan, Jaya Prakash and Partha Pratim Sahu. 2008. *Transnationalization of Indian Pharmaceutical SMEs*. New Delhi: Bookwell.

Roderick, Peter, Rushikesh Mahajan, Patricia McGettigan and Allyson M. Pollock. 2014. 'India Should Introduce a New Drugs Act', *The Lancet* 383(9913): 203–6.

22

The Case for Health Insurance Regulation and Its Evolution in India*

Somil Nagpal

The health insurance industry in India has come a long way since its humble origins in 1986 when the first standardized commercial health insurance product, Mediclaim, was introduced by the government-owned insurance companies. Several hundred commercial health insurance products have been introduced in India since 2001, when the insurance industry reopened its gates to new entrants, and has seen the entry of over 50 new insurance companies in India since then. Not surprisingly, health insurance has been the fastest growing segment in the Indian insurance industry over the last decade and a half—and in fact, one of the fastest growing segments in the country's financial services industry as a whole. A large variety of innovative health insurance policies is now available for consumers to choose from, but the choices are not easy to make. The product itself is complex, given the many possible permutations and combinations of policy features on offer. Then there is the added complexity of stakeholder interests and stakeholder interactions which are common in the health insurance space in any market, and have been specially pronounced in the rapidly growing and evolving context in India. Such high complexity needs regulatory oversight for managing stakeholder interests in the best long-term interest of the consumer.

India's health insurance industry is regulated by the federal insurance regulator Insurance Regulatory and Development Authority of India (IRDAI, known earlier as IRDA). In addition to the regulatory provisions that apply to the insurance industry as a whole, and thereby also to the health insurance segment, there are some specific regulations promulgated by IRDAI that are primarily aimed at the health insurance segment, and these include the IRDAI (Health Insurance) Regulations, 2016 and the IRDAI (Third Party Administrators—Health Service) Regulations, 2016. The sections that follow discuss the concept of health insurance regulation and the need for such regulation, as well as some specific details of how the sector is regulated in the Indian context.

*This chapter has been adapted for the Indian context from Gottret and Nagpal (2010). Content in this chapter uses a descriptive framework based on 'Private Voluntary Health Insurance—Customer Protection and Prudential Regulation' and the IC27 course of Insurance Institute of India.

NEED FOR HEALTH INSURANCE REGULATION

It is widely recognized that the health insurance market has several imperfections. These imperfections (listed further) are among the key causes that make the nature of health insurance very complex, and also the reason that they require regulatory intervention to ensure that the health insurance sector itself remains sustainable.

1. *Information asymmetry*: It operates at the end of the insurer as well as the insured, with neither having the full picture about the other. An insurer does not necessarily know the health status of the prospective insured, while a customer will also find it very difficult to fully understand the fine print and provisions in the health insurance coverage.
2. *Risk selection* by insurers: In the absence of regulation insurers may not want to continue coverage for those who are now unwell and may need frequent healthcare.
3. *Adverse selection* of insured: When healthy and young, the perceived need and interest in health insurance may be much lesser, than when a real health risk is perceived by the individual.
4. *Moral hazard*: This can be demand side (insured) or supply side (healthcare providers)—whereby the consumer or the provider may overuse the services covered by insurance.

Another reason for regulation is to ensure that any insurer has the required financial, managerial and technical capacity to manage risks. Insurance is the business of managing risks, and a health insurance company does manage the insurance risk transferred to it through the insurance contract, but this is not the only uncertainty managed by it. There are various other types of risks which a health insurer is required to manage in addition, and to ensure that the insurers have the capacity and intent, as well as actually do their task effectively, requires regulatory oversight. These are:

- *Insurance risk*: This arises from underwriting practices and risk appetite of the insurer. In health insurance, each risk by itself is not very large but there still exists the risk of 'concentration' and reckless underwriting can create trouble for the insurer.
- *Investment risk*: This depends on how the collected funds are used and what is the mix of investment options chosen by the insurer, as also the overall environment in the economy. Even if the insurer holds good quality assets, holding long-term debt can lead to liquidity risk. Complex investment products may be very risky and have actually led to large insurance companies collapsing in the 2008 meltdown of financial markets.
- *Credit risk*: As in any other business with financial dealings, there is risk of default by business associates such as providers, suppliers, and reinsurers.
- *Liquidity risk*: Even if the insurer is profitable, it can still have a mismatch in its cash flows, and in its current assets and liabilities, reducing the insurer's ability to arrange adequate cash to pay its liabilities at a short notice.
- *Business environment risk*: The insurer may be exposed to changes in the policy environment and the economic environment which may affect them adversely.
- *Operational and other risks*: This includes risk of frauds, risk of not keeping up with technology, and the risk of losing key human resources.

All these risks are not discrete—they overlap and interplay, and thus require the insurer's management to be actively managing these risks, which needs regulatory oversight for effectiveness. While self-regulation has been stated as an option, the incentives to manage risk are different from a regulator's perspective, and so an independent regulator is more effective. Self-regulation often falls short of what a statutory regulator is able to achieve, as the incentives for industry bodies to self-regulate are weak and often there are not enough penal provisions either. For example, in India's own regulatory experience in the health insurance context, the self regulatory measures adopted by the General Insurance Council for adequacy of group health insurance pricing had only limited effect. As a result, as IRDAI's annual reports have illustrated over the years, the group health insurance portfolio of the industry continued to be making losses for several years after this self-regulatory guidance was adopted in the mid-2000s. Likewise, in a non-health experience in India, the life insurance industry was unable to self-regulate on the issue of inadequate information to consumers around certain high risk products linked to stock markets (unit-linked insurance), and a strong regulatory response to address this issue in late 2000s affected the industry's prospects for several years thereafter.

Institutional failures are, in general, caused by lax management, weak corporate governance, poor central controls and supervision, unsound accounting systems, and other infrastructure failures compounded by weaknesses in the legal framework (IAIS 1999). A study of 21 companies in financial trouble found that management issues were at the root of the problem (Lorent 2008 citing Ashby, Sharma, and McDonnell 2002). Moreover, the complexity of health insurance business, the multiple risks which health insurers manage, and the market failures in the sector, all require a very effective top management role. When regulator mandates a particular level of corporate governance, level of regulatory involvement can decrease. Mechanisms like independent directors, actuaries, internal auditors and so on are often required (but that alone too did not work in the case of AIG in 2008). Thus, the complexity of health insurance business makes it very vulnerable to the effects of poor corporate governance. Regulation monitors and brings about corrective changes in time to reduce the risk of institutional failure.

Regulation also serves to harmonize the activities of different players, helping achieve the desired social objectives from health insurance, most notable of which is equitable access to health insurance which regulators can play a major role in. In any country, health remains an important social objective for governments, and this often extends to expectations from how health insurance sector contributes (or does not contravene) these social objectives. When regulating private health insurance, such expectations often take the form of requirements to keep access to health insurance relatively open, to expect continued renewals and sometimes even explicit mechanisms to cross-subsidize groups such as the elderly. Regulators generally take on a strong customer protection focus too—ensuring that customers are treated fairly. Health insurance is ultimately a promise, and regulation is the key to the customer's confidence in the 'promise' of health insurance. If an insurer fails, people may lose their confidence in the entire health insurance system, which is a key mandate for the regulator to preserve and protect as its mandate.

Also, in health insurance, the policyholder has longer term expectations for continued coverage. It is always more difficult to switch insurers as that may entail loss of benefits. Policyholders who are already ill and in need of ongoing medical care may lose coverage because of the insurer's failure. New insurers can decline those who present a higher chance of making claims or exclude certain conditions and give them poorer coverage than they already had. Even otherwise, health insurance coverage becomes richer as the person keeps being continuously insured, as the waiting periods are met and so the one-year, two-year and four-year exclusions then stand covered. If a person switches insurers, he/she may then have to start these waiting periods all over again. Such issues primarily affect individual or family policies rather than corporate or group health insurance covers where such exclusions may be waived. For this reason, such a continuity of insurance cover is particularly relevant for India, where individual or family health insurance is about half of the total health insurance market, in contrast with most other countries where group health insurance is the predominant part of commercial health insurance business.

ORIGIN AND EVOLUTION OF INSURANCE REGULATION IN INDIA

IRDAI began its journey in India as the interim Insurance Regulatory Authority in 1996, taking over the regulatory role hitherto served by the office of the Controller of Insurance in the Ministry of Finance. After the passage of the IRDA Act in 1999, it started its statutory role as the regulator for insurance in India. At this point, the voluntary health insurance market was synonymous with the hospitalization indemnity product Mediclaim, sold by the four government-owned insurance companies that constituted the entire non-life insurance market in India. The lone life insurer then, the government owned Life Insurance Corporation of India, had a large portfolio of riders (supplements to a base life insurance cover) covering defined 'critical illnesses', such as cancers, strokes, and heart attacks, but health insurance was primarily seen as a non-life product.

From 2001, private non-life insurance companies entered the market and started offering new variants of health insurance policies. Slowly but steadily, the variety of options available in the market grew, but also created difficulties for the consumers in understanding the insurance cover, or to compare offerings across insurers. Limited access to health insurance for those who were already senior citizens also emerged as a concern. It was increasingly clear that the regulator needed a closer watch over the health insurance space, and a specialized department for health insurance was established in 2007, initially headed by an external official with domain knowledge in the subject, seconded from the Government of India to IRDA.

Formal instructions on themes such as consumer protection and submission of data to the regulator soon followed, and the myriad instructions and circulars were consolidated into Health Insurance Regulations in 2013, which were then revised and reissued in 2016. Supported by a steady regulatory environment, the sector continued to grow at a very fast pace, and remained the fastest growing sub sector in the insurance industry.

KEY CHARACTERISTICS OF HEALTH INSURANCE REGULATION IN INDIA

Statutory Base

Legal sanctity for the regulatory function, an independent source of financing and adequate 'teeth' for the regulator to take penal action are an important statutory base for the regulator. In India, the IRDA Act, 1999, creates the statutory base for the insurance regulatory functions exercised by the IRDAI—though the insurance industry itself is governed by the Insurance Act, 1938, as amended from time to time.

Administrative Location

A health insurance regulator can be housed within a health ministry or in an insurance regulatory agency. In the context of a small country with limited regulatory manpower, or in a case where the regulator is dealing with integrated insurers which also have non-health businesses, having a health insurance regulator within the overall insurance regulatory structure is an option. An independent health insurance agency located outside the health ministry and also outside the regulatory mechanism for non-health insurance entities is also an option, which is indeed the case in several countries. Cases where resources for supervision are scarce, and a cadre of supervisory professionals is being developed, the argument that all the relevant human capital should be concentrated in a single organization becomes particularly strong. This may involve the creation of a specialist unit within an integrated agency to focus on private voluntary health insurance, for example, as was done in India, by the creation of a specialized health insurance unit within the IRDAI, the statutory insurance sector regulator for the country.

Licensing and Registration

Licensing and registration are a regulator's tools to ensure that they can check the management background and their integrity, financial strength, and business plans before granting the insurance license to any entity. These aspects can be important in ensuring the safety of large amounts of public money which the insurers will be managing once they have a licence. India has a rigorous licensing regimen in place for its insurance industry, laid down in the Insurance Act, 1938, (as amended) and the IRDA (Registration of Indian Insurance Companies) Regulations, 2000. The requirements include an insurer to bring in an initial capital of INR 100 crore (or 1 billion), and requires a multi-stage scrutiny of each application before a licence is awarded. Incidentally, as a developmental measure, these laws provide preference for insurers aiming to serve the health insurance sector, too. India does not allow composite licences, that is, life and non-life insurance licences are separate, but either of these licence types allows health insurance line of business, and both life and non-life insurance companies can offer health insurance policies. In practice, most health insurance products are offered by non-life insurance companies and standalone health insurance companies, while life insurance companies have focused on health savings[1] and critical illness[2] products.

Financial Regulation

Regulators usually lay down prudential accounting regulations and rules, financial reporting requirements, and undertake constant monitoring of the financial position of the insurance companies to ensure that they stay solvent and their accounting statements are true and fair. The Indian regulatory system has laid down regulations in terms of prudential accounting norms, which include the IRDA (Preparation of Financial Statements and Auditor's Report of Insurance Companies) Regulations, 2000, as well as the more recent IRDAI (Assets, Liabilities, and Solvency Margin of Life Insurance Business) Regulations, 2016 and the IRDAI (Assets, Liabilities, and Solvency Margin of General Insurance Business) Regulations, 2016.

[1] Health savings type of products allow the contributions to be accumulated and be available for healthcare needs of the individual in the future (along with growth on the invested amounts, as applicable). Several life insurers in India now offer such products.

[2] Critical illness products typically cover a small number of rare, very high-cost medical conditions, and offer a fixed, lump sum payout if such an illness occurs. This is a very common life insurance industry product in India, often sold as an add-on (or 'rider') to a life insurance policy.

Product Regulation

Regulators lay down filing or approval requirements for health insurance products, which include transparency and fairness requirements to take care of the information asymmetry from the insurer's side. In India, IRDAI requires a 'File and Use' procedure for the non-life insurance industry, which is de facto an approval procedure for each product. Products need to comply with regulatory requirements, be fairly priced, and need to have a design that protects the interests of the policyholders. These are among the areas for the regulator's review of the product documentation.

Price Regulation

In certain situations, regulators may also regulate the prices (and increases thereof) of health insurance products. IRDAI monitors product pricing in India but it does not micromanage or prescribe the pricing. The more a regulator enters into prescribing product pricing, the deeper it will need to manage the content and clauses of the insurance product itself, too.

Other Regulatory Approaches

In some countries, including India, an insurer with either a life or non-life insurance licence can offer health insurance, while in other countries there may be a completely separate category for licensing or health insurance may be restricted to one class of insurers, life or non-life. In India, non-life companies have historically played a predominant role in the health insurance space, even though both life and non-life companies can offer health insurance products. Since 2006, a third category has also emerged comprising non-life licences restricted to conduct of health insurance business, thus creating standalone health insurers in the country. The Health Insurance Regulations, 2016, have reduced the overlap in the type of health insurance products that life and non-life insurers can offer, limiting indemnity or reimbursement type of products to the non-life industry, while longer term products for the life insurance industry, in line with the respective strengths of these categories of insurers.

ENFORCEMENT OF REGULATIONS

Ensuring enforcement is the essence of health insurance regulation, as all regulations and monitoring systems could be meaningless without enforcement. Drafting and promulgation of regulations is not enough, and enforcement is key to achieving regulatory objectives.

Enforcement begins with careful off-site monitoring supplemented by on-site visits as necessary. Effective action for breaches or violations is key to prevention of such breaches or violations by the same and other entities shows that the regulator 'means business' and serves as a deterrent to similar breaches in future. Regulatory actions for breaches or violations can include:

- Restricting business activity or activities by the insurers
- Levying fines and penalties on the insurers
- Ordering removal/change of personnel
- Issuing warnings to the insurer
- Appointing liquidator/observer/administrator, and so on

MONITORING BY THE REGULATORS

Off-Site Monitoring

This is done at the regulator's office itself, without actually going to the offices of the insurance companies, and includes detailed examination of various documents such as:

- management information system (MIS) reports;
- accounts;
- reinsurance contracts; and
- outsourcing arrangements.

Information technology systems can play a very important role in off-site monitoring as several of the processes can be automated and attention of the regulator can be immediately drawn if any unexpected or adverse information flows through the system. This remains a regular practice for insurance regulation in India where financial statements of insurers are reviewed by the regulator's team. Requirements for submission of insurance and claims data also exist in India, which in theory allow electronic monitoring using business intelligence tools, though the use of electronic monitoring of insurance industry's policy and claims data currently seems to be limited in the Indian context. However, aggregate analysis of health insurance data is undertaken regularly. This analysis was published earlier by an entity called Tariff Advisory Committee (which existed until the late 2000s) and is now brought out by the Insurance Information Bureau of India, both of which are (or were, in the case of Tariff Advisory

Committee) closely related to IRDAI and chaired by the IRDAI chairman.

On-site Inspections

These are done to verify the reports submitted by the insurers, check their internal controls, and also examine the market conduct aspects of the insurers. These are supplemental and not a substitute of good off-site monitoring. Special IRDAI teams are constituted periodically to undertake on-site inspection at insurer's offices in India for such supplementary on-site supervision.

REGULATION FOR CONSUMER PROTECTION

Health insurance requires several areas where regulators may need to ensure that the customer's interests are protected. Some of the customer protection areas for regulatory intervention, and their application in the Indian context, are discussed in the next few paragraphs.

Access

Regulators may impose requirements such as guaranteed issue or variants thereof, for some or all products in the market. Alternatively, they may impose disclosure requirements to inform policyholders the reason for being denied insurance. India does not impose guaranteed issuance, but the Protection of Policyholders' Interests Regulations, 2017, lay down access expectations, and Health Insurance Regulations, 2016, further require insurers to make products available for an entry age of up to 65 years.

Renewability and Cancellation

Regulators may lay down certain provisions so that insurers cannot arbitrarily decline renewals or cancel policies, especially where they do so with the intention of 'cream skimming'.[3] The measures possible include requirements for guaranteed renewability, or for certain disclosures on renewability provided upfront to the consumers to enable them to make an informed decision. The Health Insurance Regulations, 2016, formalize previous instructions issued in 2008, and require health insurance products to be 'ordinarily renewable'—that is, they cannot be arbitrarily denied renewals. Further, the regulator expects lifetime renewability of the products.

Portability

This, across insurers, including creditable coverage from earlier insurers, may also be a regulatory requirement. This, however, poses practical limitations where the products are not similar. There are several dimensions of portability now available in India such as waivers of waiting periods when moving across similar products. While portability is explicitly required as per Health Insurance Regulations, 2016, the practical use of this option does not appear to have reached its potential, and may need continued regulatory efforts.

Product Terms and Conditions

These are also often regulated. There may be requirements such as:

- Standard products or minimum benefit coverage mandates
- Standardization of definitions and terms
- Caps on waiting periods and cost-sharing provisions
- Requirements for fairness, transparency, and disclosures

In the Indian context, while there are no minimum benefit coverage mandates or regulator-prescribed caps on cost sharing provisions, there are several efforts at standardization of definitions and terms, and a focus on fairness, transparency, and disclosures.

Prevention of Mis-selling

Prescribing the correct qualifications, background, and market conduct requirements for intermediaries are another area where regulators lay down the requirements and help prevent mis-selling and other market conduct issues. In India, all distribution intermediaries in the insurance industry are also closely regulated, including brokers and agents, who have specific licensing requirements before they can start transacting insurance business.

[3] 'Cream skimming' refers to a practice where the insurer tries to enroll and maintain healthier persons in their portfolio and to not enroll or renew, or reduce the coverage for the less healthy. For example, an insurer may try to stop renewing policies for a customer who has been diagnosed with an illness that is likely to create more claims in the future.

Handling Consumer Grievances and Ensuring Fair Treatment

Often multiple channels exist for an aggrieved insurance consumer to take up a grievance with, which can include:

- Insurer's internal review and grievance mechanism
- Regulator's review and monitoring mechanisms
- External reviews or ombudsman mechanisms
- Consumer law, competition laws, and company laws
- Contract law and judicial mechanism

In addition to the arbitration mechanisms provided in insurance contracts, the judicial route, the ombudsman mechanism, and grievances to the regulator, Indian consumers of insurance services can also approach district, state, and national consumer commissions that function as quasi-judicial forums to address healthcare-related consumer complaints. Unfortunately, backlogs have arisen in the consumer courts in addition to the delays experienced in the Indian courts as well.

Often, regulators take upon the onus to coordinate amongst these grievance mechanisms, to monitor the data flowing from grievances, and also intervene where necessary. Grievance redressal is important for consumers' confidence in insurance and the grievance channels also serve as 'eyes and ears' of the regulator to take action towards the causes of such grievances. IRDAI often receives grievances of policyholders too, and takes these up with the relevant insurers and intermediaries concerned for resolution in addition to the other channels that are available to policyholders.

INTERMEDIARIES AND EXTERNAL STAKEHOLDERS IN HEALTH INSURANCE

Health insurance, as mentioned above, is a complex undertaking. On the one hand, it is the expected set of insurance intermediaries such as agents and brokers who promote and distribute health insurance products or provide information about product options, and help connect the industry with the consumer. On the other hand, there are a few stakeholders that are unique to the health insurance setting—the providers of care such as hospitals, and entities which help process claims or help create networks of hospitals for insurers, known as Third Party Administrators, or TPAs. And finally, the nature of the health service provided is itself fairly complex. For example, in the health insurance space, the choice of what exactly will be 'consumed' (a procedure, a test, or a medicine, for instance), is effectively made more often by the service provider than the consumer (or the patient). Regulators for health insurance often have jurisdiction over some of the intermediaries in the insurance market, and so can take measures, for example, to prevent mis-selling of insurance products. However, the regulatory onus for other stakeholders in the health insurance space such as doctors, pharmacists, hospitals, and so on is generally with other entities, often multiple ones at that. In a federal, decentralized context this becomes even more challenging. For example, there is no single registry of hospitals in India—something that insurance industry would much benefit from, and so the initiative to create a unique 'Hospital ID' did not have a natural home until the task was taken up by the Insurance Information Bureau of India. To achieve optimal impact, the health insurance regulatory system has to find ways to manage these complexities, and to coordinate better with other regulatory bodies in the sector, which is of course easier said than done.

WAY FORWARD AND RECOMMENDATIONS

The health insurance regulatory system in India has evolved rapidly since the mid-2000s, supporting the organized development of an industry which has had a trailblazing record of growth, innovation, and influence. Notably, commercial health insurance in India has provided the initial platform or modality which was used by government to deliver publicly funded health insurance programmes for the poor, such as the Rashtriya Swasthya Bima Yojana and several other state government health insurance programmes. The regulatory regime kept its focus on protecting the interests of policyholders, while also encouraging the industry to innovate on products that would meet the needs of more consumers. Health was also the sector where the regulator's efforts on standardization of data submission and creation of a data warehouse were the most evolved before this initiative was extended to other segments of insurance business.

The next phase of regulatory and developmental measures for health insurance in India would need to sustain this momentum, but also fathom new frontiers that are increasingly becoming necessary. Some suggested themes for the future of health insurance regulation in India could include:

1. A greater coordinated future among the multiple regulators in the health sector with the insurance

regulator working closely with the federal and state ministries of health, as well as other bodies such as hospital accreditation bodies, that may be important to achieve the optimal quality and value of health services being 'purchased' by the insurance industry. Platforms/mechanisms for regular interaction and coordination among the regulators could be a good starting point, and IRDAI could even take the initiative in discussions around this platform.

2. Much greater analytical firepower being deployed by the regulatory system using the insurance and claims data collected over nearly two decades to help create better predictive models for costs and utilization, to help reduce and mitigate fraud, and to identify areas for better product development or where there is need for stronger regulatory oversight, as some illustrations of what this 'big data' analytics can achieve for the India's health insurance sector.
3. Creating a stronger and unified purchasing power to boost efficiency and quality of services. The insurance industry is a very large player, especially for hospitalization, but ironically it is also very fragmented at the level of a hospital. Because more than 50 entities from the industry could be potentially interacting with every large hospital (counting all active non-life insurers and TPAs), each individual insurance company or TPA becomes a relatively small entity for a hospital. The combined purchasing power of the insurance industry, if consolidated by the regulator in some way, could help achieve economies of scale as well as a much stronger leverage to contain costs and improve quality of services.
4. Making more information on products available to the consumer in an easy-to-understand format. The regulator may need to continue innovating ways to have more and better information with the consumers to help make their choice of health insurance products easier and more effective.
5. Coordinate more with publicly funded health insurance programmes as India has invested considerably in innovative health insurance programmes for the poor. At the commencement of these programmes, most were delivered through commercial health insurers, leveraging the industry's hospital networks, IT processes, cashless payment systems, and understanding of the space. This space has grown rapidly and maybe something for the regulatory system to closely engage with. Even when these publicly funded programmes are not offered through the same insurance companies or TPAs that make up the IRDAI's regulatory space, they are using the same hospital networks and there are potential synergies in closer coordination.

REFERENCES

Ashby, Simon, P. Sharma, and W. McDonnell. 2003. 'Lessons about risk: Analysing the causal chain of insurance company failure', *Insurance Research and Practice* 18: 4–15.

Brunner, Greg, Pablo Gottret, Birgit Hansl, Vijayasekar Kalavakonda, Somil Nagpal, and Nicole Tapay. 2012. `Private voluntary health insurance: consumer protection and prudential regulation (English)', World Bank, Washington, DC. Available at http://documents.worldbank.org/curated/en/774881468149697802/Private-voluntary-health-insurance-consumer-protection-and-prudential-regulation, last accessed on 12 December 2019.

Gottret, P. and S. Nagpal. 2010. 'Regulating Private Health Insurance', Presentation made for the flagship course on Health Financing, World Bank, Washington, DC, 7–11 March.

IAIS (International Association of Insurance Supervisors) Technical Committee. 1999. 'Principles Applicable to the Supervision of International Insurers and Insurance Groups and Their Cross-Border Business Operations' (Insurance Concordat), Basel.

Insurance Institute of India. 2011. IC27: Health Insurance. Mumbai: Insurance Institute of India.

IRDAI (Insurance Regulatory and Development Authority of India). See www.irdai.gov.in.

Lorent, Benjamin. 2008. 'Risks and regulation of insurance companies: is Solvency II the right answer?', Working Papers CEB 08-007, Universite Libre de Bruxelles, Brussels.

23

Medical Ethics

The Indian Context

Shah Alam Khan and Neha Faruqui

Among all fields of science and technology known to man, there are few which have shown such a rapid pace of change as medical sciences. Medicine and its allied branches have undergone a huge change over the last 100 years or so. With advancements in different aspects of medicine, it became important for the healthcare providers and health researchers to focus on issues pertaining to ethics. Thus, the evolution of medical ethics as a science (or rather art) within the purview of medical sciences has been enthralling. Ethical issues have influenced all aspects of medicine ranging from organ transplantation and patient consent-taking to care of end of life issues in sick patients. There is hardly any subspecialty of medical sciences which has remained untouched by issues of ethics. Hence it becomes very important that ethical issues are discussed at length by healthcare providers and medical researchers. India is a signatory to the World Trade Organization (WTO) and as a signatory country it became fully compliant to the TRIPS Agreement (or the Agreement for Trade Related Intellectual Property Rights) in January 2005. Thus, between 2005 and 2009, clinical trials sprung out like wild weeds throughout the length and breadth of the country. There was an overwhelming torrent of contract research organizations (CROs) and the sponsors of such trials in the country.

During this peak in clinical trial numbers in India, it was revealed (in 2009) that there was an enrolment of 24,000 girls in the Human Papilloma Virus (HPV) vaccination trial which, when investigated, was found to have irregularities in informed consent, a key component of all clinical trials. It is believed that between 2005 and 2012 about 2,800 patients have died across the country during participation in all clinical trials conducted by pharmaceutical companies (Khan 2017a). This was an extremely important revelation in the Indian context and the debate over medical ethics further intensified. Besides ethical issues in research, ethics in clinical practice in India is another area which needs extensive discussion and rectification. Horror stories of clinical malpractices, acts of omission and commission riddle the Indian healthcare system. This chapter shall deal with similar issues of medical ethics in the Indian context.

WHAT IS MEDICAL ETHICS?

Simply speaking, medical ethics includes a set of moral principles which govern medical practice. The origin of medical ethics dates back to between third and the fifth centuries BC when the Hippocratic Oath was described by the Greek philosopher and physician Hippocrates. It is important to note that though described in absolute terms, principles of medical ethics are not absolute. The principles are applicable as per the prevalent situations.

Principles of Medical Ethics and Importance in Indian Context

Medical ethics is based on four main principles which were best described by Tom Beauchamp and James Childress in 1979 (Beauchamp and Childress 2013):

1. Principle of respect for autonomy
2. Principle of non-maleficence
3. Principle of beneficence
4. Principle of justice

The basic essence of these four principles is the fact that these are non-hierarchical which means that one principle is not superior to the other. All four have their own equal importance in the realm of bioethics (Gillon 1994: 184–7). But their application in countries like ours is tricky most of the times. Autonomy forms an important concept in patients' ability to make an independent decision for himself/herself but this principle of autonomy is a dual sword in the Indian context. For example, if a 12-year-old child is brought to the emergency by her parents and if the parents refuse blood transfusion despite an urgent need for the same, it is a dilemma how the physician can maintain an ethical judgement. Some states in the US give the physician the right to decide for the child despite a contrary view held by the parents. The decision of the physician to salvage the life of a minor is ethical and is given preference. The problem is compounded in underdeveloped countries such as India where rampant illiteracy and ignorance affect patients' ability to make decisions. Also, there is no consensus on major issues of ethics in the country with poor legislative support. Thus, the principles of medical ethics, though well established and understood, have limitations within countries such as India not only because of intrinsic flaws but because of other socioeconomic factors which govern the society. It is thus important to realize that the principles of ethics are non-malleable but the social environment in which these operate is an important determinant of their application and feasibility. Medical organizations operating in resource challenged environments like ours should understand and keep this in mind when formulating laws and regulations.

MEDICAL ETHICS IN INDIA

As mentioned earlier, issues in medical ethics have not only been poorly understood but also poorly applied in India. Poor and flimsy quality controls in healthcare have led to an overall attrition in healthcare delivery. This in turn has led to a gradual erosion of ethics not only in healthcare delivery by professionals but also in medical research. In this chapter, we discuss the application of ethical issues in India from the perspective of clinical practice, research, and the pharmaceutical industry. Each aspect comes with its own problems of moral issues and needs to be clarified through examples and recommendations.

Ethical Issues in Clinical Practice

Healthcare in India is delivered by two entirely contrasting systems, namely public and private. Unfortunately, over the years, private healthcare providers have become important and contribute to more than 78 per cent of healthcare in the country (Khan 2016). This is in striking contrast to other countries in the region (for example, Sri Lanka where more than 90 per cent healthcare is still delivered by the public health system). The gradual takeover of healthcare by private players in India has caused significant ethical issues. Abhay Shukla and Arun Gadre (2016) discuss the important ethical issues arising out of unregulated, rampant privatization of healthcare in the country. Unfortunately, healthcare ethics are not only problematic at the private healthcare delivery level but are also flawed in the government health setups. It is an open secret that doctors and other health personnel are involved in malpractices both in the private and public healthcare setups. In a paper on corruption in Indian healthcare, Chattopadhyay (2013) mentions that corruption practices are multi-dimensional and can be classified into various groups namely bribes and kickbacks, thefts and embezzlements, intentional damage to public goods for private gain, absenteeism, informal payments, use of human subjects for financial gains, and institutionalized corruption. All the aforesaid practices are in abject violation of medical ethics and are remarkably common in one or the other form throughout the Indian healthcare system. Thus, factors promoting unethical medical practice are operational at multiple levels in our country. Lack of ethics in clinical practice is not only detrimental for the patients but also puts into jeopardy both the national and state level programmes of healthcare which can only be run through an active participation of the on-field health personnel. A classic example of this is the corruption scam unearthed in the National Rural Health Mission (NRHM) in the north Indian state of Uttar Pradesh in 2012 (*New Indian Express* 2012). Funds of the tune of USD 1.6 billion were siphoned off by corrupt bureaucrats and politicians. The failure of a good programme like the NRHM was thus ensured in a state which has infant mortality rates comparable to those in the sub Saharan Africa (Bhalla 2012).

The lack of ethical practices in clinical practice in India are well known throughout the country, although there is a paucity of objective data on such malpractices. Some authors have tried to address the problem. Drug prescription malpractices are the commonest means to fleece patients off their money both in public and private setups. In a qualitative study conducted by Roy, Madhiwalla, and Pai (2007), the range of promotional practices influencing drug usage in Mumbai were evaluated. They conducted open-ended interviews with 15 senior executives in drug companies, 25 chemists, and 25 doctors, and held focus group discussions with 36 medical representatives. The study provided a picture of what might be described as an unholy alliance between manufacturers, chemists, and doctors and how they conspire to make profits at the expense of consumers and the public's health, even as they negotiate with each other on their respective shares of these profits. Misleading information, incentives, and unethical trade practices were identified as methods to increase the prescription and sale of drugs. Medical representatives provide incomplete medical information to influence prescribing practices. An interesting and ironic aspect of the problem is that many doctors agree that the said practices are unethical yet they indulge in these malpractices overwhelmingly. For example, many doctors in the state of Karnataka were of the common opinion that taking 'cuts' (share of earnings) from diagnostic laboratories (a common practice in India) in lieu of patient referral to the lab is unethical (*Deccan Herald* 2017).

Clinical mishaps due to unethical practices in private and public hospitals is also a common occurrence in the country. The case of handing over a presumably dead (but actually alive) premature newborn to their parents in plastic bags at a corporate hospital in Delhi in December 2017 is an astounding violation of ethical principles (Jha 2017). If we see such open violation of medical ethics in the heart of Delhi, we can very well imagine the degree of abortion of ethical practices in the rural hinterlands of the country. Overuse of prescription drugs, under treatment of serious ailments, unnecessary operations such as hysterectomies, knowingly prescribing substandard drugs, lack of practicing safe health-related procedures, and so on are some of the common unethical practices which have come to the fore now and then. The unfortunate part of the story of medical ethics in India is that there has been a larger than life presence of legislative control on issues of malpractice in the clinical setup but this has failed to provide accountability. For example, the principles of standard of care were laid down by the Supreme Court of the country in the case of *Dr Laxman Balakrishna Joshi* v *Dr Trimbark Babu Godbole* AIR 1969 SC 128 and *A.S Mittal* v *State of UP* AIR 1989 SC 1570. Varied kinds of negligence were proved in all these cases and the cases became benchmarks for medical negligence but not much changed on the ground. In a commentary published by the *British Medical Journal* on tackling corruption in medical practice in India, the author Aniruddha Malpani has mentioned that traditional solutions have not worked in tackling corruption in medical practice in India. The author feels that regulation is doomed to fail because the regulators themselves are often corrupt. Exhorting doctors to become more ethical is not helpful—good doctors do not need to be told, and bad doctors will not improve because we preach to them (Malpani 2014).

The lack of ethical practices in small hospitals and nursing homes throughout the country have been under discussion for long. There is a consensus among professionals that besides big corporate hospitals, the smaller health establishments are the ones that need to be better regulated. In mid-2017, the government of West Bengal brought in a new legislation called the West Bengal Clinical Establishments (Registration, Regulation and Transparency) Act, 2017, to regulate the working of private clinical establishments in the state. The provisions in this version of the act call for stringent action against hospitals which stray from patient care. The act has led to the creation of the West Bengal Clinical Establishment Regulatory Commission (WBCERC), which is a watchdog that will take care of hospitals not towing the ethical line. Although a good method to ensure accountability of ethics in private hospitals in the country, the said legislation drew flak from multiple corners, but mainly from private clinical establishments with equal support for and disapproval of the act. The spirit of the WBCERC is not against doctors per se, but against private clinical establishments only. Such an act will hopefully help in apprehending erring doctors, but it does not, in its provisions, specify methods to take direct action against doctors. Unfortunately, on a downside, the onus of an act of commission or omission will finally rest at the doorstep of the doctor. The doctors thus feel that hospitals, in cases of neglect, will nonchalantly wash their hands off, leaving the doctors to face the music. So even when a good piece of legislation can be brought in by the government, its use as an accountability tool for ethical practice remains doubtful (Khan 2017b).

In most countries, the presence or rather the absence of ethical clinical practice is governed by a central agency. One such central agency in India is the Medical Council of India (MCI). It will not be wrong to conclude that there has been a gradual dwindling of the influence of the MCI over the last decade or so thereby further necessitating the need of acts like the WBCERC. Embezzlement within the MCI by its past presidents and other officials (some of whom were found guilty by the courts) is one of the worst tragedies in Indian medical practice. Not surprisingly, the muck within the MCI was so deep that the highest court had to intervene, undermining the role of an ethical body which is supposed to give 'certificates of good standing' to its own doctors. The MCI, unlike its counterpart the General Medical Council (GMC) of the UK, has failed both in safeguarding the interests of its patients and in regulating its doctors. There have been instances when the GMC has issued warnings to doctors for driving cars without proper insurance, as this is unbecoming of a responsible doctor. Compare that to the MCI, which has a very passive role in monitoring acts of neglect which are reported so often in this country (Khan 2017b).

Ethics of Pharmaceutical Practices in India

India is the world's pharmaceutical hub for generic drug production, which accounts for 20 per cent of global exports and an expected growth rate projection of USD 55 billion by 2020 (IBEF 2017). The research and development (R&D) interest in biotechnology and slow shift in manufacturing products more for treating non-communicable diseases (NCDs) than infectious diseases, has seen companies increasingly align their portfolios to match the current trends in demand. While this development may be noteworthy, there lies an array of ethical challenges stemming from the bottom to top tiers of the health system.

India lacks comprehensive drug regulations amongst its many Drug Acts and Schedules and has a decentralized form of authority shared between state and central governments (Shivam, Govind, and Arun 2012). This results in poor uniformity of standards with invested stakeholders lacking clarity in the laws that govern drug manufacturing, marketing, pricing, and quality. The recent ad hoc legal framework implemented by the current government in a bid to push doctors in prescribing low-cost generic medicines is a classic example of fragmented drug regulation. The law demands that doctors can no longer prescribe branded medicines and any generic names prescribed should be written in legible handwriting with capital letters. While these may be corrective measures for 'pro-underprivileged' causes, the repercussions mean the 'decision-making' is left up to the pharmacist or retailer. Drug brands can be suggested by someone behind the counter who may have poor scientific knowledge and more importantly, have vested interests in profit-making by selling the more expensive brands. Obviously, no regulation can measure whether retailers have the best interests of the patient in mind, but certainly, sensibility and fairness in reflection to the principle of justice is neglected.

At the doctor's end, despite such a regulation, unethical practices may as well be prevalent due to lack of stringent audit systems. Usually, the doctor becomes a mediator (and consumer) between a drug producer and a patient through strong field force such as use of medical representatives. Marketing involves strategies influencing the doctor's recognition of a brand such that it retains the doctor's awareness by sparking a conflict of interest and eventually boosting commercial sales. In fact, between 290 per cent and 1,025 per cent is spent more on marketing than R&D amongst the top Indian pharmaceutical companies (Soneji and Banerjee 2004). In fact, the R&D of major pharmaceutical firms in India hovers around 4 per cent of sales (Joseph 2011). Some of the influential sales strategies are through free samples, educational material, cash, meals, and gifts. Even though the practice 'dwindled down' since the MCI banned doctors from accepting gifts (Code of Ethics amendment in 2009), the contact between pharmaceutical industries and healthcare providers still remains strong for such purposes. In fact, the 2010 India Health Report's 'Ethics' chapter covered the same issue, but a decade later we are still highlighting such practices. In 2016, results of a questionnaire-based survey that assessed this influence between both parties showed that most doctors only considered 'expensive' gifts such as dinners and holidays as unethical, despite

72 per cent of consultants and 28 per cent of residents being aware of the amended MCI code of ethics (Joseph 2011). Marketing tactics lead to an understanding of mutual reciprocation where the doctor's integrity of putting patient first is questioned, as they have to choose between the most efficacious drug or a sponsored weekend trip (Munshi, Singh, and Thakkar 2016).

How certain are we that professional objectivity and patient compromise is not at risk even with new government regulations? Moreover, how transparent is the private healthcare sector in abiding to these government frameworks? There is also no availability of any third-party investigative authority such as an ombudsman in the Indian pharmaceutical scenario to provide ethical transparency. The patient bears the brunt of such practices, especially the poor. They not only suffer from debilitating diseases but are at the mercy of the doctor and pharmacist in the hope of being provided fair and adequate treatment, without detrimental out-of-pocket expenditures.

Ethics in Indian Health Research Practices

Strengthening health research in India is one of the aims of the National Health Policy, 2017. Healthcare services planning, improvements in monitoring and evaluation systems, generation of new evidence for risk factors, and disease associations are all benefits of investing in health research. India has been a source of observational and experimental studies from both clinical and non-clinical arenas through local and international funding. Nationwide programmes through the Indian Council of Medical Research (ICMR) under the Ministry of Health and Family Welfare (MoHFW) demonstrate that indeed the overall budget allocation for R&D is poor and majority of health research spending does not adequately meet the demands of growing disease burden such as the rise of non-communicable diseases (NCDs). In addition to such financial barriers, medical research is also lagging due to unreliable regulatory systems and frameworks which deter clinical trials, interventional studies and the like from securing better investment in the future. There have been numerous loopholes for such studies to unethically pass by ill-defined guidelines and regulations.

Just like the development of various ethical guidelines from the Nuremberg Code to Declaration of Helsinki, India has its own share of ethics policy evolvement. Controversial research practices are one of the main reasons the ICMR continually develops new guidelines. A study carried out in the 1970s to 1980s in Delhi on 1,158 women having various stages of cervical dysplasia is one of the earliest documented examples of unethical research practices, which formulated the 'Ethical Guidelines for Biomedical Research on Human Subjects' through Schedule Y (Munshi, Singh, and Thakkar 2016). Not only was informed consent improperly taken, but the women were left untreated to see if any progression to cancer occurred over time. At the end of the study, 71 women developed malignancies and nine of them had lesions of invasive cancer (Chakravarty and Bhavan 2017). Another example of controversial trials due to loopholes in unregulated guidelines was the use of mepacrine, an anti-malarial compound inserted into more than 30,000 Indian women as a means of female sterilization (Chakravarty and Bhavan 2017). This method was deemed illegal and untested, where even western countries banned it. However, distribution to medical practitioners continued up to five years in some regions, for example rural Bengal, despite a Supreme Court ban (Dasgupta 2005). In yet another example, an investigation into the trials in the Indian state of Telangana was conducted and it was found that volunteers from Hyderabad and Karimnagar had participated in over 30 studies in a decade, and to have broken rules to make a quick buck. This included hopping from one trial to another without a three-month gap in between, drinking alcohol, and hiding one's health history. Countries such as France and the UK have a national registry of volunteers participating in clinical trials. India with its lower levels of income and awareness, has none (Pulla 2017).

India needs more stringent rules in testing and application of such trials to any population instead of embarking on more innovative and modernized ventures. An example of this disastrous catapult can be seen in the readiness to invest in genome editing, where new species of plants and animals can be created in forms of 'designer babies', or genetically modified crops. Stem cell therapy use for conditions other than blood disorders such as for knee replacements are also new ways of unethically experimenting on patients who are unaware of this violation.

Some 'non-clinical' research studies also demonstrate a grey area of ethical practice within community settings. For example, the Million Death Study (Jha et al. 2006) was one of the largest studies for premature mortality in the world conducted in India. It was ethically carried out by local and international collaborators and used a technique called verbal autopsy (VA). However, this technique is sometimes overlooked from an ethics standpoint by other researchers. VA is used to assign cause of death in settings where postmortem examinations cannot be conducted. Information on circumstances preceding death is obtained by a relative or caregiver of the deceased, where sensitivity around distressed respondents must be considered while collecting data. For this reason, the International Committee of Medical Journal Editors mandates all authors to publish VA studies conducted according to ethical standards. India remains a hotbed for such studies given the inadequate medical expertise in rural areas for conducting postmortem examinations. A 2017 published systematic review of ethical standards in global VA studies (including India) showed that only 48 per cent of studies reported having Institutional Review Board clearance, confidentiality of data was only explained in 14 per cent of all studies, 18 per cent did not report the type of respondent interviewed, and only 62 per cent of studies reported whether interviewers collecting data were trained (Joshi et al. 2018). While taking informed verbal/written consent and providing participant information sheets may seem as the 'basics' of ethical practices, such reports highlight other fundamental principles not being honoured by researchers.

Over the years, the government and the ICMR have taken steps to ensure ethical practices in research studies is guided appropriately. By formally recognizing medical institutions that act in accordance with current guidelines and empowering local ethics committees, there have been minor improvements. A most recent example is the ICMR development of the 'National Ethical Guidelines for Biomedical Research Involving Children 2017'. The physiology and disease manifestation in children is different than in adults. The adverse effects of drugs and age-appropriateness of medications are some of the factors why separate guidelines are required. These guidelines stipulate ethical points such as the need for a prerequisite of expertise in investigators dealing with children, safety testing, and indications of efficacy of drugs in adults before administration in children and research being conducted in child-friendly environments. However, there still exists a huge gap in design and implementation of ethics in research practices, whereby such guidelines developed by the government or ICMR should turn into stringent laws and not remain merely as guidelines.

***

1. Medical ethics is based on four non-hierarchical principles which are never to be compromised but should always be considered in conjunction with the local socioeconomic factors.
2. In the Indian context, there have been numerous examples of unethical practice in healthcare and research. Ethical guidelines have continually been revised but generally poorly regulated. The lure of money has eroded the ethical base of clinical practice in the country and a non-corruptible regulatory authority is a need of the hour. Acts and legislatives can also be helpful but the ambit of their jurisdiction need to be clearly specified.
3. The pharmaceutical industry governs a large chunk of medical practice in India. Pharmaceutical lures need to be cut and monitoring and regulation of this growing industry is mandatory. Governing bodies such as the MCI in conjunction with ICMR should intervene with jurisdiction mitigating the pharma industry's negative consumerism impact on health systems.
4. India's tryst with clinical trials in the past has been fragmented and riddled with fraud and deceit. There is an urgent need of better regulation of clinical trials in the country. Organizations like the ICMR need to be proactive in regulating clinical trials to prevent unnecessary mortality and morbidity arising out of such trials and affecting the vulnerable sections of society.

POLICY RECOMMENDATIONS

1. To promote principles of ethical practice at the undergraduate level in medical, dental and other allied schools so that a culture of ethical practice can be promoted from an early age. Including medical ethics as a subject in the medical curriculum will go a long way in achieving this goal.
2. To strengthen the regulatory procedures around medical research so that false research, poorly conceived research, and research with malice intent can be curtailed. A step towards this has been taken by the development of the Clinical Trials Registry by the ICMR. This needs to be updated and implemented more rigorously across the country.
3. Developing stringent regulatory authorities to check doctor–industry nexus. This has been one of the weakest links in the present regulatory mechanisms. Its strengthening will be useful in curtailing malpractice.
4. To bring legislations which are doable but at the same time harsh enough to control malpractices and promote a healthy medical working environment.

5. Developing a core faculty of health workers, research personnel, lawyers, and public health experts in formulating guidelines whenever an ethical body is constituted. This is necessary as most regulatory bodies work with a vertical approach limiting themselves to a particular sphere. Presence of a pool of national faculty on ethics will be useful in receiving vital inputs whenever such bodies are reformulating guidelines or introducing newer practice conditions.

REFERENCES

Beauchamp, T, and J. Childress. 2013. *Principles of Biomedical Ethics*, 7th Edition. New York: Oxford University Press.

Bhalla, A. 'How they made the NRHM sick', Tehelka.com, 17 March. Available at http://old.tehelka.com/how-they-made-the-nrhm-sick/, last accessed on 20 January 2020.

Chattopadhyay, S. 2013. 'Corruption in Healthcare and Medicine: Why Should Physicians and Bioethicists Care and What should They Do?' *Indian Journal of Medical Ethics* 10(3): 153–9.

Chakravarty, A., and A. Bhavan. 2017. 'Unethical Clinical Trials in India: A Selective Preliminary Overview', *Eubios Journal of Asian and International Bioethics* 27(2): 66–8.

Dasgupta, R. 2005. 'Quinacrine Sterilization in India: Women's Health and Medical Ethics still at Risk'. Hampshire College. Available at http://sites.hampshire.edu/popdev/quinacrine-sterilization-in-india-womens-health-and-medical-ethics-still-at-risk/, last accessed on 15 November 2019.

Deccan Herald. 2017. 'Docs Agree it's Unethical of Them to Refer Patients to Labs for a Cut'. Available at http://www.deccanherald.com/content/646179/docs-agree-its-unethical-them.html, last accessed on 18 June 2019.

Gillon, R. 1994. 'Medical Ethics: Four Principles Plus Attention to Scope'. *British Medical Journal*, 309(16): 184–7.

India Brand Equity Foundation (IBEF). 2017. *Indian Pharmaceutical Industry 2017*, report. Available at: https://www.ibef.org/industry/ pharmaceutical-india.aspx.

Jha, Durgesh Nandan. 2017. 'Hospital Declares Live Baby Dead, Gives it to Parents in Plastic Bag'. *Times of India*, 2 December. Available at https://timesofindia.indiatimes.com/city/delhi/hospital-declares-live-baby-dead-gives-it-to-parents-in-plastic-bag/articleshow/61887252.cms, last accessed on 18 December 2019.

Jha, Prabhat, Vendhan Gajalakshmi, Prakash C. Gupta, Rajesh Kumar, Prem Mony, Neeraj Dhingra, Richard Peto. 2006. 'Prospective Study of One Million Deaths in India: Rationale, Design, and Validation Results'. *PLOS ONE* 3(2): e18.

Joseph, Reji K. 2011. 'The R&D Scenario in Indian Pharmaceutical Industry', RIS Discussion Papers no 176, Research and Information System for Developing Countries, New Delhi.

Joshi, R., N. Faruqui, S. Nagarajan, R. Rampatige, A. Martiniuk, H. Gouda. 2018. 'Reporting of Ethics in Peer-Reviewed Verbal Autopsy Studies: A Systemic Review'. *International Journal of Epidemiology* 47(1): 255–79.

Khan, S.A. 2016. 'A Low Priority Called Health', *The Indian Express*, 30 September. Available at: http://indianexpress.com/article/opinion/columns/health-care-hospitals-doctors-expensive-india-private-poverty-aiims-treatment-3056856/, last accessed on 9 June 2019.

———. 2017a. 'Clinical Trials in India Need Better Regulation', *The Wire*, 22 June. Available at https://thewire.in/149913/clinical-trialsin-india-need-better-regulations/, last accessed on 18 December 2019.

———. 2017b. 'Unless Morality and Medicine Combine, Regulating Private Medical Establishments is a Must'. *The Wire*, 30 July. Available at: https://thewire.in/162971/private-medical-establishments-regulation-healthcare/, last accessed on 15 January 2020.

Malpani, A. 2014. 'Use Patient Power to Tackle Medical Corruption in India'. *British Medical Journal*, 349(14): g5156.

Munshi, R.H., K.R. Singh, and A.D. Thakkar. 2016. 'Understanding the Degree of Awareness among Medical Professionals regarding the Ethics of Pharmaceutical Marketing Activities in Context of Revised Medical Council of India Code of Ethics'. doi:10.18203/2319-2003.ijbcp20160653.

The New Indian Express. 2012. 'Mayawati Misused Funds for Rural Health: PM'. Available at http://www.newindianexpress.com/nation/2012/feb/17/mayawati-misused-funds-for-rural-health-pm-341095.html, last accessed on 16 November 2019.

Pulla, P. 2017. 'Lured by Blood Money: Serial Volunteers Set a Disturbing Trend'. *The Hindu*, 30 December. Available at http://www.thehindu.com/opinion/op-ed/lured-by-blood-money-clinical-trials/article22328296.ece, last accessed on 18 December 2019.

Roy, N., N. Madhiwalla, and S. Pai. 2007. 'Drug Promotional Practices in Mumbai: A Qualitative Study', *Indian Journal of Medical Ethics*, 4(2): 57–61.Shivam, V., S. Govind, and N. Arun. 2012. 'A Comparative Study in Regulatory Trends of Pharmaceuticals in Brazil, Russia, India and China (BRIC) Countries', *Journal of Generic Medicines*, 9(3): 128–43.

Shukla, A and A. Gadre. 2016. *Dissenting Diagnosis*. New Delhi: Random House.

Soneji, H. and A. Banerjee. 2004. 'Indian Pharma Major Prefer Brand Promotion over R&D', *The Economic Times*, 15 December. Available at http://economictimes.indiatimes.com/articleshowarchive.cms?msid=959093, last accessed on 10 January 2020.

24

Corruption in Indian Healthcare

Going Beyond Scandal

Sanjay Nagral, Samiran S. Nundy, and Sunil Pandya

Although corruption in healthcare is a global phenomenon, it has reached alarming proportions in India, especially over the last few years. It has become everyday news. This may partly be an apparent rise due to increasing interest from the media but corruption is being increasingly driven and legitimized by the presence of new market forces in India's healthcare sector. There is no doubt, however, that it is a critical issue in the Indian subcontinent as it further erodes what is already a dysfunctional healthcare system. It has a significant impact on the quality of care and, in a sense, on human lives. Hence it needs urgent attention, analysis, and intervention.

Corruption in healthcare can be analysed at multiple levels. The focus could be on the individual with frameworks such morality and professional values or could be broad based in the realm of political economy of health and societal corruption. The difficulty in a rigorous analysis of healthcare corruption in India is not only the lack of solid data but also the lack of clarity of what precisely constitutes corruption. For example, many practices which a few decades ago would be labelled as 'corrupt' are now considered to be acceptable business practices. An example of this is the phenomenon of private capitation medical colleges, which now outnumber state-run colleges or the widely prevalent practice of fee splitting or commissions, which has now become the norm rather than the exception.

Healthcare in India has recently been rocked by several large scandals, which reek of systematic and well-entrenched corrupt practices. Some well-known examples include the Vyapam scam involving admissions to medical colleges in Madhya Pradesh, several scams involving drug procurement, the sordid saga of the Medical Council of India (MCI) and the sting operations on commissions and cut practice. We have discussed some of these later in the chapter. In public perception, healthcare is now seen as one of the most corrupt areas of Indian society, and trust, which is a necessary precondition for a good doctor–patient relationship, is being rapidly eroded. It may also be one of the reasons behind the increasing spate of violence against healthcare workers, which is unprecedented in comparison to the global scenario, thereby forcing many states to enact special laws for this purpose.

One simplistic and innocent way of rationalizing healthcare corruption is to label it as being just a part of the larger corrupt ecosystem in India. In fact, there is a common refrain amongst healthcare workers especially medical professionals, which goes something like this: 'There is corruption in all strata of Indian society—ministers, bureaucrats, judges, lawyers, tax officials, the police, those running schools and colleges, and property builders and owners, and now even in our armed forces. How can you then expect only doctors to remain free from this practice?' There are, of course, several valid arguments against this line of thought. The medical profession is unique because its ministrations and decisions often make the difference between death and life. Healthcare workers, especially doctors, are highly privileged. They have undergone years of instruction in schools, colleges, and medical colleges. They deal with individuals and families racked by pain and anxiety. The profession's historical social contract with society includes a certain commitment to ethical behaviour in return for recognition of its monopoly to practice medicine. Whilst these are indeed powerful arguments, we must, however, admit that it is indeed a challenge to counter healthcare corruption in isolation from the pervading environment in the rest of society.

In this chapter we try and address only some of the many factors that we believe contribute to malpractice and healthcare corruption and focus on some of its manifestations. Some of it is anecdotal but is based on our personal observations whilst working in India's mainstream healthcare sector over many decades. We have attempted to describe the changes in medical education and practice that we have observed.

We first look at some of the commonly discussed practices, which constitute both malpractice and corruption. We then go onto analyse some of the drivers of corruption and finally suggest some ways in which these issues could be tackled in future.

CUTS, COMMISSIONS, AND KICKBACKS

Commissions for referrals (colloquially called 'cuts' or 'kickbacks' or fee split) are a longstanding and widespread practice in Indian healthcare (Nagral and Nundy 2017). They often involve payment of money in cash and without public knowledge from a section of healthcare workers or institution to another in order to lure or to compensate for patient referrals. This practice has been observed globally and is not peculiar to India. However, it seems to us that in India it has now been mainstreamed and legitimized to the point of becoming the norm. Though much discussed, it has gone largely unpunished leading to huge conflicts of interests, increase in costs, and impacting the quality of care.

In the current dominant model of healthcare in India, since income is generated from individual patients, ensuring a steady stream of patients to the doctor's clinic or a hospital is essential. Awaiting patients who seek treatment on the basis of the clinician's reputation is time consuming as renown is earned over time. Also, there is cutthroat competition and intense saturation especially in urban India.

The quick and easy solution is to resort to payments—to touts such as taxi drivers, especially those who frequent airports and stations where long-distance trains terminate; to family physicians; and to fellow consultants. In most cities and towns, this system of 'cut practice'—to use a common descriptive term for this system of added commissions is well-entrenched. The recent attempt by a cardiac surgeon in Mumbai to highlight this practice in Mumbai by putting up hoardings stating that their hospital does not offer commissions and the subsequent plan of a law in Maharashtra to curb commission practice is being watched with interest. However, in the absence of a critical mass of healthcare professionals offering internal resistance, it is debatable whether just a law by one state will make any significant impact (Nagral and Nundy 2017).

Parting with a portion of the income from individual patients to others is no longer restricted to the individual practitioners of medicine. Nursing homes, hospitals, pathology laboratories, imaging centres, and other institutions, that are no longer places for healing but healthcare businesses, also indulge in this practice to attract more patients and produce greater incomes.

Its obvious fallout, harmful to the patient's interests, is that the patient referral is governed, not by proven competence, but by the sum paid by the clinician, laboratory, imaging centre, or hospital. Fee-splitting also indirectly pushes up the costs of healthcare. It is also a completely opaque monetary transaction where the unsuspecting patient is completely unaware of money exchanging hands on his or her investigations or treatment.

The MCI's ethics guidelines clearly define fee-splitting as unethical but the practice continues unabated and in fact, is taking newer and interesting forms. Thus, a few years back, a leading hospital in Mumbai had begun a scheme titled the 'elite forum' to provide 'rewards' to doctors for referring patients. The rewards ranged from INR 100,000 for 40 admissions per annum, to INR 250,000 for 75 admissions. Those joining the scheme needed to sign and stamp a statement. This was perhaps a clever attempt by some bright marketing manager to 'formalize' the kickback system. Even a hospital of this scale, which had spent crores in advertising campaigns, had to seek recourse to a well-entrenched trade practice. On receiving a show-cause notice from the Maharashtra Medical Council, the hospital hastily withdrew the scheme. When the hospital responded to questions about its kickback scheme, it had an interesting explanation. Its letter said, 'The offering of incentives to doctors, as pointed out in your letter, was a case of over enthusiasm by the Marketing Department' (Nagral 2014).

TESTS—USE AND MISUSE

The purpose for performing a medical test could be twofold. It may be used to confirm the diagnosis made by a doctor after clinical examination. The test helps to zero in onto the single correct diagnosis. An example is the examination under the microscope of a tissue from a swelling in the neck to differentiate between tuberculosis and cancer. It may also be used to determine a course of action. An example is a computerized tomography (CT) scan to determine whether a suspected blood clot between the skull and brain in an elderly person is large enough to need drainage through an operation or is small enough to be treated by drugs.

What vexes many is a demand for tests where the doctor treats the results with indifference. It is not unusual to see 'routine' tests being carried out on patients, especially after admission to hospital, the results of which lie undisturbed in the patient's file. Worse, abnormal results are missed and appropriate treatment on the basis of these findings delayed or not provided at all.

Vested interests also dictate the demand for tests. Many patients have experienced the following scenario: they have undergone several expensive tests at the request of their primary physician and now await the consultant's advice. After a cursory review of the reports, the consultant demands the same tests be redone and adds additional set of tests to the list with a command that they be performed from a particular laboratory. Such an action often raises a suspicion in the minds of patient and family members on the actual reason for the new tests. Doctors have been found to be on the payroll of the particular imaging centres and laboratories that they have been referring patients to for such tests.

Yet another worrying phenomenon is that of ordering tests in a manner similar to shotgun therapy, that is, spraying out a large number of pellets in the hope that at least a few will hit the target. Shotgun tests follow intellectual dishonesty or laziness—both equally discreditable in a physician. It is now increasingly commonplace for a patient calling a consultant for an appointment to be asked, 'Please tell me your symptoms.' Should the answer be, 'headache', he/she may well be told, 'Go to XYZ imaging centre, get an X-ray film of the chest, plain and contrast CT scan done. After this go to ABC Laboratory and get the following tests done on your blood and urine. After you get the reports, come and see me tomorrow at X p.m.' Imagine the patient's discomfiture when the findings on all these tests are negative and he learns that his headache is actually due to his blood pressure being abnormally high.

Conflict of interests either due to direct ownership and investment in laboratories or imaging centres combined with kickbacks is leading to an epidemic of over investigation which leads to an increased financial burden on an already challenged patient and family.

IRRATIONAL CARE

In the not-too-distant past, the physician faced with a patient with fever would often adopt an expectant attitude once his examination showed no cause for anxiety. He would prescribe a gentle drug to bring down the fever, keep the patient comfortable, and watch her progress. If the fever persisted or worsened, the physician would check for likely causes such as malaria or typhoid and only after confirmation of this suspicion, prescribe appropriate treatment. Where necessary, the physician would identify the germ causing the illness and prescribe an antibiotic only after confirming that the germ was susceptible to it.

These days a doctor is more likely to prescribe drugs to bring down fever, abolish pain, facilitate sleep, and add one or more antibiotics without any evidence that the latter are needed. Such a step not only adds to the cost or treatment but also leads to the development of resistance of the germs to the simpler antibiotics. The defense offered by the treating doctor for such an action is that patients are very impatient and demand rapid resolution of their symptoms.

The unusually high rates of Caesarian sections (C-sections) in India especially in the private sector have been well documented (Neumann 2014). Part of the fault lies with a section of society demanding such operations for reasons of comfort or convenience or in order to ensure that birth occurs at an exact, auspicious time. However, there is no denying the unworthy motive of the doctor who wishes to perform the delivery at a time that is convenient for them or the fact that an operation yields a greater income than the supervision of a normal delivery.

It is shocking but not surprising that when large state-funded mass insurance schemes covering surgical procedures were launched in some states of India, it led to a huge increase in procedures such as hysterectomy and appendicectomy. Thus, a lot of prescriptions, investigations, and interventions, including surgery, are being driven by commercial interest rather than need. One could debate whether this constitutes a fallout of bad practice or market medicine whose primary aim is profit, but it also constitutes corruption as it involves lack of transparency and underhanded dealings.

THE DOCTOR–PHARMA/INDUSTRY NEXUS

Industry thrives on progressive increases in profit and manufacturers of drugs, medical equipment and instruments are no exception. Their legitimate source of profit should be the sale of their products and there lies the rub. Prescriptions by doctors and purchases by clinics and hospitals influence their sales. Instead of relying on the quality of their products, they too resort to misinformation, bribery, and corruption.

It is well known that in industry circles, doctors are classified on the basis of their prescriptions. A sophisticated system links medical representatives of pharmaceutical companies to pharmacies in the vicinity of individual doctors to facilitate tracking of drugs prescribed and those actually purchased by patients. These representatives as well as doctors earn rewards based on the quantities of very expensive drugs, which are sold on the basis of such prescriptions.

The industry has not shied away from blatant means of bribery. Here are some examples. Such companies pay business or first class air fare when 'important' doctors travel to national and international destinations. Their hotel accommodation is paid for and chauffeur-driven vehicles are provided at each halt during such travels. Gifts to such doctors have included automobiles, air conditioners, and refrigerators. The less influential hoi polloi in the profession are provided laptop computers, office utilities, medical books, and subscriptions to journals.

Manufacturers of drugs and medical equipment are also huge donors to organizers of medical conferences. The budgets of most national conferences now cost millions of rupees. In return, organizers accept nominees of drug companies as speakers who will extol the virtues of their products, arrange seminars on their proprietary formulations, and ensure that slides on their products are projected on to the screen at every opportunity between scientific sessions. They are also permitted to set up stalls and enhance their sales.

Periodic efforts at curbing such practices are publicized by medical councils and the government. Thus far, the results from these efforts do not appear to be substantial. Many countries in the world have tried to tackle this problem by enforcing strict codes of conduct both for the medical profession and industry. The principle of disclosure about any relationship between these two players has been codified and enforced. And top doctors have been sacked and punished for violations. This, however, continues to be a global problem. Though there have been sporadic exposes, the Indian situation continues to be opaque and murky. In 2010, the Medical Council of India (MCI) amended its code of ethics to enumerate ethical violations and prescribed punishments. At that time it was felt that this amendment and its adoption by medical associations would be seen as the medical profession's contribution to a larger process of transparency, accountability, and professionalism which is manifesting in some sectors of Indian industry (Nagral and Roy 2010). However that has not happened.

THE DRIVERS OF CORRUPTION

Early Education

The impressionable experiences of a growing child are based on the credo that governs the acts of parents and other senior family members. Next comes teachers during early schooling. Virtues of honesty, contentment, ethical behaviour, and the spirit of service and fair play often need emphasis at an early age. The current failure on this front has many reasons. Nuclear families and the need for both parents to earn a livelihood has resulted in a considerable reduction of the time they spend with their children. The exceptional teacher, dignified, with all her acts governed by integrity and concern for the children under her care, finds it difficult to counter the examples set by those who barely teach in school but advocate attendance at their private tuition classes instead.

A career in the professions including medicine is no longer seen as a scientific pursuit or a social commitment but primarily a means to acquire wealth and status. The goalposts are thus set every early and, to use a cliché, the means justify the ends. This is perpetuated during medical school where success is being increasingly defined in monetary terms. At some stage in India's history, emphasis on teaching in vernacular languages also created a handicap in medical education as most teaching and textbooks are in the English language.

Medical Education

In the days when medical colleges were exclusively run by the state, education was largely imparted by teachers committed to imparting education and patient care. They communicated the art and science of medicine to students in classes and during clinics and taught its practice by example. In the immediate post-Independence period there was a certain idealism in the practice of medicine. There was minimal scope for political interference, caste, creed, or any other extraneous factors in the selection process. Teachers in medical colleges were generally good role models of patient-centric care.

There has, unfortunately, been a progressive deterioration over time. The dominant role models amongst medical teachers and practising professionals are now different. With the growth of the private sector and the intermingling of medical teachers with market medicine, the definition of successful doctors is now closely linked with their monetary status. The goalposts of success in medicine have changed as they have in the rest of our social lives.

The entire focus of medical education has shifted towards somehow obtaining the right marks in the right exams to get the right degree and has largely become end-oriented.

Shockingly, a system of tuition classes in medical subjects has grown and flourished. Since these classes—away from the college and hospital—can never provide medical education of any quality, all that the students learn is how to obtain more marks in the professional examinations. Standards have progressively fallen as a consequence.

Any analysis of corruption in Indian medicine must acknowledge the role of private medical college industry. Besides establishing a poor benchmark for fairness and honesty, these colleges also push students to recover their enormous investment after they start practice, fuelling unethical practices in an already commercial scenario (Nagral and Nundy 2017).

Elsewhere in the world, a new medical college and teaching hospital can only be set up if they aim to be considerably superior to those extant in the city or state and after there is demonstrable proof of the necessity for them based on a systematic study. In our country, on the other hand, medical colleges and hospitals have been sanctioned on the basis of political power and connections and through corruption in the MCI. From being at the fringe, private medical colleges now dominate the scene. In fact, of the 398 colleges offering the Bachelor of Medicine, Bachelor of Surgery (MBBS) degree throughout India, 215 are private and churn out about 27,000 graduates a year, outnumbering those from government colleges that churn out 25,000 (Nagral 2015).

Teachers in medical colleges, from senior professors to lecturers, have to perform multiple tasks like caring for their patients, teaching students and resident doctors, and researching diseases of local, regional, and national importance. Each of these demands effort and time. If all three are to be performed well, eight-hour working days are often inadequate.

Several states in India have now permitted private practice by their senior staff members including academic staff (professors, associate professors, and assistant professors). The ostensible reason was to enable these senior doctors to live comfortably despite the relatively low salaries paid to them by the government or municipal corporations running their institutions. The consequences have, however, been unfortunate. Many senior professors are now found to be operating or seeing patients in private hospitals at all hours of the day and rarely in the teaching capacities.

Big Hospitals and Corporate Medicine

Newspapers and television channels are currently full of news about overcharging in large corporate hospitals. There is a range of big hospitals from those traditionally called charitable to the more recent corporate chains. Though there is some variation, in general these hospitals share some common characteristics including their size and focus on specialized care. The current media glare is on their making huge profits from drugs and consumables used during treatment. Hospitals purchase these at considerable discounts. At times, the discounts on drugs from pharma companies to hospitals can be as high as 60 per cent of the maximum retail price (MRP). When billing patients, not only is the full MRP charged but an additional service charge of 5 per cent to 10 per cent is also added. This is an area where the pharmaceutical industry colludes to bolster their sales.

Stents, used to keep vital arteries open, especially those in the heart, have also been in the news. Whilst the cost of these stents, especially after being imported, is high to start with, hospitals have been known to add their own charges to the detriment of the patients' finances.

Hospitals have also been known to reuse items intended for single use. There is a however, a case for such reuse in a country such as India with huge multitudes of the poor with several studies showing that after careful cleansing and re-sterilization, many of these items can be reused safely. The problem is with charging each patient as if a new item has been used. Surely, when an item is reused, the charge should merely relate to the cost of cleansing and sterilization—a small fraction of the original cost of the item.

Such practices have been public knowledge for a long time but governments have turned a blind eye to them, as have the statutory regulatory bodies such as the Drugs Controller of India, the Food and Drug Administration, the various medical councils and national associations of doctors such as the Indian Medical Association (IMA).

Whether the currently publicized moves by government agencies will improve matters for patients and their families remains to be seen. But there is certainly increased public and media awareness of the issue. Individual patients or their family members are putting up valiant fights including going up to the Supreme Court for justice.

Regulatory Failure and the Medical Councils

India's healthcare system inherited a self-regulatory model of governance from the British in the form of a central and state medical councils. The MCI, which was meant to be the apex body, has a comprehensive ethics code which is binding on all practitioners of modern medicine and has powers to even suo motu look into unethical and corrupt practices. This body, which was supposed to enforce ethical standards has itself been plagued by severe corruption. It is no surprise that finally the central government has just dissolved the MCI and has announced the formation of an alternative body called the National Medical Commission.

In 2009, a review written by some of us about the functioning of the MCI and the role of the doctor, Ketan Desai, who was later arrested on the charges of corruption, was published in the *Indian Journal of Medical Ethics* (Pandya 2009). The gist of the essay was summed up in one line: 'It (MCI) is plagued by inefficiency, arbitrariness and lack of transparency.' The next year it was highlighted in an editorial in the same journal about the consequence were the MCI to follow its present course—perdition. One of the points made was that individuals like Desai thrived only due to the permissiveness and complicity on the part of their subordinates and peers.

The most damning and, in a sense, official indictment of the MCI came from the Parliamentary Standing Committee of Health and Family Welfare in 2016 (Parliamentary Committee Report, Pandya 2016). Numerous deficiencies were highlighted and condemned. Here are some excerpts from the report:

> The Medical Council of India, when tested on the above touchstone, has repeatedly been found short of fulfilling its mandated responsibilities.... [T]he MCI, as presently elected, neither represents professional excellence nor its ethos. The current composition of the Council reflects that more than half of the members are either from corporate hospitals or in private practice. The Committee is surprised to note that even doctors nominated under Sections 3(1)(a) and 3(1)(e) to represent the State Governments and the Central Government have been nominated from corporate private hospitals which are not only highly commercialised and provide care at exorbitant cost but have also been found to be violating value frameworks.... [T]he current composition of the MCI is biased against larger public health goals and public interest. (Vol. 1: 87–8)
>
> The Committee observes that the oversight of professional conduct is the most important function of the MCI. However, the MCI has been completely passive on the ethics dimension which is evident from the fact that between 1963–2009, just 109 doctors have been blacklisted by the Ethics Committee of the MCI. (Vol. 1: 102)
>
> The Committee is shocked to find that compromised individuals have been able to make it to the MCI, but the Ministry is not empowered to remove or sanction a Member of the Council even if he has been proved corrupt.... Such a state of affairs is also symptomatic of the rot within and points to a deep systemic malice. Otherwise how could it happen that the MCI, which has laid down elaborate duties and responsibilities of the 'Physician' under the MCI Code of Ethics Regulations, 2002, could have at its very top a person who was arrested on charges of corruption in 2010. The former Union Health Minister, who must have an insider's view of the functioning of the MCI, making scathing comments about corruption in the MCI, speaks volumes of the decay in the MCI and is an eye-opener on the need for urgent reforms in the structure and functioning of MCI. (Vol. 1: 76)

In an analysis, it was concluded that optimism may not be justified despite the clear statement of facts in the

Parliamentary Report and strong recommendations, as quoted further:

> Recommendations of earlier committees, when found unpalatable by the government or when conflicting with vested interests of those in power have been rendered ineffective by the simple measures of either shelving them or, worse, referring them to yet another committee for study and recommendations. A state that could transfer the then Health Secretary Mr Keshav Desiraju in order to facilitate Dr Ketan Desai's entry into the MCI through the backdoor of a recommendation by a pliant university in Ahmedabad and which could accept the replacement of Dr Ketan Desai by someone else from the same state does not generate confidence.
>
> We appear to be incapable of learning from institutions in other countries, such as the General Medical Council in Britain, that are performing duties similar to those entrusted to MCI honestly, openly, and efficiently. (Pandya 2016)

The Free Market Link

Encouraged by the liberalization of the economy in the early 1990s, the growth rate of the private sector in healthcare has hugely widened in its sweep and scale. Deliberate or otherwise, this has been accompanied by an enormous retreat of public medicine. India's emerging middle class has embraced the private sector and there is no substantive political opposition to the collapse of public health (Nagral 2016). This larger and more systemic change has impacted on the nature of healthcare in India. It has mainstreamed and given legitimacy to several trade and business practices, many of which border on corruption.

The medical profession has embraced the increased opportunities and monetary benefits this shift has created. The private sector offers a certain freedom from bureaucracy, a feeling of independence, and technology and has caught the imagination of medical professionals. This has also manifested in an entrepreneurial energy with doctors becoming healthcare investors. Of course, all this has led to severe conflict of interest scenarios, which are now throwing up their own problems.

This is not to say that public medicine and government hospitals are free of corrupt practices. Petty corruption is in fact rampant in India's state-run health services. Bribes to lower level staff for facilitating advancement of outpatient queues, patient admittances, and investigations are frequent. But large-scale privatization and acceptance of the market logic actually gives an ideological cover to many such corrupt practices.

COMBATING HEALTHCARE CORRUPTION

The cancer of corruption in Indian healthcare has now spread to a very advanced stage and eroded deep into the body politic of the system. There are enormous, well-entrenched conflicts of interest, which encourage corrupt business practices. One response is to call for more regulation, transparency, and exemplary punishment for the guilty. In the last few decades there have been an increasing number of regulatory frameworks concerning healthcare in India put into place.

There was a strong historical legacy of self regulation, which the medical profession in India enjoyed through the structure of medical councils. This opportunity has largely frittered away. Also whistleblowing from those inside the system is rare. For that matter, a significant section of the profession benefits and is hence complicit in many of the practices. For example, private medical colleges offer employment to medical teachers and other healthcare workers. Commissions are a way to quickly attract patients and recover investments. There is no substantive compulsion for self-correction beyond the nebulous ethical dimension.

Due to this failure of self-regulation, an increasing number of special laws and acts have been promulgated by the Indian state to curb specific malpractices in areas such as organ trade, female foeticide, and surrogacy. Whether external regulation can effectively curb some of the practices continues to be a matter of debate, but given the complete failure of internal consensus and regulation this currently seems to be the only way out.

Given the fear and awe on the one hand and the information asymmetry on the other, which is intrinsic to a healthcare encounter, it is unrealistic to expect individual citizens to offer resistance to some of the practices. Even the state and judiciary are partly in awe of the profession. Professional organizations such as the IMA have behaved more like guilds and resisted attempts at regulation. The unwillingness of many states to promulgate the central clinical establishment act and the recent fracas over the Karnataka Private Medical Establishment bills are testament to this tension (Krishna 2017).

Political forces, civil society groups, consumer welfare agencies, non-governmental organizations, and the media, working in coordination, can engage with the situation by monitoring practices and spreading information based on their findings. They can strive to raise existing standards, reward the ethical and efficient and make life difficult for the rest.

Highlighting malpractices and the means to identify them, spreading awareness of honest and ethical individuals and institutions in the community, and publicizing low-cost but efficient service providers are some of the ways to empower the public. Community-based healthcare organizations have partly succeeded in doing this.

Self-help groups of patients and families formed to deal with specific diseases learn much from their experiences. They wear the badge of suffering and are therefore especially valuable sources of information and suggestions for amendment. Such measures may enable accountability amongst service providers.

The Lokayukta and Right to Information (RTI) law are two other means towards uncovering wrongdoing and seeking justice. RTI is being increasingly used to uncover healthcare corruption.

It may be best to keep recourse to consumer and other courts as last resorts. Proceedings in these halls of justice are time-consuming and delays of years and even decades are not unknown. The cost in terms of time, energy, and expense may not be compensated by the ultimate judgment.

RECENT INITIATIVES BY THE STATE AND JUDICIARY

Partly as a result of failure of self-regulation by medical councils and professional associations, and partly in response to public pressure, the State and judiciary in India have had to increasingly intervene by promulgating special laws and acts. These provide guidelines but are focused on curbing malpractice in specific areas of medical activity in India. The Human Organs Transplant Act of 1994, the Pre-Conception and Pre-Natal Diagnostic Techniques (PCPNDT) Act of 1994, as well as the more recent Surrogacy Regulation Bill of 2016 and the stem cell therapy guidelines are all examples of this phenomenon.

Following the damning report of the Parliamentary Standing Committee on the MCI and the recommendations of the Ranjit Roy Chaudhary Committee as well as a Parliamentary committee, the National Medical Council Bill (NMC) was recently passed by the Parliament in 2019. This paves the way for the abolition of the MCI in the near future. It also sets up fee regulation for private medical colleges and provides for greater proportion of those outside the profession to be part of an ethics board. However, the final NMC bill is on the one hand being opposed by medical associations notably the IMA and is being seen as too watered down by activists campaigning for reform on the other.

In addition there now seems to be an increasing willingness from the State, the Centre, and Parliament to tighten regulations for infrastructure and staffing and even enter the arena of price capping. The Clinical Establishments Act (CEA) of 2010 seeks to ensure that the operative functioning of healthcare delivery systems in states is in compliance with prescribed, transparent guidelines and keep any form of regulatory malpractices in check (related to drug pricing, licensing provisions or procurement, for instance). States such as Himachal and Arunachal Pradesh and more recently Kerala have implemented it but many others are yet to accept it. On the other hand, West Bengal recently passed its own legislation called the West Bengal Clinical Establishments (Registration, Regulation and Transparency) Act, 2017. This aims to streamline the procedures of registration of clinical establishments, medical licensing systems, and accounting for criminal offences related to medical practice under a prescribed adjudicating, regulatory body called the West Bengal Clinical Establishment Regulatory Commission.

Maharashtra has been sitting on its version of the CEA which has been lying with them for the last two years, but it has announced its intention to promulgate a special law called 'The Prevention of Cut Practices in Healthcare Services Act 2017'. This act prescribes severe punishment to all those proven to indulge in any form of commission transaction in healthcare. However this act has not yet been passed. Finally, in a rather unprecedented and much publicized move, the central government has in the recent past directly intervened to cap the prices of coronary stents as well as joint replacement implants. Thus, it seems that we are all set for increasing State and judicial interventions in healthcare regulation many of which will hopefully deter corrupt practices.

THE FUTURE

The biggest continuing healthcare crisis in India is not corruption but the lack of access to quality and timely healthcare to the vast majority of its population. Corruption aggravates this huge fault line. In other ways, corruption is also a direct outcome of market medicine and its desperate efforts to generate profit from illness in what has been historically recognized as a case of market failure.

Thus, some serious self-reflection that, unlike many other countries, we have been complicit in pushing something as important as healthcare into the market paradigm is necessary. When the outrage against corruption leads to outrage against our collective failure to protect healthcare from the ravages of the market, we will move closer to effective steps in the right direction. Or else much like the one-point-agenda anti-corruption crusades in recent Indian political history (such as the India against Corruption movement), which have either lost steam or got co-opted we are afraid this will meet the same fate.

The question is who will lead the crusade for resisting corruption in Indian healthcare. Those stakeholders who have a vested interest in corrupt practices are unlikely to do it. These incidentally are also groups who reap the benefits of market medicine which include sections of the medical profession. Answers may also lie outside the world of medicine. Orgnizations such as People for Better Treatment (an organization set up by an expatriate Indian doctor whose wife died after a medical mishap) has campaigned to hold the medical profession accountable and filed multiple cases in the Supreme Court including the landmark judgment offering the largest ever compensation for medical negligence in India (*Financial Express* 2013).

We are afraid that this will have to be done by a broad coalition of forces from outside the sector aligning with a section from within. As for the consumers of healthcare, the poor have too many burdens to open yet one more front. However, the more affluent who seek private healthcare can, and they are slowly beginning to raise these issues. There is also increasing evidence that the political class is getting restless about some healthcare practices and see some political mileage in interventions and regulations. Some of the recent State interventions on issues related to generic medicine prescription, capping of stent prices, and laws such as the ones in West Bengal, Karnataka, and Maharashtra are evidence that the State and political class, which have been so far bowing to popular pressure, are now willing to step into regulating healthcare corruption even at the cost of taking on powerful stakeholders including those in the medical profession (*Firstpost* 2017; *The Hindu* 2018). This may be a potential game-changer.

Healthcare corruption in India is like an infection in a patient already ill with another severe disease. If the infection can be tackled we may be able to control the rest of the disease better. Also, if we can defeat healthcare corruption in India it creates hope to tackle it for the benefit of millions of people in other countries with similar health ecosystems (Jain, Nundy, and Abbasi 2014). Though difficult, it is an urgent task to be taken up, for it concerns every citizen's health and well-being, you and us included.

POLICY RECOMMENDATIONS

1. Increase spending on health as promised in multiple policy documents and move towards universal health coverage and care. This will reduce the dependence of citizens on the private sector, the unbridled growth of which is one of the major drivers of corruption.
2. Strengthen currently existing regulatory frameworks for the health sector. Implement the CEA across the country and create mechanisms for public participation and grievance.
3. The functioning of NMC, should be completely transparent. It should have representatives from civil society groups with proven track records.
4. Increase the number of public medical colleges especially in underserved areas and curtail the growth of the private medical college industry.
5. Implement mechanisms for digital and transparent transactions in appointments and procurement of drugs and equipment.
6. Enact and implement a strict code for ethical marketing by the pharmaceutical and equipment industry.

REFERENCES

IANS. 2017. 'West Bengal Passes Stringent Bill Against Medical Negligence in Private Hospitals', *Firstpost*, March. Available at https://www.firstpost.com/india/west-bengal-passes-stringent-bill-against-medical-negligence-in-private-hospitals-3313814.html, last accessed on 18 November 2019.

Jain, A., S. Nundy, and K. Abbasi. 2014. 'Corruption: Medicine's Dirty Open Secret Doctors Must Fight Back against Kickbacks', *British Medical Journal* 348: g4184. doi:10.1136/bmj.g4184.

Krishna, Navmi. 2017. 'What Is the KPME (Amendment) Bill and Why Are Private Doctors in Karnataka up in Arms against It?' *The Hindu*, 16 November. Available at http://www.thehindu.com/news/national/karnataka/what-is-the-kpme-amendment-bill-and-why-are-private-doctors-in-karnataka-up-in-arms-against-it/article20492020.ece.

Nagral, S. 2014. 'Corruption in Indian Medicine Or "Overenthusiasm of the Marketing Department"', *Economic and Political Weekly* 49(29).

Nagral, S. 2015. 'We Need to Discuss India's Reliance on Private Medical Colleges'. *BMJ*, 350: h237. doi:10.1136/bmj.h237.

Nagral, S. 2016. 'Medical Council of India under Parliament Scrutiny: Symptoms Documented, but What about the Disease?'. *Economic and Political Weekly* 51(14): 18–21.

Nagral, S., and S. Nundy. 2017. 'We need to end "cut" practice in Indian healthcare', TheBMJOpinion, 7 July. Available at http://blogs.bmj.com/bmj/2017/07/07/we-need-to-end-cut-practice-in-indian-healthcare, last accessed on 18 November 2019).

Nagral, S., and N. Roy. 2010. 'The Medical Council of India Guidelines on Industry–Physician Relationship: Breaking the Conspiracy of Silence'. *National Medical Journal India* 23(2): 69–71.

Neuman, M., G. Alcock, K. Azad, A. Kuddus, D. Osrin, N.S. More, N. Nair, et al. 2014. 'Prevalence and Determinants of Caesarean Section in Private and Public Health Facilities in Underserved South Asian Communities: Cross-sectional Analysis of Data from Bangladesh, India and Nepal'. *BMJ Open*, 4:e005982. doi:10.1136/bmjopen-2014-005982.

Pandya, S. 2009. 'Medical Council of India: The Rot Within'. *Indian Journal of Medical Ethics* 6(3):125–31.

Pandya, S. 2016. 'The Functioning of the Medical Council of India Analysed by the Parliamentary Standing Committee of Health and Family Welfare'. *Indian Journal of Medical Ethics* 1(2): 68–71.

Parliament of India. 2016. *Ninety-Second Report: The Functioning of the Medical Council of India*. Available at 164.100.47.5/newcommittee/reports/EnglishCommittees/Committee%20on%20Health%20and%20Family%20Welfare/92.pdf.

Press Trust of India. 2013. 'AMRI Hospital Medical Negligence Case: Supreme Court Awards Highest-ever Compensation', *Financial Express*, 25 October. Available at https://www.financialexpress.com/archive/amri-hospital-medical-negligence-case-supreme-court-awards-highest-ever-compensation/1186781/.

About the Editors and Contributors

EDITORS

Ali Mehdi is a senior fellow and leads the Health Policy Initiative at the Indian Council for Research on International Economic Relations (ICRIER), New Delhi. Among his recent books are: *A Shot of Justice: Priority-Setting for Addressing Child Mortality* (Oxford University Press) and *Freedoms, Fragility and Job Creation: Perspectives from Jammu and Kashmir, India* (Springer), both published in 2019, and both adopting a multidisciplinary orientation to explore the issue of human freedoms.

S. Irudaya Rajan is a professor at the Centre for Development Studies (CDS), Thiruvananthapuram, Kerala. With more than three decades of research experience at the CDS, Kerala, he has coordinated eight major migration surveys in Kerala since 1998 (with K.C. Zachariah). He is editor of the annual series *India Migration Report* published by Routledge since 2010 and the founder and editor-in-chief of the Journal, *Migration and Development,* published by Taylor and Francis, since 2012.

CONTRIBUTORS

Mohammed K. Ali is Vice Chair of Family and Preventive Medicine and an associate professor at Emory University's School of Medicine and Rollins School of Public Health in Atlanta. He has led or contributed to large surveillance, cohort, and intervention studies focused on cardiometabolic diseases in India continuously since 2008. He has served as an advisor for the Centers for Disease Control and Prevention since 2010 and contributed to expert committees for the World Health Organization, World Bank, and National Academy of Medicine.

Gulrez Shah Azhar is a senior fellow with IHME at the University of Washington. Previously, he has been an assistant policy researcher at the RAND Corporation and assistant professor at Indian Institute of Public Health, PHFI. He has MBBS, MD, MPH, and PhD degrees and interned at WHO headquarters. His interests are in health, environment and development.

Kalpana Balakrishnan is Professor and Director of the ICMR Center on Air Quality, Climate and Health at SRIHER, Chennai, India. She serves on the MoHFW-constituted National Steering Committee on Air Pollution Related Issues and as Chair, Environmental Risk Factors Group for the India State-level Burden of Disease Initiative.

Rama V. Baru is Professor at the Centre of Social Medicine and Community Health, Jawaharlal Nehru University, New Delhi. She has authored two books - *Private Health Care in India: Social Characteristics and Trends* and *School Health Services in India: The Social and Economic Contexts*. She is currently on several research committees for the Indian Council for Medical Research, Department of Health Research, and the All India Institute of Medical Sciences.

Lawton Robert Burns is the James Joo-Jin Kim Professor, Professor of Health Care Management, and Professor of Management at the Wharton School, University of Pennsylvania. He is also Director of Wharton Center for Health Management and Economics, and Co-Director of Roy & Diana Vagelos Program in Life Sciences and Management. Besides holding several academic positions, Burns has extensively worked on the analysis of physician–hospital integration, and has written a volume on India's healthcare industry, published by Cambridge University Press (2014).

Abhijit Das is managing trustee of the Centre for Health and Social Justice, New Delhi, and clinical associate professor at the Department of Global Health, University of Washington, Seattle. He is currently co-convenor of COPASAH, a global health rights and social accountability network. Das is a doctor with training in public health and evaluation research.

Neha Faruqui is a global health researcher with a background in Chemical Engineering. Her PhD focused on access to care for children with cancer in India and the implications for Universal Health Coverage. She continues to contribute to various global health system and policy projects through the University of Sydney.

Rohit Gupta joined Fidelity International as an Investment Analyst in Singapore in July 2019. He completed the MBA program at The Wharton School in 2019. Prior to that, he worked as an Investment Analyst at Everstone Capital ($5Bn AUM) where he was part of the investment team for several healthcare transactions. He is also a 2013 graduate from IIT Delhi where he completed BTech in Chemical Engineering.

Aditi Iyer is a senior research scientist and adjunct associate professor at the Public Health Foundation of India's Ramalingaswami Centre on Equity and Social Determinants of Health in Bangalore. Her multi-disciplinary academic background includes a PhD in Public Health from the University of Liverpool, UK, and undergraduate and master's degrees in Sociology and Social Work. She is a research affiliate of the Institute for Intersectionality Research and Policy, Simon Fraser University, Vancouver, Canada.

Anoop Jain is a postdoctoral research fellow at the Woods Institute for the Environment at Stanford University. He received his Doctor of Public Health from U.C. Berkeley. His primary research interests are the social determinants of access to water, sanitation, and hygiene in India, and the social determinants of child health outcomes. Jain is also the founding director of Sanitation and Health Rights in India, a non-profit that improves access to sanitation in Bihar and Jharkhand.

Roger Jeffery has been Professor of Sociology of South Asia at the University of Edinburgh, UK, since 1997. His work has included research on issues of public health and health policy, especially maternal and reproductive health, access to medicines, clinical trials, and the transformations of public health and medical services in South Asia since 1980.

William Joe is Assistant Professor at the Population Research Centre (PRC), Institute of Economic Growth, Delhi and Bernard Lown Scholar, Harvard-Chan School of Public Health, Harvard University, US. He has a PhD in Economics from Jawaharlal Nehru University with research interests in Health Economics, Demography and Development Economics. In 2017, he was Visiting Scientist at Department of Social and Behavioural Sciences, Harvard-Chan School of Public Health, Harvard University.

Pallavi Joshi is a research associate at Health Policy Initiative (HPI), ICRIER. Under the various research programmes of HPI, she has been working on governance and regulatory issues, with a special focus on health sector and pharmaceutical industry, and has contributed to several publications. She has also worked with Competition Commission of India, where she was involved in analysing competition issues in pharmaceutical industry.

Amir Ullah Khan is a health economist and Professor at the MCRHRDI of the Government of Telangana. He is a visiting professor at TISS, ISB, and at NALSAR in Hyderabad. Khan is a business columnist for the LiveMint and senior fellow at RGICS. Khan is a former senior advisor at the Gates foundation and former director at the India Development Foundation.

Shah Alam Khan is a professor in the Department of Orthopaedics at AIIMS, New Delhi. Khan received his medical training in India and abroad and is particularly interested in orthopaedic oncology and paediatric orthopaedics. He has played an instrumental role in developing protocol-based practices for neglected paediatric conditions. Dr Khan has authored three books and more than a hundred journal articles. He is member of the ICMR Task Force on Bone and Soft Tissue Sarcomas.

Richard Kingham is a senior counsel assigned to the Washington, DC, and London offices of Covington & Burling LLP, whose practice focuses on regulation of drugs in the US and EU. He is an adjunct professor at the Georgetown University Law Center and has taught medicines law at the University of Virginia Law School and graduate programmes of pharmaceutical medicine at Cardiff University and King's College London in the UK. He has served on committees of the Institute of Medicine of the US National Academy of Sciences and the National Institutes of Health.

Akshat Kumar is an attending physician at Penn Medicine and MBA student at the Wharton School, University of Pennsylvania. Kumar earned his MD from Kasturba Medical College in India and completed his residency in Internal Medicine at St Peter's University Hospital in New Jersey. He is also proactively engaged in *WellUHealth*, a health start-up involved in helping Medicare patients stay away from hospitals by better managing their chronic diseases by using technology.

Alissa McCaffrey is a manager at Leavitt Partners, based Washington, DC. She supports clients and health care coalitions through policy analysis and project management, and serves as an advisor to RxGPS, the alliance for global pharmaceutical serialization. McCaffrey's work is focused on issues related to public health, value-based healthcare, and pharmaceutical supply chain security.

Santosh Mehrotra is Professor of Economics at the Centre for Informal Sector and Labour Studies, Jawaharlal Nehru University, New Delhi. Previously, he was Director General of National Institute of Labour Economics Research and Development, the only research institute of the erstwhile Planning Commission. Mehrotra has extensively engaged with international organizations as a technical expert. His research on labour/employment, skill development, child poverty, and the economics of education has been translated into several international languages.

N.R. Madhava Menon (late), acclaimed as the 'father of Modern Indian Legal Education' has been the longest serving educator in India, and the Founding Director/Vice Chancellor of National Law School of India University, National University of Juridical Sciences, and National Judicial Academy. He is the recipient of several awards for education, law and public service including Padma Shri from the Government of India in 2003.

Sanjay Kumar Mohanty is working as a professor at International Institute for Population Sciences (IIPS), Mumbai. Mohanty was C.R. Parekh Fellow, 2009-10, at Asia Research Centre, London School of Economics, and Visiting Scientist at Harvard School of Public Health from September 2014 to August 2015. He has authored more than 60 research papers in international and national peer-reviewed journals and guided several students for their maiden research work.

Rahul Mongia is a clinical research professional with expertise in clinical trial regulations, GCP, and global pharmaceutical policy landscape. He has been a research scholar at the Centre for Studies in Science Policy, JNU, India and his PhD thesis focused on the evolving state of anomalously persistent combination pharmaceuticals in India. He regularly voices his opinions through several columns in national dailies and blogs.

Venkatanarayana Motkuri based at Hyderabad (India) is a Research Consultant in Development Studies and currently working as Senior Research Analyst (SRA) at Commission of Inquiry on Conditions of Muslims, Govt. of Telangana. He got his PhD from the Jawaharlal Nehru University through CDS, Trivandrum. He has been working in the field of research in Development Studies for last twelve years. His areas of interest include human and social capital, education, health, poverty, agriculture, and regional disparities.

Somil Nagpal is the cluster lead for the World Bank's health and nutrition programs in Indonesia and Timor Leste, having served recently in a similar capacity for Cambodia and Lao PDR. Prior to joining the World Bank in 2009, Nagpal has been a civil service officer in India and served the Ministries of Health and Finance. He was deputed by the Government of India to the IRDA between 2007 and 2009, when he was responsible for conceptualizing and setting up the specialized health insurance department of the Authority.

Sanjay Nagral is a surgeon specializing in hepatobiliary surgery and liver transplantation. He trained and worked at the KEM Hospital, Mumbai, till 1999 when he was associate professor of surgery, and then at the King's College Hospital in London. Currently he is the Director of the Department of Surgical Gastroenterology at Jaslok Hospital and also heads the Department of General Surgery at the KB Bhabha General Hospital. He is the publisher of the *Indian Journal of Medical Ethics*.

K.M. Venkat Narayan is currently Ruth and O.C. Hubert Chair of Global Health, Director, Emory Global Diabetes Research Center, Professor of Medicine and Epidemiology at Emory University, Atlanta. He was the chief of the diabetes science branch at the US Centers for Disease Control and Prevention (CDC). He has been involved in several national and international multicenter epidemiological studies, translational research and intervention studies.

Samiran S. Nundy was a medical undergraduate in Cambridge and Guy's Hospital London and then trained in medicine and later in surgery at Guy's, Addenbrooke's Cambridge, the Hammersmith and the Massachusetts General Hospital in Boston. He has taught at the Universities of Cambridge, London, and Harvard and returned to the All India Institute of Medical Sciences in 1975 where he eventually became Professor and Head of the Department of Gastrointestinal Surgery. Currently, Nundy is a Gastrointestinal Surgeon in Sir Ganga Ram Hospital, New Delhi.

Basant Kumar Panda is a doctoral research scholar at the International Institute for Population Sciences (IIPS), Mumbai. He has completed his M.Sc. and MPhil in Statistics from Utkal University, Bhubaneswar and Master's in Population Studies (MPS) from IIPS, Mumbai. His current research interests include ageing, health expenditure, maternal and child health and health inequality.

Sunil Pandya was appointed Professor of Neurosurgery at Seth Gordhandas Sunderdas Medical College and King Edward VII Memorial Hospital, Mumbai in 1975 and retired on superannuation in 1998. An alumnus of Grant Medical College and Sir J.J. Group of Hospitals, Mumbai, he obtained his MBBS from the University of Bombay in 1961 and MS (General Surgery) in 1965. Pandya is a life member of the Neurological Society of India and the Asiatic Society of Bombay.

Shivani A. Patel is Rollins Assistant Professor in the Hubert Department of Global Health, Emory University, Atlanta. Her research is guided by an overarching interest in describing, understanding, and addressing disparities in chronic disease morbidity and mortality globally, with a particular focus on South Asia. She actively collaborates on cohort and intervention studies focused on cardiometabolic disease in India.

D. Prabhakaran is Vice President, Research and Policy, at the Public Health Foundation of India; Executive Director at the Centre for Chronic Disease Control, New Delhi; and Professor of Epidemiology at the London School of Hygiene and Tropical Medicine. Prabhakaran is a cardiologist and epidemiologist by training. His work spans from understanding the causes of higher predisposition to cardiovascular diseases (CVD) among Indians, to developing solutions for CVD through translational research.

Anurag Priyadarshi is a postgraduate from Centre for Informal Sector and Labour Studies, Jawaharlal Nehru University. His interests include economic policy and human development. He is also a sports enthusiast. He currently lives in New Delhi.

Sunil Rajpal is an assistant professor at Institute of Health Management Research, IIHMR University, Jaipur. He has a PhD in economics from Central University of Gujarat and was an ICSSR Doctoral Fellow at the Institute of Economic Growth, Delhi. His research interests include health economics, development economics and demography. Currently he is pursuing research on social determinants of nutrition and household healthcare financing.

Sujatha Rao joined the Indian Administrative Service in 1974. She worked in the Ministry of Health and Family Welfare, Government of India as Director, Joint Secretary, DG Department of AIDS Control and retired in December 2010 form the post of Union Secretary. In 2004 she served as Member Secretary of the National Commission on Macroeconomics which was co-chaired by Union Ministers' of Health and Finance.

Saravanan V.S. is Senior Researcher in Department of Social and Cultural Change at the Center for Development Research, University of Bonn. He leads water and health research at the Center and specializes in new institutionalism, systems approach, geo-statistical analysis, integrated water management and socio-epidemiology. His research projects have involved the assessment of water-related health risks in rapidly growing economies and the impact of water management on human health in South and Central Asia.

Gita Sen is Distinguished Professor and Director of the Ramalingaswami Centre on Equity and Social Determinants of Health at Public Health Foundation of India, and is adjunct professor of Global Health and Population at Harvard University. Her work addresses gender and intersectional inequalities as key social determinants of health. She has received honorary doctorates from the University of Edinburgh, the University of Sussex, the Open University, the Karolinska Institute, and the University of East Anglia.

Abusaleh Shariff is Chief Scholar at the US-India Policy Institute, Washington and Founder President, Centre for Research and Debates in Development Policy, New Delhi. He also worked as Senior Research Fellow at the Food Policy Research Institute, Washington, DC. He was advisor to the Indian Prime Minister during 2004-6 and the Ministry of Home Affairs, Government of India during 2010–11, He was also nominated to the 13th (Indian) Finance Commission by the Finance Ministry, Government of India.

Amit Sharma is an independent economist currently associated as a consultant with NCAER, New Delhi. In the past, he has been associated as full time researcher with NCAER for more than six years and with World Bank, Copenhagen Consensus Center (on collaborative work with Tata Trusts) as a consultant. He received his bachelor's degree in engineering and master's degree in economics from BITS, Pilani.

Kirk R. Smith is Professor of Global Environmental Health, School of Public Health, University of California Berkeley; and Director, Collaborative Clean Air Policy Centre, New Delhi, and was founder and head of the Energy Program of the East-West Center before moving to Berkeley. He participated in the IPCC's 3rd and 4th assessments for which he shared the 2007 Nobel Peace Prize and was Convening Lead Author for Climate and Health for the 5th Assessment.

Smita Srinivas holds a PhD from MIT and focuses on industry dynamics including in cancer care, and other vaccines and diagnostics. She is the Founder Director of the Technological Change Lab (TCLab); Professorial Fellow in Economics and Development, Open University UK; Visiting Professor NCBS, TIFR India; and Honorary Professor at STEaPP, University College London. She received the EAEPE Myrdal Prize for *Market Menagerie: Health and Development in Late Industrial States* (Stanford University Press, 2012).

Nikhil Tandon is a Professor in the Department of Endocrinology at the All India Institute of Medical Sciences, New Delhi. He is a clinician-researcher with interest in chronic disease epidemiology across the life course and has extensive experience of managing large clinical and implementation trials.

Kenneth Thorpe is the Robert W. Woodruff Professor and Chair of the Department of Health Policy and Management at the Rollins School of Public Health at Emory University, Atlanta. He also serves as the Chairman of the Partnership to Fight Chronic Disease (PFCD). In addition to holding a number of faculty positions, Thorpe was Deputy Assistant Secretary for Health Policy in the U.S. Department of Health and Human Services from 1993 to 1995.

Leela Visaria is an honorary professor and a former director of Gujarat Institute of Development Research, Ahmedabad, Gujarat. She has worked extensively on historical demography, health, education and demographic transition. She was awarded National Professorship during 2009–10 by the Indian Council for Social Science Research, which is a parent body of social science research institutes in India. She served as the first president of Asian Population Association for two years 2009–10.

Vasudha Wattal is a doctoral candidate in economics at the University of East Anglia, UK. Her current research explores the economics of competition in the pharmaceutical sector. Prior to this, she was affiliated with the Delhi-based policy think tank—Indian Council for Research on International Economic Relations (ICRIER). Previously, she has worked on competition issues in India's healthcare sector while interning at the Competition Commission of India.

Susan Winckler is the Chief Risk Management Officer of Leavitt Partners and advisor to RxGPS, the alliance for global pharmaceutical serialization. Susan is the former chief of the staff for the U.S. Food and Drug Administration (FDA) within the Department of Health and Human Services (HHS) and former president and CEO of the Food and Drug Law Institute, a non-profit organization based in Washington, DC, which provides a marketplace for discussing food and drug law issues.